Review and Resource

Family Nurse Practitioner, 5th Edition

Volume 1

NURSING CERTIFICATION REVIEW MANUAL

CONTINUING EDUCATION SOURCE

CLINICAL PRACTICE RESOURCE

Courtney Reinisch, DNP, RN, FNP-BC, DCC

NURSING
KNOWLEDGE
CENTER

Library of Congress Cataloging-in-Publication Data

Names: Reinisch, Courtney, editor. | Nursing Knowledge Center, publisher.
Title: Family nurse practitioner review and resource manual / edited by
    Courtney Reinisch.
Other titles: Family nurse practitioner (2009)
Description: 5th edition. | Silver Spring, MD : Nursing Knowledge Center,
    American Nurses Association, [2016]- | Preceded by: Family nurse
    practitioner review manual / edited by Elizabeth Blunt and Courtney
    Reinisch. Fourth edition. [2013] | Includes bibliographical references.
Identifiers: LCCN 2016043988| ISBN 9781935213901 (pbk.) | ISBN 9781935213918
    (ePDF) | ISBN 9781935213925 (epub) | ISBN 9781935213932 (prc)
Subjects: | MESH: Family Nursing | Nurse Practitioners | Examination Questions
Classification: LCC RT73 | NLM WY 18.2 | DDC 610.7306/92076--dc23 LC record available at
https://lccn.loc.gov/2016043988

The American Nurses Association (ANA) is the only full-service professional organization representing the interests of the nation's 3.4 million registered nurses through its constituent member nurses associations and its organizational affiliates. ANA advances the nursing profession by fostering high standards of nursing practice, promoting the rights of nurses in the workplace, projecting a positive and realistic view of nursing, and by lobbying the Congress and regulatory agencies on healthcare issues affecting nurses and the public.

ISBNs

Volume 1:
print   978-1-935213-90-1
ePDF   978-1-935213-91-8
EPUB   978-1-935213-92-5
PRC   978-1-935213-93-2

Volume 2:
print   978-1-935213-94-9
ePDF   978-1-935213-95-6
EPUB   978-1-935213-96-3
PRC   978-1-935213-97-0

NOTE ABOUT THIS TWO-VOLUME SET

Thank you for purchasing the *Family Nurse Practitioner Review and Resource Manual, 5th Edition*. Please note that this book is printed in two volumes; one volume alone does not contain information covering the entire test content outline for this exam. You will need to purchase both volumes in order to be eligible to obtain the continuing education for this manual. You can contact revmanuals@ana.org with any questions.

FAMILY NURSE PRACTITIONER REVIEW AND RESOURCE MANUAL, 5TH EDITION
2016

Please direct your comments and/or queries to: revmanuals@ana.org

The healthcare services delivery system is a volatile marketplace demanding superior knowledge, clinical skills, and competencies from all registered nurses. Nursing autonomy of practice and nurse career marketability and mobility in the new century hinge on affirming the profession's formative philosophy, which places a priority on a lifelong commitment to the principles of education and professional development. The knowledge base of nursing theory and practice is expanding, and while care has been taken to ensure the accuracy and timeliness of the information presented in the *Family Nurse Practitioner Review and Resource Manual, 5th Edition*, clinicians are advised to always verify the most current national guidelines and recommendations and to practice in accordance with professional standards of care used with regard to the unique circumstances that apply in each practice situation. In addition, every effort has been made in this text to ensure accuracy and, in particular, to confirm that drug selections and dosages are in accordance with current recommendations and practice, including the ongoing research, changes to government regulations, and the developments in product information provided by pharmaceutical manufacturers. However, it is the responsibility of each nurse practitioner to verify drug product information and to practice in accordance with professional standards of care. In addition, the editors wish to note that provision of information in this text does not imply an endorsement of any particular products, procedures, or services.

Therefore, the authors, editors, American Nurses Association (ANA), American Nurses Association's Publishing (ANP), and the Nursing Knowledge Center cannot accept responsibility for errors or omissions, or for any consequences or liability, injury, and/or damages to persons or property from application of the information in this manual and make no warranty, express or implied, with respect to the contents of the *Family Nurse Practitioner Review and Resource Manual, 5th Edition*. Completion of this manual does not guarantee that the reader will pass the certification exam. The practice examination questions are not a requirement to take a certification examination. The practice examination questions cannot be used as an indicator of results on the actual certification.

Published by

The Nursing Knowledge Center
8515 Georgia Avenue, Suite 400
Silver Spring, MD 20910-3402
https://www.nursingknowledgecenter.org

CONTENTS

VOLUME 2

INSTRUCTIONS FOR OBTAINING CONTINUING EDUCATION CREDIT FOR STUDY OF THE *FAMILY NURSE PRACTITIONER REVIEW AND RESOURCE MANUAL, 5ᵀᴴ EDITION*

The Nursing Knowledge Center offers continuing nursing education contact hours (CE) to those who review and study this manual and successfully complete an online module. To obtain CE credit you must purchase and review the manual, pay required fees to enroll in the online module, and complete all module components by the published CE expiration date including disclosures, pre- and post-tests, and the course evaluation. The continuing nursing education contact hours online module can be completed at any time prior to the published CE expiration date and a certificate can be printed from the online learning management system immediately after successful completion of the online module. To purchase the online module for this manual visit the Nursing Knowledge Center's online catalog at https://learn.ana-nursingknowledge.org/. Please contact online support with any questions about the CE or module.

Inquiries or Comments

If you have any questions about the content of the manual please e-mail revmanuals@ana.org. You may also mail any comments to Editorial Project Manager at the address listed below.

Nursing Knowledge Center
Attn: Editorial Project Manager
8515 Georgia Avenue, Suite 400
Silver Spring, MD 20910-3492
Fax: (301) 628-5342

CE Provider Information

ANA's Center for Continuing Education and Professional Development is accredited as a provider of continuing nursing education by the American Nurses Credentialing Center's Commission on Accreditation.

ANCC Provider Number 0023.

ANA is approved by the California Board of Registered Nursing, Provider Number CEP6178.

Disclaimer

Review and study of this manual and successful completion of the online module do not guarantee success on a certification examination. Purchase of this manual and completion of the online module are not required to obtain certification.

ACKNOWLEDGMENTS

The authors would like to thank the following contributors for their invaluable advice and feed-back during the development of this manual:

Ranbir Mangat Bains, PhD, MSN, APRN, CPNP (Chapter 19)
Pediatric Nurse Practitioner
Barnard Environmental Magnet School-Based Health Center/Yale-New Haven Hospital, New Haven, CT

Susan D. Boulware, MD (Chapters 12 and 18)
Assistant Clinical Professor in Pediatrics
Pediatric Endocrinology & Metabolism
Yale University School of Medicine/School of Nursing, New Haven, CT

Elizabeth A. Doyle, DNP, APRN, CDE, BC-ADM
Yale Diabetes Center
Yale New Haven Hospital, New Haven, CT

Kimberly J. Erlich, MSN, RN, MPH, CPNP, PMHS (Chapter 16)
Nurse Practitioner and Project Coordinator
Mills-Peninsula Health Services & Palo Alto Medical Foundation, Palo Alto, CA

Therese Harrison, MSN, APRN, CPNP, PMHS-BC (Chapter 19)
Director of Medical Services
St. Christopher's Inc., Dobbs Ferry, NY

Katherine Myint-Hpu, MSN, MPH, PPCNP-BC, CRNP (Chapter 17)
National Institutes of Health
The Clinical Center's Pediatric Consult Service, Bethesda, MD

Meara Peterson, DNP, RN, CPNP (Chapter 12)
North County Health Services, San Marcos, CA

Nancy Rollinson, MSN, PPCNP-BC (Chapter 9)
Inpatient Coordinator, Pediatric Arrhythmia and Pacemaker Services
Yale University/Yale-New Haven Hospital, New Haven, CT

CHAPTER 1

TAKING THE CERTIFICATION EXAMINATION

When you sign up to take a national certification exam, you will be instructed to go on-line and review the testing and review handbook (http://www.nursecredentialing.org/GeneralTestingRenewalHandbook). Review it carefully and be sure to bookmark the site so you can refer to it frequently. It contains information on test content and sample questions. This is critical information; it will give you insight into the nature of the test. The agency will send you information about the test site; keep this in a safe place until needed.

GENERAL SUGGESTIONS FOR PREPARING FOR THE EXAM

Step One: Control Your Anxiety

Everyone experiences anxiety when faced with taking the certification exam.

- ▶ Remember, your program was designed to prepare you to take this exam.

- ▶ Your instructors took a similar exam, and have probably talked to students who took exams more recently, so they know how to help you prepare.

- ▶ Taking a review course or setting up your own study plan will help you feel more confident about taking the exam.

Step Two: Do Not Listen to Gossip About the Exam

A large volume of information exists about the tests based on reports from people who have taken the exams in the past. Because information from the testing facilities is limited, it is hard to ignore this gossip.

- ▶ Remember that gossip about the exam that you hear from others is not verifiable.

- ▶ Because this gossip is based on the imperfect memory of people in a stressful situation, it may not be very accurate.

- ▶ People tend to remember those items testing content with which they are less comfortable; for instance, those with a limited background in women's health may say that the exam was "all women's health." In fact, the exam blueprint ensures that the exam covers multiple content areas without overemphasizing any one.

Step Three: Set Reasonable Expectations for Yourself

▶ Do not expect to know everything.

▶ Do not try to know everything in great detail.

▶ You do not need a perfect score to pass the exam.

▶ The exam is designed for a beginner level—it is testing readiness for *entry-level* practice.

▶ Learn the general rules, not the exceptions.

▶ The most likely diagnoses will be on the exam, not questions on rare diseases or atypical cases.

▶ Think about the most likely presentation and most common therapy.

Step Four: Prepare Mentally and Physically

▶ While you are getting ready to take the exam, take good physical care of yourself.

▶ Get plenty of sleep and exercise, and eat well while preparing for the exam.

▶ These things are especially important while you are studying and immediately before you take the exam.

Step Five: Access Current Knowledge

General Content

You will be given a list of general topics that will be on the exam when you register to take the exam. In addition, examine the table of contents of this book and the test content outline, available at www.nursecredentialing.org/cert/TCOs.html.

▶ What content do you need to know?

▶ How well do you know these subjects?

Take a Review Course

▶ Taking a review course is an excellent way to assess your knowledge of the content that will be included in the exam.

▶ If you plan to take a review course, take it well before the exam so you will have plenty of time to master any areas of weakness the course uncovers.

▶ If you are prepared for the exam, you will not hear anything new in the course. You will be familiar with everything that is taught.

▶ If some topics in the review course are new to you, concentrate on these in your studies.

▶ People have a tendency to study what they know; it is rewarding to study something and feel a mastery of it! Unfortunately, this will not help you master unfamiliar content. Be sure to use a review course to identify your areas of strength and weakness, then concentrate on the weaknesses.

Depth of Knowledge

How much do you need to know about a subject?

► You cannot know everything about a topic.

► Remember that the depth of knowledge required to pass the exam is for entry-level performance.

► Study the information sent to you from the testing agency, what you were taught in school, what is covered in this text, and the general guidelines given in this chapter.

► Look at practice tests designed for the exam. Practice tests for other exams will not be helpful.

► Consult your class notes or clinical diagnosis and management textbook for the major points about a disease. Additional reference books can be found online at http://nursecredentialing.org/Exam22-FamilyNP-TRL.

► For example, with regard to medications, know the drug categories and the major medications in each. Assume all drugs in a category are generally alike, and then focus on the differences among common drugs. Know the most important indications, contraindications, and side effects. Emphasize safety. The questions usually do not require you to know the exact dosage of a drug.

Step Six: Institute a Systematic Study Plan

Develop Your Study Plan

► Write up a formal plan of study.

  ▷ Include topics for study, timetable, resources, and methods of study that work for you.

  ▷ Decide whether you want to organize a study group or work alone.

  ▷ Schedule regular times to study.

  ▷ Avoid cramming; it is counterproductive. Try to schedule your study periods in 1-hour increments.

► Identify resources to use for studying. To prepare for the examination, you should have the following materials on your shelf:

  ▷ A good pathophysiology text

  ▷ This review book

  ▷ A physical assessment text

  ▷ Your class notes

  ▷ Other important sources, including: information from the testing facility, a clinical diagnosis textbook, favorite journal articles, notes from a review course, and practice tests

► Know the important national standards of care for major illnesses

► Consult the bibliography on the test blueprint. When studying less familiar material, it is helpful to study using the same references that the testing center uses.

► Study the body systems from head to toe.

▶ The exams emphasize health promotion, assessment, differential diagnosis, and plan of care for common problems.

▶ You will need to know facts and be able to interpret and analyze this information using critical thinking.

Personalize Your Study Plan

▶ How do you learn best?

▷ If you learn best by listening or talking, attend a review course or discuss topics with a colleague.

▶ Read everything the test facility sends you as soon as you receive it and several times during your preparation period. It will give you valuable information to help guide your study.

▶ Have a specific place with good lighting set aside for studying. Find a quiet place with no distractions. Assemble your study materials.

Implement Your Study Plan

You must have basic content knowledge. In addition, you must be able to use this information to think critically and make decisions based on facts.

▶ Refer to your study plan regularly.

▶ Stick to your schedule.

▶ Take breaks when you get tired.

▶ If you start procrastinating, get help from a friend or reorganize your study plan.

▶ It is not necessary to follow your plan rigidly. Adjust as you learn where you need to spend more time.

▶ Memorize the basics of the content areas you will be required to know.

Focus on General Material

▶ Most of what you need to know is basic material that does not require constant updating.

▶ You do not need to worry about the latest information being published as you are studying for the exam. Remember, it can take 6 to 12 months for new information to be incorporated into test questions.

Pace Your Studying

▶ Stop studying for the examination when you are starting to feel overwhelmed and look at what is bothering you. Then make changes.

▶ Break overwhelming tasks into smaller tasks that you know you can do.

▶ Stop and take breaks while studying.

Work with Others

▶ Talk with classmates about your preparation for the exam.

▶ Keep in touch with classmates, and help each other stick to your study plans.

▶ If your classmates become anxious, do not let their anxiety affect you. Walk away if you need to.

▶ Do not believe bad stories you hear about other people's experiences with previous exams.

▶ Remember, you know as much as anyone about what will be on the next exam!

Consider a Study Group

▶ Study groups can provide practice in analyzing cases, interpreting questions, and critical thinking.

▶ You can discuss a topic and take turns presenting cases for the group to analyze.

▶ Study groups can also provide moral support and help you continue studying.

Step Seven: Strategies Immediately Before the Exam

Final Preparation Suggestions

▶ Use practice exams when studying to get accustomed to the exam format and time restrictions.

   ▷ Many books that are labeled as review books are simply a collection of examination questions.

   ▷ If you have test anxiety, such practice tests may help alleviate the anxiety.

   ▷ Practice tests can help you learn to judge the time it should take you to complete the exam.

   ▷ Practice tests are useful for gaining experience in analyzing questions.

   ▷ Books of questions may not uncover the gaps in your knowledge that a more systematic content review text will reveal.

   ▷ If you feel that you don't know enough about a topic, refer to a text to learn more. After you feel that you have learned the topic, practice questions are a wonderful tool to help improve your test-taking skill.

▶ Know your test-taking style.

   ▷ Do you rush through the exam without reading the questions thoroughly?

   ▷ Do you get stuck and dwell on a question for a long time?

   ▷ You should spend about 45 to 60 seconds per question and finish with time to review the questions you were not sure about.

   ▷ Be sure to read the question completely, including all four answer choices. Choice "a" may be good, but "d" may be best.

The Night Before the Exam

▶ Be prepared to get to the exam on time.

   ▷ Know the test site location and how long it takes to get there.

   ▷ Take a "dry run" beforehand to make sure you know how to get to the testing site, if necessary.

- ▶ Get a good night's sleep.
- ▶ Eat sensibly.
- ▶ Avoid alcohol the night before.
- ▶ Assemble the required material: two forms of identification, admission card, pencil, and watch. Both IDs must match the name on the application, and one photo ID is preferred.
- ▶ Know the exam room rules.
- ▶ You will be given scratch paper, which will be collected at the end of the exam.
- ▶ Nothing else is allowed in the exam room.
- ▶ You will be required to put papers, backpacks, etc., in a corner of the room or in a locker.
- ▶ No water or food will be allowed.
- ▶ You will be allowed to walk to a water fountain and go to the bathroom one at a time.

The Day of the Exam

- ▶ Get there early. You must arrive to the test center at least 15 minutes before your scheduled appointment time. If you are late, you may not be admitted.
- ▶ Think positively. You have studied hard and are well prepared.
- ▶ Remember your anxiety reduction strategies.

Specific Tips for Dealing with Anxiety

Test anxiety is a specific type of anxiety. Symptoms include upset stomach, sweaty palms, tachycardia, trouble concentrating, and a feeling of dread. But there are ways to cope with test anxiety.

- ▶ There is no substitute for being well prepared.
- ▶ Practice relaxation techniques.
- ▶ Avoid alcohol, excess coffee, caffeine, and any new medications that might sedate you, dull your senses, or make you feel agitated.
- ▶ Take a few deep breaths and concentrate on the task at hand.

Focus on Specific Test-Taking Skills

To do well on the exam, you need good test-taking skills in addition to knowledge of the content and ability to use critical thinking.

All Certification Exams Are Multiple Choice

- ▶ Multiple-choice tests have specific rules for test construction.
- ▶ A multiple-choice question consists of three parts: the information (or stem), the question, and the four possible answers (one correct and three distracters).
- ▶ Careful analysis of each part is necessary. Read the entire question before answering.

▶ Practice your test-taking skills by analyzing the practice questions in this book and on the ANCC Web site.

Analyze the Information Given

▶ Do not assume you have more information than is given.

▶ Do not overanalyze.

▶ Remember, the writer of the question assumes that this is all the information needed to answer the question.

▶ If information is not given, it is not relevant and will not affect the answer.

▶ Do not make the question more complicated than it is.

What Kind of Question Is Asked?

▶ Are you supposed to recall a fact, apply facts to a situation, or understand and differentiate between options?

▶ Read the question thinking about what the writer is asking.

▶ Look for key words or phrases that lead you (see Figure 1–1). These help determine what kind of answer the question requires.

Read All the Answers

▶ If you are absolutely certain that answer "a" is correct as you read it, mark it, but read the rest of the options so you do not trick yourself into missing a better answer.

▶ If you are absolutely sure answer "a" is wrong, cross it off or make a note on your scratch paper and continue reading the options.

▶ After reading the entire question, go back, analyze the question, and select the best answer.

▶ Do not jump ahead.

▶ If the question asks you for an assessment, the best answer will be an assessment. Do not be distracted by an intervention that sounds appropriate.

▶ If the question asks you for an intervention, do not answer with an assessment.

▶ When two answer choices sound very good, the best one is usually the least expensive, least invasive way to achieve the goal. For example, if your answer choices include a physical exam maneuver or imaging, the physical exam maneuver is probably the better choice provided it will give the information needed.

avoid	initial	most
best	first	significant
except	contributing to	likely
not	appropriate	of the following
most consistent with		

FIGURE 1–1.
EXAMPLES OF KEY WORDS AND PHRASES

▶ If the answers include two options that are the opposite of each other, one of the two is probably the correct answer.

▶ When numeric answers cover a wide range, a number in the middle is more likely to be correct.

▶ Watch out for distracters that are correct but do not answer the question, combine true and false information, or contain a word or phrase that is similar to the correct answer.

▶ Err on the side of caution.

Only One Answer Can Be Correct

▶ When more than one suggested answer is correct, you must identify the one that best answers the question asked.

▶ If you cannot choose between two answers, you have a 50% chance of getting it right if you guess.

Avoid Changing Answers

▶ Change an answer only if you have a compelling reason, such as you remembered something additional, or you understand the question better after rereading it.

▶ People change to a wrong answer more often than to a right answer.

Time Yourself to Complete the Whole Exam

▶ Do not spend a large amount of time on one question.

▶ If you cannot answer a question quickly, mark it and continue the exam.

▶ If time is left at the end, return to the difficult questions.

▶ Make educated guesses by eliminating the obviously wrong answers and choosing a likely answer even if you are not certain.

▶ Trust your instinct.

▶ Answer every question. You are not penalized for a wrong answer.

▶ Occasionally a question will remind you of something that helps you with a question earlier in the test. Look back at that question to see whether what you are remembering affects how you would answer that question.

About the Certification Exams

The American Nurses Credentialing Center Computerized Exam

The ANCC examination is given only as a computer exam, and each exam is different.

The order of the questions is scrambled for every test, so even if two people are taking the same exam, the questions will be in a different order. The exam consists of 175 multiple-choice questions.

▶ Only 150 of the 175 questions are part of the test, which means that how you answer them will count toward your score; 25 are included to refine questions and will not be scored. You will not know which ones count, so treat all questions the same.

▶ You will need to know how to use a mouse, scroll by either clicking arrows on the scroll bar or using the up and down arrow keys, and perform other basic computer tasks.

▶ The exam does not require computer expertise.

▶ However, if you are not comfortable with using a computer, you should practice using a mouse and computer beforehand so you do not waste time on the mechanics of using the computer.

Know What to Expect During the Test

▶ Each ANCC test question is independent of the other questions.

  ▷ For each case study, there is only one question. This means that a correct answer on any question does not depend on the correct answer to any other question.

▶ Each question has four possible answers. There are no questions asking for combinations of correct answers (such as "a and c") or multiple-multiples.

▶ You can skip a question and go back to it at the end of the exam.

▶ You cannot mark key words in the question or right or wrong answers. If you want to do this, use the scratch paper.

▶ You will get your results immediately, and a grade report will be provided upon leaving the testing site.

Internet Resources

▶ ANCC Web site: www.nursecredentialing.org

▶ ANA Bookstore: www.nursesbooks.org. Catalog of ANA nursing scope and standards publications and other titles that may be listed on your test content outline

▶ National Guideline Clearinghouse: www.ngc.gov

CHAPTER 2

IMPORTANT FACTORS INFLUENCING THE NURSE PRACTITIONER ROLE

Elizabeth Blunt, PhD, MSN, FNP-BC

LEGAL DIMENSIONS OF THE ROLE

Legal Authority for Practice

State Nurse Practice Acts—Rules and Regulations

▶ Authority for nurse practitioner (NP) practice is found in state legislative statutes and in rules and regulations. The Nurse Practice Act of every state customarily authorizes a Board of Nursing to establish statutory authority to define who may be called an NP (title protection), what they may do (scope of practice), restrictions on their practice, the requirements an NP must meet to be credentialed within the state as an NP (education, certification, etc.), and disciplinary grounds for infractions. See www.ncsbn.org for a listing of state nursing board requirements. In many states, legislative acts may specifically require that an NP develop a collaborative agreement with a physician, describe what types of drugs might be prescribed, or define some form of oversight board for NP practice.

▶ Statutory law is implemented in regulatory language. The rules and regulations for each state may further define scope of practice, practice requirements, and/or restrictions.

▶ In 1999, the National Council of State Boards of Nursing (NCSBN) began implementation of an interstate compact for nursing practice to reduce state-to-state discrepancies in nursing requirements for practice. The Advanced Practice Registered Nurse (APRN) Compact addresses the need to promote consistent access to quality advanced practice nursing care within states and across state lines. The Uniform APRN Licensure/Authority to Practice Requirements, developed by NCSBN with APRN stakeholders in 2000, establishes the foundation for this APRN Compact. Similar to the existing Nurse Licensure Compact for recognition of registered nurse (RN) and licensed practical nurse (LPN) licenses, the APRN Compact gives states the mechanism for mutually recognizing APRN licenses/authority to practice. To be eligible for the APRN Compact, a state must either be a member of the current nurse licensure compact for RN and LPN or choose to enter into both compacts simultaneously. To see which states participate, view the state compact map at https://www.ncsbn.org.

Nurse Practitioner Professional Practice

Licensure

▶ Licensure is "[a] process by which an agency of state government grants permission to individuals accountable for the practice of a profession to engage in the practice of that profession and prohibits all others from legally doing so" (Committee for the Study of Credentialing in Nursing, 1979; U.S. Department of Health, Education and Welfare [DHEW], 1971).

▶ The purpose of licensure is to protect the public by ensuring a minimum level of professional competence.

> Licensure benefits both the public and the individual nurse because essential qualifications for nursing practice are identified; a determination is made as to whether or not an individual meets those qualifications; and an objective forum is provided for review of concerns regarding a nurse's practice when needed. Licensure benefits nurses because clear legal authorization for the scope of practice of the profession is established. Licensure also protects the use of titles. Only a licensed nurse is authorized to use certain titles (i.e., registered nurses [RNs], licensed practical/vocational nurses [LPN/VNs], advanced practice registered nurses [APRNs], etc.) or to represent themself as a licensed nurse. (National Council of State Boards of Nursing [NCSBN], 2011)

Certification

▶ Certification is "[a] process by which a non-governmental agency or association certifies that an individual licensed to practice as a professional has met certain predetermined standards specified by that profession for specialty practice" (DHEW, 1971).

▶ The purpose of certification is to assure the public that a person has mastery of a body of knowledge and has acquired the skills necessary to function in a particular specialty. Some certifications are required for entry into practice (e.g., for licensure within a state) and thus have a regulatory function; some certifications denote professional competence and recognize excellence.

Accreditation

▶ Accreditation is "[t]he process by which a voluntary, non-governmental agency or organization appraises and grants accreditation status to institutions and/or programs or services [that] meet predetermined structure, process and outcome criteria" (DHEW, 1971). The purpose is to assure that the organization has met specific standards.

Scope of Practice

▶ *Scope of practice* defines a specific legal scope determined by state statutes, boards of nursing, educational preparation, and common practice within a community. For example, adult nurse practitioners (ANPs) are not legally authorized to care for children. The state might require an NP to have formal educational preparation in pediatrics. There is broad variation from state to state.

▶ General scope of practice is specified in many published professional documents (e.g., *Scope and Standards of Advanced Practice Registered Nursing*, ANA, 1996). In addition, many organizations have completed role delineation studies that attempt to qualify the core behaviors that all advanced practice nurses (APNs) must possess, as well as the core knowledge and behaviors required of persons in a particular specialty. For example, core knowledge for a pediatric nurse practitioner (PNP) is inherently different from that for a geriatric nurse practitioner (GNP). It is critical that these statements about specific scope and standards exist so that everyone—including nurses—will have access to materials to which they can refer when there are specific questions related to role. This is especially important when the traditional role of nurses is changing or "advancing" at an uneven rate through changes in state law. As the NP role has expanded into new practice settings, including hospice, acute care hospitals, and home care, it is important that core knowledge and state law protecting NPs in these practice settings also expand, providing the legal authorization and title protection necessary for these practice settings.

▶ Prescriptive authority is recognized as within the scope of practice for nurse practitioners in all 50 states, although there is major variability from state to state. This variability has created inherent difficulty in collecting data related to NP prescribing practices. The *Nurse Practitioner Journal* publishes a comprehensive update of legislative requirements and recent changes in its January issue each year. Data collected by Nurse Practitioner Alternatives, Inc., since 1996 has documented stability within prescribing patterns by NPs. Data from 2004 documents that the majority of NPs possess their own Drug Enforcement Administration (DEA) numbers (72%), write between 6 and 25 prescriptions in an average clinical day (79%), recommend between 1 and 20 over-the-counter (OTC) preparations in an average clinical day (90%), and manage between 25% and 100% of their patient encounters independently (97%; Nurse Practitioner Alternatives, Inc., 2004).

Standards of Practice

▶ Standards of practice are authoritative statements by which the quality of practice, service, or education can be judged (e.g., *Scope of Practice for Nurse Practitioners*, NONPF, 2013; *Code of Ethics for Nurses*, ANA, 2015).

▶ Professional standards focus on the minimum levels of acceptable performance as a way of providing consumers with a means of measuring the quality of care they receive. These standards may be written at the generic level to apply to all nurses (e.g., following universal precautions) as well as to define practice by each specialty.

▶ The presence of accepted standards of practice may be used to legally describe the standard of care that a provider must meet. These standards may be precise protocols that must be followed or recommendations for more general guidelines.

▶ *Healthy People 2020 Objectives* and the World Health Organization's "Health for All" are, respectively, national and international policy statements that describe objectives to be met to help all people obtain a level of health that will permit them to lead socially and economically productive lives. Eventually, these objectives are expected to form the basis for international standards of practice.

▶ The National Organization of Nurse Practitioner Faculties (NONPF; www.nonpf.com), in partnership with the American Association of Colleges of Nursing (www.aacn.nche.edu), developed nurse practitioner competencies: *Nurse Practitioner Primary Care Competencies in Specialty Areas: Adult-Gerontology Primary Care Nurse Practitioner Competencies* (2010) and *Psychiatric-Mental Health Nurse Practitioner, Family/Across the Lifespan, Neonatal, Pediatric Primary Care, and Women's Health/Gender-Related NP Competencies* (2012). Most recently, NONPF developed *Nurse Practitioner Core Competencies with Suggested Curriculum Content* (2014). Acute care nurse practitioner population-focused competencies are also available. These documents outline what an NP in each specialty area should be able to do (NONPF, 2012).

Patient Rights

Confidentiality

▶ The patient and family have a right to assume that information given to the health-care provider will not be disclosed; that is, their information will be kept confidential. This has several dimensions.

▶ *Verbal information*: Healthcare providers shall not discuss any information given to them during the healthcare encounter with anyone not directly involved in providing this care without the patient's or family's permission.

▶ *Written information*: Confidentiality of the healthcare encounter is protected under federal statute through the Health Insurance Portability and Accountability Act of 1996 (HIPAA). The Administrative Simplification provisions of HIPAA require the Department of Health and Human Services to establish national standards for electronic healthcare transactions and national identifiers for providers, health plans, and employers. The provisions also address the security and privacy of health data. Information may be accessed at http://www.cms.gov/regulations-and-guidance/hipaa-administrative-simplification/hipaageninfo/thehipaalawandrelated-information.html. The person's right to privacy is to be respected when requesting or responding to a request for a patient's medical record.

▶ The statute requires that the provider discuss confidentiality issues with patients (parents in the case of a minor), establish consent, and clarify any questions about disclosure of information.

▶ The provider is required to obtain a signed medical authorization and consent form to release medical records and information.

▶ Exceptions to guaranteed confidentiality occur when society determines that the need for information outweighs the principle of confidentiality. Examples might be when records are released to insurance companies, to attorneys involved in litigation, or in answering court orders, subpoenas, or summonses; in meeting state require-ments for mandatory reporting of diseases or conditions; in cases of suspected child abuse; or if a patient reveals an intent to harm someone.

Informed Consent

▶ *Informed consent* is the right of all competent adults (age 18 or older) and emancipated minors (age 17 or younger who are married, a parent, or self-sufficiently living away from the family domicile) to accept or reject treatment by a healthcare provider. (Some states have laws concerning birth control or abortions that apply to patients younger than 18.)

▶ The clinician has the duty to explain relevant information to the patient so the patient can make an appropriate decision. This information usually includes diagnosis, nature and purpose of proposed treatment or procedure, risks and benefits, prognosis, alternative methods of treatment along with risks and benefits, and even the remote possibility of serious harm.

▶ It must be documented in the medical records that this information has been provided.

▶ Informed consent does not absolve the NP from allegations of malpractice, should it occur.

Care of Minors

▶ In most jurisdictions, minors under the age of 18 cannot receive healthcare services without permission of a competent adult who is his or her parent or legal guardian.

▶ Exceptions to this rule may be made in some jurisdictions in the case of an emancipated minor, a pregnant minor, or in matters pertaining to sexually transmitted diseases and birth control.

Advance Directives

▶ When a patient is incapable of making decisions, the person's preferences may be expressed in a written living will or a healthcare durable power of attorney created when the patient was still competent. Such documents are called *advance directives*.

▶ *Living wills* are written documents prepared in advance in case of terminal illness or nonreversible loss of consciousness.

▶ Their provisions go into effect when:

  ▷ The patient has become incompetent, and

  ▷ The patient is declared terminally ill, and

  ▷ No further interventions will alter the patient's course to a reasonable degree of medical certainty.

Durable Power of Attorney for Health Care

▶ People can identify in writing an agent to act on their behalf, should they become mentally incapacitated. The decisions of the designated agent are:

  ▷ Binding,

  ▷ Not limited to the circumstances of terminal illness,

  ▷ Flexible enough to carry out the patient's wishes throughout the course of an illness, and

  ▷ Often accompanied by a durable power of attorney over financial issues as well.

Ethical Decision-Making

▶ Moral concepts such as advocacy, accountability, loyalty, caring, compassion, and human dignity are the foundations of ethical behavior.

▶ The ethical behavior of nurses has been defined for professional nursing in an American Nurses Association policy statement (ANA, 2015).

▶ Ethical behavior incorporates respect for the person and his or her autonomy. Thus, no decision is truly ethical if the caregiver does not involve the patient in decision-making to the full extent of the patient's capacity.

▶ Duty to help others (beneficence), avoidance of harmful behavior (nonmaleficence), and fairness are also foundational components of ethical behavior.

Quality Assurance

▶ *Quality assurance* (QA) is a system designed to evaluate and monitor the quality of patient care and facility management.

▶ Formal programs provide a framework for systematic, deliberate, and continuous evaluation and monitoring of individual clinical practice.

▶ Programs promote responsibility and accountability to deliver high-quality care, assist in the evaluation and improvement of the patient's care, and provide for an organized means of problem-solving.

▶ A good program identifies educational needs, improves the documentation of care, and reduces the clinician's overall exposure to liability.

▶ Programs identify components of structure, process, and outcomes of care. They also look at organizational effectiveness, efficiency, and client and provider interactions.

   ▷ QA may be implemented through audits, utilization review, peer review, outcome studies, and measurements of patient satisfaction.

Quality & Safety Education for Nurses (QSEN)

▶ Quality & Safety Education for Nurses (QSEN) was funded by the Robert Wood Johnson Foundation to address the knowledge, skills, and attitudes necessary to ensure the quality and safety of the healthcare systems in the nation.

▶ The Institute of Medicine (IOM), along with numerous professional organizations representing nursing, identified competencies to be used in the education, certification, and continuing education of advanced practice nurses.

▶ Areas identified that affect advanced practice include

   ▷ Patient-centered care focus,

   ▷ Teamwork and collaboration,

   ▷ Use of evidence-based practice,

   ▷ Continuous quality improvement,

   ▷ Safety to minimize harm to patients and providers, and

   ▷ Use of informatics.

Nurse Practitioner Legal and Financial Issues

Liability

► NPs should be aware of liability issues or exposure to legal risk, which include

▷ Patients, procedures, and

▷ Quality of medical records.

► There are methods of risk reduction or management:

▷ Activities or systems have been designed to recognize and intervene to reduce the risk of injury to patients and subsequent claims against healthcare providers.

▷ Malpractice insurance does not protect clinicians from charges of practicing outside their legal scope of practice. All clinicians carry their own liability insurance coverage to ensure their own legal representation by an attorney to advocate for them.

► Malpractice

▷ Malpractice involves negligent professional acts of persons engaged in professions requiring highly technical or professional skills.

▷ The plaintiff has the burden of proving the four elements of malpractice.

    ► *Duty*: The clinician does not exercise reasonable care when undertaking and providing treatment to the patient when a patient–clinician relationship exists.

    ► *Breach of duty*: The clinician violates the applicable standard of care in treating the patient's condition.

    ► *Proximate cause*: There is a causal relationship between the breach in the standard of care and the patient's injuries.

    ► *Damages*: There are permanent and substantial damages to the patient as a result of the malpractice.

▷ Types of malpractice insurance

    ► *Claims-made policy*: covers a claim only as long as both the incident and the claim take place while the policy is in force

    ► *Occurrence-based policy*: covers any claim that results from an incident that occurs during the term of the policy, regardless of how long it takes before the claim is made

    ► *Tail coverage*: additional or supplemental insurance that covers the provider for incidents that occurred during the term of a claims-made policy but are not brought forward until after the policy has expired

► National Practitioner Data Bank (NPDB)

▷ The Health Care Quality Improvement Act of 1986 established a databank to scrutinize members of the healthcare profession and list those practitioners who have had malpractice claims asserted against them.

▷ Currently, few NPs are listed in the National Practitioner Data Bank, but the number of NPs who have malpractice claims filed against them is increasing as the number of NPs in practice increases.

Reimbursement

▶ NPs are reimbursed for their services as primary care providers under Medicare, Medicaid, the Federal Employees Health Benefits Program, TRICARE (formerly known as CHAMPUS), veterans' and military programs, and federally funded school-based clinics.

▶ Medicare: People age 65 and over are eligible for Medicare.

▷ Medicare A: Hospital insurance that requires no premium. Part A covers inpatient care, including hospitals, skilled nursing facilities (not custodial or long-term care), hospice, and eligible home healthcare services.

▷ Medicare B: Outpatient insurance that requires a premium. Patients may decline coverage. Part B covers outpatient services, durable medical equipment, physical and occupational health services, home health care, and eligible preventive care services.

▷ Medicare C: Combines Part A and Part B of Medicare.

▷ Medicare D: Covers prescription drugs; usually requires a premium. Patient may decline coverage.

▷ Medicare E: Offers incentive/reimbursement for providers participating in electronic prescribing.

▶ Incident to billing: Medicare regulation. Pays 100% of the physician charge to an NP who provides care to patients under specific guidelines (see the Centers for Medicare & Medicaid Services [CMS] website for full guidelines):

▷ Services are furnished as an integral, though incidental, part of the physician's care.

▷ Physicians must provide the initial service and regular subsequent visits.

▷ A physician must be present in the office but not necessarily in the exam room.

▷ Services are billed under the physician's provider number at 100% of the physician rate.

▶ Medicaid

▷ Individual states administer and make the rules for Medicaid.

▷ States must adhere to CMS rules and regulations when directing the Medicaid program.

▷ By federal law, Medicaid will cover services of family and pediatric NPs.

▷ If a state has applied to CMS for a Medicaid waiver, it is important that NPs are allowed to be primary care providers.

▷ NPs must apply to state Medicaid for Medicaid provider numbers.

▷ Full CMS guidelines are available at www.cms.gov.

▶ Private insurance plans may elect to reimburse for NP services even if not mandated to do so by state law. In some states, however, the insurance code may be interpreted rigidly to exclude reimbursement of NPs.

▶ Managed care organizations (MCOs) have frequently excluded NPs from being designated as primary care providers carrying their own caseloads. Thus, in many

MCOs, the only option for NPs is to be salaried employees. As salaried employees, the NP contributions are often not visible and may be credited to their collaborating physicians, giving them a "ghost" provider status. Without a legitimate method to document services provided and revenue generated, the NP can find that job security is often at risk. Many state NP organizations have recently focused legislative activity on enacting state laws allowing NPs to function as primary care providers in both health maintenance organizations (HMOs) and preferred provider organizations (PPOs). These efforts have led to opposition from state medical organizations.

▶ There is considerable flux in state and national policy on what services and procedures NPs may bill for and whether they will be paid directly. Incorrect billing places healthcare providers at risk of fraud and abuse charges, regardless of whether they knowingly violate the law or are just ignorant of the regulations.

▶ NPs must be aware of specific regulations and policies for patient care services. Resources include CMS bulletins, among others (www.cms.hhs.gov/).

▶ Coding and billing practices are a responsibility of the NP provider, and knowledge of the regulations for payors is a requisite competency.

▶ Specific rules and regulations for Medicare and Medicaid can be found at www.cms.hhs.gov.

Performance Assessment

▶ The National Practitioner Data Bank (NPDB) and Health Integrity and Protection Data Bank (HIPDB) are maintained by the U.S. Department of Health and Human Services, Health Resources and Services Administration, Bureau of Health Professions, Division of Practitioner Data Banks. Developed as a result of the Health Care Quality Improvement Act of 1986, the NPDB and HIPDB are flagging systems intended to facilitate a comprehensive review of healthcare practitioners' professional credentials, with a goal of improving the quality of health care. The information contained in the NPDB includes a practitioner's licensure, professional society memberships, malpractice payment history, and record of clinical privileges. An NP may perform a self-query by visiting the site at www.npdb-hipdb.com/.

▶ Other programs monitoring and comparing health quality include the Healthcare Effectiveness Data and Information Set (HEDIS), developed by the National Committee on Quality Assurance. HEDIS is a set of standardized performance measures designed to ensure that purchasers and consumers have the information they need to reliably compare the performance of managed healthcare plans (www.ncqa.org/).

Health Records

Currently, CMS is preparing for an electronic health record (EHR) system that would allow ready access to medical records at a national level for more definitive monitoring of the effectiveness and outcomes of interventions. The data collected will be used to assist in determining the most effective clinical interventions and establishing effective guidelines for healthcare providers.

▶ Centers for Medicare & Medicaid Services and Electronic Health Records

▷ CMS is promoting the use of electronic health records (EHRs) to assist in attaining national healthcare accuracy and efficiency and better meet established goals.

▷ The term "meaningfully" is being used for the EHR to assess the efficiency of an electronic system. The 2009 American Recovery and Reinvestment Act delineates three essential components for meaningful use of EHRs for electronic prescribing, exchange of information, and measurement of clinical quality. In 2011, the first of the three stages was implemented, with the final stage implemented in 2015. The program is voluntary and requires application according to established guidelines. Reimbursement for program participation is based on specific criteria, such as benchmarks for recording accurate vital signs, height, body mass index (BMI), immunizations, and other healthcare interventions.

▷ Benefits for the patient include receiving reminders for appointments by email, accessing portions of the medical record to review lab work, and leaving messages for providers. Specifics may be found on the CMS website at https://www.cms.gov/Regulations-and-Guidance/Legislation/EHRIncentivePrograms/index.html?redirect=/ehrincentiveprograms.

▷ E-scribe: Electronically submitting prescriptions is now common practice, and specific laws regarding e-scribing vary slightly from state to state. Refer to specific state laws for accurate rules regarding the use of e-scribing by means of certified EHR.

Current Trends and Topics in Nurse Practitioner Education and Practice

NP Education

The IOM report *The Future of Nursing: Leading Change, Advancing Health* and IOM and Robert Wood Johnson Foundation studies are landmark documents that assessed and are transforming the nursing profession:

▶ Report published October 2010

▶ Advocates for nurses to practice to the full extent of their education without barriers

▶ Four key messages:

▷ Nurses should practice to the full extent of their education and training.

▷ Nurses should achieve higher levels of education and training through an improved education system that promotes seamless academic progression.

▷ Nurses should be full partners, with physicians and other healthcare professionals, in redesigning health care in the United States.

▷ Effective workforce planning and policy-making require better data collection and information infrastructure.

▶ Recommendations

▷ Remove scope-of-practice barriers

▷ Expand opportunities for nurses to lead and diffuse collaborative improvement efforts.

▷ Implement nurse residency programs.

▷ Increase the proportion of nurses with a baccalaureate degree to 80% by 2020.

▷ Double the number of nurses with a doctorate by 2020.

▷ Ensure that nurses engage in lifelong learning.

▷ Prepare and enable nurses to lead change to advance health.

▷ Build an infrastructure for the collection and analysis of inter-professional healthcare workforce data.

▶ Impact on NP practice and role

▷ There is a focus on NP practice as cost-effective, quality care providers for patients in a variety of settings.

▷ There should be increased public and legislative awareness of the NP role.

▷ The report challenges barriers to NP practice.

▷ The report supports continued and lifelong learning, including achieving Doctor of Nursing Practice (DNP) or other doctoral education.

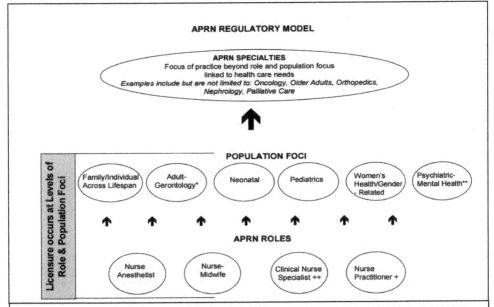

FIGURE 2–1.
APRN REGULATORY MODEL

Reprinted from *Consensus Model for APRN Regulation: Licensure, Accreditation, Certification, & Education* (p. 10), by the APRN Consensus Work Group and the National Council of State Boards of Nursing APRN Advisory Committee, 2008. Retrieved from https://www.ncsbn.org/Consensus_Model_for_APRN_Regulation_July_2008.pdf

Consensus Model for Advanced Practice Registered Nurse (APRN) Regulation: Licensure, Accreditation, Certification, and Education

▶ Consensus document from more than 40 nursing and advanced practice organizations and the NCSBN APRN Advisory Committee

▶ Published July 2008

▶ Provides a national baseline for APRN licensure, accreditation, certification, and education (LACE)

▶ Defines APRN practice, describes APRN regulatory model, identifies titles to be used, defines specialty, describes emergence of new roles and population foci, presents strategies for implementation

▶ Key issues:

  ▷ Goal is standardization of APRN education, licensure, and practice across all states and territories

  ▷ Limits APRN title to four roles: nurse practitioner, nurse anesthetist, nurse midwife, and clinical nurse specialist

  ▷ Identifies six population foci, with potential for more as practice changes

  ▷ Provided for elimination of separate geriatric and adult NP role and certification, replaced with combined ANP-GNP role, education, and certification

Doctor of Nursing Practice (DNP)

▶ 2004: American Association of Colleges of Nursing (AACN) members approve DNP Position Statement and 2015 target implementation date.

▶ 2006: *The Essentials of Doctoral Education for Advanced Nursing Practice* is published.

▶ Doctor of Nursing Practice (DNP) is the degree associated with practice-focused doctoral nursing education.

▶ The goal is to prepare graduates for the highest level of nursing practice beyond initial preparation in the discipline.

▶ It includes, but is not limited to, the four current APN roles: clinical nurse specialist, nurse anesthetist, nurse midwife, and nurse practitioner.

▶ The degree may be entry into practice or post-master's degree.

▶ It includes eight essentials of doctoral education for advanced nursing practice:

  ▷ Scientific Underpinnings for Practice

  ▷ Organizational and Systems Leadership for Quality Improvement and Systems Thinking

  ▷ Clinical Scholarship and Analytical Methods for Evidence-Based Practice

  ▷ Information Systems/Technology and Patient Care Technology for the Improvement and Transformation of Health Care

  ▷ Healthcare Policy for Advocacy in Health Care

  ▷ Inter-Professional Collaboration for Improving Patient and Population Health Outcomes

▷ Clinical Prevention and Population Health for Improving the Nation's Health

▷ Advanced Nursing Practice

▶ It is endorsed by APRN organizations but has no required entry-into-practice date established for NPs.

▶ In 2014, DNP programs were offered at more than 250 schools nationwide, with an additional 64 in the planning stages.

▶ From 2013 to 2014:

▷ The number of students enrolled in DNP programs increased from 14,688 to 18,352.

▷ The number of DNP graduates increased from 2,443 to 3,065.

▶ Recognition of the need to ensure the quality of NP education, faculty, and curricula has led to efforts by the National Organization of Nurse Practitioner Faculties (NONPF) and the AACN to promulgate core competency statements. These can be viewed at http://www.nonpf.org/displaycommon.cfm?an=1&subarticlenbr=14.

▶ In addition, NONPF, AACN, numerous NP professional organizations, NP accrediting bodies, and educational organizations have jointly promulgated criteria for evaluating nurse practitioner programs. In combination with accreditation standards for graduate programs and specialty areas, the criteria provide a basis for evaluating the quality of nurse practitioner programs. Documents may be viewed at http://www.nonpf.org/displaycommon.cfm?an=1&subarticlenbr=15.

▶ AACN, working with NONPF (and with input from other groups), has developed a practice doctorate in nursing. In the future, the practice doctorate is expected to be the graduate degree for advanced nursing practice preparation, including but not limited to the four current APN roles: clinical nurse specialist, nurse anesthetist, nurse midwife, and nurse practitioner.

▶ The Board of NONPF regards the practice doctorate of nursing as an important evolutionary step for the preparation of nurse practitioners (NPs). We anticipate that the practice doctorate degree will become the standard for entry into nurse practitioner practice; however, much like with the movement of educational preparation of NPs from the post-basic certificate to a master's degree, this evolution will be gradual. NONPF does not support any finite deadline by when NP programs should be at doctoral level preparation but instead encourages NP educators to continue to sustain the highest quality programs to prepare NPs for clinical practice. (NONPF, 2006)

▶ In 2006, NONPF published *Practice Doctorate Nurse Practitioner Entry-Level Competencies,* replaced in 2011 by a single set of nurse practitioner core competencies. This document may be viewed at http://c.ymcdn.com/sites/www.nonpf.org/resource/resmgr/competencies/npcorecompetenciesfinal2012.pdf.

Practice Environment

1. *Health disparities:* There is growing recognition of disparities in the health services and outcomes of different populations in the United States. The National Institute on Minority Health and Health Disparities at the National Institutes of Health (NIH) is a government organization with a mission to promote minority health and to lead, coordinate, support, and assess the NIH effort to reduce and ultimately eliminate health disparities (for more information, visit http://ncmhd.nih.gov/).

2. *Health literacy:* Now recognized as one of the largest contributors to health outcome is the ability of a patient and family to understand and act on health information. Both the IOM and the Agency for Healthcare Research and Quality (AHRQ) have launched efforts to quantify and offer solutions to the problems that result from inadequate health literacy. The IOM report may be viewed at http://www.iom.edu/Reports/2010/The-Future-of-Nursing-Leading-Change-Advancing-Health.aspx. The AHRQ study can be found at http://www.ahrq.gov/research/findings/factsheets/literacy/healthlit/.

3. *Research:* FNPs need to understand research methods and be able to translate research into practice:

   ▷ Research Ethics: The American Nurses Association and other organizations provide Codes of Ethics related to research activities.

   ▷ Quantitative vs. Qualitative Research

      ▶ Quantitative research: research that uses objective measurements to provide numerical and statistical information and data in the form of numbers, percentages, and ratios; may include interventions and treatments

      ▶ Qualitative research: investigation of a problem using inquiry methods and developing conclusions based on observations, quotes, and themes

   ▷ Translational Research

      ▶ Understanding research methodology and bio-statistical data in order to evaluate, interpret, and implement research findings

      ▶ Identification of evidence-based research and use of critical thinking to implement new research findings and ideas into practice

   ▷ FNPs must be prepared to be

      ▶ Lifelong learners: identifying research problems, participating in research activities, and using and applying research findings

      ▶ Scholars: providing outcomes research data through various dissemination modes such as publications, speaking engagements, and professional presentations

4. *Assurance of Safe Practice*

   ▷ A system to evaluate and monitor the quality of patients' care and facility management.

   Formal programs that provide a framework for continuous, consistent monitoring and evaluation:

      ▶ Structure, process, and outcomes of care

      ▶ Client interactions

      ▶ Clinical competence

      ▶ Performance assessment

         ▷ Knowledge of standards of care and clinical guidelines

         ▷ Minimizing clinical errors and complications by using risk-reducing tools such as smart phones and tablets, flow sheets, and electronic resources

         ▷ Promoting a safe work environment using principles of QSEN

    ▷ Evaluation of clinical outcomes using

        ▶ Continuous Quality Improvement (CQI),

        ▶ Peer review, and

        ▶ Audit.

Coordination of Transcultural Care

Cultural Diversity

▶ Culture: Common beliefs, values, practices, and behaviors shared by multiple sub-groups or individuals

▶ Rapidly shifting demographics in the United States—the melting pot

▶ U.S. census data estimates:

    ▷ 2010: White 72%, Black 12%, Hispanic 12%, Asian 4%

    ▷ 2050: White 52%, Black 15%, Hispanic 25%, Asian 8%

▶ Immigrant populations change the needs of communities.

▶ Most immigrants (60%) cluster in large, mostly coastal metropolitan areas: Los Angeles, New York, San Francisco, Chicago, Miami, Houston, and Washington, DC.

▶ Cultural diversity is not just about race or language; it also includes country of origin, cultural practices and beliefs, food, religion, and values.

▶ Diversity presents challenges to all aspects of life: education, literacy, communication, access to care, transportation, and cultural assimilation.

Role of the FNP

▶ Prevent personal biases from interfering with the delivery of quality care

▶ Help patients of diverse cultures gain access to quality care

▶ Address the influence of culture, ethnicity, and spirituality on the mental and physical health of the individual and family in varied healthcare settings

▶ Provide culturally sensitive care across the life span:

    ▷ Access to appointments and services in appropriate language

    ▷ Translators for visits

    ▷ Written instructions in appropriate language

▶ Incorporate cultural preferences, values, health beliefs, and behaviors into the management plan

▶ Help patients and families meet their spiritual needs and incorporate patients' spiritual beliefs into care

▶ Ensure healthcare resources are available to people from diverse backgrounds:

    ▷ Identify other services and facilities (lab, radiology, nursing home, hospital, etc.) that can provide culturally sensitive care

▶ Facilitate the development of healthcare systems that address the needs of culturally diverse populations, providers, and communities

Disaster and Emergency Care and Planning

Attention is increasingly being paid to preparing registered nurses to assume emergency roles during a time of mass casualties from either natural disasters or terrorist attacks. Because other countries have had more experience in dealing with terrorism, the International Nursing Coalition for Mass Casualty Education has been established, headquartered at the Vanderbilt University School of Nursing, to help U.S. nurses profit from others' experience and to identify the educational competencies for registered nurses responding to mass casualty incidents. The coalition desires to improve the ability of all nurses to respond safely and effectively to mass casualty incidents through identification of existing and emerging roles of nurses, ensuring appropriateness of education for mass casualty incidents, and helping to understand response frameworks and ensure collaborative efforts. All NPs are expected to prepare themselves to play a larger role in delivery of care during a time of disaster. Information on the objectives and work that has been done toward a uniform curriculum in this area may be obtained at http://www.nursing.vanderbilt. edu/advantage/emergency.html. Additionally, the Emergency Nurses Association, with endorsement from NONPF, has published specialty competencies for the NP who practices in emergency care (2008). These competencies can be found at http://c.ymcdn.com/sites/www.nonpf.org/ resource/resmgr/competencies/compsfornpsinemergencycarefinal.pdf. The Centers for Disease Control and Prevention also maintains emergency preparedness resources for healthcare providers. These can be found at http://emergency.cdc.gov/.

Complementary and Integrative Health

There is greater recognition of the use of complementary and integrative modalities by patients. The National Center for Complementary and Integrative Health is the federal government's lead agency for scientific research on complementary and integrative health (https://nccih.nih.gov).

Definitions (NCCIH)

NCCIH uses the following terms:

"Complementary health approaches" is used when discussing practices and products of nonmainstream origin.

"Integrative health" is used when discussing practices that incorporate complementary approaches into mainstream health care.

If a practice is nonmainstream and used together with conventional medicine, it's considered "complementary."

If a practice is nonmainstream and used in place of conventional medicine, it's considered "alternative."

Demographics

▶ More than 30 percent of adults and 12 percent of children use complementary or alternative approaches to health care

▶ Many drug–herb interactions have been identified.

▶ 68% of clinically significant drug–herb reactions are related to five herbs:
  ▷ Kava
  ▷ Garlic

TEN MOST COMMON COMPLEMENTARY HEALTH APPROACHES IN USE BY ADULTS IN THE UNITED STATES	
17.7%	Natural products
10.9%	Deep breathing
10.1%	Yoga, tai chi, or qi gong
8.4%	Chiropractic or osteopathic manipulation
8.0%	Meditation
6.9%	Massage
3.0%	Special diets
2.2%	Homeopathy
2.1%	Progressive relaxation
1.7%	Guided imagery

Source: *Trends in the use of complementary approaches among adults: United States, 2002– 2012. National health statistics reports no. 79*, by T. C. Clarke, L. I. Black, B. J. Stussman, P. M. Barnes, and R. L. Nahin, 2015, Hyattsville, MD: National Center for Health Statistics.

 ▷ Ginkgo biloba

 ▷ St. John's wort

 ▷ Valerian

 ▶ The prescription medications most frequently affected:

 ▷ Warfarin

 ▷ Sedative/hypnotics

 ▷ Antidepressants

 ▷ Insulin

 ▷ Oral antidiabetic agents

 ▷ Hepatotoxic medications

 ▷ Oral contraceptives

Role of Nurse Practitioner

 ▶ NPs should be aware of current evidence-based research and resources concerning CAM interventions.

 ▶ Be nonjudgmental and maintain an unbiased attitude about patient's choice of CAM.

 ▶ Proactively ask all patients about their use of and response to CAM:

 ▷ Have patients bring their supplements (bottles, tubes, containers, packaging, etc.) to visits.

 ▷ Ask about alternative therapies.

 ▷ Document all CAM information and referrals in patient's record.

 ▷ Use caution with women of childbearing age—many herbals are category C.

TABLE 2–1.
NCCIH TYPES OF COMPLEMENTARY HEALTH APPROACHES

APPROACH	EXAMPLES
Natural Products*	Vitamins and minerals, probiotics, herbs (also known as botanicals)
Mind and Body Practices	Acupuncture, relaxation techniques, guided imagery, tai chi, gi qong, healing touch, hypnotherapy, movement therapies, yoga, chiropractic, meditation, massage therapy
Other Complementary Health Approaches	Homeopathy, traditional healers, Ayurvedic medicine, naturopathy, traditional Chinese medicine,

*Herbal products, probiotics, and vitamins are not approved by the FDA and are considered food supplements.

Source: National Center for Complementary and Integrative Health (NCCIH). Retrieved from https://nccih.nih.gov/health/integrative-health#term

TABLE 2–2.
SELECT DRUG–HERB INTERACTIONS

HERB	DRUG(S)	EFFECT
Garlic	Warfarin	Decreased blood concentrations
Ginkgo biloba	Anticoagulants, aspirin, NSAIDs	Increased risk of bleeding with warfarin
	Thiazide diuretic	Increased blood pressure
	Trazodone	Coma
	Anticonvulsants, TCAs	Decreased seizure threshold
Kava	Benzodiazepines	Additive CNS depression
	Levodopa	Increased "off" periods in Parkinson patients
St. John's wort	Warfarin and related anticoagulants, cyclosporin, amitriptyline, digoxin	Decreased blood concentrations
	Piroxicam, tetracyclines	Increased phototoxicity
	Antidepressants, CNS stimulants	Additive effects
	Theophylline	Decreased xanthine levels
Valerian	CNS depressants	Additive CNS depression

Note. NSAIDs = nonsteroidal anti-inflammatory drugs; TCAs = tricyclic antidepressants; CNS = central nervous system.

Caring for People with Disabilities

Definitions

- ▶ Americans with Disabilities Act (ADA), 1990
  - ▷ A person with a disability has a physical or mental impairment that substantially limits one or more major life activities, *or* a record or history of such an impairment, *or* is regarded/ perceived by others as having such an impairment.
- ▶ World Health Organization
  - ▷ Disability is an umbrella term, covering impairments, activity limitations, and participation restrictions.

▷ Disability is a complex phenomenon, reflecting an interaction between features of a person's body and features of the society in which he or she lives.

▶ International Council of Nurses (ICN), 2010

▷ A disability is a physical, mental, sensory, or social impairment that, in the long term, adversely affects one's ability to carry out normal day-to-day activities.

▷ ICN advocates for

▶ Programs designed to integrate people with disability (PWD) in all aspects of daily life (family, school, workplace, and community),

▶ Ensuring that nursing education addresses competencies needed for the prevention of disability and the care and rehabilitation of PWD, and

▶ Assistance, support, and advocacy for PWD and their families to access education, information, and support services that allow them to lead fulfilling lives.

▶ Another view of disability (Kirschner & Curry, 2009): Disability is a universal experience that affects nearly everyone without exception at some time in their lives.

▶ Significance of definitions of disability—NPs must determine:

▷ Who is eligible for services,

▷ What services are "allowed,"

▷ Our views about and perceptions of PWD, and

▷ How we interact with and treat PWD in all education, clinical practice, and community sites and settings.

Demographics

▶ 60 million people in the United States and more than 1 billion worldwide live with one or more disabilities.

▶ 1 in every 4 people lives with one or more disabilities.

▶ Disabilities occur across the life span:

▷ 13.9% of children

▷ 11.0% of people age 18 to 44

▷ 23.9% of people age 45 to 64

▷ 51.8% of those ≥ 65 years

▶ Reasons the population of PWD is increasing in size:

▷ Advances in health care and survival of people with disabilities across the life span (very low birth weight babies, adults who are chronically critically ill, etc.)

▷ Increase in number of people with chronic disease

▷ Increased survival after trauma and war

▷ Increased number of elderly and frail elderly

Models of Disability

▶ Medical model: views disability as a problem of the person

▶ Rehabilitation model: sees PWD as having deficiencies or defects

▶ Social model: views disability as socially constructed and due to failure of able-bodied society to provide access and accommodations

▶ Biopsychological model: addresses health from a biologic, individual, and social perspective

▶ Interface model: most favored by PWD

  ▷ Based on the life experience of the person with a disability

  ▷ Views disability at the intersection (i.e., interface) of health issue and environmental barriers

  ▷ Considers, rather than ignores, the health issue or medical problem

  ▷ Only model of disability developed by a nurse who had a disability

Characteristics of Disabilities

▶ Disabilities vary in severity:

  ▷ Very mild (inconvenience)

  ▷ Moderate (interfere with some activities)

  ▷ Severe (need assistance for instrumentals [IADL] and activities of daily living [ADL])

  ▷ Very severe (need technology for survival)

▶ Disabilities vary in type:

  ▷ Physical

  ▷ Sensory (vision and hearing)

  ▷ Psychiatric or mental health

  ▷ Cognitive or intellectual

  ▷ Communication

▶ Disabilities vary in visibility:

  ▷ Not at all visible to others

  ▷ Visible to informed others

  ▷ Visible to all

▶ Issues for providers

  ▷ Access and care

    ▶ People with disabilities encounter serious barriers to receiving quality health care, including preventive care and screening and reproductive care.

    ▶ Healthcare providers are often unable to address sexuality, pregnancy, childbearing, and common health problems in people with disabilities.

    ▶ People with disabilities have received lower quality of care and less aggressive treatment and are offered few choices.

    ▶ People with disabilities have reported being refused care.

      ▷ Poor communication is a major barrier to care for people with disabilities.

▷ Barriers include

- ▶ Lack of awareness and knowledge about specific disabilities and of disability in general,

- ▶ Lack of sensitivity to and knowledge about the effect of disability on health issues and the effect of health issues on disability,

- ▶ Lack of awareness and sensitivity to the need for "disability etiquette,"

- ▶ General disregard of the experience and expertise of people with disabilities about their disability,

- ▶ Lack of accountability of healthcare providers for providing needed accommodations to enable people with disabilities to receive health care,

- ▶ Lack of knowledge about the law or disregard for the legal mandates, and

- ▶ An often erroneous assumption that people with disabilities are dependent on others and incapable of making their own decisions.

▷ Consequences of lack of access and care

- ▶ Negative encounters, often resulting in people with disabilities avoiding healthcare providers unless and until absolutely necessary

- ▶ Inadequate health care, including preventive screening

- ▶ Delay in treatment or lack of treatment

- ▶ Low level of participation in health promotion activities

- ▶ Poor health status, isolation, and psychological issues

▷ Strategies to address health-related disparities

- ▶ Increase our own awareness, sensitivity, and knowledge about disability, health issues of this population, and disparities related to disability

- ▶ Identify our own attitudes, biases, and prejudices

- ▶ Adopt "person-first language"

- ▶ Use disability etiquette in interaction with people with disabilities

- ▶ Assume that people with disabilities are the experts on their own disabilities

- ▶ Attend programs on disability in practice and education

- ▶ Involve people with disabilities in teaching you and others

- ▶ Provide accommodations (large print, Braille, pictures, tapes, etc.) to address disabled patients' learning needs

▶ Remember that PWDs are often the experts on their disability and their response(s) to it.

▶ Practice the concept of "nothing about us without us" and the concept that no policy should be decided by a group or representative without participation of the members of the group affected.

Genetics and Genomics

Overview

▶ Genetic and genomic science is redefining the understanding of the continuum of human health and illness. Recognition of genomics as a central science for health professional knowledge is essential.

▶ The human genome project was completed in April 2003.

▶ This science is number one on the list of the 10 most important medical advances in the first decade of the 21st century.

▶ Care for all people, across the life span, will increasingly require familiarity with genetic and genomic information related to

▷ Prevention,

▷ Screening,

▷ Diagnostics,

▷ Prognostics,

▷ Selection of treatment,

▷ Monitoring of treatment effectiveness,

▷ Referral, and

▷ The International HapMap Project (haplotype map).

     ▶ Genetic databank allows exploration of relationships between genetic differences and diseases

     ▶ A global catalog of common human genetic variants

     ▶ Contains a description of each variant, identifies where it occurs in human DNA, describes variation and distribution within and across populations

     ▶ Links genetic markers with human traits (e.g., celiac disease) and/or the presence or absence of disease

Definition

▶ *Genetics:* The study of individual genes and their impact on relatively rare single-gene disorders

▶ *Genomics*: The study of all the genes in the human genome together, including their interactions with one another, the environment, and the influence of psychosocial and cultural factors

Role of the FNP

▶ Understand the relationship of genetics and genomics to health, prevention, screening, diagnostics, prognostics, selection of treatment, and monitoring of treatment effectiveness

▶ Facilitate access to genetic specialists

▶ Develop a family history

▷ Complete detailed family history, including genetic and environmental risk factors

▷ Use these mnemonics to identify "red flag" issues:

- ▶ SCREEN
  - ▷ Some concern
  - ▷ Reproduction
  - ▷ Early disease, death, or disability
  - ▷ Ethnicity
  - ▷ Nongenetic
- ▶ Family GENES
  - ▷ Family: multiple affected siblings or persons in multiple generations
  - ▷ G: groups of congenital anomalies
  - ▷ E: extreme or exceptional presentation of common conditions
  - ▷ N: neurodevelopmental delay or degeneration
  - ▷ E: extreme or exceptional pathology
  - ▷ S: surprising laboratory values
- ▶ Pharmacogenomics
  - ▷ Drug metabolism is orchestrated by complex interactions among dozens of different genes.
  - ▷ There is potential for safer drugs, more effective prescribing, more accurate dosing, targeted vaccines, and reduced cost (e.g., warfarin).
- ▶ Lifestyle
  - ▷ Lifestyle risk factors are known to affect overall health (sedentary lifestyle, obesity).
  - ▷ Biologic processes are complex and poorly understood.
  - ▷ Findings in telomere studies identify some impact of lifestyle on the life of the gene.
  - ▷ Further genetic research may identity genetic components to lifestyle risk.
- ▶ Genetic counseling and screening
  - ▷ Multidisciplinary healthcare team provides counseling and screening
  - ▷ Considerations for genetic counseling and/or screening:
    - ▶ Those who have, or are concerned that they might have, an inherited disorder or birth defect
    - ▶ Women who are pregnant or planning to be after age 35
    - ▶ Couples who already have a child with an inherited disorder, undiagnosed disease, or birth defect
    - ▶ Couples whose infants have a genetic disease diagnosed by routine newborn screening
    - ▶ Women who have had three or more miscarriages or babies who died in infancy

- ▶ People concerned that their jobs, lifestyles, or medical histories may pose a risk to the outcome of pregnancy (common causes of concern include exposure to radiation, medications, illegal drugs, chemicals, or infections)
- ▶ Couples who would like testing or more information about genetic conditions that occur frequently in their ethnic groups
- ▶ Couples who are first cousins or other close blood relatives
- ▶ Pregnant women whose ultrasound examinations or blood testing indicate that their pregnancies may be at increased risk for certain complications or birth defects

- ▶ Prenatal testing
  - ▷ Began in 1970s with alpha fetal protein testing
  - ▷ Quad screen with ultrasound can identify approximately 90% of trisomy 21
  - ▷ Markers help identify risk pregnancies such as preeclampsia, fetal growth restriction, fetal demise, and abnormal placentation

- ▶ Gene therapy
  - ▷ This is a technique for correcting defective genes responsible for disease development. All require "carrier molecule" or vector to carry therapeutic gene to patient's target cells; most common vector is a genetically adapted virus. Several approaches:
    - ▶ Most common: normal gene inserted into a nonspecific location within the genome to replace a nonfunctional gene
    - ▶ Abnormal gene could be switched with normal gene through homologous recombination
    - ▶ Abnormal gene repaired through selective reverse mutation that returns gene to its normal function
    - ▶ Gene regulation (the degree to which a gene is turned on or off) could be altered
  - ▷ The Food and Drug Administration (FDA) has not yet approved any human gene therapy product for sale; all are still experimental.
  - ▷ Ethical questions and opinions about gene therapy abound.
  - ▷ NPs need to become increasingly familiar with pharmacogenomics and the most recent indications for medication prescribing.

End-of-Life Care

All patients are entitled to counsel regarding end-of-life care to ensure that patients have input and can involve their families with their care at the end of life. Advance care directives assure that the patient's desires are known and followed when the patient is no longer able to communicate. NPs play a unique role in this care delivery process in both the inpatient and outpatient settings.

- ▶ Palliative care is comprehensive and coordinated, using all resources available within the community, with no exclusions regarding curative therapy.
- ▶ Hospice care is more focused on keeping patients comfortable at the end of life and generally does not include treatment intended to be curative.

▶ Palliative care

▷ Comprehensive care for short- or long-term illnesses, including incurable conditions

▷ Multidisciplinary approach

▷ Includes pain and symptom management

▷ Addresses social, psychological, and spiritual needs as well as physical (including pain management)

▷ Information available from the Hospice and Palliative Nurses Association (http://www.hpna.org/) and the Center to Advance Palliative Care (www.getpalliativecare.org)

▶ Hospice care

▷ Available when all curative treatment options are exhausted or refused

▷ Multidisciplinary approach

▷ Focuses on pain control and comfort measures

▷ Stresses quality of life

▷ Provides family support

▷ Exclusions regarding therapeutic interventions delineated before patient enters hospice care

Direct-to-Consumer Advertising

Patients frequently present to the office already having formed their diagnosis and wanting specific treatments. NPs must become knowledgeable about the newest products on the market and how they are marketed to consumers to appropriately counsel and treat patients. NPs must critically read clinical studies and make evidence-based decisions about the appropriateness of medications and therapies based on individual patient presentation.

Telehealth

With rapidly expanding technology, the use of telecommunications in healthcare delivery is ever-changing. Telehealth in part includes "use of information and technologies that are emerging, as well as the ability to move the caregiver and information to where the patient is rather than moving the patient to centralized places to deliver health services and information." (Huston, 2013) Areas to be included in these advances:

▶ High-quality video conferencing between provider and patient

▶ Medical records

▶ Surgical robots

▶ Remote monitoring of implanted medical devices such as pacemakers, defibrillators, and some pain medication delivery systems

Since the release of the IOM report *To Err is Human: Building A Safer Health System* (1999). increased attention has been paid to changes all healthcare providers should make to reduce medical errors. In response, The Joint Commission (formerly known as JCAHO, or The Joint Commission on Accreditation of Healthcare Organizations, www.jointcommission.org/) has issued a list of abbreviations that should not be used in health care. In addition, the Institute for Safe Medication Practices has published a list of dangerous abbreviations related to medication use that it recommends should be explicitly prohibited (http://www.ismp.org/). The list of banned abbreviations includes many symbols traditionally used in patient charts and writing prescriptions.

Therapeutic Communication

Overview

▶ *Therapeutic communication* is a transaction between the sender and the receiver. Both parties participate simultaneously.

▶ In the transactional model, both participants perceive each other, listen to each other, and simultaneously engage in the process of creating meaning in a relationship, focusing on the patient's issues.

▶ Both patient and provider bring preexisting conditions and bias to the exchange that influences the intended message and its interpretation.

▶ Interactions must be viewed in the context of both the patient and the provider:

▷ Values, attitudes, and beliefs

▷ Gender

▷ Age or developmental level

▷ Culture or religion

▷ Social status

▷ The environment

▶ Requirements for therapeutic relationships:

▷ Rapport

▷ Trust

▷ Respect

▷ Honesty

▷ Empathy

▶ Therapeutic communication involves actively listening to what the patient says, both verbally and nonverbally.

▷ Nonverbal

    ▶ Body language

    ▶ Affect and demeanor

▷ Verbal

    ▶ Giving broad openings—offering general leads

    ▶ Using silence—accepting

    ▶ Giving recognition—restating

    ▶ Reflecting—focusing

    ▶ Exploring—seeking clarification and validation

▶ Nonverbal behaviors to promote active listening:

    ▷   **S**—Sit squarely facing the patient

    ▷   **O**—Observe an open posture

    ▷   **L**—Lean forward, toward the patient

    ▷   **E**—Establish eye contact

    ▷   **R**—Relax

Therapeutic Boundaries

▶ The therapeutic relationship is a planned, goal-directed, and contractual relationship between the provider and the patient for the purpose of providing care to the patient to meet his or her physical, emotional, and spiritual healthcare needs.

▶ Therapeutic relationships occur along a dynamic continuum.

▶ The provider is accountable and takes responsibility for setting and maintaining the boundaries of a therapeutic relationship, regardless of the client's actions or requests.

▶ Professional boundaries identify the parameters of the therapeutic relationship.

▶ Boundary crossing is a conscious or unconscious decision by the provider to deviate from established ethical and professional boundaries, including these examples:

    ▷   Accepting gifts

    ▷   Self-disclosure by the provider

    ▷   Embarking on a social relationship with a patient

    ▷   Sexual misconduct

    ▷   Exploiting the therapeutic relationship for the emotional, financial, sexual, or personal advantage or benefit of the provider

▶ Conclusions

    ▷   Effective communication is a core skill in primary care.

    ▷   Establishing, maintaining, and communicating professional boundaries to the patient is imperative to the therapeutic relationship.

Teaching Strategies/Group Dynamics/Literacy

Patient education is essential to successful clinical interventions. Busy clinical settings hinder patient education. Opportunities for education are essential for each clinical visit, with encouragement for further education outside the clinical exam room. Literacy levels differ considerably within the clinical setting. The average literacy level for patients is estimated to be at the fifth-grade level, and inadequate functional health literacy may be as high as 80% in some clinical settings. Healthcare expenses escalate considerably in the lower-literacy populations.

▶ Teaching strategies include using written patient education material in the patient's primary language, and multimedia approaches such as audio and video that are specific to the literacy level of the patient.

▶ Group dynamics may alter the efficacy of group teaching and require considerable time on the part of the clinician.

▶ Improving patient education using multimedia computer programs and touch screens is rapidly becoming a more feasible option, followed by one-on-one interaction with the instructor and/or smaller group interaction.

Professional Organizations

▶ Participation in professional organizations is important because nurse practitioners, acting as a unified group, can influence the direction of the profession and of
healthcare policy in the United States. All NPs should be involved and active in their
professional organizations at the national, state, and local levels.

▶ State organizations work diligently to monitor and affect laws and regulations affecting NP practice and health policy. In addition, these associations provide a group of
peers for discussion and continuing education. Many state NP organizations have
local chapters.

▶ National organizations

▷ American Association of Nurse Practitioners (AANP): In January 2013, the
American Academy of Nurse Practitioners and the American College of Nurse
Practitioners joined to create the largest full-service national professional
membership organization for NPs of all specialties (www.aanp.org). The mission
of AANP is to lead NPs in transforming patient-centered health care with a
vision of "providing high-quality health care for all by the patient's provider of
choice" (AANP, 2013).

▷ The National Organization of Nurse Practitioner Faculties (NONPF) is an
organization of nurse practitioner educators who are instrumental in setting
standards for nurse practitioner education. NONPF has developed core
competencies describing the domains of practice with critical behaviors that
should be exhibited by all entry-level NPs. Originally written in 1995, the revised
edition of the core competencies became available in 2000 to reflect the current
NP practice (www.nonpf.com). The NP core competencies were last updated in
2012.

THEORY AND PRINCIPLES OF FAMILY-FOCUSED CARE

The traditional family nurse practitioner (FNP) provides primary and secondary preventive care to
persons across the life span living as singles or in nuclear or extended family networks. Today's
family consists of those who identify themselves as family members, not limited by walls, genetics, or legally defined relationships. Friedman (2002) defines family as "two or more persons
who are joined together by bonds of sharing and emotional closeness and who identify themselves as being part of the family" (p. 9).

Family members may live either together or within close proximity in a common community
and participate in educational, social, and religious experiences together. Families may form as
an outgrowth of kinship bonds with others in the community or as a result of culturally specific
extended family networks. Due to changes in society, family members may share multiple
instrumental and expressive tasks that are often overlapping and subject to communication and
negotiation (Kaakinen, Coehlo, Steele, Tabacco, & Hanson, 2015). Family forms are varied—the
FNP will interact with nontraditional and multicultural family forms such as the gay and lesbian
family, the single-parent family, the extended family, and adoptive or step-parent families, as well
as traditional families.

Family-focused care is the specialized role of the family nurse practitioner. FNPs acknowledge
that the family process is an interaction among members that serves to promote mental
and physical health, prevent disease, and restore health in times of illness. FNPs provide a

comprehensive psychosocial approach to caring for people that fosters health-promoting life-styles among family members. The FNP interacts across the interdependent roles of individual, family, and community to act as advocate, case manager, coordinator, counselor, and expert provider of care.

The FNP assesses family structure and dynamics to help people maximize their health, given the realities of their personal and family health histories, psychosocial histories, genetic makeups, cultural and religious values, traditions, and social and economic contexts. FNPs teach family members to recognize the influences of their family health patterns and risks, use family members as resources for knowledge and support during periods of health, maintain psychosocial ties with their family of origin, and assume functions that help optimize health in family members by using resources in the community.

The FNP role is interpreted as a unique NP role. It is not, as some would suggest, an adult NP plus pediatric NP plus geriatric NP role, but it requires mastery of a unique constellation of knowledge and tasks involving the care of an individual within a family context. The FNP is not expected to have the depth of knowledge of NPs practicing in the specialty areas but is expected to know something about many different diseases and processes affecting the person through-out the life span. As such, the FNP works closely with physician colleagues in the diagnosis and development of the initial treatment regimen and is prepared to refer frequently to specialists.

Family Theory—Assessment and Intervention

In general, family theory serves as a basis for assessing and coming to understand the structure, development, and function of families through the process of family assessment. Authors such as Friedman (2002), Kaakinen et al. (2015), and Wright and Leahey (2012) have developed family assessment tools. Family theory is grounded in general systems theory, including structural functional theory, family systems theory (Bowen), family development theory (Duvall, 1977), child development theory (Erikson; Havinghurst), and other social science theories, including communication, stress, and interactional theory.

Theoretical Basis for Family Theory—General Systems Theory

General systems theory provides a framework that explains the dynamic structure and function of the family within the context of a unified whole. The family performs activities reflected by the actions of interacting parts or subsystems. Any *system* is defined as "a bounded set of inter-related elements exhibiting coherent behavior as a trait" (Constantine, 1986, p. 67). Families are considered systems because they are made up of interrelated elements or objectives, exhibit coherent behaviors, have regular interactions, and are interdependent on one another.

These are the major principles of systems theory adapted from Friedman (2002), Kaakinen et al. (2015), and Wright and Leahey (2012):

- ▶ Each system has its own characteristics, and the whole is greater than the sum of the parts, rather than just the sum of the characteristics of individual parts of a system.

- ▶ All parts of the system are dependent on one another, even though each part has its own role within the system.

- ▶ Families are organized in a way that enables the interdependence and interactivity of its members.

▶ Each family system has mechanisms for exchange of information within the system and between the system and the broader environment.

▶ Boundaries that are open, closed, or operate at random exist within family systems.

▶ Family systems change over time as both individuals and the whole respond to change in the internal and external environments. With change, families become more complex, reflecting adaptation and differentiation of their members.

▶ Change occurs through feedback processes that allow for circular interaction within the family system, rather than a linear cause-and-effect pattern.

▶ A change affecting one part of a family manifests itself as change in the whole family system.

▶ Families strive for homeostasis or a predictable steady state that reflects a balance between change and stability.

The value of systems theory lies in understanding that families are composed of interacting parts in constant interaction with one another and the larger environment, and that change in one part of the family is reflected in change in the family as a whole. As families expand and grow and experience stress and illness, their ability to be changed and yet maintain homeostasis reflects the health and coping strategies of the family to adapt. Families with poor coping strategies may resist change or be unable to restore homeostasis after change. Stress and illness may trigger dysfunctional coping patterns or disequilibrium. Families with closed boundaries may resist help from outside resources during periods of disequilibrium.

Structural Functional Theory

▶ Families are social systems that form interdependent and independent relationships, referred to as *subsystems* both within and outside of the family. Structure describes relationships within families, such as the husband–wife subsystem, parent–child subsystem, sister–brother subsystem, and so on.

▶ Internal family subsystems function as a microcosm of society, reflecting the larger sphere of human needs. Rank order within families is a component of structure, such as the ordering of children by birth in the family or by ages if they are adopted or stepchildren.

▶ Function includes the tasks that families carry out to provide members with safety, reproduction, education, parenting, sexual expression, economic security, transfer of cultural traditions and inheritance, social support, play, relaxation, and health promotion opportunities.

▶ Supra-systems form outside the family and reflect functional needs not met within the family. Relationships with teachers, schools, religious and civic organizations, the healthcare system, and friends are examples of supra-systems that meet needs not fulfilled by interactions within the family system. Multiple relationships are formed through supra-systems that reflect family values, beliefs, and emotional boundaries. By developing an ecomap, the FNP can visualize family members' relationship with systems outside the family system (Wright & Leahey, 2012).

▶ These are the principles of structural functional theory adapted from Friedman (2002), Hanson et al. (2005), and Wright and Leahey (2012):

▷ Families are social systems with instrumental and expressive functions that include activities of daily living, communication, social support, role acquisition, values, beliefs, problem-solving, and relationships.

▷ In optimally functioning families, members take on predictable roles that meet the instrumental and expressive needs of their members.

▷ Families are composed of small numbers with characteristics of small-group behavior.

▷ Families are social systems that carry out functions necessary to meet the need for orderly transfer of wealth, procreation, and education of members of society.

▷ People adopt norms, values, and cultural traditions that are learned as part of the process of family socialization.

▶ Disease or ill health can interfere with the family's ability to carry out its internal functions and meet the responsibilities it has formed in relationships with systems outside the family. Families with multiple unmet needs may experience guilt, stress, dysfunction, and poor coping strategies during periods of stress and illness.

Family Developmental Theory

▶ Developmental theory explains human growth and development according to theorists such as Erikson, Piaget, and Havinghurst. Duvall (1977) and Duvall and Miller (1985) further applied the concept of development to the sociological study of families. The model outlines the eight consecutive stages in the family life cycle, offers a predictive overview of the activities that occur in families over time, and serves as a basis for anticipatory guidance when assessing and teaching families.

▶ According to Duvall (1977), families pass through eight chronological stages; as in child development theory, success in one task sets the stage for success in subsequent tasks. Failure in one task leads to frustration or delays in subsequent tasks or stages in the family life cycle. These stages are supported by Duvall's model and adapted from Friedman (2002):

▷ Beginning family

▷ Childbearing family (oldest child up to 30 months of age)

▷ Family with preschool children (oldest child 2½ to 5 years of age)

▷ Family with schoolchildren (oldest child 6 to 12 years of age)

▷ Family with adolescents (oldest child 13 to 20 years of age)

▷ Launching center family (grown children leaving the home)

▷ Family with middle-aged parents (empty nest, up to time of retirement)

▷ Family with old age and retirement

▶ Underlying assumptions (Adapted from Friedman, 2002; and Hanson et al., 2005)

▷ Families change over time because of the influence of environmental conditions.

▷ Developmental tasks are the aims, although they are not completed at one time and may overlap with other developmental tasks.

▷ Families demonstrate different forms of membership across developmental stages that perform age-related functions.

> ▷ Families bring with them an experience of their pasts, as well as current circumstances.

> ▷ Families share common developmental processes with other families.

> ▷ Families express developmental milestones in a variety of ways.

Communication Theory

As described by Friedman (2002), Hanson et al. (2005), and Wright and Leahey (2012):

▶ Communication theory emphasizes the interaction of people that includes both verbal and nonverbal communication among members of a family.

▶ Communication functions include emotional support, shared information, and instruction.

▶ The content of messages is time-bound and must be appreciated within the context of the sender.

▶ Communication that lacks clarity may lead to family dysfunction or poor coping strategies.

▶ Communication conveys values and beliefs between members and the external environment.

▶ Communication with clarity and congruence promotes positive behavior within the family.

CASE STUDIES

Case 1

Joan graduated from a family nurse practitioner program 5 years ago and has worked part-time in a college health center since graduation. She is now accepting a job as an FNP in a family practice setting and was asked to cover the prenatal clinic 1 day a week, in addition to providing regular family practice care. The collaborating physician assures her that he will provide her with direct supervision during the first 6 to 8 weeks of her experience and that he will be present in the clinic while she is seeing patients.

1. Is Joan legally authorized to provide care to prenatal women? To children?
2. Should she accept this assignment? Why or why not?
3. What standards of care should she follow in providing care to prenatal patients?

Case 2

Lee Ann is a 14-year-old who presents in the clinic for a physical exam and immunizations. She is alone and reports that her mother is working and does not know that she has come to the clinic. Lee Ann reports that she must have the exam and immunizations for school. The school has advised you in writing that Lee Ann's immunizations are not up-to-date, and she cannot return to school until a record is provided to validate her updated immunization history.

1. What are the legal issues presented in this case?
2. What ethical principles will guide you in making a decision regarding this case?

Case 3

Alice is a 49-year-old Black mother and grandmother. She has three children living at home, and the oldest daughter, in high school, now has a baby. Alice reports that she is very angry with her adolescent daughter, who does not want to help out around the house or care for her baby. Alice feels like there is chaos all the time, and she complains of having frequent stress-related headaches.

1. What theoretical model will assist you in planning an intervention for Alice?
2. What additional information would you like to obtain?
3. How can you best help Alice and her daughter today?

CASE STUDIES DISCUSSION

Case 1

1. Is Joan legally authorized to provide care to prenatal women? To children?

   If her certification has been maintained as a family nurse practitioner, she is legally authorized to provide care.

2. Should she accept this assignment? Why or why not?

   She is legally authorized and she can accept this assignment because adequate supervision will be provided to her during this training period.

3. What standards of care should she follow in providing care to prenatal patients?

   Standards of care are developed by professional organizations such as the American Nurses Association, which has created the Standards for Advanced Practice Nursing, and the American Association of Colleges of Nursing (AACN) and the National Organization of Nurse Practitioner Faculties (NONPF), which have created population-focused Nurse Practitioner Primary Care Competencies. The NP should use established guidelines and standards of practice that guide safe and appropriate care for prenatal patients.

Case 2

1. What are the legal issues presented in this case?

   The main legal issue is the provision of care to minors without the consent of a parent or legal guardian. This patient is a minor and does not have a life-threatening illness. Thus, the patient should return with her mother/guardian for treatment or the NP should contact the mother by phone to receive authorization for care before initiating any interventions. Informed consent is necessary to provide care.

2. What ethical principles will guide you in making a decision regarding this case?

   You will involve Lee Ann in the decision-making process by asking whether she would like to call her mother and making a new appointment with her mother present. In this way, you are using the principle of beneficence—duty to help others—as well as compassion and caring. You also can speak with the mother and call the school nurse to clarify the need for Lee Ann's absence from school.

Case 3

1. What theoretical model will assist you in planning an intervention for Alice?

   The developmental model proposes that families progress through developmental processes that are predictable. Because this is a nontraditional family, Alice may be experiencing some disappointment that she cannot enjoy just being a mother in the launching phase of family life but instead must also assume the role of grandmother and caretaker for her daughter's child. In addition, the daughter's developmental stage of adolescent carries with it several developmental tasks that are not being met when caring for a child. Alice's daughter may be exhibiting conflict over not being able to finish high school and the need to care for her child rather than spend time with her peers. Conflict over development processes is apparent.

2. What additional information would you like to obtain?

    What coping mechanisms and support systems does Alice have for handling stress? Who else would be considered part of the family—does Alice have a partner? What about the baby's father? What roles do other members of the family assume? What are the financial resources? What are the strengths of the family? Are there any safety issues for the baby, Alice, or her daughter? What is the developmental stage and anticipatory guidance needs of the adolescent daughter?

3. How can you best help Alice and her daughter today?

    Acknowledge the stress in Alice's life and treat her headaches. Ask about her willingness to engage a counselor for additional help for both her and her daughter, either alone or in family therapy. Identify and strengthen Alice's coping skills. Encourage Alice to see that she, her daughter, and the baby maintain regular health promotion visits. Consult with social services for a referral to a program for teenage mothers for Alice's daughter and for needed resources for the baby.

REFERENCES

Alligood, M. R., & Tomey, A. M. (2010). *Nursing theorists and their work* (7th ed.). Philadelphia: Elsevier-Health Sciences Division.

American Association of Colleges of Nursing. (2011). *The essentials of master's education in nursing.* Retrieved from http://www.aacn.nche.edu/education-resources/mastersessentials11.pdf

American Association of Colleges of Nursing. (2015). *Fact sheet: The doctor of nursing practice (DNP).* Retrieved from http://www.aacn.nche.edu/media-relations/fact-sheets/dnp

American Association of Nurse Practitioners (2013). Strategic focus. Retrieved from https://www.aanp.org/about-aanp/strategic-focus

American Nurses Association. (2010b). *Nursing's social policy statement: The essence of the profession.* Silver Spring, MD: Nursesbooks.org.

American Nurses Association. (2015). *Nursing: Scope and standards of practice* (3rd ed.). Silver Spring, MD: Nursesbooks.org.

American Nurses Association. (2015). *Code of ethics for nurses with interpretive statements.* Silver Spring, MD: Nursesbooks.org.

American Psychological Association. (n.d.). Psychology & aging: Addressing the needs of older adults. Washington, DC: APA. Retrieved from https://www.apa.org/pi/aging/resources/guides/aging.pdf

American Recovery and Reinvestment Act (ARRA) of 2009. (2009). Pub. L. No. 111-5, 123 Stat. 115, 516. Retrieved from http://www.govtrack.us/congress/bills/111/hr1

Americans with Disabilities Act of 1990. Retrieved from http://www.ada.gov/pubs/ada.htm

APRN Consensus Work Group & the National Council of State Boards of Nursing APRN Advisory Committee. (2008). *Consensus model for APRN regulation: Licensure, accreditation, certification, & education.* Retrieved from http://www.aacn.nche.edu/education-resources/aprnrport.pdf

Berger, K. S. (2014). *The developing person through the life span* (9th ed.). New York: Worth.

Buppert, C. (2014). *Nurse practitioners' business practice and legal guide* (5th ed.). Sudbury, MA: Jones & Bartlett.

Butts, J. B., & Rich, K. L. (2013). *Nursing ethics across the curriculum and into practice* (3rd ed.). Sudbury, MA: Jones & Bartlett.

Clarke T. C., Black, L. I., Stussman, B. J., Barnes, P. M., & Nahin, R. L. (2015). *Trends in the use of complementary health approaches among adults: United States, 2002–2012.* National health statistics reports, no 79. Hyattsville, MD: National Center for Health Statistics.

Committee for the Study of Credentialing in Nursing. (1979). *Credentialing in nursing: A new approach.* Kansas City, MO: American Nurses Association.

Constantine, L. (1986). *Family paradigms: The practice of theory in family therapy.* New York: Guilford Press.

Duvall, E. M. (1977). *Marriage and family development* (5th ed.). Philadelphia: Lippincott.

Duvall, E. M., & Miller, B. C. (1985). *Marriage and family development* (6th ed.). Philadelphia: Lippincott.

Edmunds, M. W., & Mayhew, M. S. (2013). *Pharmacology for primary care providers* (4th ed.). St. Louis, MO: Mosby.

Facchiano, L., & Snyder, C. H. (2012). Evidence-based practice for the busy nurse practitioner: Part one: Relevance to clinical practice and clinical inquiry process. *Journal of the American Academy of Nurse Practitioners, 24,* 579–586.

Federation of State Medical Boards of the United States. (1988). *Non-physician duties and scope of practice* (Position Statement 210.003, July). Dallas, TX: Author.

Ford, L. C. (1992). Advanced nursing practice: Future of the nurse practitioner. In L. H. Aiken & C. M. Fagin (Eds.), *Charting nursing's future: Agenda for the 1990s.* Philadelphia: Lippincott.

Friedman, M. (2002). *Family nursing: Research, theory, and practice* (5th ed.). Upper Saddle River, NJ: Prentice Hall.

Geisler, C., Cheung, C., Steinhagen, S. J., Neubeck, P., & Brueggeman, A. D. (2015). Nurse practitioner knowledge, use, and referral of complementary/alternative therapies. *JAANP, 27*(7), 380–388.

Giger, J. N. (2013). *Transcultural nursing* (6th ed.). St Louis, MO: Mosby.

Glanz, K., Rimer, B. K., & Viswanath, K. (Eds.). (2015). *Health behavior and health education: Theory, research, and practice* (4th ed.). Hoboken, NJ: John Wiley & Sons.

Gray, B., & Orrock, P. (2014). Investigation into factors influencing roles, relationships, and referrals in integrative medicine. *Journal of Alternative and Complementary Medicine, 20*(5), 342–346.

Health Insurance Portability and Accountability Act of 1996 (HIPAA). Pub. L. 104–191.

HealthIT.gov. (2015). EHR incentives & certification. Retrieved from http://www.healthit.gov/ providers-professionals/meaningful-use-definition-objectives

Huston, C., (2013) The impact of emerging technology on nursing care: Warp speed ahead. *OJIN: The Online Journal of Issues in Nursing, 18*(2), Manuscript 1. DOI: 10.3912/OJIN. Vol18No02Man01

Institute of Medicine. (2012). *The role of telehealth in an evolving health care environment: Workshop summary.* Washington, DC: National Academies Press. Available from http://iom. nationalacademies.org/reports/2012/the-role-of-telehealthin-an-evolving-health-care-environment.aspx

Institute for the Future. (2003). *Health & health care 2010: The forecast, the challenge.* Hoboken, NJ: John Wiley & Sons.

Institute of Medicine. (1999). *To err is human: Building a safer health system.* Available from http://nationalacademies.org/hmd/reports/1999/to-err-is-human-building-a-safer-health-system.aspx

Institute of Medicine. (2010). *The future of nursing: Leading change, advancing health.* Available from http://nationalacademies.org/hmd/reports/2010/the-future-of-nursing-leading-change-advancing-health.aspx

International Council of Nurses. (2000). *ICN position statement: Prevention of disability and the care of people with disabilities.* Retrieved from http://www.icn.ch/images/stories/documents/publications/position_statements/A16_prevention_disability_care.pdf

Kaakinen, J. R., Coehlo, D. P., Steele, R., Tabacco, A., & Hanson, S. M. H. (2015). *Family health care nursing: Theory, practice, and research* (5th ed.). Philadelphia: F. A. Davis.

Kirschner, K. L., & Curry, R. H. (2009). Patients with disabilities. *JAMA, 302*(12), 1334–1335.

Josen, A. R., Winslade, W. J., & Siegler, M. (2015). *Clinical ethics: A practical approach to ethical decisions in clinical medicine* (8th ed.). Columbus, OH: McGraw-Hill.

Mason, D. J., Leavitt, J. K., & Chaffee, M. W. (2015). *Policy & politics in nursing and health care* (7th ed.). Philadelphia: Elsevier.

Mullen, F., Politzer, R. M., Lewis, C. T., Bastacky, S., Rodak, J. Jr., & Harmon, R. G. (1992). The National Practitioner Data Bank: Report from the first year. *JAMA, 268*, 73–79.

Murray, R. B., Zentner, J. P., & Yakimo, R. (2009). *Health promotion strategies through the life span* (8th ed.). Upper Saddle River, NJ: Prentice Hall.

Nahin, R. L., Stussman, B. J., & Herman, P. M. (2015). Out-of-pocket expenditures on complementary health approaches associated with painful health conditions in a nationally representative adult sample. *Journal of Pain, 16*(11), 1147–1162.

National Center for Complementary and Integrative Health. (2015). *Herbs at a glance.* Retrieved from https://nccih.nih.gov/health/herbsataglance.htm

National Council of State Boards of Nursing. (1993). *Regulation of advanced nursing practice* (National Council Position Paper, 1993). Chicago, IL: Author.

National Council of State Boards of Nursing. (2011). *What you need to know about nursing licensure and boards of nursing.* Retrieved from https://www.ncsbn.org/Nursing_Licensure.pdf

National Council of State Boards of Nursing. (2007). *A nurse's guide to the importance of appropriate professional boundaries.* Chicago: Author. Retrieved from https://www.ncsbn.org/ProfessionalBoundaries_Complete.pdf

National Hospice and Palliative Care Organization. (2015). **Hospice and palliative care.** Retrieved from http://www.nhpco.org/about/hospice-care

National Institutes of Health: National Center for Complementary and Integrative Health. (2011). *Children and the use of complementary health approaches.* Retrieved from https://nccih.nih.gov/health/children#key

National Institutes of Health: National Center for Complementary and Integrative Health. (2015). **Complementary, alternative, or integrative health: What's in a name?** Retrieved from https://nccih.nih.gov/health/integrative-health

National Institutes of Health: Office of Dietary Supplements. (n.d.). **Dietary supplement fact sheets.** Retrieved from http://ods.od.nih.gov/

National Organization of Nurse Practitioner Faculties. (2010). *Position on Clinical Hours for Nurse Practitioner Preparation in Doctor of Nursing Practice Programs. In NONPF, Clinical education issues in preparing nurse practitioner students for independent practice: An ongoing series of papers* (pp. 7–15). Washington, DC: Author. Retrieved from http://c.ymcdn.com/sites/www.nonpf.org/resource/resmgr/imported/clinicaleducationissuespprfinalapril2010.pdf

National Organization of Nurse Practitioner Faculties. (2012). *Criteria for evaluation of nurse practitioner programs.* Washington, DC: Author.

National Organization of Nurse Practitioner Faculties. (2013). *Population focused nurse practitioner competencies.* Washington, DC: Author.

National Organization of Nurse Practitioner Faculties. (2014). *Nurse practitioner core competencies.* Washington, DC: Author.

Papero, D. V., & Kerr, M. E. (1997). *Bowen family systems.* Upper Saddle River, NJ: Allyn & Bacon.

Pearson, L. J. (2015). *The Pearson Report.* Burlington, MA: Jones & Bartlett.

Pohl, J. M., Nath, R., Zheng, K., Rachman, F., Gans, D. N., & Tanner, C. (2013). Use of a comprehensive patient safety tool in primary care practices. *Journal of the American Academy of Nurse Practitioners, 25*(8), 415–418.

Quinlan, E., & Robertson, S. (2013). The communicative power of nurse practitioners in multidisciplinary primary healthcare teams. *Journal of the American Academy of Nurse Practitioners, 25,* 91–102.

Robert Wood Johnson Foundation. (2010). *Quality and safety education for nurses.* Retrieved from http://qsen.org/about-qsen/

Saba, V. K., & McCormick, K. A. (2015). *Essentials of nursing informatics* (6th ed.). New York, NY: McGraw-Hill.

Sand-Jecklin, K., Murray, B., Summers, B., & Watson, J. (2010). Educating nursing students about health literacy: From the classroom to the patient bedside. *Online Journal of Issues in Nursing, 15*(3). Retrieved from http://www.medscape.com/viewarticle/729395

Tsai, H. H., Lin, H. W., Pickard, A. S., Tsail, H. Y., & Mahady, G. B. (2012). Evaluation of documented drug interactions and contraindications associated with herbs and dietary supplements: A systematic literature review. *International Journal of Clinical Practice, 66*(11), 1056–1078.

U.S. Department of Health and Human Services. (n.d.). *National practitioner data bank.* Retrieved from http://www.npdb-hipdb.hrsa.gov/

U.S. Department of Health and Human Services. (2003). *OCR privacy brief: Summary of the HIPAA privacy rule.* Washington, DC: U.S. Dept. of Health & Human Services Office for Civil Rights.

U.S. Department of Health and Human Services. (2010). *Healthy People 2020* (3rd ed.). McLean, VA: International Medical Publishing Inc.

U.S. Department of Health and Human Services. (2014). *Healthy People 2020 leading health indicators progress update.* McLean, VA: International Medical Publishing Inc.

U.S. Department of Health, Education and Welfare. (1971). *Report on licensure and related health personnel credentials* (DHEW Pub. No. (HSM) 72-11). Washington, DC: Author.

U.S. Food and Drug Administration: U.S. Department of Health and Human Services. (2015). *Questions and answers on dietary supplements.* Retrieved from http://www.fda.gov/Food/DietarySupplements/UsingDietarySupplements/ucm480069.htm

U.S. Office of Technology Assessment. (1986). *Nurse practitioners, physician's assistants and certified nurse midwives: A policy analysis.* Washington, DC: U.S. Government Printing Office.

Villaseñor, S., & Piscotty, R. J. (2015). The current state of e-prescribing: Implications for advanced practice registered nurses. *AANP.* Online preview 5-5-2015. Retrieved from http://onlinelibrary.wiley.com/doi/10.1002/2327-6924.12263/full

Wright, L. M., & Leahey, M. (2012). *Nurses and families: A guide to family assessment and intervention* (6th ed.). Philadelphia, PA: F. A. Davis.

CHAPTER 3

HEALTHCARE ISSUES
Michael A. Carter, DNSc, DNP, FAAN, DCC

GENERAL APPROACH

▶ All countries throughout the world have financial limits on their abilities to support healthcare systems.

▶ The United States spends about 50% more per person than any other country in the world (National Center for Health Statistics, 2013).

▶ Healthcare access and health disparities in the United States continue even after passage of the Affordable Care Act.

▶ There are 6,234 primary care Health Professional Shortage Areas (HPSAs) representing the underserved with limited access to care.

▶ The leading causes of infant mortality in the United States are congenital malformations, disorders of short gestation and low birth weight, and sudden infant death syndrome.

▶ A resurgence of previously controlled infections and the emergence of newer infections, coupled with antibiotic resistance and an increasingly global environment, make infectious disease a persistent threat to people at either end of the age spectrum.

▶ Current healthcare trends support greater emphasis on disease prevention, risk reduction, health promotion, and chronic disease management care rather than exclusive disease management.

▶ There is increased emphasis on evidence-based practice (the use of current and best evidence to make decisions about care) and early translation of the best evidence into practice to improve healthcare quality and outcomes of care.

▶ There is increasing healthcare complexity through technological advances, particularly in healthcare information systems.

RED FLAGS

▶ *Health disparities*: the difference in the incidence, prevalence, mortality, and burden of disease and other adverse conditions that exist among specific population groups in the United States (National Institute on Aging, 2008)

▶ *Access*: the availability (or lack thereof) of healthcare services to all

▶ *Medically underserved community*: a setting with a shortage of primary care, dental, and/or mental health services

▶ *Vulnerability*: open to physical, emotional, and/or socioeconomic harm

▶ *Disadvantaged*: inhibited from knowledge, skills, and abilities to participate in the healthcare system as a provider and/or a receipt of health care because of economic, social, ethnic, or racial background, and/or physical or mental impairment

▶ *Underrepresented minorities*: racial and ethnic populations whose representation among the health professions is lower than their proportion of the general population

▶ *Social determinants of health*: defined by the World Health Organization as "conditions in which people are born, grow, live, work, and age, and the wider set of forces and systems shaping the conditions of daily life" (WHO, 2015)

THE PATIENT PROTECTION AND AFFORDABLE CARE ACT

▶ Patient Protection and Affordable Care Act (ACA) became law in 2010 (U.S. Department of Health and Human Services, n.d.).

▶ Persons are now required to have insurance under the ACA, but 11.4% of U.S. citizens are still without insurance in March 2015 (Obamacare Facts, 2015).

▶ ACA ended preexisting condition exclusions, keeps adults under 26 years old on parents' plan, and ended lifetime limits.

▶ ACA requires insurers to offer preventive care with no copayment.

NATIONAL HEALTH PREVENTION STRATEGY

The National Prevention Strategy (Centers for Disease Control & Prevention, n.d.) presents evidence-based recommendations designed to reduce the burden of the most-common preventable causes of disease and death. The aim of this initiative is to guide the nation in the most effective and achievable ways to improve health and well-being. The strategic directions include healthy and safe community environments, clinical and community preventive services, empowered people, and the elimination of health disparities. Here are the priority areas:

▶ Tobacco-free living

▶ Preventing drug abuse and excessive alcohol use

▶ Healthy eating

▶ Active living

▶ Injury- and violence-free living

▶ Reproductive and sexual health

▶ Mental and emotional well-being

MODEL EPIDEMIOLOGIC PRINCIPLES

Definition

▶ The study of how disease is distributed in populations

▶ Includes factors that influence this distribution (Gordis, 2014)

Natural History of Disease

The course of disease is one of development, expression, and progression in a person over time. Several stages appear to be universally descriptive:

▶ Stage of susceptibility (pre-pathological)

▶ Stage of pre-symptomatic disease (subclinical)

▶ Stage of clinical disease

▶ Stage of disability (or death)

Prevention of Disease

The goal is to intervene as early as possible to prevent disease or disability.

Primary Prevention

▶ Interventions at the stage of susceptibility, directed at preventing disease from occurring

▶ Education, exercise, nutrition, water fluoridation, immunizations, food-handling regulations, pollution control

Secondary Prevention

▶ Interventions at the subclinical stage, directed at early detection of the illness or problem to reduce the progress and severity of the disease

▶ Genetic testing in newborns, lead screening, vision and hearing screening, smoking cessation programs, cholesterol screening, and mammography

Tertiary Prevention

▶ Interventions at the clinical stage of disease, directed at treatment and rehabilitation of the illness to prevent or minimize progression of the disease or its sequelae, such as disability

▶ Use of inhaled steroids in the management of asthma and penicillin prophylaxis in patients with sickle cell anemia

Etiology

The cause or the web of causation of a disease or problem:

▶ Any factors (direct or indirect) that increase the likelihood of disease

▶ Prevalence rates describe the number of persons who have a condition in the population at a specific time divided by the number of people in the population.

▶ Incidence rates describe the number of new cases that occur during a specified time in a group at risk. See Table 3–1, which identifies the leading causes of death per age group.

TABLE 3–1.
LEADING CAUSES OF DEATH BY AGE GROUP

AGE	CAUSE OF DEATH
Under 1 year	Congenital anomalies
	Short gestation
	Maternal complications
	Sudden infant death syndrome (SIDS)
	Unintentional injuries
	Placenta, cord, or membranes
	Bacterial sepsis
	Respiratory distress
	Circulatory system disease
	Neonatal hemorrhage
1–4 years	Unintentional injuries
	Congenital anomalies
	Homicide
	Malignant neoplasm
	Heart disease
	Influenza and pneumonia
	Chronic lower respiratory disease
	Septicemia
	Benign neoplasm
	Perinatal period
5–9 years	Unintentional injuries
	Malignant neoplasm
	Congenital anomalies
	Homicide
	Chronic lower respiratory disease
	Heart disease
	Influenza and pneumonia
	Cerebrovascular disease
	Septicemia
	Benign neoplasm
10–14 years	Unintentional injuries
	Malignant neoplasm
	Suicide
	Congenital anomalies
	Homicide
	Heart disease
	Chronic lower respiratory disease
	Influenza and pneumonia
	Cerebrovascular disease
	Benign neoplasms

AGE	CAUSE OF DEATH
15–24 years	Unintentional injuries Suicide Homicide Malignant neoplasm Heart disease Congenital anomalies Influenza and pneumonia Diabetes mellitus Complicated pregnancy Chronic lower respiratory disease
25–34 years	Unintentional injuries Homicide Suicide Malignant neoplasm Heart disease Diabetes mellitus Liver disease HIV Cerebrovascular disease Influenza and pneumonia
35–44 years	Unintentional injuries Malignant neoplasm Heart disease Suicide Homicide Liver disease Diabetes mellitus Cerebrovascular disease HIV Influenza and pneumonia
45–54 years	Malignant neoplasms Heart disease Unintentional injuries Liver disease Suicide Diabetes mellitus Cerebrovascular disease Chronic lower respiratory disease Septicemia HIV

(CONTINUED)

AGE	CAUSE OF DEATH
55–64 years	Malignant neoplasms
	Heart disease
	Unintentional injuries
	Chronic lower respiratory disease
	Diabetes mellitus
	Liver disease
	Cerebrovascular disease
	Suicide
	Septicemia
	Nephritis
65 years and older	Heart disease
	Malignant neoplasm
	Chronic lower respiratory disease
	Cerebrovascular disease
	Alzheimer's disease
	Diabetes mellitus
	Influenza and pneumonia
	Unintentional injuries
	Nephritis
	Septicemia

Adapted from "10 Leading Causes of Death by Age Group, United States – 2013," by Centers for Disease Control and Prevention, 2013. Retrieved from http://www.cdc.gov/injury/wisqars/pdf/leading_causes_of_death_by_age_group_2013-a.pdf

Risk Factors

▶ Age, sex, social, cultural, familial, racial/ethnic, genetic, occupation, and lifestyle history represent potential sources of problems and diseases that may be difficult or impossible to alter.

▶ Risk reduction programs may be established to decrease the vulnerability of persons to certain problems by modifying some risks.

Communicable or Infectious Diseases

Illnesses caused by organisms that attack and invade vulnerable persons

▶ Involve identification of causative agents,

▶ Rely on microbiology principles in understanding life cycle of organism,

▶ Focus on intervention at vulnerable phases in course of disease or life cycle of organism, and

▶ Use selected infectious disease definitions (Box 3–1).

Reservoirs of Infection

▶ Cases and carriers

▶ Animal carriers (lower vertebrate animals)

BOX 3.1

INFECTIOUS DISEASE DEFINITIONS

General Definitions

- *Infection*: colonization and multiplication of an organism in the host, typically producing an immune response but no signs or symptoms
- *Disease*: Stage when an infection produces signs and/or symptoms (including pathologic changes). Certain organisms (such as influenza virus) are capable of infection with or without producing disease; other organisms (such as measles virus) always produce disease in susceptible persons. Disease may vary in severity.
- *Colonization*: The organism invades the host at a particular site, multiplies, and acts as a parasite but does not produce infection, immune response, or disease.
- *Carrier state*: persistence of an organism in a host; this stage may follow infection, disease, or colonization and may be infective to others

Agent (Organism) Properties

- *Infectivity*: Ability of an organism to invade and multiply in a susceptible host. Varicella is highly infective, rhinovirus is intermediate, and tubercle bacilli are of low infectivity.
- *Pathogenicity:* Ability of an organism to produce disease. Rabies, rhinovirus, and varicella are highly pathogenic; adenovirus and rubella are intermediate; and tubercle bacillus is low.
- *Virulence*: Severity of disease that an organism can produce, measured by criteria such as number of days in bed or the frequency of serious sequelae including death (fatality rate). Rabies virus is highly virulent (nearly 100% fatality rate); poliovirus is moderately virulent; varicella and rhinovirus are of low virulence (almost zero fatality rate).
- *Immunogenicity*: Ability to produce a lasting and effective immunity. Rhinovirus, which primarily acts locally, results in a poor systemic immune response. Systemic viral infections such as measles produce lasting immunity.

Agent–Host Relations

- *Latent infection*: The organism is not shedding or obtainable (likely hidden in host cells).
- *Patent infection:* The organism is shedding and/or obtainable from such areas as feces, urine, blood, or respiratory tract. Certain infections may remain permanently patent (some cases of hepatitis B) or be intermittently patent (herpes virus), or, after being latent for a long time, reactivate and produce disease (tuberculosis and herpes zoster).
- *Period of communicability*: the time when sufficient numbers of organisms are shed to cause transmission; usually concurrent with disease but not always
- *Incubation period*: the time from exposure to the onset of disease

▶ Invertebrate hosts (insects)

▶ Inanimate objects: Some infectious agents are free-living in the environment, multiplying on inanimate objects (such as *Salmonella* in food, *Legionella* in pools of water, and *Histoplasma* in oil).

Mechanisms of Transmission of Infection

▶ Direct: through touching, kissing, sexual intercourse, childbearing, breastfeeding, transfusions

▶ Indirect: through air, vector (insects, animals), vehicle (food, water, towels)

Control Measures

▶ Measures directed against the reservoir: isolation, quarantine, insect spraying

▶ Measures that interrupt the transmission of organisms: water purification, milk pasteurization, barrier protection during sexual intercourse

▶ Measures that reduce host susceptibility: immunization, appropriate use of antibiotics, improved nutrition

Concepts of Epidemic vs. Endemic Infections

▶ *Generation time:* interval between receipt of infection and the maximal communicability of the host; applied to both subclinical and clinical infections (incubation period applies only to clinical cases); used to describe and analyze the spread of infectious diseases (i.e., common vehicle, single-exposure epidemic, determined by the incubation or generation time)

▶ *Herd immunity:* resistance of a group to invasion and spread of an infectious agent because a large portion of the group is immune; decreases the likelihood of an epidemic in an area

▶ *Endemic:* a disease or infectious agent that is usually present in a population

▶ *Epidemic:* occurrence of disease in excess of what is normally expected in a population

▶ *Morbidity:* occurrence of illness in a population

▶ *Mortality:* occurrence of death in a population

HUMAN DEVELOPMENT

Definition

▶ Most development is patterned and orderly, with both a purpose and a direction.

▶ Development is continuous throughout life, although the degree of change in many areas decreases after adolescence.

▶ Development may occur simultaneously in several areas, such as physical and social, but the rate of change in each area varies.

▶ The pace of development varies among persons.

▶ Physical and mental stress during periods of critical developmental change, such as puberty, may make a person particularly susceptible to outside stressors.

▶ Anticipatory guidance is an important component of patient and family education throughout the life span.

Infant and Child Development

▶ Assessment of growth is determined by routine monitoring of height, weight, head circumference (until age 2), dental development, and appearance of secondary sex characteristics.

▶ Adequacy of growth is determined by comparison with normal growth parameters (see Tables 3–2 through 3–5) and/or plotting the measurements of height, weight,

TABLE 3–2.
NORMAL GROWTH PARAMETERS FOR HEIGHT AND WEIGHT

AGE	WEIGHT*	HEIGHT*
Newborn	95% of newborns weigh 5–10 lbs Approximately 5%–10% of body weight is lost in first few days, then birth weight is regained in 7–10 days.	95% of newborns are between 18 and 22 in. long.
Birth–6 months	Weekly gain 140–200 g (5–7 ounces). Birth weight doubles by 6 months.	Monthly gain is 2.5 cm (1 in.).
6–12 months	Weekly gain 85–140 g (3–5 ounces). Birth weight triples by age 1 year.	Monthly gain is 1.25 cm (0.5 in.). Birth length increases by approximately 50% by age 1 year.
Toddlers	Yearly gain 2–3 kg (4½–6½ lbs).	Growth is approximately 12 cm (5 in.) between ages 1 and 2 years; 6–8 cm (2½–3½ in.) between ages 2 and 3 years. Approximately 50% of adult height is reached by age 2 years.
School age	Yearly gain approximately 2–3 kg (4½–6½ lbs).	Growth is approximately 5–6 cm (2–2½ in.) per year. Birth length doubles by age 4 years and triples by age 13 years.
Puberty—girls (10–14 years)	Weight gain 15–55 lbs (mean 38 lbs).	Growth is approximately 5–25 cm (2–10 in.). 95% of adult height is achieved by menarche (skeletal age of 13 years).
Puberty—boys (11–16 years)	Weight gain 15–65 lbs (mean 52 lbs).	Growth is approximately 10–30 cm (4–12 in.). 95% of adult height is achieved by skeletal age of 15 years.

*These measurements are averages.
Adapted from "CDC Growth Charts," by National Center for Health Statistics, 2010. Retrieved from http://www.cdc.gov/growthcharts/

and head circumference on a standard National Center for Health Statistics (NCHS) (2010) growth chart.

▶ There are two periods of rapid growth: infancy and adolescence; in between, growth is steady but slower.

▶ The growth of most body tissues parallels physical growth, which is most rapid in the first 2 years; lymph tissue growth is rapid in the preschool and early school-age years; growth of reproductive organs remains slow until puberty.

Patterns of Development

▶ The sequence of development is basically the same in all children, but the rate varies.

▶ Attainment of developmental landmarks in one area does not always run parallel to another area of development.

▶ Development is dependent on maturation of the nervous system.

▶ Generalized activity precedes specific movements (a young infant kicks and waves arms with excitement, whereas an older infant reaches out and grasps).

▶ Development occurs in a cephalocaudal direction (head control develops before walking) and a proximal-to-distal direction (shoulders before fingers).

▶ Certain primitive reflexes must be lost before the corresponding voluntary movement is acquired (grasp reflex lost before deliberately grasping objects can occur).

Tooth Eruption

▶ Deciduous teeth usually begin at 6 months of age with the central incisors and move laterally.

▶ All 20 deciduous teeth are usually in place by 2½ to 3 years of age.

▶ Delayed dentition is considered when no teeth have erupted by 13 months of age.

▶ Shedding of deciduous teeth begins at about 6 years of age and continues through age 12.

▶ Eruption of the first permanent teeth occurs with the first molars, at about age 6 years.

▶ Eruption of all 32 permanent teeth may not be complete until ages 17 to 21, with third molars.

Developmental Landmarks and Milestones

▶ Development typically assessed in four areas: gross motor, fine motor, language, and social skills

▶ Purpose is to identify children in need of further assessment and determine if a developmental disability exists

▶ All states required to have a system to identify and treat developmental disabilities in children ages 3 to 5 years; most states have voluntarily extended this age range

Interpreting Results

▶ Attainment of milestones is in ranges.

▶ A significant finding in any developmental assessment is the loss of developmental milestones previously achieved or lack of key milestones by certain age (see Table 3–3).

▶ Language and fine motor skills are sensitive indicators of intellectual development.

▶ Early attainment of gross motor skills is not a significant indicator of advanced intellectual development, but does usually preclude the diagnosis of intellectual disability. Developmental warning signs can be found in Table 3–4.

▶ No child is intellectually disabled if delayed in one area but normal in all others.

Adolescent Pubertal Changes

Boys

▶ Average age of onset is 10.5 to 16 years

▶ Precocious puberty is the development of secondary sex characteristics before age 9 and is often associated with a pathological etiology in boys.

▶ Delayed puberty is lack of changes by age 14 years.

TABLE 3–3.
DEVELOPMENTAL MILESTONES

TASKS	AVERAGE AGE (RANGE)*
GROSS MOTOR SKILLS	
Moves head from side to side	2 weeks
Lifts shoulders while prone	2 months
Rolls over	4 months (2–6 months)
Head control (no bobbing)	4 months
Sits alone	6 months (5–9 months)
Pulls to stand	9 months (6–10 months)
Crawls (reciprocal)	9 months (8–11 months)
Cruises	9 months (8–13 months)
Walks alone	12 months (9–15 months)
Runs, walks upstairs holding rail	18 months (14–21 months)
Throws ball overhand	19–20 months (16–24 months)
Pedals tricycle	28 months (21–36 months)
Balances on one foot	28–30 months (22–38 months)
Hops on one foot	4 years (3–4½ years)
Tandem walk	5 years (3½–5 years)
Skips	5 years
FINE MOTOR SKILLS	
Unfists	3–4 months
Holds objects placed in hand	3–4 months (2½–5 months)
Reaches for objects	4 months (3–5 months)
Transfers objects	6 months (4½–7 months)
Ulnar raking	6 months (5–7 months)
Inferior pincer	9–10 months
Mature pincer	11–12 months
Deliberate throw	12–13 months
Spontaneous scribble	14–16 months (12–16 months)
Tower of 2	15 months (12½–20 months)
Tower of 4	18 months (16–20 months)
Tower of 6	24 months (17–30 months)
Imitates line	24 months (19–30 months)
Tower of 10	36 months
Copies circle	36 months (2½–3½ years)
Uses scissors	3 years
Copies square	4 years (4–5 years)
Draws 3-part figure	4 years (3½–5 years)
Copies triangle	5 years
Draws 6-part figure	5½ years (4½–6 years)
LANGUAGE (RECEPTIVE AND EXPRESSIVE)	
Localizes sound	4–9 months
Babbling vowels	5–6 months
Babbling consonants	6–7 months
"Dada"/"mama"—nonspecific	9–10 months
"Dada"/"mama"—specific	10–12 months

(CONTINUED)

TASKS	AVERAGE AGE (RANGE)*
LANGUAGE (RECEPTIVE AND EXPRESSIVE) (CONTINUED)	
13 words	11–13 months
Follows one-step command	11–15 months
10–15 words, 25% intelligible	15–18 months
Points to named pictures when asked "show me"	18–24 months
Approximately 50-word vocabulary; 2-word combinations	21–24 months
Approximately 100-word vocabulary by 2nd birthday; says "me" and "mine" (As a rule, the number of words in a sentence equals the child's age [2 by age 2, 3 by age 3]) 2- to 3-word phrases	2 years
Follows 2-step commands without gesture	30 months
Few possessives ("my ball") and progressives (the –ing: "I playing")	30 months
Concept of "I" questions	30 months
Knows few colors, pronouns, plurals, full name, age, approximately 250-word vocabulary, 3–4 word sentences (75% intelligible)	36 months
Counts to 4, can say a nursery rhyme, asks and answers why, how, when, knows opposite analogies, and uses past tense	4 years+
Uses complex sentences, understands meaning of words, counts to 10, has fluent speech, uses future tense	5 years
SOCIAL, INTERACTIVE, VISION	
Regards face	0–1 month
Smiles responsively	1–1½ months
Hand regard	4–5 months
Smiles at mirror image	5 months
Plays peek-a-boo	5½–8½ months
Plays pat-a-cake	10 months
Waves goodbye	10 months (7–14 months)
Indicates wants	12 months (10–14 months)
Imitates housework	15 months (13–18 months)
Washes and dries hands	22 months (19 months–2½ years)
Puts on clothing	22 months

*Ages will vary with different tests.

Adapted from "Child Development," CDC, 2016. Retrieved from http://www.cdc.gov/ncbddd/childdevelopment/index.html

▶ First change is testicular enlargement, followed by pubic hair development at the base of the penis (adrenarche); testicular size larger than 2 to 2.5 cm indicates puberty has begun.

▶ Penile growth occurs approximately 6 to 12 months after testicular enlargement; penis grows from a prepubertal size of 3.5 to 5.5 cm to an adult length of 12 cm (7.5 to 15.5 cm).

TABLE 3–4.
DEVELOPMENTAL WARNING SIGNS

6 weeks	Absence of auditory alertness
	Lack of visual fixation (focusing)
	Excessive head lag on pulling-to-sitting position
6 months	Persistence of hand regard
	Failure to follow 180° (for both near and far objects)
	Persistent fisting
	Preference of one hand
10 months	Absence of babble
	No smiling or social responsiveness
	Absence of weight-bearing while hand held
	Failure to sit without support
18 months	No spontaneous vocalizations
	No single words
	No pincer grasp
	Inability to stand without support
2 years	No recognizable words
	No walking

▶ Growth spurt begins about 1 year after the first testicular changes (average age 12.5 years), peaks after 1.5 years, and lasts 2 to 4 years.

▶ Accompanying changes, such as axillary and facial hair and deepening voice, occur later in puberty.

Girls

▶ Average age of onset is 11 years, with a range of 8 to 13 years.

▶ Precocious puberty is the onset of changes before 8 years of age or menarche before age 10 years.

▶ Delayed puberty is no breast development by age 13 years or no menses by 15 to 16 years.

▶ First pubertal change is usually breast budding under the areola and pubertal fine hair over the mons pubis (adrenarche or pubarche).

▶ Menarche occurs at an average age of 12.5 years (range 10 to 15).

HEALTH MAINTENANCE

Current factors support greater emphasis on health promotion and disease prevention.

Healthy People 2020 (U.S. Department of Health and Human Services, n.d.):

▶ A set of goals and objectives based on annual targets to guide the nation's health promotion and prevention efforts

▶ National objectives that emphasize disease prevention and define leading health indicators necessary to measure health; as a group, reflect major health concerns in United States in 21st century

▶ Emphasizes social determinants of health and promotion of health across all stages of life and use of technology, such as interactive websites, as main vehicle of dissemination of evidence-based resources for implementation

▶ Leading health indicators selected on the basis of their ability to motivate action, availability of data to measure progress, and importance as public health issues. They include:

▷ Access to health services

▷ Clinical preventive services

▷ Environmental quality

▷ Injury and violence

▷ Maternal, infant, and child health

▷ Mental health

▷ Nutrition, physical activity, and obesity

▷ Oral health

▷ Reproductive and sexual health

▷ Social determinants

▷ Substance abuse

▷ Tobacco

HEALTH MAINTENANCE PRACTICE

Lifestyle/Health Behaviors

Routine counseling and chemoprophylaxis in primary prevention may prevent certain conditions (see Table 3–5). Specific health behaviors that are amenable to intervention can be found in Table 3–6.

Exercise

▶ Recommendation is 30 minutes of moderate physical activity on most days of the week; does not have to be continuous

▶ Recommendation is as important for children as for adults

Child and Adolescent Pre-Participation Sports Assessment

▶ Children and adolescents participating in sports should have a pre-participation evaluation (PPE). Almost all states require medical clearance before sports participation, although no standardization of PPEs exists and evaluations may vary. The American Academy of Pediatrics and the American Association of Sports Medicine Physicians each have developed guidelines.

▶ The PPE should involve parents for athletes younger than 18 years of age.

▶ The goal of the PPE is to identify those who may need conditioning or rehabilitation, need further evaluation for clearance, and should be excluded from participation. Particular attention should be directed at the cardiopulmonary and musculoskeletal systems.

TABLE 3–5.
CHEMOPROPHYLAXIS FOR DISEASE PREVENTION

CONDITION	RATIONALE	RECOMMENDATIONS
PREVENTING PRIMARY DISEASE		
Neural tube defects	Disorders of the cranium, spine, and nervous system that occur when the neural tube fails to close. Folic acid supplementation has resulted in more than 50% reduction in these birth defects. The average North American diet includes less than half of the recommended dietary intake of folic acid.	All women of childbearing years, whether pregnant or not, should take 0.4 mg daily of folic acid either alone or as part of a multivitamin supplement. The dose is increased with pregnancy.
Hemorrhagic disease of the newborn	Newborn gut lacks the bacteria necessary to synthesize vitamin K, which is used for coagulation.	Vitamin K (phytonadione), 1 mg, is administered once immediately after birth.
Ophthalmia neonatorum	Primary purpose is the prevention of gonococcal and *Chlamydial* conjunctivitis in the neonate. Silver nitrate is not effective against *Chlamydia*.	Instilled immediately postpartum: a single application of 1% silver nitrate ophthalmic drops, 0.5% erythromycin ophthalmic ointment, or 1% tetracycline ophthalmic ointment
Group B *Streptococcus* (GBS) (prevention in the newborn)	In the early 1970s, GBS was a primary cause of neonatal sepsis and meningitis. Prevention strategies began to screen women for GBS and provide antibiotic prophylaxis for women who were positive or had specific risk factors.	Screen pregnant women for GBS in one of two ways: • Obtain vaginal and rectal cultures at 35–37 weeks' gestation. • If no culture results are available, the decision for chemoprophylaxis is based on the presence of one or more risk factors: delivery at 37 weeks' gestation or less, membranes ruptured for more than18 hours, intrapartum fever of 38° C or higher, or mother had a previous infant with GBS disease or had GBS bacteriuria herself. Whichever screening method is used, the treatment is the same: IV penicillin G, 5 million units, followed by 2–5 million units every 4 hours until delivery. Treatment is most effective if at least two doses of penicillin are given.
Dental caries	Reduction of dental caries can be accomplished with fluoride and sealants. Excess fluoride will cause fluorosis (mottling of the teeth).	Dose of fluoride is dependent on fluoride concentration in the water and age of the child. Sealants are plastic coverings applied by the dentist for secondary molars.

(CONTINUED)

CONDITION	RATIONALE	RECOMMENDATIONS
DISEASE PREVENTION IN HIGH-RISK PEOPLE		
Respiratory syncytial virus (RSV)	RSV is responsible for the majority of lower respiratory tract infections in children. RSV is a paramyxovirus that produces fusion of human cells in tissue. RSV attacks the upper and lower respiratory tracts, often causing life-threatening pneumonia and bronchiolitis. Bronchiolitis may begin as a mild upper respiratory tract infection that progresses to difficulty breathing with a cough and wheeze. RSV causes potentially life-threatening airway obstruction.	Treatment is focused on symptom relief. Airway management with bronchodilators, hydration, and antivirals may be used to manage RSV.
Infective endocarditis (IE) or subacute bacterial endocarditis (SBE)	SBE prophylaxis with antibiotics is recommended for people with specific cardiac conditions who are undergoing procedures that may induce a transient bacteremia. *High-risk conditions* include prosthetic valves, most congenital heart malformations, rheumatic heart disease, hypertrophic cardiomyopathy, mitral valve prolapse with regurgitation, and previous bacterial endocarditis. *High-risk procedures* include most type of dental work (tooth extractions, cleaning, and surgery) and operations within the oropharynx, gastrointestinal, and genitourinary tract. Failures may occur even with adherence to recommendations.	Recommended prophylaxis: oral amoxicillin, 50 mg/kg (maximum 2 grams) 1 hour prior to the procedure. If allergic to penicillin, use cephalexin (50 mg/kg, maximum 2 grams) or azithromycin or clarithromycin (15 mg/kg, maximum 500 mg). Post-procedural antibiotics are no longer recommended.
Streptococcus pneumoniae (pneumococcal disease)	Extended (possibly lifelong) antibiotic prophylaxis is recommended for those persons at risk for developing fulminant pneumococcal disease, particularly patients with sickle-cell disease and asplenia. Pneumococcal vaccine may change these recommendations, but currently antibiotics are recommended even if vaccine is given.	Penicillin G or V Younger than 5 years of age, 125 mg b.i.d. Older than 5 years of age, 250 mg b.i.d.

CONDITION	RATIONALE	RECOMMENDATIONS
PREVENT RECURRENCES OF DISEASE		
Acute rheumatic fever (ARF)	Continuous antibiotics effective against Group A streptococcus are provided for persons who have a documented history of acute rheumatic fever to prevent recurrences. Antibiotic prophylaxis should begin as soon as the diagnosis of ARF is made and continue through life.	Benzathine penicillin IM every 4 weeks or daily oral antibiotics: • Penicillin V, 125–250 mg b.i.d., or • Erythromycin 250 mg b.i.d., or • Sulfadiazine More than 60 pounds, 1 g daily Less than 60 pounds, 0.5 g daily
Urinary tract infections (UTIs)	Children (infants to adolescents) with recurrent UTIs (more than 2 to 3 episodes) may be candidates for antibiotic prophylaxis to prevent recurrences.	Daily antibiotic therapy, usually with nitrofurantoin or trimethoprim-sulfamethoxazole, is given for various lengths of time: • Children with normal urinary tracts are usually treated until infection-free for 6–12 months. • Children with vesiculoureteral reflux are treated until reflux resolves. • Children with urinary tract abnormalities are often on long-term therapy.
PREVENT DISEASE AFTER EXPOSURE		
Meningitis (*Neisseria meningitidis* or *Haemophilus influenzae*)	Antibiotic prophylaxis is recommended for household members and child-care contacts of infected person.	Administer rifampin within 24 hours of identifying the person at 10 mg/kg every 12 hours x 2 days (four doses) for *Neisseria*; for *Haemophilus*, use a 4-day regimen.
Pertussis	Household contacts of infected person should receive antibiotic prophylaxis.	Administer erythromycin estolate (some experts use azithromycin) at 40–50 mg/kg/day (maximum 2 g/day) for 14 days.
Sexually transmitted diseases	Symptomatic or asymptomatic persons exposed to partners with *Chlamydia*, gonorrhea, or syphilis are treated with appropriate antibiotics.	Same treatment regimen is used for the infected and the exposed person.

▶ Sports physicals should not replace the routine physical exam, but may include preventive healthcare teaching on topics such as the use of supplemental aids and prevention of injuries.

▶ Results of the PPE may allow for full participation (the majority), temporary deferral (due to illness or injury), partial deferral (i.e., no contact or collision sports), recommendation for an appropriate sport for certain conditions, and/or exclusion.

TABLE 3–6.
SPECIFIC HEALTH BEHAVIORS AMENABLE TO INTERVENTION

FACTOR	STRENGTH OF EVIDENCE	BENEFIT	AGE FOR WHICH RECOMMENDED	RECOMMENDATION
Exercise	Good evidence	Many, including preventing cardiac disease, death	All ages	Individualize
Nutrition	Simple, focused intervention can be effective	Help with many chronic conditions	No upper limit	Counseling about adequate diet
Calcium	Good evidence in high-risk patients	Reduce risk of osteoporosis	Postmenopausal women	1,000–1,500 mg/day for women; no recommendation for men
Cholesterol	Diet not shown sufficient to reduce cholesterol level; normal levels protect young to middle-aged men	Reduce hyperlipidemia, atherosclerotic cardiovascular disease (ASCD)	No support for screening and treatment over age 75	Total cholesterol under 200, LDL depends on risk factors
Weight loss	Well-documented in adults up to 65	Reduce risk factor for atherosclerotic coronary disease	Not studied in elderly	Maintain ideal body weight
Stop smoking	Strongest recommendation, simple interventions can have 5%–10% quit rate	Reduce risk for cardiovascular, pulmonary, gastrointestinal diseases and malignancies	Quitting at any time improves pulmonary function and decreases risk of myocardial infarction (MI) and death	Ask about and encourage cessation at each visit
Alcohol	Cessation difficult to achieve in alcoholics	Reduce risk for falls and confusion in the elderly	No age limit to improve safety	Ask about, counsel to use in moderation
Drugs	Well documented	Reduce many risks of polypharmacy: adverse reactions, drug interactions, death in the elderly	Never too late	Check medications at each visit; ask about over-the-counter and herbal remedies; use only medications that are medically necessary
Safety, injury/ abuse prevention	Little data on prevention effectiveness	Reduce risk of falls, sixth leading cause of death	Different focus in the elderly	Home safety evaluation

FACTOR	STRENGTH OF EVIDENCE	BENEFIT	AGE FOR WHICH RECOMMENDED	RECOMMENDATION
Aspirin	Evidence in middle-aged men; few studies in elderly, look promising	Primary and secondary prevention of cardiovascular and cerebrovascular disease	Recommended for men over 40 or 50	Low dose: 81 mg/d for cardiovascular health
Estrogen	Well-documented; weigh risks (such as increased risk of breast cancer) versus benefits	Reduce risk of osteoporosis	Postmenopausal women with no contraindications	Progestin reduces risk of endometrial cancer, increases risk of breast cancer
IMMUNIZATION				
Influenza	Well-documented	Reduce incidence, severity of influenza	65+ years	Annually
Pneumonia	60% efficacy	Prevent *Streptococcus pneumoniae* infection	65+ years	Once; may repeat in 5 years
Tetanus	Well-proven	Prevent tetanus	No age limit	Every 10 years

Exercise Recommendations for Adults

▶ Focus on fundamental fitness and not sport-specific skills

▶ Goal: Sustain target heart rate for 30 minutes for maximum cardiopulmonary conditioning

  ▷ Subtract patient's age from 220

  ▷ Multiple result by 0.8 for target heart rate

  ▷ A 40-year-old patient's target heart rate is 144 bpm

▶ Before prescribing an exercise program for any patient, conduct a history and physical examination and evaluate:

  ▷ Fatigue, shortness of breath, chest pain

  ▷ Risk factors for thromboembolic disease

  ▷ Excessive bruising

  ▷ Cardiac murmurs, clicks, hums

  ▷ Carotid bruits

  ▷ Other physical indicators of undiagnosed vascular disease

  ▷ Current medications

▶ Decrease intensity or components of exercise program if the patient

  ▷ Is unable to talk while exercising,

    ▷   Is fatigued for more than 1 hour after finishing, or

    ▷   Develops swelling or pain.

▶ Increase intensity and/or time as patient develops tolerance

General Nutrition

▶ Goal: maintain or achieve ideal body weight and supply all essential body nutrients to maintain or regain health

▶ Normal growth requires appropriate intake of protein, fat, carbohydrates, water, vitamins, minerals, and trace elements.

▶ Recommended dietary allowances (RDA) are estimates of safe and adequate amounts of nutrients recommended to be consumed daily to maintain health. The RDA is the amount of nutrient needed to meet the known nutrient requirements of approximately 97% of the population.

▶ U.S. Department of Agriculture (USDA, n.d.) MyPlate suggests:

    ▷   Make half your plate of fruits and vegetables

    ▷   Switch to fat-free or low-fat (1%) milk

    ▷   Make at least half your grains whole

    ▷   Compare sodium, sugars, and saturated fats in foods and choose the foods with lower numbers

Infant/Childhood/Adolescent Nutrition

Diet planning

▶ Energy requirements can be determined using charts or the calculations in Table 3–7.

▶ Adolescents who have completed their growth and wish to lose weight will need to reduce calorie intake by 500 calories per day for each pound they wish to lose each week.

▶ No more than 2 pounds should be lost per week.

▶ Weight loss is not recommended for growing children (except under special circumstances and with close supervision).

▶ For children older than 2 years, 55% to 60% of calories should come from carbohydrates, 10% to 15% from protein, and no more than 30% from fat (with saturated fat 10% or less), and less than 300 mg of cholesterol per day.

TABLE 3–7.
DETERMINING ENERGY REQUIREMENTS

AGE	AVERAGE KCAL/KG/DAY
0–6 months	110–120
7–12 months	90–105
1–10 years	80
Adolescence	30–55

Ex: 9-month-old infant weighing 8 kg requires approximately 800 calories/day (8 kg x 100 kcal/kg/day = 800)

▶ Fat and cholesterol should not be restricted in the first 2 years of life.

▶ Recommended fiber intake is 0.5 g/kg/day, to a maximum of 35 g/day.

Recommended Nutritional Supplements

▶ Vitamin K, 1 mg IM, given at birth to all newborns to prevent hemorrhagic disease

▶ Vitamin D, 200 units/day, recommended for all breastfed infants until they are ingesting a minimum of 500 mL/day of vitamin D-fortified formula or milk

▶ Ferrous sulfate, 2–3 mg/kg/day (max 15 mg/day), recommended for breastfed preterm infants by 2 months old

▶ Iron-fortified cereals starting by 6 months of age in all infants to replace iron stores, which are depleted by the time the infant doubles birth weight at approximately age 4 to 5 months

▶ Fluoride supplements to reduce susceptibility to dental caries

▶ No fluoride supplements before 6 months of age and where water fluoride content is higher than 0.6 ppm, to avoid fluorosis (excessive mottling of the teeth; see Table 3–8)

Infant Nutrition

▶ Breast milk and/or formulas are sufficient to meet the nutrient needs of infants up to 4 to 6 months of age (exceptions noted above); see Table 3–9.

▶ Advantages of breast milk: nutritionally balanced, contains antibodies and macrophages, allergic reactions are rare, savings on time and money

▶ Possible disadvantages: milk supply may be insufficient, mechanical difficulties such as inverted nipples may occur, medications and infectious organisms may pass to infant, nutritional deficiencies in the mother may affect infant

▶ All FDA-approved infant formulas meet minimum nutrient standards and are 20 calories/ounce except for those specifically labeled as higher in calories (e.g., Enfamil 24).

▶ Evaporated milk formula not recommended, although it may be used in extenuating circumstances (e.g., unable to breastfeed and/or cannot afford formula). It is made by mixing one can of evaporated milk (13 ounces) with 19½ ounces of water and 3 tablespoons of corn syrup. These infants must also receive a multivitamin with iron; dosage varies with age.

Food Introduction

▶ Guidelines have been directed more by tradition than by science.

▶ May be introduced when infant is able to sit with support and has good neuromuscular control of head and neck, typically around 4 to 6 months of age

TABLE 3–8.
RECOMMENDED FLUORIDE DOSES WHEN WATER HAS 0.3–0.6 PPM

AGE	< 0.3 PPM	0.3–0.6 PPM
6 months–3 years	0.25 mg	0
3–6 years	0.5 mg	0.25 mg
6–11 years	1.0 mg	0.5 mg

TABLE 3–9.
INFANT FORMULAS

	COW'S MILK–BASED	SOY PROTEIN ISOLATE	PROTEIN HYDROLYSATES
Examples	Enfamil, Similac, Good Start	Isomil, ProSobee	Nutramigen, Pregestimil, Alimentum
Composition comments	Casein/whey ratio varies with manufacturer Lactose is usual carbohydrate (CHO) source; lactose-free formulas using corn syrup and/or fructose now widely available Available in iron-fortified and low-iron preparations; low-iron formulas not recommended	CHO—sucrose and/or glucose Methionine added to all soy formulas to correct deficiencies All are iron-fortified	Partially hydrolyzed protein that results in peptides that do not elicit an immunologic response Most are lactose-free
Uses	Routine use in well infants	Infants with lactose intolerance Infants with cow's milk protein sensitivity (approximately 20% of infants allergic to cow's milk also allergic to soy)	Infants with cow's milk and soy sensitivity
Contraindications	Milk protein sensitivity Lactose intolerance Galactosemia	Soy protein allergy Preterm infants—CHO, protein, mineral absorption of soy formulas in preterm infants is not adequately documented and American Academy of Pediatrics (2004) does not recommend their use; soy formulas specifically developed for preterm infants available Infants with renal disease	None reported

▶ Tradition has held that cereals are a good place to begin; use a spoon, avoid adding to bottle.

▶ Start with single-ingredient foods and add one new food at a time, with up to 4 to 7 days between foods to identify intolerances.

Food/Formula Cautions

▶ No low-iron formula use

▶ No cow's milk in the first year of life

▶ No honey before age 1 year because of possible development of infantile botulism

▶ Avoid foods high in salt or sugar, such as canned or processed foods; RDA for sodium for infants is 17.6 mg/kg/day.

▶ Avoid foods that are easily choked on, such as grapes, popcorn, hot dogs, raisins, nuts, candy, and peanut butter.

▶ Home preparation of foods such as spinach, beets, carrots, or collard greens may have enough nitrates to cause methemoglobinemia and are therefore not recommended in infancy.

▶ Foods considered highly allergenic, such as eggs, wheat, seafood, and nuts, have traditionally been withheld in the first year of life to avoid a possible allergic reaction, but the validity of this practice is uncertain.

Adult Nutrition

▶ Calculate body mass index (BMI) to determine overweight and obesity: weight in lbs ÷ height in inches^2) x 703. BMI of 25 or higher is considered overweight according to CDC, Assessing Your Weight (n.d.).

▶ An online BMI calculator can be found at www.cdc.gov/nccdphp/dnpa/bmi/adult_BMI/english_bmi_calculator/bmi_calculator.htm

  ▷ Normal weight: BMI 18.5–25

  ▷ Overweight: BMI 25–30

  ▷ Class I obesity: BMI 30–34.9

  ▷ Class II obesity: BMI 35–39.9

  ▷ Class III obesity: BMI > 40

Losing Weight

▶ In establishing realistic weight goals, calculate relationship of current weight compared to ideal body weight:

▶ Determine IBW

▶ Divide IBW by current body weight

▶ Multiply by 100

▶ Subtract 100

▶ Result gives percent over or under ideal body weight

Diet Planning

▶ Determine caloric needs by adding basal calories (IBW x 10) and activity calories (IBW x 3) for sedentary people, IBW x 5 for moderately active people, or IBW x 10 for people involved in strenuous activity.

▶ Example: IBW = 120 lbs for sedentary person

▶ 120 x 10 = 1,200 basal calories; 120 x 3 = 360

▶ 1200 + 360 = 1,560 total calories needed per day

▶ People who wish to lose weight will need to reduce calorie intake by 500 calories per day for each pound they wish to lose each week.

▶ Diets should limit fat to 30% or less of total calories, carbohydrates to 55% to 60% of calories, and the rest of calories from protein.

Geriatric Nutrition

▶ Goal: Supply all essential body nutrients to maintain or regain health

▶ Maintain, gain, or lose weight if necessary

▶ Adequate calcium intake: 1,000–1,500 mg a day

▶ Adequate vitamin D intake: 800 IU a day but consider higher deficiency levels in home-bound

▶ Frail elderly at risk for malnutrition—low albumin levels

Safety

Childhood Injuries

▶ Injury is the number one cause of death among children ages 16 and younger.

▶ Motor vehicle accidents, suffocation, drowning, poisoning, fires, and falls are some of the most common ways children are hurt or killed.

▶ Many injuries are preventable (see Table 3–10).

Injury Prevention in Adults/Geriatrics

▶ Home safety evaluation for fall prevention

▷ Bathrooms are the site of most falls.

▷ Throw rugs are dangerous.

▷ Use contrast lighting to reduce hazards.

▷ Sufficient lighting is needed both inside and outside the home.

▷ Safe and appropriate assisting devices are important.

▶ Driving evaluations for safety

▷ Driving is essential for independence, making patients reluctant to give it up.

▷ Driving can be impaired due to dementia, impaired vision, slowed reflexes, or musculoskeletal disorders.

▷ Seat belts are necessary for safety.

▶ Smoke and carbon monoxide detectors

▶ Safety locks on firearms

▶ Tips for environmental safety can be found in Table 3–11.

Assessment for Violence and Abuse

▶ Clinicians should ask about and watch for signs of physical abuse during encounters with patients.

▶ Patients will often admit to problems, but only if they are asked.

▷ Know and use state laws in determining requirements for reporting suspected abuse.

▷ Learn state requirements for a sexual assault examination.

TABLE 3–10.
INJURY AND PREVENTION

TYPE OF INJURY	EPIDEMIOLOGY	PREVENTION
Motor vehicle accident (MVA)	MVAs account for about half of all unintentional injury deaths; infants and adolescents usually injured as occupants, school-age children predominantly injured as pedestrians.	Use of child restraints and seat belts is the most effective way to prevent occupant injuries. There are four basic types of restraints: 1. Infant/toddler (birth to 2 years): Place semi-inclined and backward-facing in the back seat. 2. Toddler/preschool: Convertible seats and forward-facing seats with harnesses as long as possible up to the weight or height limit by the manufacturer. 3. School-aged: Belt positioning booster seat. Place preferably in the back seat. An infant or toddler car seat fits if the child's ears are below the top of the seat's back and shoulders are below the seat strap slots. 4. Older children: Use lap and shoulder belts. All children younger than 13 years should be restrained in rear seats. A shoulder strap should not be used if it goes across the face or throat. Child should be in booster seat to keep shoulder strap in proper place. See https://www.healthychildren.org/English/safety-prevention/on-the-go/Pages/Car-Safety-Seats-Information-for-Families.aspx Car seat adaptations are available for premature infants and patients in casts, on ventilators, or with special medical conditions such as spina bifida.
Drowning	Drowning is the second leading cause of accidental death for children 1 to 4. Poor supervision plays a key role in drowning of young children and infants. Adolescent drowning is often associated with alcohol use. Approximately 75% of drowning occurs in bodies of water that are part of the person's home, particularly bathtubs and pools. Infants can drown in inches of water and in unusual ways, such as in pails of water and toilet bowls. Approximately one-third of all survivors of drowning will suffer irreversible brain injury.	Supervision is the key to prevention: 1. Leave no children unattended in or near water and observe closely. 2. Keep the bathroom door closed. 3. Empty all pails of water. 4. Keep swimming pools completely fenced with a locking gate. 5. Make life jackets a must. 6. Teach children to swim and to behave safely around water, such as using life preservers. Infant swim lessons are not recommended because of the risk of water intoxication.

(CONTINUED)

TYPE OF INJURY	EPIDEMIOLOGY	PREVENTION
Fire and burns	More than 300 children between the ages of 0 to 19 are treated in emergency rooms daily for burn-related injuries. More than 1 million burn injuries occur per year and as many as 30,000 people younger than 15 years of age are hospitalized yearly for burns. Approximately 75% of all burns are scalds that occur in the kitchen. Bathtub water can cause burns if hotter than 120°F. Skin damage rarely occurs at temperatures below 110°F, but a full-thickness burn can occur in 1 second in water 160°F. Approximately 85% of all deaths from fire are due to smoke inhalation during house fires.	Keep smoke alarms on each floor of the house and check the batteries every month. (All three types—heat, photoelectric, and ionization—are effective.) Keep pot handles turned inward on the stove. Keep an ABC-rated fire extinguisher in the kitchen. Do not allow children to sit in adult laps when drinking hot liquids. Teach children fire escape route and rules, and practice escapes. Keep water temperature at 120°F.
Asphyxiation and choking	This type of injury accounts for approximately 40% of all unintentional deaths in children younger than1 year of age. Food items commonly choked on are hot dogs, candy, nuts, grapes, raisins, and raw vegetables. Nonfood items that children choke on include balloons, undersized infant pacifiers, small toys such as balls and jacks, coins, pop-tops, and safety pins. Asphyxiation occurs from situations such as hanging from drapery cords or bibs tied around neck; crib strangulations (head entrapment); toy chest lids falling on a child's head and neck; or when the nose and mouth are covered in a soft pillow, beanbag, or waterbed.	Do not feed small, round, hard foods to children less than 2 to 3 years of age. Do not allow children to run with food. No balloons before age 3 years and then monitor. Keep small objects out of the reach of children; evaluate all toys for safety. Encourage parents to learn the Heimlich maneuver. Tie up all cords. Use bibs with Velcro instead of ties. Use cribs with slat spacing 2 3/8 in. or less. Do not place infants on any soft or enveloping surfaces.

TYPE OF INJURY	EPIDEMIOLOGY	PREVENTION
Poisoning	The American Association of Poison Control Centers estimates that there are 1.2 million poisonings in children younger than 6 years annually. Although the number of pediatric poisonings is high, the fatality rate is low—much less than 0.1%. Toddlers are at the greatest risk. Children 6–12 years account for a very small percentage. Adolescent exposures are usually intentional (suicide or abuse) or occupational. More than half of pediatric poisonings involve nondrug products—commonly, cosmetics, personal care products (deodorants), cleaning substances, and plants. Pharmaceutical preparations comprise the remainder of ingestion poisonings with vitamins (particularly iron-containing products), analgesics, cold/cough medications, and antibiotics being the most common agents.	Childproofing the home should include putting all medications and other substances out of reach and/or behind locked doors. Use child-resistant medication containers. Keep the phone number of poison control readily available. Syrup of ipecac no longer recommended.
Falls	Falls are the fifth leading cause of death in children and result in enormous morbidity. Approximately 13,000 deaths occur annually due to falls. A disproportionately large number of fall injuries are caused by falling down stairs in infant walkers and falls from bunk beds, playground equipment, skateboards, and trampolines.	Never leave infants or toddlers unattended on elevated surfaces. Do not use crib with rails that lower. Avoid walker use. Gates should be placed in front of all staircases. Windowsills and bunk beds should never be used as play areas. Use window guards. Do not allow children to participate in activities beyond their physical abilities, such as skateboarding down steep hills. Discourage the use of any trampolines. Use protective gear (helmets, pads) for bike riding, skateboarding, and sports.

Adapted from *Guide to clinical preventive services,* by Agency on Healthcare Research and Quality. (2014). Washington, DC: Department of Health and Human Services. Retrieved from http://www.ahrq.gov/professionals/clinicians-providers/guidelines-recommendations/guide/index.html

TABLE 3–11.
PREVENTION OF ENVIRONMENT-RELATED HEALTH PROBLEMS

SAFETY HAZARD	RISK	RECOMMENDATIONS
Secondhand smoke	Increased risk of respiratory problems and cancer	No smoking in the home, car, or around children
Carbon monoxide exposure	Ranges from chronic flu-like symptoms to death	Use acceptable carbon monoxide detector in home; properly use and maintain fuel-burning devices
Radon	Increased risk of cancer	Test home for radon with a home test kit; if level exceeds 4pCi/L, identify and seal basement leaks
Lead	Lead poisoning—neurological damage, anemia	Do not use lead-containing utensils for cooking or eating. Renovations done with proper precautions Employment in high-risk places/occupations—use precautions

Adapted from *Guide to clinical preventive services,* by Agency on Healthcare Research and Quality. (2014). Washington, DC: Department of Health and Human Services. Retrieved from http://www.ahrq.gov/professionals/clinicians-providers/guidelines-recommendations/guide/index.html

Geriatric Abuse and Neglect

▶ Risk factors include age over 84; social isolation; lack of support; cognitive impairment; and physical, emotional, and financial dependency.

Stress

▶ Stress is the emotional and physical response to an increase in the environmental demands beyond the resources of a person to cope with those demands.

▶ Small amounts of stress may add excitement and variety and increase the quality of life. Large amounts of stress may be overwhelming and lead to disease.

▶ The goal is to find the right balance of stress in life.

▶ People often seem to have vulnerability to stress in one system (e.g., hypertension, ulcer, mental problems).

Management

Stress may be managed through various techniques:

▶ Avoid unnecessary change during stressful times.

▶ Manage time by keeping to predetermined goals and priorities.

▶ Avoid stressful triggers (people, activities, etc.) when possible.

▶ Create habits or routines to decrease stress.

▶ Develop alternative activities or friendships that increase pleasure.

▶ Physical exercise often decreases stress.

▶ Participate in religious, motivational, or service projects that increase self-esteem or change focus to helping others.

▶ Use biofeedback, tension-relaxation exercise, yoga, or imagery to control stress reactions.

Interpersonal Support

▶ High-quality interactions with others help persons maintain or regain health (Pender, 1996).

▶ Types of supporting behaviors (Friedman, 1998)

▷ Instrumental support gives direct assistance and service.

▷ Informational support uses advice, suggestions, and information in solving problems.

▶ Emotional support comes when love, care, empathy, and trust are provided through relationships.

▷ Appraisal support uses feedback and affirmation to help people evaluate themselves.

Stressors in the Elderly

▶ A common myth about the elderly is that they do not tolerate change.

▶ The elderly do face major life changes, especially losses—death of spouse and/or friends, having to move, retiring or losing jobs, ability to do many activities, etc.; these changes cause major stress in the elderly.

Dependency

▶ A common personality tendency that, in its extreme form, causes a person to rely on other people or activities, such as eating food, drinking alcohol, having sex, gambling, or other activity, to try to satisfy an emotional hunger

▶ Action begun voluntarily but, through repetition, becomes involuntary

▶ Becomes addiction when there is loss of control (compulsivity), continuation despite adverse consequences, and obsession or preoccupation with the activity

▶ Treatment may be complex and require long-term therapy.

Pharmacology in the Geriatric Population

▶ Polypharmacy of five or more drugs at one time is a common problem with potential drug interactions.

▶ Age-related changes increase risk of drug toxicities.

▷ Absorption is slower, delayed onset

▷ Distribution in tissues affected by change in fat-to-muscle ratio

▷ Metabolism slowed, increasing toxicity by drugs metabolized by the P450 system

▷ Excretion through the kidney may be decreased due to reduced renal function

▶ Drug toxicities are more common and more serious in the elderly.

▷ Use lower doses, titrate up slowly.

▷ Monitor over-the-counter drug use closely.

Health Maintenance

Child Health Supervision

▶ The general health of children can be significantly improved through the effective use of healthcare supervision (e.g., disease prevention, early detection and intervention of disorders, providing anticipatory guidance).

▶ Health supervision should be done at regularly scheduled well visits and should include obtaining a history and physical exam; vital signs; assessment of growth and development; obtaining age-appropriate screening tests; and counseling about nutrition, safety, and other topics.

▶ Recommended ages for well visits are at 2 weeks; 2, 4, 6, 9, 12, 15, 18, and 24 months; yearly from ages 3 to 6 years; every other year from ages 6 to 11 years; and yearly during adolescence.

▶ Additional visits may be needed for children with some variations of normal, for sports physicals, and for presurgical procedures.

Pediatric Health Screening

▶ Purpose: early detection of treatable conditions (see Table 3–12)

▶ Not all abnormal results are identified on screening tests, so continual monitoring of patient's condition and repeat testing may be necessary.

▶ Use of screening tests will change as incidence of disease changes (e.g., lead testing) and as technology improves (e.g., newborn hearing tests).

▶ Screening tests may be recommended primarily for high-risk groups (e.g., lead, cholesterol) at certain ages; others are universal tests for all children (anemia).

Adult/Geriatric Health Screening and Supervision

▶ Routine periodic health supervision visits have not been established for adults.

▶ Routine screening recommendations are established by the U.S. Preventive Services Task Force and are updated for asymptomatic persons, based on evidence supporting the effectiveness of preventive measures (see Table 3–13).

▶ Various specialty groups, such as the American Cancer Society, National Cancer Institute, American College of Obstetricians and Gynecologists (ACOG), and American Academy of Family Physicians, also make recommendations, and these may not agree with the U.S. Preventive Services Task Force.

▶ Clinicians should be prepared to clearly identify and document the basis for their preventive practices because there is not always agreement among the recommending bodies.

GERIATRIC ASSESSMENT

Nonspecific presentation of illness

▶ The elderly often present with vague complaints or deterioration in functional independence as an early subtle sign of illness.

▶ This generally occurs in the absence of classical (typical) symptoms and signs of disease.

TABLE 3–12.
PEDIATRIC SCREENING RECOMMENDATIONS

SCREENING TESTS	AGES FOR SCREENING	TESTING AND INTERPRETATION
Neonatal, metabolic, and genetic screening (PKU test)	All full-term infants before discharge and in 1–2 weeks	All states screen for phenylketonuria (PKU) and hypothyroidism; most screen for galactosemia. Other tests are determined on a state-by-state basis and may include sickle-cell disease, maple syrup urine disease, homocystinuria, congenital toxoplasmosis, adrenal hyperplasia, and cystic fibrosis. All positive screening results require immediate confirmation and/or referral.
Hearing screening	All newborns	Newborns to be screened appropriately for hearing impairment.
Hearing screening	3, 4, 5, 10, 12, 15, and 18 years of age	Audiometric screening: Minimal evaluation should be 20 dB HL with frequencies of 1, 2, and 4 kHz. Any unheard frequency is a failure and the child should be retested at a later date. Failure again requires a referral.
Anemia screening	Hgb and Hct for asymptomatic children 6–12 months who are at increased risk of iron-deficiency anemia	Hgb is sensitive for iron-deficiency anemia but not mild deficiency states.
Lead screening	Selectively obtain blood lead levels (BLLs) of at-risk children at 9–12 months and possibly again at 2 years old. BLLs > 10 mg/dL require retesting and possible further evaluation and treatment, depending on the level.	1. Screen children who live in communities where: 27% of housing was built before 1950 or 12% of 1–2-year-olds have BLLs > 10 mcg/dL. (Such information is provided by state health officials.) 2. In all other communities, screen children who live in or regularly visit homes/facilities built before 1950, or 1978 if renovated in the past 6 months, or who have siblings/playmates with elevated BLLs. 3. Screen all children where community and home information is unknown. 4. Any child may be screened if other risk factors for lead exposure exist, such as cultural practices (use of lead pottery or lead-containing folk medicines), parent occupation, or adoption from countries where lead poisoning is prevalent, or where elevated BLLs may be contributing to a problem such as developmental delay.

(CONTINUED)

SCREENING TESTS	AGES FOR SCREENING	TESTING AND INTERPRETATION
Tuberculin (TB) skin test	Annual testing, with Mantoux (PPD) skin test for children at high risk. For children with no risk factors who live in high-prevalence regions or who lack a clear history, do periodic testing at ages 1, 4–6, and 11–16 years of age (suggested; can be any age). IGRA blood test may be used in place of skin test.	Children at high risk include those who: 1. Have contacts with infected adults 2. Have clinical or X-ray findings suggestive of TB 3. Are immunosuppressed (HIV) 4. Have chronic illness (diabetes, renal disease) 5. Come from high-prevalence countries (or their parents did) 6. Have or had frequent exposure to high-risk adults: HIV positive, homeless, drug abuser, poor health, nursing home resident, malnutrition or migrant worker Induration considered positive if: Larger than 5 mm: risk factors 1–3 (see above) Larger than 10 mm: risk factors 4–6, or any child less than 4 years old Larger than 15 mm: all other people
Vision screening	Obtain visual acuity (V/A) and binocular vision by age 3–5 years.	Test V/A with the Snellen chart standardized at 20 feet. Use a Tumbling E or Lea chart (uses symbols—apple, circle, square, and house) if letters cannot be recognized. A failed test is V/A 20/40 or greater in either eye, or if there is a two-line discrepancy between the eyes (e.g., 20/20 in one eye and 20/40 in another). All children should be tested once for color blindness. Make referrals for all failures.

Adapted from *Guide to clinical preventive services,* by Agency on Healthcare Research and Quality. (2014). Washington, DC: Department of Health and Human Services. Retrieved from http://www.ahrq.gov/professionals/clinicians-providers/guidelines-recommendations/guide/index.html

▶ Acutely ill older adults often present with

  ▷ Confusion or delirium,

  ▷ Increased difficulty performing activities of daily living (ADLs),

  ▷ Incontinence, or

  ▷ Falls.

TABLE 3–13.
ADULT/GERIATRIC SCREENING RECOMMENDATIONS

PROBLEM OR ISSUE	GENERALLY ACCEPTED RECOMMENDATIONS
Asymptomatic heart disease	Do not screen asymptomatic adults at low risk for coronary heart disease.
Breast masses	Women 50–74 years every 2 years with mammography. Diagnostic exam if positive or with mass.
Cervical cancer	Screening women ages 21–65 with Pap smear every 3 years. Ages 30–65 screen with Pap smear every 3 years or contesting with cytology and HPV every 5 years.
Colon cancer	Screen with high-sensitivity fecal occult blood testing (FOBT) every year, sigmoidoscopy every 5 years, with FOBT every 3 years or colonoscopy every 10 years in adults 50–75.
Vision	Screen visual acuity with Snellen testing and refer people at high risk for glaucoma to eye specialists.
Dental/oral	Yearly exam and counseling
Hearing	Assess hearing through physical exam and refer as needed.
Hyperlipidemia	Men older than 34 and women older than 44 who are at increased risk for coronary heart disease. Screening for others has lower level evidence.
Hypertension	Blood pressure screening every 2 years in normotensive patients older than 21
Menopause	Counsel all perimenopausal and postmenopausal women about potential risks and benefits of hormone replacement.
Osteoporosis	Counsel all women about the risks and benefits of hormone replacement therapy, dietary calcium, vitamin D, weight-bearing exercise, and smoking cessation. Bone density measurement for women older than 65, earlier in women at increased risk. Optimal intervals not established.
Prostate cancer	No recommended routine screening for prostate cancer such as digital rectal examinations, prostate-specific antigen (PSA), or transrectal ultrasound. Potential harm is greater than benefit.
Testicular cancer	No evidence supports routine screening of asymptomatic men.
Hypothyroidism	Evidence does not recommend screening with TSH in asymptomatic persons.
Skin cancer	Counsel about minimizing exposure to ultraviolet radiation. Screening not recommended for general population.
Dementia, functional impairment	Not recommended in asymptomatic persons
Sexually transmitted diseases	Offer high-intensity counseling for adults at increased risk for STIs.

Adapted from *Guide to clinical preventive services,* by Agency on Healthcare Research and Quality. (2014). Washington, DC: Department of Health and Human Services. Retrieved from http://www.ahrq.gov/professionals/clinicians-providers/guidelines-recommendations/guide/index.html

Functional Assessment

▶ Assessment tools provide standardized data to follow trends and evaluate response to treatment.

▶ Cognitive and functional assessments are the keystone to providing geriatric care.

▶ Many assessment tools are available.

Normal Changes of Aging

▶ What is normal becomes less uniform as patients age.

▶ Normal changes usually mean less functional reserve.

▶ It is often difficult to differentiate among normal aging, chronic disease, medication effect, and disuse.

IMMUNIZATION

▶ Recommended for various age groups to prevent the spread of disease and to reduce the mortality and morbidity related to diseases that are responsive to vaccines

▶ Immunization schedules change from time to time, so the advanced practice nurse must review update schedules annually, as well as stay apprised of schedule and vaccine changes for all age groups. This information is located on the Centers for Disease Control's Prevention Vaccine and Immunization website (http://www.cdc.gov/vaccines/schedules/hcp/index.html).

▶ Most children are immunized by the time they enter school, but many remain unimmunized until that time, leaving them at unnecessary risk for infections or considered risks to other children.

▶ Many adults are inadequately immunized from lack of immunization as children, failure to get boosters, or have not received newly recommended immunizations for adults.

▶ Some categories of workers may require additional immunizations such as food handlers, those working with animals, and travelers.

▶ Older adults are the largest age group acquiring tetanus.

Immunization Guidelines

▶ All states require children entering school and licensed day care are required to have vaccines. To check individual state laws, refer to the Immunization Action Coalition (http://immunize.org/laws/index.htm).

▶ The immunization schedule must be modified when immunization has not begun in early infancy or was interrupted. Previously given vaccines do not need to be repeated.

▶ The child is considered not immunized if the vaccine status is unknown.

▶ Preterm infants should be immunized with regular doses according to postnatal chronological age.

▶ Adverse effects: Common to almost all the vaccines are local injection-site reactions such as pain, tenderness, and erythema that are mild and transient, and mild to moderate fevers and myalgias for 24 to 48 hours.

▶ General contraindications to vaccinations include hypersensitivity reactions (urticaria, shock, wheezing) and prior encephalopathy within 7 days of pertussis vaccine; undefined illnesses where administering vaccines may confuse the diagnosis; and prior severe reactions where administering the vaccine would be more harmful than withholding.

▶ Not contraindications: minor illnesses, family history of seizure disorders, sudden infant death syndrome, presence of a pregnant woman in the household

▶ There is no contraindication to simultaneous administration of the routine vaccines.

▶ Informed consent from parent/guardian prior to vaccination with information provided regarding the disease to be prevented, risks and benefits of the vaccine, and potential adverse effects

▶ Additional vaccines may be indicated or recommended for specific illnesses and/or disorders, travel, geographical area, and/or special circumstances. Adult vaccines are listed in Table 3–14.

▶ Free vaccines are available through the Vaccines for Children program for uninsured and Medicaid-eligible children, and Native American and Alaskan Native children.

Other Disease-Prevention Programs

Back to Sleep Program

▶ For the prevention of SIDS, the most common cause of death in children under 1 year of age

▶ Risk factors for SIDS: sleep position, exposure to cigarette smoke, low birth weight, and prematurity; highest incidence in Black people and Native Americans, lowest in Asian people

▶ Recommends positioning infants on the back or side for sleeping. Incidence of SIDS has decreased dramatically with these sleeping positions.

Smoking Cessation

▶ More than 40% of U.S. children are exposed to environmental tobacco smoke in their own homes.

▶ Teenage smokers experience a decrease in physical fitness and lung function and, later, an increase in the risk of lung cancer and heart disease.

▶ Encourage cessation of smoking first without pharmacologic interventions; if unsuccessful, may educate regarding products available for assistance.

TABLE 3–14.
IMMUNIZATION GUIDELINES FOR ADULTS

Please visit http://www.cdc.gov/vaccines/schedules/hcp/imz/adult.html for the latest vaccination guidelines as the recommendations change frequently.

TYPE OF IMMUNIZATION	RECOMMENDATIONS FOR ADULTS
Hepatitis A	Two doses if another risk factor is present (medical, occupation, or lifestyle indication)
Hepatitis B	All people 12–25 years with no history of infection or previous immunization; high-risk adults
Human papillomavirus (HPV)	Women through age 26 years, men through age 21 years; men who have sex with men and men who have compromised immune systems including HIV through age 26
Influenza	Pregnant women; annually for all adults 50+ years of age; others if at high risk or household contacts of those at high risk. Healthy, ages 2–49, and nonpregnant women, can receive either intranasally administered live, attenuated influenza vaccine (LAIV), (FluMist), or IIV. Annually for healthcare workers, particularly those who care for severely immunocompromised people (i.e., those who require care in a protected environment); should receive IIV rather than LAIV.
Measles, mumps, and rubella (MMR)	Administer one or two doses to anyone over 18 years of age born after 1957 with no documented proof of immunity. Contraindicated in pregnancy or immunocompromising conditions
Meningococcal	College freshmen living in dormitories and travelers to endemic areas with no history of prior infections; anyone whose spleen was damaged or removed
Pneumococcal polysaccharide (PPSV23)	Once at 65+; one or two doses over age 18 if at high risk and repeat if injection was more than 5 years ago
Pneumococcal 13-valent conjugate (PCV13)	One dose for adults over the age of 18 with another risk factor present
Rubella screen or immunization	Women of childbearing age
Tetanus, diphtheria, pertussis (Tdap/DTaP/Td)	Substitute one-time dose of Tdap for Td booster, then booster every 10 years; booster at 5 years for wound management. Administer one dose of Tdap vaccine to pregnant women during each pregnancy (preferred during 27–36 weeks' gestation), regardless of number of years since prior Td or Tdap vaccination.
Varicella	Administer two doses in adults with no history of varicella or previous vaccination. Contraindicated in pregnancy and immunocompromising conditions.
Zoster	Once at 60+ for all adults with history of chicken pox infection

Adapted from *Immunization schedules,* by Centers for Disease Control and Prevention. (2015). Retrieved from http://www.cdc.gov/vaccines/schedules/hcp/index.html

Other Healthcare Considerations

Cultural Influences

▶ The healthcare provider who is sensitive to issues surrounding health care and the traditional health beliefs of the patient can provide more comprehensive healthcare.

▶ Family structure and values have an impact on the health encounter.

▶ Ethnicity is based on the race, tribe, or nation with which a person identifies and influences the person's beliefs and behaviors.

Environmental Factors

▶ General circumstances such as climate, altitude, and temperature affect all people in a region and cannot be modified unless the person relocates.

▶ Other factors such as air pollution, water fluoridation and contamination, crime, poverty, and transportation are examples of factors that might be manipulated to have a positive effect on the community.

Evidence-Based Medicine

▶ The trend today is to base decisions on evidence from randomized controlled research trials when possible but at times evidence with less confidence is used. Many sources of recommendations are available through U.S. government-sponsored websites like CDC, NIH, and AHRQ.

▶ There are conflicting guidelines among various organizations, and these must be reconciled by the practitioner.

Clinical Guidelines

▶ Standards of practice are devised from research by experts in the field to guide and standardize practice across the nation. Nurse practitioners should know how to analyze clinical guidelines to determine those that are written by objective scholars and are without organizational, professional, or pharmaceutical bias. (See the National Guideline Clearinghouse at www.guideline.gov.)

▶ Factors to consider in evaluating guidelines include source of guideline; appropriateness of methodology used to develop guideline such as randomized trials; use of expert opinion/clinical experience in decision-making; public policy issue considerations; feasibility issues; use of peer preview; and congruence with other practice guidelines, timeliness, and funding source.

CASE STUDIES

Case 1

Emily, 2 months old, has been brought by her parents to the clinic for her well baby exam. Her gestation and birth history are unremarkable. She was born at 39 weeks with a birth weight of 7 pounds, 8 ounces (3.4 kg) and length of 20.5 inches. She is breastfed on demand, about every 3 to 4 hours. She has not had any immunizations.

1. What vaccines will Emily need today?
2. What developmental milestones would you assess for in a 2-month-old?
3. There is no fluoride in the tap water at her home. When should you start Emily on fluoride? How much will you give her each day?
4. Emily's mother is thinking about discontinuing breastfeeding and starting infant formula. What information should you provide to her that might encourage her to continue to breastfeed?

Case 2

Travis, a 4½-year-old, comes to the clinic for a school physical. His last checkup was at 3 years of age. He is 40 pounds and 39 inches. His immunization records indicate he has had four DtaP, three IPV, one MMR, two hepatitis B, and three HiB vaccine shots.

1. What vaccines would he need today?
2. What anticipatory guidance and safety issues would you discuss with Travis and his parents?

Case 3

Josh, Travis's 14-year-old brother, needs a pre-participation sports physical. Josh weighs 225 pounds and is 5 feet, 8 inches tall.

1. What would be the focus of your assessment examination?
2. What counseling does Josh need?
3. What immunizations might Josh need?

Case 4

You have been asked to set up a health fair for a large computer company. The company would like to focus on employees, their families, and retired workers. You research the company and find out that equal numbers of employees with young children, single employees, and retired employees plan to attend the health fair.

1. What primary prevention topics would you address for parents of young children?
2. What secondary prevention topics would you address for adults ages 18 to 50?
3. What secondary prevention topics would you address for adults 50 and older?
4. How would you educate the participants about stress management?

Case 5

Jose M. is a 65-year-old man who has scheduled his "Welcome to Medicare" exam with you. He has recently moved to this community to be closer to his children and is new to your practice. He is particularly interested in remaining healthy and wants to do what is appropriate in screening and prevention.

1. What are the age and gender-specific screening tests that you would recommend?
2. What vaccines would you recommend?
3. What specific counseling would you recommend?

Case 6

Ms. J. is a 45-year-old Black woman who has been told she has Type 2 diabetes mellitus and that she should attempt to reduce her weight. She is 68 inches tall and weighs 237 pounds.

1. What is her BMI? What is a desired BMI for her?
2. She reports that she has seen Internet advertisements for weight-loss programs that guarantee she will lose 5 pounds in the first week and that some people have lost over 100 pounds on this plan. She asks for your advice on enrolling on this plan. What is your recommendation?

CASE STUDIES DISCUSSION

Case 1

1. What vaccines will Emily need today?

    DTaP, IPV, HBV, HIB, PCV, rotavirus

2. What developmental milestones would you assess for in a 2-month-old?

    Begins to smile at people, coos, makes gurgling sounds; begins to follow things with eyes; can hold head up

3. There is no fluoride in the tap water at her home. When should you start Emily on fluoride? How much will you give her each day?

    Begin at 6 months with 0.25 mg per day

4. Emily's mother is thinking about discontinuing breastfeeding and starting infant formula. What information should you provide to her that might encourage her to continue to breastfeed?

    Ask why she is considering the change. Breastmilk is nutritionally balanced and contains antibodies and macrophages, which are important to immunity and wound healing. Allergic reactions are rare. Breastfeeding may save money.

Case 2

1. What vaccines would he need today?

    DtaP, IPV, MMR, hepatitis B, and varicella; depending on time of year, add influenza and give hepatitis A, if not given

2. What anticipatory guidance and safety issues would you discuss with Travis and his parents?

    Recreational sports protection gear (helmets, pads); swimming safety; automobile (street safety, seatbelts); knows his address, phone number, how to call 911; smoke alarms in the house; access/storage of guns in the home

Case 3

1. What would be the focus of your assessment examination?

    History, immunization status, vital signs, pubertal development, musculoskeletal and cardiopulmonary systems

2. What counseling does Josh need?

    Weight management (his BMI is 34.2), safety (seatbelts, recreational protective gear)

3. What immunizations might Josh need?

    Assure he completed the series Tdap, hepB, varicella, MMR, IPV, MCV, and hepA. Tdap and MCV if he did not have at age 11 to 13 years. HPV series to begin at age 11.

Case 4

1. What primary prevention topics would you address for parents of young children?

    Nutrition, iron intake, fluoride, safety (car seats, falls, poisonings, drowning), immunizations, sunscreen, access/storage gun safety

2. What secondary prevention topics would you address for adults ages 18 to 50?

    Exercise, weight management, stop smoking, influenza prevention, mammography, Pap smears

3. What secondary prevention topics would you address for adults 50 and older?

    Mammography, Pap smears, colon screening, avoid UV radiation

4. How would you educate the participants about stress management?

    Large amounts of stress can lead to disease. Discuss stress management techniques (relaxation, imagery, time management). Seek out support. Recognize sources of stress for the geriatric clients—loss.

Case 5

1. What are the age- and gender-specific screening tests that you would recommend?

    Some form of colon screening, lipids screening, blood pressure

2. What vaccines would you recommend?

    Flu every year, Tdap booster every 10 years, zoster, PCV13, PCV23. hepA and hepB series if he has not had these. Others depend on his medical history.

3. What specific counseling would you recommend?

    Depends on his risk factors; general counseling for exercise, balanced diet, avoiding ultraviolet radiation, STIs if at risk

Case 6

1. What is her BMI? What is a desired BMI for her?

    Her BMI is 36. A desired BMI is between 18.5 and 25.

2. She reports that she has seen Internet advertisements for weight-loss programs that guarantee she will lose 5 pounds in the first week and that some people have lost over 100 pounds on this plan. She asks for your advice on enrolling on this plan. What is your recommendation?

    Plans that propose more than 1 or 2 pounds of weight loss per week are difficult to sustain. Advertised programs are often expensive and may not consider the needs of people with diabetes. She will need to lose over 70 pounds to reach her desired BMI, and this may take a year or more to achieve and sustain.

REFERENCES

Agency on Healthcare Research and Quality. (2014). *Guide to clinical preventive services.* Washington, DC: Department of Health and Human Services. Retrieved from http://www.ahrq.gov/professionals/clinicians-providers/guidelines-recommendations/guide/index.html

Berul, C. (2000). Cardiac evaluation of the young athlete. *Pediatric Annals, 29*(3), 163.

California Health Care Almanac. (July 2014). *Health care costs 101: Slow growth persists.* Retrieved from http://www.chcf.org/~/media/media%20library%20Files/pdf/pdf%20H/pdf%20healthcarecosts14.pdf

Centers for Disease Control and Prevention. (n.d.). Assessing your weight. Retrieved from http://www.cdc.gov/healthyweight/assessing/index.html

Centers for Disease Control and Prevention. (n.d.). National prevention strategy: America's plan for better health and wellness. Retrieved from http://www.cdc.gov/features/preventionstrategy/

Centers for Disease Control and Prevention. (2013). 10 leading causes of death by age group, United States – 2013. Retrieved from http://www.cdc.gov/injury/wisqars/pdf/leading_causes_of_death_by_age_group_2013-a.pdf

Centers for Disease Control and Prevention. (2015). Immunization schedules. Retrieved from http://www.cdc.gov/vaccines/schedules/hcp/index.html

Friedman, M. (2003). *Family nursing: Research, theory, and practice* (5th ed.). Norwalk, CT: Appleton & Lange.

Gordis, L. (2014). *Epidemiology* (5th ed.). Philadelphia, PA: Elsevier.

Hockenberry, M. J., & Wilson, D. (2014). *Wong's nursing care of infants and children* (10th ed.). St. Louis, MO: Elsevier.

Immunization Action Coalition. (n.d.). State mandates on immunization and vaccine-preventable diseases. Retrieved from http://www.immunize.org/laws/

James, P., Oparil, S., Carter, B., Cushman, W., Dennison-Himmelfarb, C., Handler, J., . . . Ortiz, E. (2014). 2014 evidence-based guideline for the management of high blood pressure in adults. *Journal of the American Medical Association, 311*(5), 507–520.

Jarvis, C. (2015). *Physical examination and health assessment* (7th ed.). St. Louis, MO: Elsevier.

Marcdante, K. J., & Kliegman, R. M. (2014). *Nelson essentials of pediatrics* (7th ed.). Philadelphia, PA: Elsevier.

National Center for Health Statistics. (2010). CDC growth charts: United States. Retrieved from http://www.cdc.gov/nchs/data/ad/ad314.pdf

National Center for Health Statistics. (2013). Health expenditures. Retrieved from http://www.cdc.gov/nchs/fastats/health-expenditures.htm

National Institute on Aging. (2008). Health disparities toolbox. Retrieved from http://www.nia.nih.gov/about/features/links-minority-research-training-fall-2008

Obamacare Facts. (2015). Percentage uninsured in the U.S. by quarter. Retrieved from http://obamacarefacts.com/sign-ups/obamacare-enrollment-numbers/

Pender, N., Murdaugh, C., & Parsons, M. A. (2014). *Health promotion in nursing practice* (7th ed.). Upper Saddle River, NJ: Prentice Hall.

Tanner, J. M. (1962). *Growth of adolescents* (2nd ed.). Oxford, England: Blackwell Scientific.

U.S. Department of Agriculture. (n.d.). MyPlate and historical food pyramid resources. Retrieved from https://fnic.nal.usda.gov/dietary-guidance/myplate-and-historical-food-pyramid-resources U.S. Department of Health & Human Services. (n.d.). Affordable Care Act. Retrieved from http://www.hhs.gov/healthcare/rights/law/index.html

U.S. Department of Health and Human Services, Office of Disease Prevention and Health Promotion. (2010). *Healthy people 2020*. Retrieved from http://www.health.gov/healthypeople/default.htm

World Health Organization. (2015). What are social determinants of health? Retrieved from http://www.who.int/social_determinants/sdh_definition/en/

CHAPTER 4

INFECTIOUS DISEASES

Julie A. Lindenberg, DNP, FNP-BC, DCC
Jeffrey Kwong, DNP, MPH ANP-BC, FAANP

GENERAL APPROACH

▶ Making the correct diagnosis of infectious disease in the family setting requires familiarity with the infectious organisms *commonly* seen in each age group.

▶ Mild illness is common in children, particularly upper respiratory infections in infants and toddlers.

▶ A fever is a temperature greater than 38°C (100.4°F) rectal, 37.5°C (99.5°F) oral, and 37°C (98.6°F) axillary. The normal temperature varies throughout the circadian rhythm, being lowest in the early morning and higher in the afternoon.

▶ Transmission of infection is influenced by the type of organism, its mode of transmission, its viability in the environment, the number of organisms present in the environment, the resistance of the potential host to the organism, and the frequency of the asymptomatic or carrier state.

▶ Antibiotic resistance is a growing concern. All providers need to ensure appropriate prescribing to prevent increasing resistance in communities and populations.

▶ Evolving diseases that are now drug-resistant (such as gonorrhea and tuberculosis) add to the concern.

Assessment

▶ Obtain a thorough history of the symptoms of the present illness, as well as possible contacts and exposure to infectious illness. Inquire about patient smoking, secondhand smoke exposure, immunization status, day care attendance, and international travel history.

▶ Factors indicating possible bacterial infection include loss of appetite, dehydration, high fever, chills, significant weakness, and/or malaise.

▶ Perform a physical examination, evaluating for signs of infection, including: vital signs, skin (noting rash), eyes (noting conjunctival erythema or discharge), ears/nose/throat (noting erythema and drainage), neck (noting nuchal rigidity, adenopathy), lungs (noting dull, diminished, or adventitious breath sounds), heart (noting murmurs or rubs), abdomen (noting tenderness, change in bowel sounds, organomegaly), and musculoskeletal (noting tenderness, warmth, edema, and erythema).

▶ A neurological exam, including mental status evaluation, may be needed to exclude central nervous system (CNS) infection or complication.

▶ Rapid testing for strep, mono, flu, and other available on-site testing may be used as an initial screen to determine the best approach and course of treatment.

▶ Obtain a culture to determine causative organism(s) before treatment to prevent false-negative results.

▶ Sensitivity testing helps clarify the most appropriate antibiotic(s) to use.

Management

▶ Assess for allergies to medications and clarify type of reaction to previous antibiotic use.

▶ Be aware of drug resistance patterns in the community.

▶ Avoid treating a viral illness with an antibiotic "just in case" or because the patient or parent insists on one. Improvement with antibiotics usually occurs in 2 to 3 days for most infections. Beyond this time frame, consider reassessing the patient and treatment plan.

▶ It is important to educate the patient and document the criteria for reevaluation if the patient is not improving.

▶ Adequate hydration is important in the treatment of infectious illnesses, especially in children.

▶ 90% of respiratory infections are viral.

▶ To avoid the risk of a patient developing Reye's syndrome, do not prescribe or administer aspirin, or products containing aspirin, for viral infections to patients younger than 19 years of age.

▶ Due to decreased immune response, older adults have an increased risk of secondary bacterial infections.

▶ If the patient is pregnant, use antibiotics in pregnancy category B; be aware that most antibiotics pass into breast milk.

▶ Know local health department guidelines for reporting communicable diseases.

▶ Seek referrals to infectious disease specialists earlier rather than later in the course of unknown or unusual infection.

▶ Be alert to endemic diseases.

▶ Be alert to diseases that may be a result of international travel or bioterrorism.

RED FLAGS

▶ The very young and very old are at special risk for severe infections, as are those with compromised immune systems, such as people with a history of splenectomy or concomitant illness such as diabetes.

▶ Recognize the unique physiologic and psychological responses of older patients to infectious disease and therapy.

▶ A fever with listlessness or flaccidity requires an aggressive evaluation, no matter the patient's age.

▶ Bacteremia and sepsis may present with fever or hypothermia, chills, tachycardia, tachypnea, hypotension, or altered mental status; mortality is nearly 50% in septic shock.

▶ Consult or refer to a specialist if the illness does not respond to initial therapy or the presentation is unusual; hospitalization may be necessary if the patient is unable to take oral medication or maintain hydration, or has a severe infection requiring IV antibiotics.

▶ Know and recognize common diagnostic features of certain illnesses, such as Koplik spots in measles (rubeola), subcutaneous nodules in rheumatic fever, etc.

▶ Educate the patient and caregiver, document recommendations, and follow-up with the patient and caregiver when an infection is not resolving as expected.

PEDIATRIC ISSUES

▶ Any infant with fever who is younger than 4 weeks of age, or 1 to 3 months of age with fever and no focal sign of infection, may require admission with a workup, including urine and blood cultures, lumbar puncture, and chest X-ray.

▶ Frequent (up to 10) viral illnesses, especially upper respiratory illnesses, per year are common in infants and toddlers.

▶ To avert the risk of Reye's syndrome, the family nurse practitioner should educate the caregivers of children between newborn and 19 years of age and educate adolescents to avoid over-the-counter medications and other products that contain salicylates and other related compounds.

▶ Transmission of infections in older infants and toddlers is mainly through droplet secretions on hands and sharing toys in group settings.

▶ Children are contagious long before they are symptomatic. While it is important to exclude sick children from group settings and contact with other children, parents and day care workers need to understand that this will not necessarily reduce the spread of infection to others.

▶ Good handwashing is the single most effective tool in the prevention of illness.

▶ Washing toys may prevent the spread of illness.

2012 Childcare Exclusion List

This list applies to:

▶ All children in out-of-home childcare

▶ All students in 3-, 4-, and 5-year-old kindergarten

▶ Medically fragile students in 1st through 12th grades—those students with special healthcare needs and/or developmental delays that require close assistance with feeding or personal hygiene activities. (The parents, in concert with the child's school, will determine whether a child is considered medically fragile.)

Varicella

Children with chicken pox may return to day care or school with a parent note once all of the sores and blisters are dried or scabbed over, or, if there are no scabs, until no new sores appear.

Diarrhea

For *most kinds* of diarrhea (defined as three or more loose stools in 24 hours), students in 1st through 5th grades should stay home until diarrhea stops, or until a doctor clears the child to return to school. The child can return with a parent note when the diarrhea has stopped. Older children in 6th through 12th grades with diarrhea do not have to stay home, unless they are spreading illness in the school setting or have diarrhea with blood or mucus.

▶ Students of any age must have a medical clearance to return to school after having diarrhea that contains blood or mucus.

▶ Students who can use the restroom or whose stools are contained in diaper-type underwear do not have to be excluded if the diarrhea is known to be from a non-contagious condition, or if it continues after the child completes antibiotics for a diarrhea-causing illness.

▶ A medically fragile child or child who needs help with toileting may be excluded for fewer than three episodes of diarrhea if his or her condition makes it hard for caretakers to maintain sanitary conditions in the classroom.

Diarrhea from Campylobacter, E. coli, *Giardia, Norovirus, Rotavirus, Salmonella, or Shigella*

Students of any age are excluded for one of these infections. A child may return to school with a medical note for the following conditions:

▶ **Campylobacter**, *norovirus, rotavirus,* **Shigella**, *and most types of* **Salmonella**: after diarrhea stops

▶ *E. coli:* For the most severe type of *E. coli*, students of any age must be out of school until the diarrhea stops and two lab tests taken 24 hours apart test negative for *E. coli* O157:H7, which causes bloody diarrhea.

▶ **Giardia**: once diarrhea stops or child has taken antibiotics for at least 24 hours

▶ **Salmonella typhi** *(Typhoid fever):* after 24 hours without diarrhea and three lab tests are negative, if a doctor clears the child to return

▶ **Shigella**: after 5 days of antibiotics or a negative lab test

Fever by Itself

Infants less than 4 months old: Keep them home for rectal temperature of 101°F or higher.

▶ Children over 4 months old: Keep the child home for a fever of 101°F or higher by mouth, 100°F or higher if taken under the arm, or 102°F or higher if taken in the rectum.

▶ Children can return with a parent note when the fever has resolved.

Fever with Rash, Behavior Change, or Other Symptoms

A child should be taken to a doctor or clinic for any fever if he or she also has signs of severe illness such as a rash, change in behavior, earache, vomiting confusion, sore throat, or irritability. A medical note is required to return.

Flu/Influenza or Influenza-Like Illness (ILI)

A student with ILI or the flu will be excluded for a fever of 100°F with cough and/or sore throat until fever-free for at least 24 hours without any fever medicines.

Rubella/German Measles/3-Day Measles

Keep a child at home until 7 days after rash starts. The child may return with a medical note.

Head Lice

Children with crawling lice or nits (eggs) one fourth inch or closer to the scalp may be sent home at the end of the day if head-to-head contact with other children can be avoided. Otherwise, they may be excluded immediately. A child may return with a parent note after his or her first treatment with a school-approved lice-removal product, if there are no active lice crawling on the child's head. The school or center should check the child 7 days after treatment for any newly hatched crawling lice. If any are present, the child will have to be retreated for lice to return to school or childcare.

Hepatitis A/Yellow Jaundice

Children with acute hepatitis A may return with a medical note 1 week after the start of the jaundice.

HiB (Haemophilus influenzae Type B)

Students with proven HiB infection need to be out of school until at least 24 hours after they complete their antibiotics. A medical note is required to return.

Impetigo

A child who has dry, honey-colored, crusty sores that cannot be covered should be sent home at the end of the school day until 24 hours after starting antibiotics.

▶ If the sores are weepy, oozing, or wet or cannot be covered and kept dry, the child will be sent home immediately. The child may return after 24 hours of antibiotics, if the sores have stopped oozing and are starting to get smaller.

▶ A medical note is needed to return to school.

Rubeola/Measles/Red Measles/10-Day Measles

Children with measles can return with a medical note 4 days after the rash begins, if they have no fever and feel well enough to participate in regular school activities.

Meningitis

A student with signs of meningitis (high fever, rash, stiff neck) must remain out of school until a healthcare provider says that the student may return.

Mononucleosis (Mono)

A child's healthcare provider will decide when a child is well enough to go back to childcare or school after having mono. No contact sports, heavy lifting, strenuous activity for first 2 to 3 weeks and as long as splenomegaly persists (extend to 8 weeks).

Mumps

Children with mumps can return with a medical note 5 days after the beginning of swelling.

Conjunctivitis /Pink-Eye

Children whose eyes are red or pink, and who have eye pain and reddened eyelids, with white or yellow eye discharge or eyelids matted after sleep, should not be in school until they have been examined and treated. A medical note is required to return.

Rash

A student who has a rapidly spreading rash or a rash with fever or behavior change should be excluded from school immediately. A medical note is required to return.

Tinea Corporis/Ringworm

Children with ringworm of the scalp must remain out of school until they have begun treatment with a prescription oral antifungal medication. The child may return with a medical note. Children with ringworm of the body may return with a parent's note once they have begun oral or topical antifungal treatment, unless the affected area can be completely covered by clothing the entire time that the child is at school or in childcare.

Scabies

Children with scabies should be out of school until treatment/medication has been applied. A medical note is required to return.

Herpes Zoster/Shingles

Children who have shingles lesions/sores/blisters that cannot be covered should be kept at home. They may return with parent notes once the lesions are dried/scabbed.

Sores Inside the Mouth

Children with sores inside the mouth who also drool should stay home until their healthcare providers say that the sores are not contagious. A medical note is needed to return to school.

Staph or Strep Skin Infections (Including MRSA)

A child with a draining sore, boil, or abscess that cannot be covered, or with sores that ooze through and soak dressings, should remain home. The child may return once the draining stops, or if the drainage (oozing) can be contained in the dressing, so no one else comes into contact with the drainage.

Streptococcal Pharyngitis /Strep Throat

A child with strep throat can return to school with a medical note 24 hours after starting antibiotics if there is no fever.

Sty (or Stye)

A child with a draining/oozing sty/stye should remain home until the draining stops.

Tuberculosis (TB)

A child with TB should be kept home until the healthcare provider treating the TB writes a medical note that says the child is no longer contagious.

Vomiting

A child who has vomited two or more times in 24 hours should stay home until the vomiting stops, unless the child is known not to be contagious.

Pertussis /Whooping Cough

A child with whooping cough can return to school with a medical note after completing 5 days of prescribed antibiotics, unless directed otherwise by the local health department or the school nurse.

For more information, go to http://www.scdhec.gov/health/childteenhealth/schoolexclusion/.

VIRAL INFECTIONS

Fifth Disease (Erythema Infectiosum)

Description

► A mild, self-limiting viral disease characterized by erythematous and macular rash first appearing on the cheeks and ears, leading to a "slapped cheek" appearance

Etiology

► Caused by human parvovirus B19

► Transmitted via droplet, most often through contact with infected saliva, nasal secretions, sputum, and sometimes blood

► Communicable before onset of symptoms; not infectious after onset of rash

► Incubation period 4 to 14 days, up to 21 days; rash and joint symptoms occur 2 to 3 weeks after acquiring the infection

Incidence and Demographics

► Cases often occur as part of community outbreaks during late winter and early spring; may also occur sporadically.

► Spread to household contacts is common.

Risk Factors

► Institutional-style day care setting

► School age

► Adults without immunity

► Contact with saliva, nasal secretions, and sputum of infected persons

Prevention and Screening

▶ May reduce transmission through rigorous handwashing and careful handling of used facial tissues

Assessment

History

▶ Prodrome is usually absent; if present, includes mild fever, malaise, headache, mild pruritus, and myalgia; occurs 7 to 10 days before rash.

▶ Rash, beginning on face and ears, with circumoral pallor, leading to slapped cheek appearance; progressing to erythematous, maculopapular, "lacy" (often pruritic) rash beginning on the trunk and moving to arms, buttocks, and thighs

▶ Arthralgia and arthritis may also be present; more common in infected adults, especially women.

Physical Exam

▶ Fever is low grade, if present.

▶ Note characteristic appearance of rash on face and body (see above).

▶ Rash fluctuates in intensity with environmental changes up to weeks and months after appearance; may increase or reappear following sunlight exposure, warm bath, or vigorous play.

▶ No lymphadenopathy or focal signs of infection

▶ May also see evidence of arthralgia and arthritis; more common in infected adults, especially women

Diagnostic Studies

▶ None usually performed in uncomplicated cases

▶ White blood count (WBC) usually normal; anemia with decreased reticulocyte count is possible

▶ Detection of parvovirus B19-specific immunoglobulin (Ig) M antibody is possible to confirm diagnosis in complicated cases (persist for 2 to 4 months); IgM usually detectable 3 days after infection; IgG antibody usually detectable 7 days after infection; positive IgG antibody in the absence of IgM antibody indicates previous infection and immunity

▶ Pregnant women exposed to fifth disease in first trimester should be serologically tested for IgM and IgG antibodies; if susceptibility or a positive infection, weekly fetal ultrasounds indicated for 4 to 8 weeks after exposure or 2 to 4 weeks after infection to detect fetal hydrops.

Differential Diagnosis

▶ Undifferentiated viral syndrome before appearance of rash

▶ Other viral infections with rash

Management

Nonpharmacologic Treatment

- ▶ Symptomatic
- ▶ Isolation not indicated, but avoid pregnant women and the immunocompromised

Pharmacologic Treatment

- ▶ Acetaminophen or ibuprofen for fever, myalgia, arthralgia in patients less than 19 years of age
- ▶ Antipruritic medication, if necessary
- ▶ Intravenous immunoglobulin for chronic infection in immunocompromised patients
- ▶ If evidence of fetal hydrops, fetal transfusion may be considered

How Long to Treat

- ▶ As long as symptomatic

Special Considerations

- ▶ Infections during pregnancy may cause fetal hydrops and death, although risk is relatively low.
- ▶ The highest risk is if the mother is exposed during the first 20 weeks of pregnancy.
- ▶ B19-infected fetuses may be treated with intrauterine blood transfusions.
- ▶ Persons with sickle-cell disease or other chronic anemia are at risk for developing severe anemia, if infected.
- ▶ Immunocompromised people are at risk of serious illness, if infected.
- ▶ Aspirin and aspirin-containing products should not be administered to anyone less than 19 years of age for a viral illness to avoid risk of developing Reye's syndrome.

When to Consult, Refer, Hospitalize

- ▶ Refer to hematologist for complications—aplastic crisis, chronic anemia

Follow-Up

- ▶ None necessary in low-risk patients
- ▶ Closely with immunocompromised patients or those experiencing aplastic crisis

Complications

- ▶ Aplastic crisis, chronic anemia
- ▶ Arthritis, arthralgia in adults

Herpangina

Description

- ▶ Acute viral illness causing fever, ulcerative mouth lesions, cough, coryza, pharyngitis

Etiology

▶ Enterovirus (Coxsackie A and B)

▶ Transmitted by fecal-oral and oral-oral route

▶ Incubation 3 to 6 days

Incidence and Demographics

▶ Seen more frequently in temperate climates (summer and fall)

▶ Affects primarily children, day care through school age

Risk Factors

▶ More frequent in low socioeconomic groups

Prevention and Screening

▶ Good handwashing

Assessment

History

▶ The prodrome of fever is as high as 106°F, pharyngitis, malaise, headache, backache, anorexia, drooling, vomiting, diarrhea

Physical Exam

▶ 1–2 mm vesicles and ulcers on the anterior tonsillar pillars, soft palate, uvula, tonsils, pharyngeal wall, and posterior buccal surfaces

Diagnostic Studies

▶ Throat culture to exclude streptococcal pharyngitis

Differential Diagnosis

▶ Herpes simplex gingivostomatitis

▶ Aphthous stomatitis

▶ Hand, foot, and mouth disease

▶ Vincent's angina

▶ Streptococcal pharyngitis

Management

Nonpharmacologic Treatment

▶ Symptomatic—rest and fluids

Pharmacologic Treatment

▶ Acetaminophen or ibuprofen for fever and discomfort in patients under 19 years of age

▶ Variety of suspension—viscous lidocaine 2%, diphenhydramine, and either Maalox or Kaopectate—can be applied to lesions to relieve discomfort

How Long to Treat
▶   As long as symptomatic

Special Considerations
▶   None

When to Consult, Refer, Hospitalize
▶   Consult if symptoms persist for longer than 2 weeks or if child is unable to drink or eat.

Follow-Up
▶   None usually needed

Expected Course
▶   Resolves in 3 to 5 days

Complications
▶   Rarely myocarditis, meningitis, or encephalitis

Human Immunodeficiency Virus (HIV) Infection and Acquired Immunodeficiency Syndrome (AIDS)

Description
▶   HIV: Viral infection with the human retrovirus that destroys cells with critical immune system functions. The HIV-1 virus can infect all cells expressing the T4 (CD4+) antigen, which serves as a receptor for HIV; once in the cell, it replicates and causes cell fusion or death. The virus depends on reverse transcriptase for replication and, because the CD4+ lymphocyte directs many other cells in the immune network, infection of the CD4+ lymphocyte allows for disorder of virtually all body systems.

▶   AIDS: Disease characterized by opportunistic infections; or HIV+ persons with CD4 cell counts less than 200 cells/ μl or a CD4 % less than 14%.

Etiology
▶   Viral transmission—HIV usually transmitted through sexual intercourse; IV drug use; transfusions of blood or blood products; needle stick or mucous membrane exposures in healthcare workers; injections with unsterilized, used needles such as acupuncture, tattooing, or medical injection; perinatal; breastfeeding (mother to child)

▶   Seroconversion takes an average of 3 weeks from initial infection.

▶   Median time from infection with HIV to AIDS in persons who are not on antiretroviral treatment is estimated to be 10 years.

▶   Stages of HIV disease include acute HIV infection (acute retroviral syndrome), early infection , asymptomatic chronic infection, symptomatic HIV infection, and AIDS or advanced HIV infection.

Incidence and Demographics

▶ The cumulative number of AIDS cases in the United States reported to CDC through December 2012 was **estimated to be 1.2 million**. Sexual intercourse is the most common method of HIV transmission, followed by injection drug use.

▶ The rate of AIDS diagnosis in African Americans remains higher than in any other ethnic group.

▶ The highest new HIV infection incidence in 2012 was in 20- to 24-year-olds.

▶ Men who have sex with men (MSM) are more severely affected by HIV than any other group in the United States (CDC.gov, 2015).

Risk Factors

▶ Unprotected anal, oral, or vaginal sex with multiple partners

▶ Unprotected sex with HIV-positive person or IV drug abuser

▶ IV drug abuse or needle-stick exposure

▶ Blood transfusion outside United States, or in United States 1977–1985

▶ Unprotected sex with person with recent or past history of sexually transmitted diseases

▶ Sexually transmitted disease

▶ Children born to HIV+ women

▶ People sustaining occupational exposure to blood or bodily fluids

▶ Incarceration—high rates in prison populations who take infection back to community upon release

Prevention and Screening

▶ Incorporate and promote HIV testing as part of routine primary care, per CDC (2006) and U.S. Preventive Services Task Force (USPSTF, 2013) recommendations.

▶ Promote sexual abstinence or decrease the number of sexual partners; reduce unsafe sexual behavior; encourage condom use.

▶ Treat sexually transmitted infections.

▶ Evaluate and offer HIV preexposure prophylaxis (PrEP), if appropriate.

▶ Prevent/treat IV drug use. Counsel regarding not sharing injection drug using equipment.

▶ Test plasma, organ, and tissue donors for HIV.

▶ Provide healthcare workers with postexposure antiretroviral prophylaxis treatment.

▶ Counsel HIV+ mothers about the risks of transmission of HIV to their infants associated with breastfeeding.

▶ Screen all pregnant women.

▶ Give antiretroviral treatment (ART) to HIV+ women during pregnancy and labor; newborns should receive ART after delivery, to prevent perinatal transmission.

▶ Refer to http://aidsinfo.nih.gov/contentfiles/perinatalgl.pdf for current guidelines.

Assessment

History

▶ Index of suspicion is raised by obtaining a complete history of symptoms, risk factors, personal medical history, although the patient may remain asymptomatic for years.

▶ Complaints causing parents to seek care for their children are generalized lymphadenopathy, failure to thrive, recurrent or persistent thrush, recurrent infections.

▶ Adolescents may present with sexually transmitted infections, persistent vaginal candidiasis, or persistent "colds."

▶ Adults may present with a variety of complaints at any stage of HIV.

Physical Exam

▶ A complete physical exam is necessary.

▶ An infant born to an infected mother may be entirely normal for 1 year or more.

▶ An infant/child may show failure to gain weight (failure to thrive), generalized lymphadenopathy, hepatosplenomegaly, recurrent or persistent thrush, recurrent or chronic parotitis, recurrent infections, or infections that fail to respond to treatment; *Pneumocystis jiroveci (PCP)* infection may be first manifestation.

▶ Adolescents and adults may show a wide variety of physical findings related to STIs, serious infections, malignancies, and cardiac and neurologic dysfunction.

▶ Hairy leukoplakia of the tongue and Kaposi's sarcoma are highly linked to HIV infection.

Diagnosis by Stage of HIV

▶ Acute HIV infection: time from exposure to onset of symptoms usually 2 to 4 weeks

▶ Typical symptoms include fever (96%), adenopathy (74%), pharyngitis (70%), rash (erythematous maculopapular; 70%), myalgia or arthralgia (54%), diarrhea (32%), headache (32%), nausea and vomiting (27%), hepatosplenomegaly (14%), and thrush (12%).

▶ Early and asymptomatic infection: clinically asymptomatic or in some cases persistent generalized lymphadenopathy

▶ Symptomatic HIV infection: conditions more common and more severe in HIV infection but are not AIDS-indicator conditions

  ▷ Examples: thrush, oral hairy leukoplakia, peripheral neuropathy, cervical dysplasia, constitutional symptoms (fever, weight loss), recurrent herpes zoster, idiopathic thrombocytopenic purpura, and listeriosis

▶ AIDS (CDC definition): HIV+ persons with CD4 cell counts less than 200 cells/µl or a CD4% less than 14% or a variety of conditions such as candidiasis of esophagus, trachea, bronchi, or lungs; invasive cervical cancer; recurrent bacterial pneumonia; Kaposi's sarcoma (KS); pneumocystis pneumonia; wasting syndrome due to HIV; and others

For Diagnosis in Infants and Children

▶ Infants younger than 18 months

▶ Positive results on at least one specimen (excluding cord blood) using one or more HIV virologic (non-antibody) tests:

▷ HIV-1 nucleic acid (DNA or RNA detection)

▷ HIV-1 p24 antigen test, including neutralization assay in a child older than 1 month of age

▷ HIV isolation (viral culture)

▷ HIV nucleotide sequence (genotype)

▶ Presumptive diagnosis for children younger than 18 months: may be based on positive results of HIV virologic tests on 1 serum specimen and no subsequent negative tests or diagnosis of HIV infection based on laboratory criteria and documented in medical record by healthcare provider or presence of AIDS-defining conditions as defined by CDC

▶ Children younger than 18 months born to HIV-infected mother categorized as "not infected with HIV" if child does not meet the criteria for infection and has at least two negative HIV antibody screening tests from separate specimens at 6 months of age or older or at least two negative HIV virologic tests from separate specimens at 1 month to 4 months of age *and* no other laboratory or clinical evidence of HIV infection (definitive criteria)

▶ Presumptive criteria for children younger than 18 months born to HIV-infected mother categorized as "not infected with HIV" if child does not meet definitive criteria but has one negative HIV antibody test at 6 months of age or older and no positive HIV virologic tests *or* has one negative HIV virologic test performed at 4 months of age or older and no positive virologic tests *or* one positive HIV virologic test with at least two subsequent negative virologic tests, at least one of which is at 4 months of age older or negative HIV antibody results, at least one of which is at 6 months of age or older *and* no other laboratory or clinical evidence of infection *or* designation by healthcare provider to be "not infected" and healthcare provider has noted testing results in medical record *and* no other laboratory or clinical evidence of HIV infection is noted

▶ Children younger than 18 months born to HIV+ mothers and not meeting above criteria for HIV infection or "not infected with HIV" categorized as having perinatal exposure

▶ Children older than 18 months and adolescents diagnosed as having HIV infection if have positive screening test for HIV antibody and positive result on a confirmatory test *or* positive result of HIV virologic test *or* diagnosis of HIV infection based on laboratory tests and recorded in medical record by healthcare provider *or* presence of AIDS-defining conditions

Diagnostic Studies

▶ 4th generation HIV antigen/antibody test

▶ Negative 4th generation antigen/antibody test: does not guarantee person is HIV uninfected; window of time from infection to reactive test can be delayed by several weeks; retesting recommended 4 to 12 weeks from last high-risk exposure

▶ If acute HIV infection suspected, HIV viral load should be ordered

▷ CD4 count: used to assess degree of immune suppression.

▷ HIV viral load: used to monitor response to ART; used in conjunction with antigen/antibody test to confirm acute HIV infection

▶ Maternal antibodies: may remain present for up to 15 months so antibody tests unreliable in infants

Differential Diagnosis

▶ Cancer

▶ Endocrine diseases

▶ Malabsorption syndromes

▶ Candidiasis

▶ Tuberculosis

▶ Other infections

▶ Hepatic disease

▶ Lymphoma

▶ Enterocolitis

▶ Endocarditis

▶ Renal disease

Management

Nonpharmacologic Treatment

▶ Counsel regarding prevention of transmission through use of condoms, cleaning up blood spills, and not sharing razor blades or needles.

▶ Stress that patients must adhere to a drug regimen if it is to be helpful.

▶ Encourage a healthy lifestyle: balanced diet, smoking cessation, substance abuse cessation, decrease stress, and adequate sleep.

▶ Discuss protection from contagious disease: washing hands after contact with soil; avoiding cleaning litter box (toxoplasmosis) or rough play with kittens (cat scratch disease); maintaining food safety.

▶ Health maintenance referral: dental exam every 6 months, ophthalmology examination at diagnosis and annually; when CD4+ count is less than 50 cells/μl, refer to ophthalmologist or optometrist trained in CMV retinitis for screening

▶ Tests to determine concomitant diseases, immunity status; Mantoux PPD or Interferon Gamma Release Assay (IGRA), rapid plasma regain serum (RPR) or Treponemal specific assay, cervical Pap smear every 6 to 12 months, HBsAg, hepatitis C antibody, toxoplasmosis IgG, cytomegalovirus IgG, varicella IgG, chest X-ray

▶ Baseline labs before drug therapy: HIV viral load, CD4+ count, HIV genotype, metabolic panel, liver function, renal profile, CBC with differential and platelets, fasting lipids, fasting glucose or HgA1C, urinalysis, pregnancy testing

▶ Immunizations: annual inactivated influenza vaccine; pneumococcal vaccine (PCV13 and PPV23), consider hepatitis B (HBV; 3-dose schedule unless evidence of immunity) and *H. influenzae* B vaccines (in asplenic patients); tetanus-diphtheria (Td) vaccine should be given if the patient had not been vaccinated within the last 5 years. Substitute one time dose of tetanus-diphtheria and acellular pertussis (TDaP) at time of next booster, then Td every 10 years. If the patient has not received the primary series of Td, the patient should begin the primary series of three doses of Td with the first two doses administered 4 weeks apart and the third dose administered 6 to 12 months later. A dose of TDaP can be substituted for any of the three doses of Td. Give inactivated polio, hepatitis A (HAV; two-dose schedule unless serologic evidence of previous disease), HBV (unless evidence of immunity); Varicella zoster and MMR for asymptomatic patients with CD4 counts greater than 200 cells/μl and no evidence of immunity or significant exposure; human papillomavirus vaccine (HPV) recommended for those who have not received the three-dose series and who meet the recommended age requirements. The second dose should be given 2 months after the first and the third dose given 6 months later. Do not administer live vaccines to any patient severely immunocompromised (CD4 counts less than 200 cells/μL): MMR, varicella, zoster, BCG, LAIV (Flumist). MMR and varicella and zoster are also contraindicated in pregnant women.

Pharmacologic Treatment

▶ Antiretroviral treatment should be offered to all patients, regardless of CD4+ count or viral load.

▶ The Department of Health & Human Services Guidelines (2016) (http://aidsinfo.nih.gov) recommends the following as preferred regimens for antiretroviral (ARV)-naive patients:

　▷ Darunavir + ritonavir + *either* tenofovir alafenamide/emtriciabine (DRV/r + TAF/FTC) (AIII) *or* tenofovir disoproxil fumarate/emtricitabine (DRV/r + TDF/FTC) (AI)

　▷ Raltegravir + *either* tenofovir alafenamide/emtricitabine (RAL+TAF/TDF) (AIII) *or* tenofovir disoproxil fumarate/emtricitabine (RAL + TDF/FTC) (AI)

　▷ Elvitegravir/cobicistat/tenofovir disoproxil fumarate/emtricitabine (ELV/COBI/TDF/FTC) (AI)

　▷ Elvitegravir/cobicistat/tenofovir alafenamide/emtrictaabine (ELV/COBI/TAF/FTC) (AI)

　▷ Dolutegravir + *either* tenofovir alafenamide/emtricitabine (DTG+TAF/FTC) (AIII) *or* tenofovir disoproxil fumarate/emtricitabine (DTG + TDF/FTC) (AI)

　▷ Dolutegravir/abacavir/lamivudine (DTG/ABC/FTC) (AI) — only in persons who are HLA-B*5701 negative

▶ Selection of a regimen should be individualized on the basis of virologic efficacy, toxicity, and pill burden, dosing frequency, drug-drug interaction potential, resistance testing results, and comorbid conditions.

▶ Based on individual patient characteristics and needs, in some instances, an alternative regimen may actually be a preferred regimen for a patient.

　▷ Initiate *P. carinii* if CD4+ count is less than 200 cells/μl and M. avium prophylaxis if CD4+ count is less than 50 cells/μl.

　▷ Treat concurrent infections of disseminated tuberculosis and/or viral hepatitis.

When to Consult, Refer, Hospitalize

▶ Every HIV-infected infant, child, adolescent, pregnant woman, and older adult should be referred to and followed by an HIV specialist knowledgeable for that age group.

▶ Refer HIV patients to appropriate support groups.

▶ All 50 states; Washington, DC; and U.S. territories require reporting AIDS cases to local health authorities.

Special Considerations

▶ Always maintain patient confidentiality.

▶ In older HIV patients, it is important to differentiate between geriatric conditions and HIV symptoms (such as dementia) and be aware of potential drug interactions.

Follow-Up

▶ See U.S. Department of Health & Human Services publications for guidelines on HIV primary care, ART recommendations, and opportunistic infection prevention and treatment. ART treatment guidelines are updated at least annually.

▶ Assess for mental health issues and social isolation.

Healthcare Worker Exposures to Blood and Other Body Fluids that may Contain HIV

Description

▶ Exposure may place a healthcare worker (e.g., an employee, student, contractor, attending clinician, public safety worker, volunteer) at risk for HIV infection and therefore requires consideration for postexposure prophylaxis (PEP).

▶ Exposure is a percutaneous injury; contact with mucous membrane or non-intact skin; contact with intact skin when the duration of contact is prolonged (i.e., several minutes or more) or involves an extensive area with blood, tissue, or other body fluids; or any direct contact with concentrated HIV in a research laboratory or production facility.

Etiology

▶ Fluids with known risk of HIV transmission: blood, bloody fluids, semen, vaginal fluids, concentrated HIV materials in research labs

▶ Fluids with suspected risk of HIV transmission: pleural fluid, cerebrospinal fluid, peritoneal fluid, synovial fluid, pericardial fluid, amniotic fluid

▶ Materials with doubtful risk of HIV transmission: feces, vomitus, urine, saliva, sweat, tears (unless bloody)

Risk Factors

▶ Device visibly contaminated with patient's blood, procedure that involved a needle placed directly in a vein or artery, or deep injury

▶ After percutaneous exposure to HIV-infected blood—approximately 0.3%; mucous membrane exposure—0.09%; skin exposure less

▶ Contact with blood or other body fluids from patients in healthcare or laboratory setting

Prevention and Screening

▶ Healthcare workers should always follow CDC recommendations for universal or standard precautions.

▶ Wear gloves when contact with blood or bodily fluids is possible.

▶ Use "personal protective equipment" (masks, goggles, gowns) when engaging in procedures that involve blood or bodily fluids.

▶ Prevent needle injuries, use puncture-proof containers, use "safety" needles, and refrain from resheathing or post-use manipulation of needles.

Assessment

History

▶ Evaluate exposure: type of fluid, type of exposure (needle gauge, depth of needle-stick, visible blood, mucous membrane), and duration of exposure.

▶ Evaluate exposure-source person: prior HIV testing results, history of possible HIV exposures, and risk for HIV (IV drug use, sexual contact, acute HIV syndrome).

▶ If source person is HIV-positive, document current HIV RNA levels (viral load), CD4 levels, and current or previous antiretroviral treatment (ART) and compliance.

Physical Exam

▶ Assess site or wound, anxiety level of healthcare worker.

Diagnostic Studies

▶ Source person: If HIV serologic status is unknown, request HIV antibody after incident, provide pretest counseling and consent form; also test for hepatitis B and C.

▶ If consent cannot be obtained, follow local and state laws.

▶ If source person is HIV seronegative, no testing of worker is needed.

▶ Exposed healthcare workers: Offer HIV antibody testing for baseline evaluation with worker consent.

▶ Test healthcare workers for hepatitis B immune status.

▶ Pregnancy testing should be offered to all women of childbearing age.

▶ Maintaining confidentiality of test results and documentation is critical.

Management

Nonpharmacologic Treatment

▶ Immediately following exposure:

   ▷ Skin: Wash thoroughly with soap and water.

   ▷ Eyes: Irrigate immediately with saline or water. Tilt head back, hold eyelid open, pour water or saline over eye, and pull eyelid up and down to cleanse entire area. If wearing contact lenses, do not remove lenses while irrigating eye. After flushing the affected eye, remove contact lenses and clean thoroughly.

   ▷ Mouth or nose: Use clean water rinse/flush.

   ▷ Consider and discuss risks and benefits of postexposure prophylaxis, based on type of fluid, source risk, and type of exposure.

▷ Counsel exposed worker to follow measures to prevent secondary transmission, especially the first 6 to 12 weeks: practice sexual abstinence or use condoms; refrain from donating blood, plasma, organs, tissue, or semen; and refrain from breastfeeding if applicable.

Pharmacologic Treatment

▶ Tetanus-diphtheria (Td) vaccine should be given if the patient has not been vaccinated within the last 5 years. Patients older than 65 years of age who have never received tetanus toxoid-diphtheria and acellular pertussis (TDaP) should receive a dose of TDaP instead of Td. If the patient has completed the primary series of three doses Td, a dose of tetanus-diphtheria and acellular pertussis (TDaP) vaccine should be substituted for Td as a booster. If the patient has not received the primary series of Td, the patient should begin the primary series of three doses of Td with the first two doses administered 4 weeks apart and the third dose administered 6 to 12 months later. A dose of TDaP can be substituted for any of the three doses of Td.

▶ Hepatitis B vaccine series (if not already vaccinated and no evidence of immunity)

▶ Hepatitis B immune globulin (if source antigen positive or high risk for hepatitis B and healthcare worker not immune)

▶ After evaluation/assessment of HIV infection risk, determine need for postexposure prophylaxis

▶ Current guidelines recommend the use of a tenofovir + emtricitabine with raltegravir as the standard regimen. Consultation with an HIV expert may be required if the source patient has extensive HIV treatment history.

How Long to Treat

▶ PEP should be provided for 28 days.

Special Considerations

▶ Pregnant women

▷ Consider short- or long-term effects on fetus and newborn when offering postexposure prophylaxis.

▷ Counsel regarding potential risk for HIV transmission based on type of exposure, stage of pregnancy (first trimester = period of maximal organogenesis and risk for teratogenesis), and safety of drug combinations.

▷ Breastfeeding: Consider temporary discontinuation of antiretroviral therapy.

▷ Resistance of the source virus to antiretroviral drugs; if resistance known or suspected, consultation with an HIV expert is recommended

When to Consult, Refer, Hospitalize

▶ Consult with HIV expert; refer to current U.S. Department of Health and Human Services guidelines.

▶ The Clinician Consultation Center, (888) 488-4911, provides clinician-to-clinician guidance for PEP, nPEP.

Follow-Up

▶ Advise exposed healthcare workers to seek medical evaluation for any acute illness occurring during the follow-up period; illness characterized by fever, rash, myalgia, fatigue, malaise, or lymphadenopathy may indicate acute HIV infection.

▶ Healthcare providers with high risk exposure or exposed to HIV+ source: HIV testing with a 4th generation assay at 6 weeks, and 4 months after exposure

Complications

▶ HIV seroconversion

▶ Side effects from antiretroviral therapy such as nausea/vomiting, nephrolithiasis, hemolytic anemia, hyperglycemia, or worker unable to finish medication

▶ All FDA-approved HIV PEP medications are associated with hepatotoxicity.

Infectious Mononucleosis (IM)

Description

▶ Acute viral illness with fever, fatigue, pharyngitis, and adenopathy; some risk of complications

Etiology

▶ Epstein-Barr virus (EBV), a gamma herpesvirus, is the causative organism.

▶ The transmission is commonly oropharyngeal route (saliva); blood, semen, cervical secretions less common routes.

▶ Communicability: Respiratory tract viral shedding can occur for months after infection.

▶ Incubation is 30 to 50 days, making it difficult to pinpoint exact date of exposure.

▶ Transmission of the virus to others is possible for 3 months or longer.

Incidence and Demographics

▶ Common in high school– and college-age (no sexual predisposition)

▶ Not seasonal or cyclical

Risk Factors

▶ Living in group settings

Prevention and Screening

▶ Handwashing

▶ Avoid sharing eating or drinking utensils.

▶ Avoid close personal contact (kissing, sexual contact).

Assessment

History

▶ Fatigue, fever, swollen lymph nodes, sore throat occur in most people.

▶ Fever (rarely exceeding 102° F) lasts about 10 days; fatigue may linger for several weeks.

▶ Malaise, myalgia, and headache (50%) also frequently occur.

Physical Exam

▶ Lymphadenopathy may be significant and include posterior cervical and occipital nodes; lasts 1 to 4 weeks.

▶ Exudative pharyngitis (50%) often confused with streptococcal pharyngitis; tonsillar ulceration (20%)

▶ Petechiae of palate and eyelid edema may occur; body rash occurs in a few cases.

▶ Skin rash (maculopapular, pruritic, copper-colored or tan) in one-third of patients thought to be due to those with IM who are prescribed amoxicillin.

▶ Hepatomegaly or particularly splenomegaly may occur in about 40% of people; this is a late finding and lasts about 4 weeks.

▶ Jaundice is evident in a few.

Diagnostic Studies

▶ Mono-spot is usual screening test—rapid, nonspecific test for heterophile antibody agglutination (85% sensitive and 94% specific); should not be used beyond one month; 25% false negative within first week of symptoms

▶ Complete blood count (CBC) with differential shows lymphocytosis (greater than 50%) with 10% atypical; elevated white blood cell count (10,000–20,000 mcg/L)

▶ Abnormal liver function tests: aminotransferases (ALT, AST) and gamma glutamyl transferase (GGT) levels elevated in 80% to 90% of cases; may need to follow in severe infection

▶ Consider throat culture to R/O group A streptococcal infection.

▶ Consider EBV antibody titer (viral capsid antigen, early antigen) if diagnosis in doubt, especially in older patients or early in disease state.

Differential Diagnosis

▶ Other viral syndromes: rubella, adenovirus, toxoplasmosis, cytomegalovirus

▶ Serum sickness

▶ Leukemia

▶ Hepatitis

▶ Group A streptococcal or viral pharyngitis

Management

Nonpharmacologic Treatment

▶ Symptomatic, no isolation required, see Prevention and Screening

▶ Warm salt water gargles for pharyngitis

▶ No contact sports, heavy lifting, strenuous activity for first 2 to 3 weeks and as long as splenomegaly persists (extend to 8 weeks).

▶ Realistic schedule of rest, including bed rest

▶ Increased fluid intake

Pharmacologic Treatment

▶ Give acetaminophen or ibuprofen for fever and discomfort in patients under 19 years of age.

▶ Do not prescribe ampicillin or amoxicillin unless comorbid streptococcal pharyngitis exists; if needed, treatment may cause rash.

▶ Steroids may be given to treat pharyngitis that leads to airway obstruction or hematologic complications (5- to 7-day taper).

Special Considerations

▶ Patients with recent EBV infection should not donate blood.

When to Consult, Refer, Hospitalize

▶ Refer to hematologist, neurologist, hepatologist, etc., early if any complications suspected.

▶ Hospitalization may be necessary for complications.

Follow-Up

▶ Based on clinical course; none may be necessary if fever and symptoms resolve after 10 days; do if jaundice, hepatosplenomegaly, or complications develop

Expected Course

▶ Duration variable, 3 to 4 weeks

▶ If symptoms persist after 6 months, further evaluation should take place.

Complications

▶ Tend to occur in young or older patients

▶ CNS disorders such as aseptic meningitis, encephalitis, seizures, Guillain-Barré syndrome, optic neuritis, coma, transverse myelitis, Bell's palsy

▶ Hematologic complications such as hemolytic anemia, aplastic anemia, thrombocytopenia, hemolytic uremic syndrome

▶ Other rare complications: upper airway obstruction (1% to 5%) splenic rupture (0.5% to 1%), myocarditis, pericarditis, pleural effusion, pneumonitis, hepatitis, erythema multiform, nephrotic syndrome, uveitis, mono-arthritis

▶ Chronic fatigue is most commonly reported sequelae, occurring in up to 7% of adolescents at 12 months.

Influenza

Description

▶ Acute viral illness that occurs in epidemics, usually in the fall and winter

Etiology

▶ It is caused by an orthomyxovirus that appears in antigenic types A and B.

▶ Frequent mutations produce new strains each flu season; H1N1, prime example

Incidence and Demographics

▶ Very common

▶ Frequently leads to pneumonia in older adults, contributing to fifth leading cause of death in that population; young children also commonly affected

Risk Factors

▶ Close contact with infected people

▶ Nursing home residents

▶ Older adult patients residing with children

▶ Pregnant women

▶ Persons with chronic pulmonary, cardiovascular, renal, hepatic, hematological, metabolic, neurologic, or immunosuppressive disorders

Prevention and Screening

▶ Handwashing

▶ Influenza vaccine provides immunity to 85% (live vaccine) and 71% (inactivated vaccine) of those inoculated; however, many host factors may individually affect immunity.

▶ Protection begins about 2 weeks after vaccination and lasts several months.

▶ Vaccination recommended universally for everyone older than 6 months of age.

▶ No influenza vaccines are approved for children younger than 6 months, although pregnant and lactating women are highly targeted to receive influenza vaccine to protect their infants.

▶ Consider high-dose (four times the dose of traditional vaccine) vaccine in those age 65 and older.

▶ Administer antiviral medication such as oseltamivir 75 mg orally once a day for 5 days and zanamivir two 5 mg inhalations once a day for 5 days after exposure in influenza A or B.

▶ Live attenuated influenza vaccine (LAIV), FluMist (a flu vaccine nasal spray) may be used in all healthy people between 2 years and 49 years old without a history of asthma or wheezing; it is *not* to be administered to pregnant women, children and adolescents on aspirin therapy, persons with history of Guillain-Barré syndrome, or people with allergy to chicken eggs or nasal spray components.

Assessment

History

▶ Acute onset

▶ Malaise

▶ Headache

▶ Nausea

▶ Muscle aching

▶ Nasal stuffiness

Physical Exam

▶ Fever, chills

▶ Mild pharyngeal injection

▶ Conjunctival redness

Diagnostic Studies

▶ CBC: leukopenia common

▶ Nasal or throat swab for identifying influenza antigen

Differential Diagnosis

▶ Rhinovirus

▶ Bronchitis

▶ Pneumonia

▶ RSV

▶ Other acute febrile illnesses

Management

Nonpharmacologic Treatment

▶ Rest

▶ Encourage fluids

Pharmacologic Treatment

▶ Analgesics

▶ Cough suppressant (*Note:* Over-the-counter cough formulations are not recommended for children younger than 2 years of age)

▶ Antiviral medication must be started within 2 days of symptom onset to be effective

▶ Oseltamivir (Tamiflu) 75 mg orally twice a day or zanamivir (Relenza) two 5 mg inhalations twice a day for 5 days for influenza A or B

When to Consult, Refer, Hospitalize

▶ Patients at either extreme of age are very vulnerable and should be referred to an infectious disease specialist.

Follow-Up

Expected Course

▶ Usual duration is 1 to 7 days

▶ Often a longer and more severe course in older adults

Complications

▶ Pneumonia

▶ Death

Measles (Rubeola)

Description

▶ Acute viral disease with fever (higher than 101°F); erythematous, maculopapular rash; cough; coryza; conjunctivitis; characteristic rash of oral mucus membranes known as Koplik spots

Etiology

▶ Measles virus (RNA virus, paramyxovirus family)

▶ Transmitted by direct contact with infectious droplets, or less commonly by airborne spread; highly contagious

▶ Incubation period 7 to 21 days

▶ Communicable 1 to 2 days before symptoms begin; 3 to 5 days before rash to 4 days after rash onset

Incidence and Demographics

▶ Greater than 99% reduction in the reported incidence of measles since vaccination began in 1963

▶ Most new cases secondary to importation from other countries

▶ In 2014, the United States experienced a record number of measles cases, the highest number since measles was declared eliminated.

Risk Factors

▶ Lack of immunization; up to 5% of cases secondary to vaccine failure

Prevention and Screening

▶ Vaccine, usually given as MMR (measles, mumps, rubella) subcutaneous per routine schedule with first dose at 12 to 15 months, booster at 4 to 6 years of age

Assessment

History

▶ Prodrome of fever higher than 101°F, malaise; cough, coryza, and/or conjunctivitis—the three Cs of measles

Physical Exam

▶ Red, maculopapular rash beginning on face and neck; progressing slowly down trunk and extremities (cephalocaudal) between second and fourth days and lasting 5 to 7 days

▶ Rash begins as discrete lesions, then becomes confluent and salmon-colored (morbilliform rash); lesions initially blanch with pressure

▶ When fever subsides, rash fades to faint brown stain; skin may desquamate

▶ Koplik spots are tiny, bluish-white spots on an erythematous base, clustered on the buccal mucosa near the molars, and are pathognomonic for measles. They appear 1 to 2 days before onset of rash and may last up to 12 to 15 days.

Diagnostic Studies

▶ Acute (when rash appears) and convalescent (2 to 4 weeks) antibody titers

▶ Serum IgM antibodies peak 10 days after onset of rash, disappear after 20 to 60 days

▶ Measles virus detected from nasopharyngeal secretions, conjunctiva, blood, urine

Differential Diagnosis

▶ Rubella

▶ Scarlet fever

▶ Roseola

Management

Nonpharmacologic Treatment

▶ Symptomatic: rest and fluids

▶ Isolation for 4 days after appearance of rash

▶ Avoid bright lights (photosensitivity)

Pharmacologic Treatment

▶ Give acetaminophen or ibuprofen for fever and discomfort (no aspirin-containing products in patients under 19 years of age).

▶ Consider vitamin A (200,000 IU orally if older than age 1 year; 100,000 IU orally for infants 6 to 12 months old) in children at high risk for complications such as pneumonia (e.g., immunodeficiency, malabsorption, malnutrition); repeat in 24 hours and in 4 weeks if any ophthalmologic evidence of vitamin A deficiency.

▶ Give to all children in communities with vitamin A deficiency, particularly in developing countries.

▶ Live measles vaccine given within 72 hours of exposure may provide protection in some cases.

▶ Immune globulin may be given within 6 days of exposure; do not give with live vaccine. Susceptible household contacts should receive immune globulin because identification of the index case usually occurs after 72 hours (American Academy of Pediatrics [AAP], 2006).

▶ Immune globulin dosing: 0.25 mL/kg body weight, IM; immunocompromised children should receive 0.5 mL/kg body weight; maximum dose 15 mL

Special Considerations

▶ Do not prescribe or administer aspirin or aspirin-related products for a viral infection or syndrome because of the risk of Reye's syndrome in patients under 19 years of age.

▶ Children between 6 and 11 months traveling outside the United States should be administered monovalent measles vaccine, or MMR if unavailable, before traveling if possible. The dose administered before 12 months of age should not count toward the MMR series (Centers for Disease Control and Prevention, 2007a).

▶ Children older than 12 months of age traveling outside the United States should receive two doses of MMR at least 28 days apart before departing (Centers for Disease Control and Prevention, 2007a).

When to Consult, Refer, Hospitalize

▶ No reason to refer in uncomplicated cases

Follow-Up

▶ Daily during acute phase, 3 to 4 days after onset of rash; more often if indicated (high-risk person, infant, presence of complications)

Expected Course

▶ Recovery within 3 to 4 days after onset of rash, resolves in 10 days

Complications

▶ Otitis media, bronchopneumonia, laryngotracheobronchitis, diarrhea, acute encephalitis (1 in 1,000 cases); subacute sclerosing panencephalitis (SSPE) very rare, may develop years after measles infection

Mumps (Parotitis)

Description

▶ Acute viral disease affecting salivary glands, primarily parotid gland

Etiology

▶ Caused by a paramyxovirus

▶ Transmitted via respiratory route (direct contact)

▶ Communicable 1 to 2 days before 5 days after onset of parotid swelling

▶ Incubation period 16 to 18 days, but cases may occur 12 to 25 days after exposure

Incidence and Demographics

▶ Fewer than 1,000 cases per year; dramatic decline since implementation of vaccination

▶ Most reported cases in children 5 to 14 years of age; declining since introduction of second MMR vaccine in early childhood

▶ May see outbreaks in immunized populations; however, most cases of parotitis in immunized children not due to mumps

Risk Factors

▶ Unimmunized people

Prevention and Screening

▶ Primary prevention through vaccination; vaccine, usually given as MMR subcutaneous per routine schedule with first dose at 12 to 15 months, booster at 4 to 6 years of age; postexposure vaccination not effective

▶ Exclusion from school or day care until 9 days from onset of parotid gland swelling

▶ During outbreaks, exclusion of unimmunized children from school or day care for 26 days after onset of parotid gland swelling of the last person with mumps in affected school or day care

Assessment

History

▶ Fever, malaise, pain in or behind ear during chewing or swallowing

▶ "Classic" symptom is extreme pain when ingesting tart or sour substances

Physical Exam

▶ Tender, swollen parotid glands, typically covering angle of jaw; may also see submaxillary and sublingual gland involvement; parotid glands may not be involved; approximately one-third of mumps cases do not have clinically apparent salivary gland swelling.

▶ Tenderness persists 1 to 3 days; swelling persists 7 to 10 days

▶ Openings of ducts of involved salivary glands may be red and swollen.

▶ Fever may be normal, slight, or high (up to 104° F).

Diagnostic Studies

▶ WBC may show leucopenia and lymphocytosis.

▶ Isolation of mumps virus in cell culture, best collected from saliva

▶ Rise in serum IgG titers or positive mumps IgM antibody test

▶ Serum amylase level increased in approximately 90% of patients with parotitis, not specific to mumps. Helpful in differentiating parotitis from cervical adenopathy.

Differential Diagnosis

▶ Parotitis from other causes, including infectious, tumor, or parotid duct obstruction

▶ Tooth infection or abscess

▶ Cervical adenitis

Management

Nonpharmacologic Treatment

▶ Supportive—encourage fluids, bed rest, warm or cold compresses to swollen areas (whichever is more soothing).

▶ Avoid tart, sour, acidic food and drink, and mucous membrane irritants such as peppermint.

▶ Wash mouth with fat-free broth or saline solution.

▶ Isolate until swelling is gone.

Pharmacologic Treatment

▶ Give acetaminophen or ibuprofen for fever and discomfort (no aspirin-containing products in patients under 19 years of age).

When to Consult, Refer, Hospitalize

▶ Refer to specialist with any suggestion of complications.

▶ Mumps must be reported to CDC.

Special Considerations

▶ International travelers are at risk for exposure to mumps. Immunization is recommended if a person is unsure of his or her immunity status. Evidence of presumptive immunity includes documentation of healthcare provider–diagnosed disease, laboratory evidence of immunity, documentation of administration of two doses of live mumps vaccine, or birth date before 1957 (MMWR, 2013).

Follow-Up

Expected Course

▶ Up to 10 days

Complications

▶ Meningitis—symptomatic in approximately 10% of patients

▶ Other CNS involvement, including cerebellar ataxia

▶ Orchitis common in infection after puberty, but sterility rare

▶ Rare: arthritis, thyroiditis, mastitis, glomerulonephritis, oophoritis, pancreatitis, myocarditis, transverse myelitis, thrombocytopenia, paresis of the facial nerve, hearing impairment

Roseola

Description

▶ Acute viral disease of infants and young children characterized by significant fever for 7 to 10 days; when resolved, followed by faint, erythematous, maculopapular rash lasting hours to days

Etiology

▶ It is caused by the human herpes virus 6 ( ).

▶ HHV-6 is a common cause of febrile illness in infants and young children, with or without rash.

▶ Roseola-like illnesses may be caused by a variety of different viruses, such as Coxsackie viruses, echoviruses, adenoviruses, and para influenza virus.

▶ Transmission is by droplet and fecal-oral route.

▶ Incubation period is 9 to 10 days.

Incidence and Demographics

▶ Affects children ages 3 months to 4 years; peak age 6 to 24 months

Risk Factors

▶ Institutional-style day care setting

Prevention and Screening

▶ Prevention difficult; should institute droplet and secretion precautions in institutional-ized patients

▶ Remove from day care until afebrile (no infectious risk after afebrile, even if rash still present).

Assessment

History

▶ Sudden onset of fever (may be sustained or spiking); fever may be as high as 106°F; fever what usually prompts parents to seek medical attention; lasts 3 to 7 days

▶ Cough, sore throat; faint rash that appears when the fever begins to drop

Physical Exam

▶ Presence of fever up to 106°F

▶ Faint blanching, erythematous, maculopapular rash beginning on day 4 (lasts 1 to 2 days)

▶ May have lymphadenopathy (suboccipital, posterior cervical, postauricular), mild pharyngitis

Diagnostic Studies

▶ None indicated; if CBC performed, may see leucopenia and lymphocytosis

Differential Diagnosis

▶ Other viral, febrile illnesses with rash

▶ Drug reaction rash

Management

Nonpharmacologic Treatment

▶ Supportive—encourage fluids in febrile phase

Pharmacologic Treatment

▶ Acetaminophen or ibuprofen for fever and discomfort in patients under 19 years of age

How Long to Treat

▶ While symptomatic

Special Considerations

▶ None

When to Consult, Refer, Hospitalize

▶ No reason to refer in uncomplicated cases

Follow-Up

Expected Course

▶ Mild, self-limiting

Complications

▶ Seizures (probably associated with high fever as opposed to viral invasion of cerebro-spinal fluid [CSF] or cerebral structures), aseptic meningitis, encephalitis, thrombocy-topenia purpura

Rubella (German Measles)

Description

▶ Mild viral disease with low-grade fever and generalized erythematous, maculopapu-lar rash; generalized lymphadenopathy, most commonly suboccipital, postauricular, cervical; high risk if contracted during pregnancy

Etiology

▶ Rubella virus (RNA virus, Togaviridae family)

▶ Transmitted by direct or droplet contact with nasopharyngeal secretions

▶ Incubation period 14 to 23 days

▶ Communicable a few days before rash onset and for 5 to 7 days after rash appears

▶ Infants with congenital rubella—may shed virus for 1 year or more

Incidence and Demographics

▶ Incidence has declined by 99% since onset of vaccination; most cases now occur in young non-immunized or inadequately immunized adults (outbreaks in colleges or occupational settings).

Risk Factors

▶ Non-immunized or inadequately immunized young adults

Prevention and Screening

▶ Administer live attenuated vaccine, usually in the form of measles/mumps/rubella vaccine (MMR), to non-immunized persons, especially women of childbearing age. Vaccine is usually given as MMR subcutaneous per routine schedule with first dose at 12 to 15 months and a booster at 4 to 6 years of age.

▶ Active immunization after exposure will not prevent infection; initiation of passive immunity with immune globulin is not helpful.

▶ Women of childbearing age should be tested for rubella antibody titer and, if titer is low, should receive vaccine; avoid pregnancy for at least 28 days after vaccination.

Assessment

History

▶ History of cough, coryza, malaise, fever, headache, possibly arthralgia

Physical Exam

▶ Maculopapular rash, beginning on face and spreading rapidly to trunk; second day, rash begins to disappear in same pattern; usually resolves by third day

▶ Fever, lymphadenopathy (suboccipital, postauricular, cervical), conjunctivitis, pharyngitis

Diagnostic Studies

▶ Virus can be detected on nasal smear.

▶ Acute (7 to 10 days) and convalescent (2 to 3 weeks) serum titers (fourfold increase or more)

▶ Determine immune status—latex agglutination immunoassay

Differential Diagnosis

▶ Other viral diseases characterized by fever and rash

Management

▶ Symptomatic—rest and fluids

▶ Isolation if in an institution

▶ Stay home from work or school for 7 days after onset of rash.

Special Considerations

▶ Maternal infection associated with high incidence of congenital anomalies and/or fetal demise

▶ Follow droplet precautions when caring for infants with congenital rubella until three or more successive negative nasopharyngeal and urine cultures are obtained.

▶ Be sure patients are immune to rubella before taking a cruise; outbreaks of rubella have been reported on cruise ships.

When to Consult, Refer, Hospitalize

▶ No reason to refer in uncomplicated cases

▶ Must be reported to CDC

Follow-Up

Expected Course

▶ Usually acute, self-limiting illness

▶ Arthritis and/or neuritis may occur in young children, more common in older children and adults.

Complications

▶ Congenital rubella is associated with congenital anomalies and/or fetal demise.

▶ Rare complications of postnatal acquired rubella include encephalitis and thrombocytopenia.

Varicella Zoster (Chickenpox)

Description

▶ Usually mild acute viral disease characterized by fever and generalized, pruritic, vesicular rash

Etiology

▶ Caused by varicella zoster virus (herpes virus family)

▶ Highly contagious; transmitted by airborne respiratory secretions from infected people

▶ Rarely spread through contact with fluid from vesicles

▶ Can be caused by contact with patients with herpes zoster (shingles) in susceptible persons

▶ Communicable 1 to 2 days before rash until vesicles are crusted, approximately 5 days after onset of rash

▶ Incubation period usually 14 to 16 days but may be 10 to 21 days

Incidence and Demographics

▶ Seen in all ages; most frequent in young schoolchildren, children attending day care

Risk Factors

▶ Unimmunized person

Prevention and Screening

▶ Vaccination is the best form of prevention (refer to the *Centers for Disease Control and Prevention Recommended Immunization Schedule for Adults Aged 19 Years and Older—United States, 2013*).

▶ Isolate infected people.

▶ Children should not return to school or day care and adults should not return to work until all lesions are crusted over.

Assessment

History

▶ Headache, mild fever, malaise

Physical Exam

▶ Rash in various stages; progresses from macules to papules to vesicles on erythematous base within 6 hours after onset

▶ Vesicles crust in 4 to 6 days.

▶ Some medical authors note vesicles appearing first on scalp and mucus membranes; others report vesicles appearing first on the trunk and back simultaneously with mucus membranes, and then spreading to scalp and extremities.

▶ Vesicles may be seen in the conjunctivae, mouth, throat, esophagus, trachea, rectum, and vagina; little scarring occurs.

▶ Vesicles rarely appear on the palms and soles.

▶ Pruritus is present in areas of crusted vesicles.

▶ Vesicles usually appear in three crops on 3 successive days.

Diagnostic Studies

▶ None indicated

▶ May see leucopenia

▶ May see WBC elevation with secondary infection

▶ May perform acute and convalescent titers

▶ Can be detected in vesicular scrapings during the first 3 to 4 days of the eruption

Differential Diagnosis

▶ Herpes simplex

▶ Papular urticaria

▶ Multiple insect bites

▶ Allergic skin reaction

▶ Scabies

▶ Smallpox

▶ Other viral fever and rash diseases

▶ Impetigo

Management

Nonpharmacologic Treatment

▶ For pruritus: calamine or Cetaphil lotion, baths with baking soda or oatmeal

Pharmacologic Treatment

▶ May administer varicella vaccine to exposed, susceptible children within 72 hours (up to 120 hours) after varicella exposure; may prevent or modify the disease

▶ Acetaminophen or ibuprofen for fever and discomfort for persons under 19 years of age

▶ Antipruritic medication such as diphenhydramine 5 mg/kg/day, divided q.6.h.

▶ Consider oral acyclovir (Zovirax) or other antiviral medication for people at high risk of severe infection (older than age 12, chronic disease, immunocompromised, long-term salicylate therapy) if initiated within 24 hours of onset of rash.

▶ Administer varicella zoster immune globulin (VZIg) within 72 to 96 hours after exposure in immunocompromised children.

Special Considerations

▶ Varicella zoster virus remains latent in nerve roots and may emerge later in life as herpes zoster (shingles).

▶ Do not prescribe or administer aspirin or aspirin-related products to persons less than 19 years of age because of associated risk of Reye's syndrome.

▶ Because of increased risk of severe disease and complications in children over 12, adolescents without reliable history of disease should be immunized.

When to Consult, Refer, Hospitalize

▶ No reason to refer in uncomplicated cases

Follow-Up

▶ Return to day care, school, or work only after all lesions are crusted.

Complications

▶ Secondary, bacterial infection of skin (impetigo)

▶ Scarring—may be a cosmetic concern

▶ Encephalitis, nephritis, hepatitis, glomerulonephritis

▶ Reye's syndrome

▶ Thrombocytopenia

▶ Pneumonia

West Nile Virus (WNV)

Description

▶ Viral infection causing febrile illness, headache, fatigue, rash, arthritis, myalgia, weakness, lymphadenopathy, and meningoencephalitis

Etiology

▶ The WNV is caused by the arbovirus of family *Flaviviridae*. The transmission cycle is spread by infected mosquitoes to birds and from infected birds to feeding mosquitoes.

▶ Human infection is primarily from the bite of an infected mosquito.

▶ Domestic animals, including horses, are sometimes infected by bites of infected mosquitoes; however, there is no documentation of spread of the disease from animal to animal or animal to human.

▶ Although rare, infection can be spread through blood transfusions, organ transplantation, and prenatal transmission.

Incidence and Demographics

▶ Reported in Asia, Africa, Europe, and United States

▶ In 2013, 48 states within the United States reported cases of WNV, according to the CDC.

▶ Incubation period 5 to 15 days

▶ Mild illness in 20% of infected people, lasting 3 to 6 days

▶ 1 in 150 develop severe neurological disease; encephalitis more than meningitis

▶ Adults older than 50 years at greatest risk for serious illness

▶ Mortality 5%; most deaths in older adults

Risk Factors

▶ Outdoor activities when mosquito activity is high

▶ Outdoor occupation

▶ Blood transfusion and organ transplant

▶ Older adults

Prevention and Screening

▶ Avoid mosquito bites: Minimize outdoor activity, wear protective clothing, and protect home and yard from breeding mosquitoes by draining standing water and maintaining window screens.

▶ When outdoors, apply insect repellent containing DEET (up to 50% strength), picaridin, or oil of lemon eucalyptus; permethrin is also recommended for use on clothing, shoes, and other gear.

  ▷ *Pediatric note:* Oil of lemon eucalyptus products should not be used on children under 3 years of age. The American Academy of Pediatrics does not recommend the use of DEET on infants younger than 2 months.

▶ Apply repellent to clothing and exposed skin, avoiding eyes and mouth; do not apply to skin under clothing—efficacy of repellent is affected by concentration, perspiration, and getting wet. Reapply repellent as needed.

▶ Communities can control vectors by public health spraying against mosquitoes.

▶ Wear gloves when disposing of dead birds.

▶ Report dead birds to local health department.

▶ Screen blood donations for WNV using nucleic acid-amplification test.

Assessment

History

▶ Determine exposure to mosquitoes.

▶ Check for history of blood transfusion or organ transplantation.

Physical Exam

▶ Nondescript fever with maculopapular or morbilliform rash on neck, trunk, arms, and legs

▶ Arthritis, myalgia, generalized weakness, and lymphadenopathy

▶ Meningitis: fever, headache, and nuchal rigidity

▶ Encephalitis: fever, headache, and altered mental status ranging from confusion to coma, with or without additional signs of brain dysfunction (paresis, flaccid paralysis, ataxia, sensory deficits, optic neuritis, seizures, and abnormal reflexes)

Diagnostic Studies

▶ CSF with IgM antibody for WNV is confirmative; CSF with pleocytosis (increased number of lymphocytes)

▶ WNV antibody in serum is presumptive of recent infection in patients with acute CNS infection; greater than a fourfold increase in antibody titers 2 to 4 weeks apart is confirmative

▶ Pleocytosis: increased number of lymphocytes in CSF

Differential Diagnosis

▶ California encephalitis

▶ Eastern equine encephalitis

▶ Western equine encephalitis

▶ Powassan encephalitis

▶ St. Louis encephalitis

▶ Colorado tick fever

▶ Dengue fever

Management and Treatment

Nonpharmacologic Treatment

▶ Supportive care

▶ Monitor for complications

Pharmacologic Treatment

▶ Appropriate treatment of complications

How Long to Treat

▶ Continue supportive care until improvement.

Special Considerations

▶ See CDC website: http://www.cdc.gov/ncidod/dvbid/westnile/index.htm /

When to Consult, Refer, Hospitalize

▶ Report West Nile virus encephalitis cases to the state health department.

▶ Immediately refer patients to an infectious disease specialist.

▶ Patients with deteriorating mental status should be referred immediately to a health-care provider for hospitalization.

▶ West Nile virus must be reported to CDC.

Follow-Up

▶ Majority have very minor illness and recovery without complications.

Complications
- ▶ Central nervous system abnormalities
- ▶ Death

BACTERIAL AND OTHER INFECTIONS

Lyme Disease

Description
- ▶ Tick-borne infection from a spirochete transmitted via deer tick bite, often begins with rash (erythema migrans), progresses to headaches, arthritis, and neurologic sequelae; up to 20% of patients have complications; most do not have permanent sequelae

Etiology
- ▶ Caused by the spirochete *Borrelia burgdorferi;* most common vector-borne disease in the United States
- ▶ Transmitted to humans by *Ixodes scapularis* tick (deer tick); not transmitted by larger dog tick
- ▶ Size of tick 2–9 mm
- ▶ Painless bite; ticks usually drop off unnoticed in 2 to 4 days; must be embedded longer than 24 hours to transmit disease
- ▶ Incubation period from bite to appearance of erythema migrans 3 to 31 days; usually 7 to 14 days

Incidence and Demographics
- ▶ 90% of cases are diagnosed in the Mid-Atlantic, Northeastern, and North Central areas of the United States.
- ▶ Preliminary results from three different evaluation methods suggest that the number of people diagnosed with Lyme disease each year in the United States is around 300,000.
- ▶ Lyme disease patients are most likely to have illness onset in June, July, or August and less likely to have illness onset from December through March (CDC, 2015).

Risk Factors
- ▶ Live in endemic region
- ▶ Spend time outdoors for recreation or occupation
- ▶ Exposed skin
- ▶ No use of repellents
- ▶ 30% to 50% of cases in children and adolescents; reported cases of Lyme disease are most common among boys aged 5 to 9

Prevention and Screening

▶ *Reduce exposed skin*: Wear light-colored clothing to see ticks; wear long pants and long sleeves; tuck shirts into pants, tuck pants into socks. When outdoors, apply insect repellent containing DEET (up to 50% strength), picaridin, or oil of lemon eucalyptus; permethrin is also recommended for use on clothing, shoes, and other gear.

▷ *Pediatric note*: Oil of lemon eucalyptus products should not be used on children under 3 years. The American Academy of Pediatrics does not recommend the use of DEET on infants younger than 2 months.

▶ Apply repellent to clothing and exposed skin, avoiding eyes and mouth; do not apply to skin under clothing—efficacy of repellent is affected by concentration, perspiration, and getting wet. Reapply repellent as needed.

▶ Walk in the middle of a path; avoid walking near tree branches, bushes, or grass; inspect skin, hair, and scalp after spending a day outside; examine clothing before coming into the house.

▶ Examine pets for ticks regularly.

▶ The Lyme disease vaccine was withdrawn from the market in 2002 by manufacturer because of low sales and is no longer commercially available.

▶ Prophylactic antibiotics are not routinely used following tick bites. However, factors to take into consideration include: Was the tick on the person for 24 hours before being removed or falling off? Has it been at least 3 days since the person removed the tick or it fell off? Is Lyme disease common in the location where the person was exposed to the tick?

Assessment

History

▶ Most unable to identify tick bite, but have history of possible exposure

Physical Exam

▶ Complete physical exam

▶ Characteristic rash (target lesion); may find tick or tick remnant in Stage 1

▶ Signs of cranial nerve palsies, meningeal signs, pericarditis, mono-arthritis in Stage 2

▶ May see recurrent tendonitis, bursitis, synovitis late in disease; memory loss; motor or sensory deficits; iritis, optic neuritis, and other eye manifestations (see Table 4–1 for descriptions of each stage of disease)

Diagnostic Studies

▶ Lyme disease is primarily a clinical diagnosis; serology has uncertain sensitivity but is used to confirm the presence of specific antibodies to *B. burgdorferi* in serum (see Table 4–2).

▶ Step 1: ELISA method is preferred: more sensitive and specific. If positive, proceed to step 2.

▶ Step 2: Western blot assay can detect both IgM and IgG and is used as a confirmatory test.

TABLE 4–1.
STAGES OF LYME DISEASE

STAGE	SYMPTOMS
Stage 1: Early localized disease (3–30 days postexposure)	• Flu-like symptoms of fever, chills, myalgia, arthralgia, headache; • 50%–90% of patients develop distinctive rash termed erythema migrans within about 1 week of tick bite: begins as red macule or papule, expands rapidly over several days to annular, erythematous patch with central clearing, >5 cm to as large as 30 cm • Resolves in 3–4 weeks without treatment; usually in area of tick bite but may occur anywhere
Stage 2: Early disseminated disease (weeks to months postexposure)	• Begins roughly 3–5 weeks after initial infection, as spirochete spreads • Wide variety of symptoms, most notably persistent fatigue • Migratory arthralgia common • Cranial nerve palsies (especially facial nerve) common • Meningitis, conjunctivitis may occur; carditis with heart block rare • Most common manifestation is multiple erythema migrans lesions, usually smaller than initial lesion
Stage 3: Late disease (months to years later)	• Months to years after initial infection, characterized by recurrent polyarticular arthritis, usually affecting large joints (knees) • Central and peripheral nervous system affected, may develop subacute encephalopathy, distal paresthesias • Memory, mood, sleep problems may be noted • Cardiac involvement

TABLE 4–2.
LABORATORY FINDINGS IN LYME DISEASE

SERUM TEST	EARLY FINDINGS	MIDCOURSE	LATE FINDINGS
	2–4 weeks after erythema migrans	6–8 weeks	4–6 months
IgM	Appears	Peaks	Declines to low levels
IgG	Negative	Appears	Peaks; remains elevated but at lower level

▶ Serologic tests are not necessary if patient has classic presentation of exposure to endemic area and erythema migrans; tests often negative early in course.

▶ For late disease, patient must have specific symptoms and objective signs before testing.

▶ Patients with Lyme disease may not have elevated titers during the first several weeks of illness (false-negative test result).

▶ Do not test patients with nonspecific symptoms for Lyme disease as there is a relatively high incidence of false positives in the general population.

Differential Diagnosis

▶ Rocky Mountain spotted fever

▶ Rheumatic fever

▶ Viral disease

▶ Fibromyalgia

▶ Other forms of arthritis

Management and Treatment

Nonpharmacologic Treatment

▶ Hydrate patients; keep skin well-lubricated.

▶ Remove tick using firm tension and fine tweezers. Clean site. Do not squeeze or puncture the tick. If the tick head or other parts are not removed, clean with antimicrobial as removing head can cause tissue damage and has no effect on risk of Lyme disease.

Pharmacologic Treatment

▶ Adults

▷ Early disease: doxycycline 100 mg twice a day orally for 14 to 21 days

▷ Late disease: same as early disease but 21 to 28 days

▷ Persistent or recurrent arthritis, carditis, meningitis, or encephalitis:

▶ Ceftriaxone (Rocephin) 2 g once daily or 1 g twice daily IV or IM for 14 to 21 days *or*

▶ Penicillin G IV 20 million units in four divided doses

▶ Pediatric

▷ Early disease: younger than 8 years of age, amoxicillin 25–50 mg/kg/day orally divided into two doses daily, not to exceed 2 g/day for 14 to 21 days

▷ Early disease: 8 years of age or older, doxycycline 100 mg twice a day orally for 14 to 21 days

▷ Late disease: same as early disease except extend treatment for 21 to 28 days

▷ Persistent or recurrent arthritis, carditis, meningitis, or encephalitis:

▶ Ceftriaxone (Rocephin) 75–100 mg/kg once daily, not to exceed 2 g/day for 14 to 21 days

▶   *or* Penicillin G IV 300,000 U/kg/day in four divided doses not to exceed 20 million U/day

How Long to Treat

▶   14 to 21 days for early disease and 21 to 28 days for late disease

▶   30 to 60 days for meningitis or encephalitis

Special Considerations

▶   Amoxicillin is recommended for children and for pregnant and lactating women.

When to Consult, Refer, Hospitalize

▶   Refer to infectious disease specialist and/or to other specialist as soon as diagnosis is suspected. Monitor for central nervous system or cardiac involvement, uncertain diagnosis, or failure to respond to p.o. medication.

▶   Consult if IV therapy is required.

▶   Lyme disease must be reported to CDC.

Follow-Up

Expected Course

▶   Most respond promptly; complete resolution of symptoms in 4 weeks

▶   Long-term outcome not clear—in one study, many had residual symptoms; however, treatment often delayed or patients undertreated

Complications

▶   Recurrent arthritis, chronic neurologic symptoms, congestive heart failure, cardiomyopathy

Pertussis

Description

▶   An upper respiratory illness characterized by a progressive cough lasting longer than two weeks with one of the following symptoms: spasms of coughing, inspiratory "whoop," or post-tussive vomiting; or in infants younger than 1 year, apnea with or without cyanosis

Etiology

▶   *Bordetella pertussis*

▶   Transmission is respiratory

▶   Incubation 6 to 20 days

▶   Communicable until 5 days after treatment initiated

Incidence and Demographics

▶   As of August 2014, a total of 17,325 cases of pertussis had been reported to the CDC for the year; this is a 30% increase compared with the same period in 2013.

Risk Factors

▶ Lack of immunization

Prevention and Screening

▶ See CDC immunization schedule for pertussis vaccine for children and adults.

Assessment

History

▶ Catarrhal stage: mild upper respiratory symptoms with cough, nasal congestion, rhinorrhea, sneezing, low grade fever and mild conjunctival injection (most contagious stage); indistinguishable from the common cold

▶ Paroxysmal stage: severe bursts of cough with inspiratory whoop followed by vomiting; fever absent or low grade (less than 101°F); cough is forceful, rapid, staccato sequence; child unable to breath between coughing attacks, which are often accompanied by emesis; face may become reddened or have petechiae; cough is worse at night

Physical Exam

▶ Depending on stage, patient may appear tired; apnea may occur in young infants.

▶ Obtain vital signs; check eyes, ears, nose, throat, lymph, respiratory, and cardiac exam to exclude other illnesses.

Diagnostic Studies

▶ PCR swab of nasal cavity or nasopharyngeal cultures in the catarrhal stage or IgA testing for *B. pertussis* to confirm diagnosis

▶ CBC will show leukocytosis.

Differential Diagnosis

▶ Bronchiolitis

▶ Bronchitis

▶ Pneumonia

▶ Other viral and bacterial upper respiratory infections

▶ Cystic fibrosis

▶ Foreign body

Management and Treatment

Nonpharmacologic Treatment

▶ Symptomatic—rest and fluids

▶ Admission for infants younger than 6 months old

Pharmacologic Treatment

▶ Erythromycin 40–50 mg/kg/day in four divided doses *or*

▶ Trimethoprim/sulfamethoxazole (Bactrim) 8mg/kg/day (trimethoprim component) given twice a day

▶ Beta-2 agonists to control paroxysmal cough

▶ Corticosteroids for severely ill patients

How Long to Treat

▶ 14 days

Special Considerations

▶ Give antibiotics early; they are not effective late in the course of illness except to deal with complications.

▶ Antibiotics do not significantly shorten the disease but do reduce transmission.

▶ The CDC recommends antibiotic treatment for everyone in close proximity to the one with pertussis illness regardless of age.

▶ Do not use cough suppressants.

When to Consult, Refer, Hospitalize

▶ Consult for infants younger than 6 months and others who present with potentially severe disease; they often require hospitalization for supportive care.

▶ Pertussis must be reported to CDC.

Follow-Up

▶ Follow via telephone contact; discourage clinic visits.

Expected Course

▶ May be 10 weeks in uncomplicated cases

Complications

▶ Pneumonia

▶ Seizures

▶ Encephalopathy

▶ Death

Rheumatic Fever (RF)

Description

▶ Serious inflammatory systemic immune process occurring 1 week to 6 months after group A beta-hemolytic streptococcal pharyngitis

Etiology

▶ Antistreptococcal antibodies cross-react with human cardiac myocytes, cartilage, and thalamic and subthalamic nuclei of the CNS, causing carditis, arthritis, and chorea.

▶ Heredity may play a role, causing a particular immune response to strep.

Incidence and Demographics

▶ Frequency and severity have decreased due to better treatment of pharyngitis.

▶ RF remains an important cause of cardiac death in 5- to 25-year-olds.

▶ Many older patients have valvular disease caused by rheumatic fever.

Risk Factors

▶ Immigrants to the United States

▶ Genetic predisposition

▶ Ages 5 to 15

▶ More common in girls and Black people

▶ Living in the Midwest or Intermountain West in the mid- to late 1980s

Prevention and Screening

▶ Timely antibiotic treatment of group A beta hemolytic streptococcal upper respiratory infection

Assessment

History

▶ May have history of recent sore throat

▶ Presents with gradual onset of fever, malaise, and joint pain (classically migratory pain and possible inflammation of large joints; disappears in 3 to 4 weeks)

▶ Fatigue, irritability, abdominal pain, epistaxis (rare)

Physical Exam

▶ Heart murmurs indicating mitral valve 75%, aortic valve 30%, tricuspid or pulmonic less than 5% involvement; occur within 2 weeks, may be permanent

▶ Pericarditis, myocarditis; may last 6 weeks to 6 months

▶ Subcutaneous nodules (painless, freely movable over extensor surfaces of elbows, knees, and wrists)

▶ Neurologic: facial grimaces and tics, chorea (purposeless, involuntary, rapid movements of trunk and/or extremities) are late findings

▶ Rash is rare; presents with erythematous, macular lesions with rounded or serpiginous margins and pale centers; transient and migratory, occurs mainly on trunk and proximal extremities

▶ Guidelines for diagnosis—Jones criteria

▷ Required: evidence of a preceding streptococcal infection such as elevated or increasing antistreptolysin-O titer or other streptococcal antibodies, positive rapid antigen detection test (RADT) or throat culture for group A streptococcus, or recent scarlet fever

▷ Also required: two major symptoms or one major and two minor (see Table 4–3)

TABLE 4–3.
JONES CRITERIA FOR RHEUMATIC FEVER

MAJOR SYMPTOMS	MINOR SYMPTOMS
Carditis (common) Polyarthritis (common) Chorea (uncommon) Erythema marginatum (uncommon) Subcutaneous nodules (uncommon)	Clinical: fever (101°F –102°F), arthralgia, previous RF or preexisting rheumatic heart disease Laboratory: acute phase reaction (leukocytosis, elevated erythrocyte sedimentation rate [ESR], abnormal c-reactive protein or prolonged PR interval or other electrocardiographic changes)

Diagnostic Studies

▶ Current strep throat: rapid antigen detection test (RADT) or throat culture; may or may not be positive

▶ Preceding strep infection: streptococcal antibody titers—obtain acute and convalescent serum titers (2 to 4 weeks)

▶ To confirm diagnosis and evaluate severity of illness:

  ▷ ESR elevation

  ▷ C-reactive protein elevation

  ▷ Prolonged PR interval on ECG

Differential Diagnosis

▶ Rheumatoid arthritis

▶ Systemic lupus erythematosus

▶ Lyme disease

Management and Treatment

Nonpharmacologic Treatment

▶ Strict bed rest until C-reactive protein has been normal for 2 weeks, ESR and temperature normal

Pharmacologic Treatment

▶ Depends on specific symptoms and severity of disease; refer to specialist

▶ Pain— codeine rather than nonsteroidal anti-inflammatory drugs (NSAIDs)

▶ Carditis—inotropic agents, diuretics, vasodilators, and corticosteroids as indicated

▶ Chorea treated with sedatives and benzodiazepines

How Long to Treat

▶ Bed rest until temperature, lab results, pulse rate (less than 100/min in adults), and ECG return to normal

▶ Antibiotics as above

Special Considerations

▶ Educate patient regarding meticulous oral hygiene to prevent bacterial seeding.

▶ Educate patient to notify healthcare providers about cardiac condition before any procedure.

▶ Treat patients who have a history of rheumatic fever prophylactically to prevent recurrence (secondary prevention). The usual antibiotic is penicillin. These patients should take a full course of antibiotic followed by a continuous prophylactic dose for 10 years if the patient had carditis; 5 years if patient did not have carditis.

▶ Prophylaxis before procedures that may cause bacteremia is important indefinitely (see Table 4–4).

▶ Patients who should receive prophylaxis:

  ▷ High-risk

    ▶ Prosthetic valve; previous bacterial endocarditis; complex, cyanotic congenital heart disease; surgically constructed systemic pulmonary shunts or conduits

  ▷ Medium- or moderate-risk

    ▶ Acute rheumatic fever (ARF) patients who have acquired valvular dysfunction but *not* for patients with previous ARF without valvular dysfunction

    ▶ Those with uncorrected cardiac congenital defects, hypertrophic cardiomyopathy, mitral regurgitation, mitral valve prolapse with murmur, and possibly men greater than 45 with mitral valve prolapse without murmur

When to Consult, Refer, Hospitalize

▶ Refer to rheumatologist and/or cardiologist for all suspected cases.

▶ Hospitalize for acute carditis and/or chorea.

Follow-Up

▶ Usually by cardiologist to monitor C-reactive protein; reevaluate every 4 to 6 weeks when patients present for prophylaxis

Expected Course

▶ Initial episodes may last months in children and weeks in adults.

Complications

▶ Recurrent acute rheumatic fever secondary to streptococcal reinfection

▶ Cardiomegaly, heart failure, pericarditis, mitral regurgitation, aortic insufficiency

▶ Death in 1% to 2%

Rocky Mountain Spotted Fever (RMSF)

Description

▶ Moderate systemic febrile illness with rash caused by vasculitis of small vessels; systemic symptoms including fever, characteristic rash; risk of severe complications and death

TABLE 4–4.
PROPHYLAXIS FOR RECURRENT RHEUMATIC FEVER

PROCEDURES FOR WHICH INDICATED	PROPHYLACTIC REGIMEN NEEDED
DENTAL* AND RESPIRATORY TRACT, ESOPHAGUS	
Periodontal surgery, scaling, professional teeth cleaning*; tonsillectomy, adenoidectomy; respiratory tract surgery, bronchoscopy	*Adults*: amoxicillin 2 g orally 1 hour before the procedure; if unable to take oral: ampicillin 2 g IV or IM 30 minutes before procedure *Children*: amoxicillin 50 mg/kg orally 1 hour before procedure; if unable to take oral: ampicillin 50 mg/kg IV or IM 30 minutes before procedure *Penicillin-allergic*: • Clindamycin (Cleocin): adults 600 mg, children 20 mg/kg, orally 1 hour before or IV 30 minutes before procedure • Cefadroxil (Duricef) or cephalexin (Keflex): adults 2 g, children 50 mg/kg, orally 1 hour before procedure • Azithromycin (Zithromax) or clarithromycin (Biaxin): adults 500 mg, children 15 mg/kg, orally 1 hour before procedure *Penicillin-allergic, unable to take oral*: • Cefazolin (Kefzol): adults 1 g, children 25 mg/kg, IM or IV 30 minutes before procedure
GASTROINTESTINAL AND GENITOURINARY TRACT	
Sclerotherapy of esophageal varices, esophageal stricture dilation, endoscopic retrograde cholangiography, biliary tract surgery, surgery associated with intestinal mucosa, prostatic surgery, cystoscopy, urethral dilation	Amoxicillin: adults 2 gm, children 50 mg/kg, orally 1 hour before procedure; IV or IM 30 minutes before *Penicillin-allergic*: • Vancomycin (Vancocin): adults 1 g, children 20 mg/kg, IV over 1–2 hours, completed within 30 minutes of procedure *If patient high-risk*: • *Adults*: ampicillin 2 g IM or IV and gentamicin 1.5 mg/kg (not to exceed 120 mg) within 30 minutes of starting the procedure; 6 hours later, ampicillin 1 g IV/IM or amoxicillin 1 g orally • *Children*: ampicillin 50 mg/kg IM or IV (not to exceed 2 g) and gentamicin 1.5 mg/kg within 30 minutes of starting the procedure; 6 hours later ampicillin 25 mg/kg IM/IV or amoxicillin 25 mg/kg orally *High-risk, penicillin-allergic*: • Adults: vancomycin 1g IV over 1–2 hours and gentamicin 1.5 mg/kg (not to exceed 120 mg), 30 minutes before procedure • Children: vancomycin 20 mg/kg IV over 1–2 hours and gentamicin 1.5 mg/kg IV/IM 30 minutes before procedure

Adapted from *The Sanford guide to antimicrobial therapy* (43rd ed.), by D. N. Gilbert, R. C. Moellering, & M. A. Sande, 2012, Hyde Park, VT: Antimicrobial Therapy, Inc.

*AHA dental prophylaxis guidelines apply to high-risk patients only (such as artificial valve).

Etiology

▶ *Rickettsia rickettsii* transmitted by bite of infected tick

▶ Tick must attach and feed for 4 to 6 hours to transmit infection

▶ No person-to-person transmission; disease confers immunity

▶ Incubation 2 to 14 days

Incidence and Demographics

▶ More than 50% of cases in South Atlantic region, predominantly in southeastern and central states; also upper Rocky Mountain states, Canada, Mexico, and South and Central America

▶ The most common tick-borne disease in the United States, approximately 250 to 1,200 cases are reported annually; peaks in late spring and summer

▶ Two-thirds of patients are younger than 15 years old.

Risk Factors

▶ Exposure to tick bites; camping or yardwork; exposed skin due to short pants, sleeves; no repellent

Prevention and Screening

▶ Avoid tick bites (see Lyme Disease).

Assessment

History

▶ Triad: headache, fever, rash (and history of tick bite, although not all present at time of initial assessment)

▶ Presents with sudden onset of fever higher than 104°F in nearly 100% of patients

▶ Severe headache unrelieved by analgesics; myalgia (particularly in calf and thigh)

▶ Rash: small, flat, pink, non-pruritic on wrists, forearms, ankles then spreads to trunk (sometimes palms and soles) turning purple and petechial

▶ Malaise, anorexia, nausea and vomiting, abdominal pain, lymphadenopathy, cough, confusion are possible

▶ History of possible tick bite or exposure

Physical Exam

▶ Characteristic maculopapular rash usually appears before the sixth day of illness, spreads from wrists and ankles to trunk, neck, and face.

▶ If untreated, rash becomes petechial in about 4 days, progresses to purpuric and coalesced.

▶ Moderate to high fever, conjunctival injection

▶ Splenomegaly in approximately 50% of patients

Diagnostic Studies
- ▶ Titers; acute and convalescent sera (fourfold increase in antibody titer) may not rise for 10 to 14 days
- ▶ Routine blood work may show nonspecific changes, identify complications: CBC with differential (thrombocytopenia, variable WBC count, mild anemia), PT and PTT (prolonged), BUN and creatinine (elevated in renal insufficiency), electrolytes (mild hyponatremia), elevated LFTs

Differential Diagnosis
- ▶ Systemic viral infection
- ▶ Bacterial sepsis
- ▶ Meningitis
- ▶ Meningococcemia
- ▶ Lyme disease
- ▶ Rubella
- ▶ Scarlet fever
- ▶ Mononucleosis
- ▶ Rheumatic fever
- ▶ Drug reaction
- ▶ Erythema multiforme
- ▶ Ehrlichiosis

Management
Nonpharmacologic Treatment
- ▶ Rest and fluids
- ▶ Isolation not indicated

Pharmacologic Treatment
- ▶ **Important to treat promptly**; treatment before day 5 of illness in children affords highest likelihood of good outcome
- ▶ Doxycycline is treatment of choice in adults who are not pregnant and children of all ages unless hypersensitive to tetracyclines
- ▶ Adults
  - ▷ Doxycycline 100 mg twice a day after loading dose of 200 mg once
  - ▷ If patient is sensitive to tetracyclines, use:
    - ▶ Amoxicillin 500 mg three times a day *or*
    - ▶ Cefuroxime (Ceftin) 500 mg twice a day
    - ▶ Late stage: ceftriaxone (Rocephin) 2 g IV once a day
- ▶ Pediatric
  - ▷ Less than 45 kg: doxycycline 2–4mg/kg/day orally in two divided doses

▷ More than 45 kg: doxycycline 100 mg orally twice a day

▶ Pregnant women

▷ Chloramphenicol (Chloromycetin) 500 mg every 6 hours

How Long to Treat

▶ 5 to 10 days or until afebrile 2 to 5 days

Special Considerations

▶ Educate patient on the tick associated with RMSF and ways to avoid the infection.

When to Consult, Refer, Hospitalize

▶ Consult with infectious disease specialist as soon as possible for potential hospitalization, any signs of complications.

▶ Rocky Mountain spotted fever must be reported to CDC.

Follow-Up

▶ See patient for follow-up every 2 to 3 days if not hospitalized, until symptoms resolved.

Expected Course

▶ Follow-up 1 to 2 days after initial visit; inform patients to return at first sign of complications.

▶ Most cases resolve without complication if treated promptly; infection can persist for 3 weeks.

▶ Refer for tertiary care as soon as complications develop or if patient has a petechial rash on first visit.

Complications

▶ Central nervous system, cardiac, pulmonary, gastrointestinal, and renal involvement; disseminated intravascular coagulation, shock, death

Scarlet Fever

Description

▶ Acute infectious disease usually associated with streptococcal pharyngitis and characterized by a vascular response to bacterial exotoxin

Etiology

▶ Toxin produced by group A hemolytic streptococcus (GAS) and occasionally produced by certain strains of staphylococci.

▶ Strep toxin usually has a pharyngeal source.

▶ Strep or staph infections from wounds or burns is rare source.

▶ Transmitted by direct projection of large droplets or physical transfer of respiratory secretions

▶ Incubation 3 to 5 days

▶ Communicable during incubation and clinical illness, 10 days; no longer communicable after 24 hours of antibiotic

Incidence and Demographics

▶ Usually occurs in children 6 to 12 years, but also occurs in adults

Risk Factors

▶ Outside-the-home day care setting

▶ School-age children

Prevention and Screening

▶ Early identification of GAS by rapid antigen detection test (RADT) or throat culture and removal from school or childcare for 24 hours after initiation of antibiotic

▶ Good handwashing

▶ Household contact screening for GAS or prophylactic treatment not effective

Assessment

History

▶ Prodrome: 1 to 2 days of fever, sore throat, headache; also may be abdominal pain and vomiting

▶ Rash appears in 1 to 5 days.

Physical Exam

▶ Initial pharyngitis is beefy red with or without exudate; white coating on tongue on days 1–2 that sheds by days 4–5 (shiny red with prominent papillae)

▶ Rash presents as fine eruptions on an erythematous bases, texture of sandpaper, blanches with pressure; initially on chest and axilla, spreads to abdomen and extremities

▶ Red streaks in skin folds of axillae and antecubital fossa (Pastia's lines)

▶ Flushed face with circumoral pallor

▶ Rash becomes generalized; desquamation begins on face after 7 to 10 days

Diagnostic Studies

▶ Rapid antigen test or throat culture for strep

▶ Antistreptolysin-O (ASO) titer to confirm recent infection with group A strep (not useful in management of acute streptococcal pharyngitis)

Differential Diagnosis

▶ Viral syndromes

▶ Mononucleosis

▶ Drug reaction

Management

Nonpharmacologic Treatment

▶ Rest and fluids

Pharmacologic Treatment

▶ Prompt therapy imperative to prevent rheumatic fever and other complications

▶ Penicillin V (Pen VEE K) 500 mg twice a day; erythromycin 250 mg every 6 hours, or cefadroxil (Duricef) 500 mg twice a day

▶ For staphylococcal scarlet fever, dicloxacillin

How Long to Treat

▶ 10 days

Special Considerations

▶ Recurrence of GAS pharyngitis may be treated with prophylactic penicillin during times of increased risk of infection (spring, late fall, and winter)

When to Consult, Refer, Hospitalize

▶ Chronic GAS pharyngitis

▶ Evidence of pneumonia, bacteremia, shock, or other severe complications

Follow-Up

▶ Repeat throat culture indicated for patients at risk for rheumatic fever

Expected Course

▶ Improvement should be seen 2 to 3 days after starting antibiotic.

Complications

▶ Otitis media, sinusitis, bacteremia, rheumatic fever, glomerulonephritis

▶ Risk is reduced with prompt diagnosis and treatment.

ILLNESSES OF UNKNOWN ORIGIN

Fever Without Localizing Signs

Description

▶ Fever 38.4°C (101.1°F) or higher at least once in 24 hours with no source of infection or cause for hyperthermia; also known as fever without focus. For children with fever longer than 10 days' duration, the term "fever of unknown origin" (FUO) is used; some experts suggest that fever should be present for 3 weeks as an outpatient or 1 week as an inpatient before the term FUO is applied.

Etiology

▶ The principal causes of FUO are rheumatologic disease, infection, and neoplasm; drug fever is uncommon.

▶ Most FUOs result from atypical presentations of common diseases.

Incidence and Demographics

▶ Fever without localizing signs or symptoms, usually of acute onset and present for less than 1 week, is a common diagnostic dilemma in children younger than 36 months of age.

▶ An infectious agent, usually viral, is identified in 70% of infants younger than 3 months of age with fever.

Risk Factors

▶ Independent of age, fever with petechiae with or without localizing signs indicates high risk of life-threatening bacterial infections such as bacteremia, sepsis, and meningitis.

Prevention and Screening

▶ Have routine wellness exams.

▶ Avoid infected people.

▶ Seek medical attention if fever does not resolve with rest, fluids, and antipyretics within 24 hours of onset.

Assessment

History

▶ Note onset of fever, degree, duration, diurnal variation.

▶ Changes in environment, foods, and/or lifestyle changes around time of fever onset, particularly history of exposure to animals (domestic and wild), travel history

▶ Uncommon dietary habits or pica, tick bites, ethnic background, family history of disease

▶ Recent sick contacts (healthcare workers or day care)

▶ Medications and transfusions

▶ Number of school days missed

▶ Family stresses

▶ Review systems; particularly note intermittent rashes, arthralgia, weight loss, behavior changes

Physical Exam

▶ May be entirely normal, or demonstrate mild findings such as clear rhinorrhea

▶ Absence of sweating: may indicate familial dysautonomia

Diagnostic Studies

▶ CBC with differential and platelets: Blood, urine, and CSF cultures should be obtained, as indicated.

▶ Consider ESR, chest X-ray, and TB skin testing.

▶ The course of action and diagnostic studies performed should be individualized based on presentation and child's age.

Differential Diagnosis

▶ Inflammatory disease

▶ Viral illness

▶ Bacterial infections

▶ Neoplasm

▶ Abscess

▶ Familial dysautonomia

▶ Hypothalamic dysfunction

▶ Drug fever

Management

Nonpharmacologic Treatment

▶ Maintain hydration, good nutrition, adequate sleep.

▶ Treat symptomatically.

Pharmacologic Treatment

▶ See Box 4–1.

Special Considerations

▶ Do not prescribe or administer aspirin or aspirin-related products to patients under 19 years of age.

When to Consult, Refer, Hospitalize

▶ All HIV-infected infants, children, adolescents, pregnant women, and adults presenting with FUO should be referred and followed by an HIV specialist knowledgeable for that age group/circumstance.

Follow-Up

▶ If not hospitalized, follow-up in 1 to 3 days, depending on age of child, degree of fever; occasionally, source of infection will become identifiable in time.

▶ If blood or CSF cultures are positive and a child is not hospitalized, admit and treat with IV antibiotics.

Complications

▶ Children with FUO have a better prognosis than do adults, depending on primary disease process, which is usually an atypical presentation of a common childhood illness.

BOX 4–1.

GUIDELINES FOR MANAGEMENT OF FEVER

Infants <1 Month of Age

- Infants may acquire community pathogens; also at risk for late-onset neonatal bacterial diseases and perinatally acquired herpes simplex virus infection
- CBC, blood culture, urine culture; consider lumbar puncture and culture
- Always treated aggressively in hospital; maintain on prophylactic antibiotics for 3 days pending culture results. Some practitioners hospitalize infants <3 months of age if no focus of infection found on PE in office.

Infants Between 1 and 3 Months of Age

- Serious bacterial disease occurs in 10%–15%, including bacteremia in 5%, of febrile infants <3 months old.
- Infants who appear generally well, have been previously healthy, have no focus for infection, total WBC 5,000–15,000 cells/mm^3, absolute band count <1,500 cells/mm^3, and normal urinalysis are unlikely to have a serious bacterial infection. The negative predictive value of these criteria for serious bacterial infection is >98%, and >99% for bacteremia.
- CBC, blood culture, urine culture; consider lumbar puncture
- Usually treated aggressively with 24-hour hospital observation and prophylactic antibiotics
- If CBC is within normal limits and adequate follow-up assured, consider treatment with IM ceftriaxone pending culture results.

Children >3 Months of Age/Adults

- Low-grade fever: Give antipyretics and observe.
- Acetaminophen 15mg/kg/dose no more than q.4.h. and no more than five doses in 24 hours
- Ibuprofen 10 mg/kg/dose if >6 months old; no more than q.6.h. and no more than four doses in 24 hours
- Fever >102°F, obtain a CBC. If WBC is >15,000/mm^3, obtain a blood culture and administer IM Ceftriaxone. Obtain urine culture in boys younger than 6 months and girls younger than 2 years; some providers obtain urine cultures on all children with high fever and no focus for infection found on exam.

▶ In many cases, no diagnosis can be established, and fever abates spontaneously.

▶ In as many as 25% of cases in which fever persists, cause of fever remains unclear, even after thorough evaluation.

Kawasaki Disease

Description

▶ Acute, self-limiting, multisystem vascular illness with rash and fever; also known as mucocutaneous lymph node syndrome

▶ Leading cause of acquired heart disease in children in the United States

Etiology

▶ Unknown; most likely infectious

Incidence and Demographics

▶ 80% of cases in children younger than 5 years old (peak age 18 to 24 months); 5% of cases in children older than 10 years old; rare over age 15

▶ 1.5:1 male-to-female ratio

▶ Recurrence low

▶ No clear genetic pattern, although incidence is lowest among White Americans and highest among Americans of Asian and Pacific Island descent

▶ Epidemics in the United States seem to occur during the winter and spring in 2–3 year intervals.

▶ No person-to-person spread, although siblings seem to be affected at higher rate.

Risk Factors

▶ Unknown

Prevention and Screening

▶ Unknown

Assessment

History

▶ May report recent history of cold, cough, or ear infection

▶ Persistent fever, red mouth and lips, and swollen hands with rash

Physical Exam

▶ Erythematous mouth and pharynx with "strawberry tongue" and red, swollen, and cracked lips

▶ Bulbar conjunctivitis without exudate

▶ Cervical lymphadenopathy—usually unilateral, involves at least one node swollen to more than 1.5 cm diameter

▶ Polymorphous, generalized, erythematous rash

▶ Induration of hands and feet

▶ Periungual and groin desquamation may occur.

Diagnostic Criteria

▶ Persistent fever plus four of the five criteria in Box 4–2 *or*

▶ Persistent fever plus three of the criteria in Box 4–2 and evidence of coronary artery abnormalities

▶ Infants—may have atypical Kawasaki disease; irritability, abdominal pain, diarrhea, vomiting may be apparent with coronary artery disease

BOX 4–2.

DIAGNOSTIC CRITERIA FOR KAWASAKI DISEASE

Adapted from *Red Book 2012*, American Academy of Pediatrics: Elk Grove Village, IL.

Persistent fever >5 days without an identifiable source, presence of four of five other clinical criteria, and unresponsive to antibiotics; diagnosis can be made if fever and only three criteria are met along with documented coronary artery disease

1. Mucous membrane involvement (erythematous mouth, pharynx; strawberry tongue; dry, fissured lips)
2. Non-purulent bilateral conjunctivitis
3. Polymorphous, erythematous, generalized rash
4. Cervical lymphadenopathy involving at least one node ≥1.5 cm in diameter
5. Polymorphous exanthema

Diagnostic Studies

▶ None available; nonspecific tests include ESR, platelet counts, serum C-reactive protein

▶ CBC with differential: WBC usually elevated with left shift (increased band forms); thrombocytosis develops in second week

▶ ECG, echocardiogram indicated to assess presence of cardiac or coronary artery disease

Differential Diagnosis

▶ Rickettsial diseases

▶ Rubella

▶ Rubeola

▶ Scarlet fever

▶ Rheumatic fever

▶ Epstein-Barr virus

▶ Drug reaction (Steven-Johnson syndrome)

▶ Lyme disease

▶ Juvenile rheumatoid arthritis

▶ Scalded skin syndrome

▶ Toxic shock syndrome

Management

Nonpharmacologic Treatment

▶ Supportive: rest, fluids, protection of skin (lubrication, good hygiene)

▶ No tart or acidic beverages

▶ Bland diet (secondary to mouth ulceration)

Pharmacologic Treatment

▶ High-dose aspirin as anti-inflammatory (80–100 mg/kg/day four times a day); dose reduced after acute phase to prevent coronary thrombosis; if coronary artery abnormalities present, continue low-dose aspirin therapy (3–5 mg/kg) indefinitely

▶ High-dose immune globulin intravenous (IGIV) therapy (2 g/kg as single dose)—initiate as soon as possible; efficacy questionable if initiated after 10th day of illness

▶ Initiation of aspirin and IGIV within 10 days of fever onset—substantially reduces prevalence of coronary artery dilation and aneurysms

▶ Hold measles and varicella immunizations for 11 months after IGIV therapy; if at high risk for measles exposure, may immunize and repeat immunization after 11 months

Special Considerations

▶ Aspirin therapy in patients under 19 years of age should be monitored closely due to risk of Reye's syndrome.

When to Consult, Refer, Hospitalize

▶ All suspected cases of Kawasaki disease are managed in a hospital.

▶ Refer all suspected cases to a cardiologist.

Follow-Up

▶ Long-term management depending on degree of cardiac involvement; echocardiogram in 6 to 8 weeks

Expected Course

▶ Without treatment, fever resolves in 12 days; other symptoms, 6 to 8 weeks after onset

▶ Myocardial infarction and sudden death may occur months to years later.

Complications

▶ Bacterial superinfection (desquamating skin)

▶ Coronary aneurysms

▶ Pericardial effusion

▶ Myocarditis

▶ Myocardial infarction

▶ Arthritis and arthralgia

▶ Jaundice, liver, and gallbladder problems

▶ Aseptic meningitis

INFECTIONS FROM BIOWEAPONS (BW)

Description

▶ Biological agents with bioweapons potential are characterized as Category A agents. These agents can be easily disseminated or transmitted from person to person, cause high mortality with potential for major public health impact, and require prompt action. Numerous viruses, several bacteria, and toxins may be used as weapons, but those that are known to have been weaponized, have effective dispersal methods, and be environmentally stable include anthrax, botulism, plague, smallpox, tularemia, and viral hemorrhagic fevers (Ebola, Marburg, Lassa, dengue, yellow fever, and others).

Etiology

▶ Naturally occurring organisms that have been altered to increase lethality

Incidence and Demographics

▶ Smallpox is no longer found in a wild form; all other potential bio-agents occur naturally. Inhalation anthrax is rare, although dermatologic infection is still found fairly often in farm workers. Large-scale outbreaks of botulism have never occurred.

Risk Factors

▶ Any population can be at risk, although bioweapons attacks are more likely to occur in densely populated, urban areas or at large, crowded events, such as sporting events.

Prevention and Screening

▶ Primary care providers must maintain an elevated level of suspicion.

▶ Family nurse practitioners must be aware of modes of transmission, incubation periods, and communicable periods of these diseases; an excellent source of information is the CDC Emergency Preparedness and Response website: http://emergency.cdc.gov/.

Assessment

History

▶ Symptoms for most agents may initially mimic those of common viral illnesses and include fever, fatigue, malaise, muscle aches, headache, cough, vomiting, diarrhea, rashes.

▶ For most agents, symptoms will quickly increase in intensity and severity.

▶ The first indication of an unannounced biologic attack is likely to be an unusual increase in number of people seeking care.

Physical Exam

▶ Ill-appearing patient, often out of proportion to degree of illness prevalent in the community

Diagnostic Studies

▶ Blood cultures, CBC, electrolytes

▶ Other studies dictated by clinical picture

Differential Diagnosis

▶ Common wild virus agents (fifth disease, coxsackie, varicella)

▶ Other potential biological agents

Management

Nonpharmacologic Treatment

▶ Rapidly isolate patient and contacts.

▶ Refer to infectious disease specialists.

▶ Rapidly notify public health authorities.

▶ Psychological and mental health problems brought on by the event will require significant expertise.

Pharmacologic Treatment

▶ See Table 4–5.

▶ Empiric therapy may be indicated if large numbers of people present with a nonspecific febrile illness in a limited time frame and location under credible threat of attack. Empiric therapy is ciprofloxacin or doxycycline orally or IV at routine recommended doses.

Special Considerations

▶ Appropriate management of postexposure prophylaxis and its complications will be critical in containing spread of infection.

When to Consult, Refer, Hospitalize

▶ Anthrax, botulism, hantavirus, plague, and tularemia must be reported to the CDC.

Follow-Up

Complications

▶ Dependent on agent

▶ Most potential agents have high lethality, 30% to 100%.

TRANSMISSION-BASED PRECAUTIONS

Contact Precautions

These are used in addition to standard precautions when caring for patients with known or suspected diseases that are spread by direct or indirect contact. These include methicillin-resistant *Staphylococcal aureus* (MRSA), vancomycin-resistant *Enterococcus* (VRE), and *Clostridium difficile*. Contact precautions include gloving and gowning when in contact with the patient, objects, and surfaces within the patient's environment. All reusable items should be cleaned and disinfected according to organizational policy, and disposable items should be thrown away immediately after being used.

TABLE 4-5.
POTENTIAL BIOWEAPONS AGENTS

BIOLOGICAL AGENT	TRANSMISSION/ INCUBATION	CLINICAL PRESENTATION	DIAGNOSIS	MANAGEMENT
Anthrax (*bacillus anthracis*): Gram-positive, spore-forming aerobic rod that causes cutaneous or pulmonary infection	Inhalation of aerosolized spores; person-to-person transmission does not occur Incubation up to 6 weeks	Biphasic, with initial prodrome of nonspecific febrile flulike illness. May be followed by brief period of improvement, then rapid onset of high fever, severe respiratory distress. Shock, death within 24–36 hours.	Chest X-ray shows mediastinal widening; Gram-positive bacilli on unspun peripheral blood smear	Ciprofloxacin or doxycycline for 60 days; standard contact precautions Prophylaxis should be offered with the same agents. A vaccine is available, but supply is limited. Raxibacumab, new drug containing antibodies which neutralize anthrax toxins
Cutaneous anthrax does not have BW potential.	1–7 days	Skin blisters	History, clinical, wound culture	7–10 day antibiotic course
Botulism: Caused by neurotoxin produced by Clostridium botulinum, a spore-forming, obligate anaerobe found in soil. Botulinum toxin is the most lethal natural poison known.	Toxin can be aerosolized; sources of entry include wounds, GI and respiratory tracts. It can also be dispensed in food. There is no person-to-person transmission. Incubation 12–36 hours.	Symmetric cranial neuropathies (e.g., drooping eyelids, weakened jaw clench, difficulty swallowing, speaking), blurred vision or diplopia, symmetric descending weakness in a proximal-to-distal pattern, respiratory dysfunction	Routine laboratory tests usually unremarkable. Definitive diagnostic testing for botulism available only at the CDC; diagnosis is primarily clinical.	Supportive care, including ventilator support Passive immunization with equine antitoxin

Plague (*Yersinia pestis*): Non-motile bacillus	Bubonic: transmitted by bites from infected fleas of rodents; most common type Pneumonic: inhalation of respiratory droplets from a human or animal with respiratory plague; may be aerosolized Secondary cases would occur from contact with infected persons. A BW attack most likely to produce pneumonic plague. Incubation 2–4 days.	Bubonic: enlarged, painful, regional lymph nodes (buboes), fever, chills, headache, malaise, GI symptoms, and prostration Pneumonic: fever, weakness, and rapidly developing pneumonia with shortness of breath, chest pain, cough, and sometimes bloody or watery sputum Can be fatal without treatment.	Clinical diagnosis important as treatment must begin in <24 hours. Large numbers of patients with severe pneumonia, particularly if accompanied by hemoptysis, must trigger prompt presumptive treatment and isolation. Prophylaxis of close contacts	Streptomycin, gentamicin, tetracycline, or chloramphenicol begun within 24 hours greatly improves prognosis; isolation and supportive care necessary Prophylactic therapy begun within 7 days is very effective in preventing infection. Vaccine under investigation.
Smallpox: Caused by a DNA virus in the orthopox-virus family	Person-to-person transmission; spread by inhalation of air droplets or aerosols. Smallpox virus is specific for humans; animal infection does not occur. Weaponized smallpox can be spread by aerosol or by bombs or missiles. Secondary infection would occur from direct person-to-person spread, via both droplet and infected fomites (clothing, bedding). Incubation 12–14 days.	High fever, malaise, severe aching pains, prostration Later, a papular rash develops over the face and spreads to the extremities, soon becomes vesicular and later, pustular. Rash is most dense on face.	Patients are most contagious from time of onset of rash until scabs form. Initial diagnosis must occur at a military facility. After confirmation of community disease, subsequent diagnoses made on basis of clinical presentation.	No known effective antiviral agents Treatment is supportive. All potentially infected persons should be hospitalized in their homes. In event of widespread outbreak, specific hospitals would be designated for treatment of smallpox patients. Widespread vaccination would be indicated; smallpox vaccine is effective only if administered within 4 days of exposure. Vaccine is available, though supply is government-controlled.

CONTINUED

BIOLOGICAL AGENT	TRANSMISSION/ INCUBATION	CLINICAL PRESENTATION	DIAGNOSIS	MANAGEMENT
Tularemia (*Francisella tularensis*): Gram-negative coccobacillus. Type A most virulent and likely to be weaponized. Very small amount (10–50) organisms can produce disease.	Naturally occurring in temperate areas of North America, Europe, and Asia. Weaponized tularemia can be delivered via aerosol, with infection occurring secondary to inhalation, skin or mucus membrane contact, or GI exposure from contaminated soil, water, food, or animals. Person-to-person transmission is not known to occur. Incubation 1–4 days, depending on virulence of strain, site, and size of inoculums.	Presentation dependent on route of administration. Inhalation most likely Symptoms include abrupt onset of fever with progression to pneumonia and respiratory disease, hilar lymphadenopathy and pleuritis. Inhalation can also cause sepsis without respiratory symptoms; this syndrome has a high fatality ratio.	No means of rapid testing is widely available. Diagnosis is initially clinical. *F. tularensis* may be identified by culture done in biological safety level (BSL) 3 labs.	Streptomycin IM or gentamicin IV for infection Ciprofloxacin or doxycycline at usual doses recommended for mass casualties or postexposure Vaccine is not widely available and immunity is incomplete.

Viral Hemorrhagic Fevers (VHFs): A group of illnesses caused by several distinct RNA viruses (Arenaviridae, Bunyaviridae, Filoviridae, Flaviviridae), including Ebola hemorrhagic fever*, Marburg virus, Lassa fever, hantavirus pulmonary syndrome (HPS)	Humans are not the natural reservoir of these viruses and are infected when they come into contact with secretions of infected hosts. Ebola, for example, is spread through direct contact with the blood or body fluids of a person who's sick with EVD or objects contaminated with the virus. However, humans can transmit some viruses to one another, after the accidental transmission from the host. Naturally occurring human cases occur sporadically. Incubation dependent on virus.	Specific signs and symptoms vary by the type of VHF; initial signs and symptoms include marked fever, fatigue, dizziness, muscle aches, loss of strength, and exhaustion. Patients often show signs of bleeding under the skin, in internal organs, or from body orifices (mouth, eyes, ears, etc.). Full-blown VHF evolves to shock and generalized bleeding from the mucous membranes.	High index of suspicion, detailed travel history important Lab findings supportive of infection vary, typically leucopenia, thrombocytopenia occur Immunoglobulin (Ig) M antibody by enzyme linked immunosorbent assays (ELISA) during the acute illness Diagnosis by viral cultivation requires 3–10 days and can only be done at BSL 4 labs (CDC, military facilities).	There is no cure or established drug treatment for VHFs, though ribavirin has been tried with Lassa fever and recent drug therapy has advanced for EVD. Therapy is supportive and barrier isolation techniques should be initiated, including guidance by the CDC for donning and doffing personal protective equipment (PPE) for healthcare workers (HCWs). Vaccines are newly available for EVD.

*Ebola virus disease (EVD) is a rare, but deadly, disease that wasn't diagnosed in the United States until 2014. Four (non-weaponized) cases were confirmed, including three healthcare workers who were exposed while caring for EVD patients in the United States and in the African nation of Guinea. Although the risk of exposure in the United States is minimal, thorough assessment and identification of persons who've traveled to parts of the world where EVD is prevalent are imperative to prevent the spread of the disease, as is strict adherence to infection control guidelines specific to EVD.

Droplet Precautions

These require the use of a surgical mask in addition to standard precautions when you're within 3 feet (6 feet for smallpox) of a patient known to have or suspected of having a disease spread by droplets. These include influenza, pertussis, and meningococcal disease. HCWs should observe droplet precautions when examining a patient with respiratory symptoms, especially if the patient has a fever. These precautions should remain in effect until it's determined that the symptoms aren't caused by an infection that requires droplet precautions.

Airborne Precautions

These are used in addition to standard precautions when in contact with patients with known or suspected diseases spread by fine particles transmitted by air currents, such as tuberculosis, measles, and severe acute respiratory syndrome (SARS). You must wear a National Institute for Occupational Safety and Health (NIOSH)–certified, fit-tested N-95 respirator just before entry into an area shared with a patient suspected or known to have one of these diseases. If eye protection is needed, wear goggles or a face shield during all contact with the patient, not just if you predict splashes or sprays.

DONNING AND DOFFING PERSONAL PROTECTIVE EQUIPMENT (PPE)

All HCWs involved in the care of EVD patients must have training in the proper use of PPE. No skin should be exposed while working in the PPE. A trained observer must supervise every step of the PPE donning/doffing procedure to ensure that the established protocol has been followed.

Donning PPE

▶ The gown should fully cover the torso from the neck to the knees, the arms to the wrists, and wrap around the back. It should be tied at the neck and waist.

▶ Nonsterile gloves should cover the wrist of the gown. They should be put on after the gown.

▶ The mask's ties should be secured at the back of the head and at the neck. The flexible noseband should be fitted to the bridge of the nose. The mask should fit snugly to the face and extend below the chin.

▶ The goggles and face shield should be adjusted to fit the face.

▶ After the PPE is in place, you should work from clean to dirty and limit the surfaces touched. Keep your hands away from your face. The equipment should be changed if torn or heavily contaminated.

▶ Perform hand hygiene before and after putting on PPE.

Doffing PPE

▶ Remove all PPE before leaving the patient room or anteroom. Remember that the outside of all equipment is considered contaminated.

▶ To remove gloves, grasp the outside of one glove in the palm of the opposite hand and peel off. Hold the removed glove in the gloved hand, while sliding fingers of the ungloved hand under the remaining glove at the wrist and peeling off.

▶ To remove goggles and face shield, handle by the clean headband or earpieces.

▶ Remove the gown by unfastening the neck and waist ties and peeling it from each shoulder toward the same hand, turning the gown inside out. Hold the removed gown away from the body, roll it into a bundle, and discard.

▶ Without touching the front of the mask, remove the mask by grasping the ties.

▶ Perform hand hygiene.

TROPICAL/GLOBAL DISEASES

See Table 4-6.

TABLE 4-6.
TROPICAL/GLOBAL DISEASES

DISEASE	TRANSMISSION METHOD	INFECTED COUNTRIES	SEVERITY/SYMPTOMS	TREATMENT/PREVENTION
Chagas disease (American trypanoso-miasis)	Parasite transmitted by infected reduviid bugs	South and Central America; now >300,000 cases in the U.S.	Skin lesion, fever, anorexia, lymphadenopathy, hepatosplenomegaly, carditis; later — dementia, heart failure, wt. loss	Benznidazole and nifurtimox Prevention: avoid buildings made of mud, adobe, and thatch
Chikungunya	Vector-borne virus (arbovirus) spreads via the Aedes aegypti and Aedes albopictus mosquitoes	Certain regions of Africa, Asia, Europe; spreading to Caribbean & Central America w/ 232 cases reported in the U.S. now	Fever, malaise, polyarthralgia, headache, myalgia, rash, lymphopenia; rarely fatal	NSAIDs, hydration, rest Antiviral agents, monoclonal antibody treatments, and several vaccines are in various stages of development.
Cholera	Bacterial infection transmitted in contaminated food or water	Developing countries with poor sanitation; more common in warm months	Perfuse, watery diarrhea, abdominal pain, vomiting lasting 1–3 days; can be fatal with profound dehydration	Tetracycline, oral rehydration Prevention: risk generally considered low to travelers and vaccine not available in U.S.
Dengue fever	Vector-borne virus (arbovirus) spreads via the Aedes aegypti	Any tropical or subtropical country, greater risk in cities	High fever, severe headache, vomiting, backache, eye pain, myalgia, arthralgia, rash x 2–7 days; rarely hemorrhagic	Acetaminophen, hydration, blood transfusions Prevention: protection against daytime mosquitoes
Japanese encephalitis	A number of different viruses carried by mosquitoes	Worldwide although high-risk areas include China, Korea, India, SE Asia	Headache, stiff neck, confusion, irritability, fever, weakness, dizziness, tremors, seizures, paralysis, lethargy, delirium, coma, death	Treatment: symptomatic only Prevention: Vaccine (Je-Vax) only recommended for rural areas in high-risk Asian countries for travel >30 days.
Leptospirosis	Exposure to the urine of animals by swimming or bathing in contaminated fresh water	Subtropical and tropical countries pose highest risk	High fever, severe headache, diarrhea, eye inflammation, internal bleeding, liver and kidney failure	Treatment: antibiotics as early as possible Prevention: Avoid fresh water activities in risk countries.
Malaria	Parasite transmitted by Anopheles mosquitoes	Found in every tropical and subtropical country in the world	Flu-like with possible nausea and vomiting, jaundice; fatal without prompt treatment Typically presents within 10–30 days of exposure but can occur up to 1 year	Treatment and prevention: mefloquine (Larium), atovaquone/proguanil (Malarone), or doxycycline Minimize mosquito exposure

Plague	Bacteria carried by rodents and transmitted by fleas	Africa, SE Asia, parts of South America and the U.S.; risk in rural, mountainous areas	Lymphadenopathy, fever, chills, headache, malaise, fatigue, and GI symptoms; can be fatal without treatment	Streptomcyin antibiotics, sulfonamides for children Prevention: insect repellents, avoid handling animals, consider preventive antibiotics Vaccine pending
Polio	Viral infection transmitted in contaminated water or food	Most developing countries in Africa, Asia, Central America, India, the Middle East, and Eastern Europe	Flu-like symptoms, fever, headache, stiff neck and back, myalgia; leading to paralysis. Can be fatal.	Treatment is symptomatic. Prevention: Universal immunization with vaccine is required in infancy. Booster necessary for adults traveling to endemic areas. Inactivated polio vaccine is used.
Rabies	Virus transmitted from exposure to saliva from an infected animal	Worldwide except Antarctica	Disease is nearly always fatal once symptoms develop.	Treatment: rabies IG after bite(s), vaccine, if not previously vaccinated (previously vaccinated only require booster vaccine); immediately clean wound thoroughly with soap and water Prevention: vaccine is available; does not eliminate need for treatment after exposure
Severe acute respiratory syndrome (SARS)	Coronavirus spread by infected droplets from coughing or sneezing	First identified in China in 2003; not currently active	High fever, cough, dyspnea, atypical pneumonia, acute respiratory distress	Supportive care Prevention: hand hygiene, avoid contact with SARS patients, vaccine in development
Typhoid fever	Bacterial infection with *Salmonella typhi* in contaminated food and water	Any region where food or water is contaminated; common after natural disasters in urban areas of poor countries	Flu-like symptoms, fever, diarrhea and/or constipation; untreated, can last up to 4 weeks and is fatal in 10% of cases; patient can remain infectious after resolution of symptoms	Antibiotics essential; ciprofloxacin is antibiotic of choice; oral rehydration. Prevention: vaccination recommended for travelers to high-risk countries >4 weeks; bottled water only
Yellow fever	Arbovirus transmitted by mosquito	African countries near the equator and in tropical parts of South America	Flu-like symptoms, headache, fatigue, fever, nausea, vomiting, constipation, jaundice, hemorrhagic fever; fatal in 23% of severe cases	Supportive care; lifetime immunity after illness Prevention: vaccination prior to traveling to endemic areas; required for entry into certain countries. Live vaccine contraindicated in pregnancy, infants, lactation, immunocompromised.

CASE STUDIES

Case 1

18-year-old male freshman complains of losing weight and fatigue x 1 month. He states he is chronically tired, can't get enough sleep, and feels feverish, but he doesn't have a thermometer in his dorm room. He has occasional aching joints. Of note is a cold a few weeks ago with a sore throat. He went to the university clinic at that time, had a rapid strep test done, and was told it was negative. He is concerned because he has missed more than eight classes this month.

PMH: Usually healthy. Few occasional colds. Was told he had a heart murmur but not sure if he still does. Chickenpox at age 8. No past surgeries or hospitalizations; not sure of his immunizations status. No current medications, NKDA.

1. Should you be concerned about measles, mumps, rubella, polio, diphtheria, or pertussis because he does not know if his immunizations are up to date?

2. What other history is needed?

Exam: No lymphadenopathy, pharynx pink without exudate, systolic murmur best heard over the 2nd ICS, no joint swelling or tenderness, no rash or skin lesions

1. What is your differential diagnosis?

2. What initial diagnostic and management plan is appropriate?

Case 2

6-year-old boy whose parents both are quite worried because his "hands are swollen and his eyes are red." Has had a low-grade fever for over 1 week; highest 101°F. Also had runny nose so mother thought he had a cold. Yesterday, his eyes were red, but they didn't notice anything about the hands. Today, eyes are very red, lips are red and swollen, and hands are swollen and beginning to peel.

PMH: No childhood illnesses; occasional colds; one or two ear infections as a baby. Bilateral hernia repair at age 9 months. Immunizations up to date.

1. What are you looking for in a physical exam?

2. What do you suspect from this child's presentation?

3. What is your management plan?

Case 3

14-month-old girl whose father states, "She had a high fever a few days ago. Now she has a rash."

HPI: Visited 4 days ago for persistent fever of 2-day history. Fever as high as 104°F. Diagnosed with viral syndrome and sent home with instructions for fever management and to push fluids. Now returns, afebrile, but has a light red rash on chest and back. Appetite poor, drinking liquids. Her face was flushed when she had the fever, but now face is pale.

PMH: History of recurrent otitis media, four episodes in 9 months. Immunizations up to date. No current medications.

1. What other history is needed?

2. What screening tests should be done?

3. What is the likely diagnosis and what management is appropriate?

CASE STUDIES DISCUSSION

Case 1

1. Should you be concerned about measles, mumps, rubella, polio, diphtheria, or pertussis because he does not know if his immunizations are up to date?

   No, it is unlikely that he has missed these immunizations because they would have been required upon entrance to college.

2. What other history is needed?

   Health of his roommates, dorm-mates, and friends; any rash, specific joint pain and swelling; how much weight has he lost; has he had any night sweats or cough; tick bite or outdoor exposure; and his sexual preference and partner history (how many, use of STI protection, any symptoms of STIs in partners), history and symptoms of STIs, any swollen glands, other associated symptoms

3. What is your differential diagnosis?

   Rheumatic fever, mononucleosis (unlikely with no lymphadenopathy), Lyme disease (dependent on history of exposure), HIV primary infection (unlikely without additional symptoms), viral illness (unusual to last this long and be unaccompanied by rash)

4. What initial diagnostic and management plan is appropriate?

   Aortic murmur is significant and rheumatic fever should be highly suspected. Immediate referral to cardiologist is essential with initiation of penicillin treatment. Initial diagnostic testing would include CBC, ESR, C-reactive protein, streptococcal antibody titer, ECG, and 2D-echocardiography.

Case 2

1. What are you looking for in a physical exam?

   Fever, cervical lymphadenopathy, rash, skin desquamation in groin; eye, ear, nose, throat exam for signs of local infection; cardiac exam for signs of pericarditis, myocarditis; neurologic exam for signs of meningitis; abdominal exam for hepatosplenomegaly; musculoskeletal exam for arthritis; skin for rash

2. What do you suspect from this child's presentation?

   Kawasaki disease

3. What is your management plan?

   Immediate referral to pediatric cardiologist

Case 3

1. What other history is needed?

   Her contact with other children and if any of them have been ill; does she seem to have a sore throat; how is she eating, sleeping; activity level

2. What screening tests should be done?

If sore throat is present, a throat swab and a CBC with differential will rule out group A B-hemolytic streptococcal infection.

3. What is the likely diagnosis and what management is appropriate?

Given the history of high fevers that relented on the onset of rash on day 4, is likely to be roseola. Expected PE findings would be a blanching erythematous maculopapular rash and may have adenopathy. Rule out otitis media. Continue supportive management.

REFERENCES

American Academy of Pediatrics. (2012). *Red book 2012: Report of the Committee on Infectious Diseases* (29th ed.). Elk Grove Village, IL: Author.

Burns, C., Dunn, A., Brady, M., Starr, N., & Blosser, C. (2009). *Pediatric primary care* (4th ed.). St. Louis, MO: Saunders.

Centers for Disease Control and Prevention. (2008a). *Preparation and planning for bioterrorism emergencies.* Retrieved from http://emergency.cdc.gov/bioterrorism/prep.asp

Centers for Disease Control and Prevention. (2008b). Summary of notifiable diseases. *MMWR: Morbidity and Mortality Weekly Report 57* (7), 179–183. Retrieved from http://www.cdc.gov/mmwr/preview/mmwrhtml/mm5707a4.htm

Centers for Disease Control and Prevention. (2012a). *Health information for the international travel,* NY: Oxford University Press.

Centers for Disease Control and Prevention. (2012b). *West Nile virus update: United States.* Retrieved from www.cdc.gov/ncidod/dvbid/westnile/index.htm

Centers for Disease Control and Prevention. (2013a). *Blood-borne infectious diseases: HIV/AIDS, hepatitis B, hepatitis C management and treatment guidelines.* Retrieved from http://www.cdc.gov/niosh/topics/bbp/

Centers for Disease Control and Prevention. (2013b). *Recommended immunization schedule for adults aged 19 years and older — United States, 2013.* Retrieved from http://www.cdc.gov/vaccines/adults/index.html

Centers for Disease Control and Prevention. (2013c). *Reported cases of Lyme disease by year, United States.* Retrieved from http://www.cdc.gov/lyme/stats/chartstables/casesbyyear.html

Centers for Disease Control and Prevention. (2015). *HIV by group.* Retrieved from http://www.cdc.gov/hiv/group/index.html

Centers for Disease Control and Prevention, Division of Global Migration and Quarantine. (2008b). *Protection against mosquitoes, ticks, fleas and other insects and arthropods.* Retrieved from http://www.cdc.gov/travel/yellowBookCh2-InsectsArthropods.aspx

Centers for Disease Control and Prevention, Division of Global Migration and Quarantine. (2013). *Lyme disease.* Retrieved from http://wwwn.cdc.gov/travel/yellowBookCh4-LymeDisease.aspx

Centers for Disease Control and Prevention, National Center for Immunization and Respiratory Diseases. (2008a). Notice to readers: Expansion of use of live attenuated influenza vaccine (FluMist®) to children ages 2–4 years and other FluMist changes for the 2007–08 influenza season. *MMWR: Morbidity and Mortality Weekly Report,* 56(46), 1217–1219. Retrieved from http://www.cdc.gov/mmwr/preview/mmwrhtml/mm5646a4.htm

Centers for Disease Control and Prevention, National Center for Infectious Disease. (2008b). *Parvovirus B19 (fifth disease).* Retrieved from http://www.cdc.gov/parvovirusb19/fifth-disease.html

Gilbert, D., Chambers, H. F., Eliopolis, G., Chambers, H., & Saag, M. (2014). *The Sanford guide to antimicrobial therapy* (44th ed.). Sperryville, VA.: Antimicrobial Therapy, Inc.

Goroll, A., & Mulley, A. (2014). *Primary care medicine: Office evaluation and management of the adult patient* (7th ed.), PA: Lippincott Williams & Wilkins.

Hamilton, R. J. (Ed.). (2015). *Tarascon pocket pharmacopoeia: 2015 deluxe lab-coat pocket edition* (16th ed.). Lompoc, CA: Tarascon (Jones & Bartlett Publishing).

Kaplan, J. E., Dominguez, K., Jobarteh, K., & Spira, T. J. (2015). Post-exposure prophylaxis against human immunodeficiency virus: New guidelines from the WHO: A perspective. *Clinical Infectious Diseases, 60*(Suppl 3), s196–s199.

Morbidity and Mortality Weekly Review (MMWR). (2013). Prevention of measles, rubella, congenital rubella syndrome, and mumps, 2013 summary recommendations of the ACIP, Vol. 62, #RR-04.

National Institutes of Health. (2013). *Recommendations for use of antiretroviral drugs in pregnant HIV-1-infected women for maternal health and interventions to reduce perinatal HIV transmission in the United States.* Retrieved from http://aidsinfo.nih.gov/guidelines

Papadakis, M. A., McPhee, S. J., & Rabow, M. W. (Eds.). *Current medical diagnosis and treatment 2015* (54th ed.), NY: Lange/McGraw-Hill.

Pickering, L. K., Baker, C. J., Kimberlin, D. W. & Long, S. S. (Eds.). *Red book: 2012 report of the Committee on Infectious Diseases* (29th ed). Elk Grove Village, IL: American Academy of Pediatrics.

South Carolina Department of Health and Environmental Control Bureau of Disease Control. (2012). *Childcare exclusion list.* Retrieved from http://www.scdhec.gov/health/childteenhealth/schoolexclusion/

U.S. Department of Health and Human Services, Food and Drug Administration. (2008). *Public health advisory: Nonprescription cough and cold medicine use in children.* Retrieved from http://www.fda.gov/CDER/drug/advisory/cough_cold_2008.htm

U.S. Department of Health and Human Services, Panel on Antiretroviral Guidelines for Adults and Adolescents. (2008). *Guidelines for the use of antiretroviral agents in HIV-1-infected adults and adolescents.* Retrieved from http://aidsinfo.nih.gov/contentfiles/AdultandAdolescentGL.pdf

U.S. Preventive Services Task Force. *The guide to clinical preventive services 2014: Recommendations of the U.S. Preventive Services Task Force.* (2014). Rockville, MD: Agency for Healthcare Research & Quality.

Wilson, W., Taubert, K. A., Gewitz, M., Lockhart, P. B., Baddour, L. M., Levison, M.,…Durack, D. T. (2008). Prevention of infective endocarditis: Guidelines from the American Heart Association. *Journal of the American Dental Association , 139* (Suppl 1), s3–s9, s11–s24. http://dx.doi.org/10.14219/jada.archive.2008.0346

CHAPTER 5

COMMON PROBLEMS OF THE SKIN
Deborah Gilbert-Palmer, EdD, MSN, FNP-BC

GENERAL APPROACH

▶ Dermatologic complaints can be indicative of a dermatological disorder or may prove to be symptomatic of a systemic problem.

▶ Dermatologic disorders can have a profound impact on the patient's self-image; psychological assessment has to be included in the history-taking and addressed in the treatment plan.

▶ Use proper terminology to describe dermatologic lesions (see Tables 5–1 and 5–2).

▶ The most important part of the assessment is a thorough history.

▶ The physical exam is best performed in a well-lit room with a penlight for illumination and shadowing (to determine if lesion is raised), a Wood's lamp for fluorescing certain types of lesions, a magnifying lens, glass slides for diascopy (to determine blanching) and skin scrapings, potassium hydroxide (KOH) solution (to illuminate hyphae), 5% acetic acid for aceto-whitening (to illuminate human papilloma virus lesions), mineral oil for suspected scabies, Giemsa or Wright stains, and a regular microscope.

▶ Assessment should also include appearance of the patient (comfortable, agitated, toxic) and vital signs, with direct admission or referral to an emergency department (ED) for the toxic patient. New comprehensive primary care initiative directs reserving ED referral unless no other inpatient facility is available.

TABLE 5–1.
MORPHOLOGIC DEFINITIONS FOR PRIMARY SKIN LESIONS

TERM	DEFINITION AND EXAMPLE	SIZE
Macule	Flat, non-palpable colored spot (freckle)	Up to 5 mm
Papule	Solid, elevated, circumscribed lesion (acne)	Up to 5 mm
Nodule	Solid, elevated, circumscribed lesion (erythema nodosum)	0.5–1.2 cm
Vesicle	Fluid-filled, elevated, circumscribed lesion (herpes simplex)	Up to 5 mm
Cyst	Encapsulated, fluid-filled mass (epidermoid cyst)	Variable
Bulla	Fluid-filled, elevated, circumscribed lesion (second-degree burn, severe poison ivy)	Larger than 5 mm
Pustule	Pus-filled, elevated, circumscribed lesion (acne)	Up to 5 mm
Wheal	A suddenly occurring transient elevation of the skin, circumscribed, may or may not be erythematous (hives, urticaria)	0.5 to 10 cm diameter
Tumor	Solid, elevated mass	Larger than 1 cm

TABLE 5–2.
MORPHOLOGIC DEFINITIONS FOR SECONDARY SKIN LESIONS

LESION	DEFINITION	EXAMPLE
Scale	Dry, greasy fragment of dead skin	Psoriasis
Crust	Dry mass of exudate	Impetigo
Ulcer	Sharply defined, deep erosion	Decubitus ulcer
Scar	Permanent skin change as a result of newly formed connective tissue	Burn scar
Lichenification	Induration and thickening of skin resulting from chronic scratching or rubbing	Eczema
Fissure	Linear split through dermis and epidermis	Cheilitis

Dermatologic Signs to Be Assessed and Documented

▶ Distribution of lesion (generalized or localized, central or peripheral, symmetric or asymmetric, predilection for certain body areas such as extensor or flexor surfaces and intertriginous areas, sun-exposed or pressure areas)

▶ Arrangement of lesions (discrete, confluent, scattered, linear, zosteriform, polycyclic, grouped, patchy, accurate, reticular, scarlatiniform)

▶ Shape or configuration of the primary lesion (annular, oval, nummular, iris, pedunculated, verrucous, umbilicated, gyrate, serpiginous)

▶ Color of lesions (erythematous, violaceous, hypomelanotic, depigmented, flesh-colored, hypermelanotic, variegated)

▶ Borders or margins of lesions (well-demarcated or ill-defined)

▶ Palpable qualities (soft, firm, mobile, fixed, hard, fluctuant, tender, hot/warm/cool, smooth, rough, indurated)

▶ Measured dimensions (diameter, width, length, elevation, depression)

▶ Descriptive terms (lichenified, atrophied, sclerosed, pigmented, friable, hyperkeratotic, weeping, crusted, mobile or nonmobile, hypertrophic/keloidal, excoriated)

▶ Morphology of primary and secondary lesions (see Tables 5–1 and 5–2)

▶ Associated symptoms involving hair, vision, nails, mucous membranes, lymphatic system, hepatosplenomegaly, and/or neurologic changes

Changes Associated with Aging

▶ Should be identified and recognized as normal, such as dermatoheliosis or photoaging of the skin evidenced by wrinkles and drying, pigment changes, pseudo scars, senile purpura, solar lentigines, alopecia, seborrheic keratoses (benign epithelial growths that occur with aging and become darkened in color; have a warty, greasy surface; and are raised papules or plaques, 1–3 cm in size, with a characteristic "stuck on" appearance; no treatment necessary unless skin cancer cannot be ruled out, then biopsy and excise)

Health Maintenance and Screening Guidelines

▶ Skin cancer is the most common cancer in the United States today.

▶ Sun exposure, especially early in life, has been identified as a risk factor.

▶ Primary prevention involves counseling patients to avoid sun exposure and to protect themselves with appropriate sunscreen and clothing.

▶ Secondary prevention involves screening for skin lesions with premalignant or malignant characteristics during routine health exams and referring patients at increased risk for melanoma to specialists.

▶ Tertiary prevention involves removal of precancerous lesions, such as suspicious moles and actinic keratoses.

▷ Actinic (solar) keratoses are due to sun exposure and may be precursors to squamous cell carcinoma. They are single or multiple, discrete, flat or slightly raised, dry, scaly, and brownish or reddish lesions up to 1.5 cm in size. They should be biopsied if inflamed or indurated. Techniques for removal include liquid nitrogen, curettage, laser ablation, or fluorouracil cream application.

Use of Topical Steroids

▶ Steroid medications should be ordered at the lowest dosage and duration.

▶ Table 5–3 ranks the topical steroids by potency.

▶ Fluorinated steroids result in thinning of the tissue when used long term; avoid using on the face and genital region.

TABLE 5–3.
COMMON TOPICAL STEROIDS (RANKED BY POTENCY, MOST TO LEAST)

GROUP	EXAMPLE
Group 1	Augmented betamethasone dipropionate ointment 0.05% (Diprolene)
	Clobetasolpropionate cream, ointment 0.05% (Topicort)
Group 2	Augmented betamethasone dipropionate cream
	Desoximetasone cream, gel, ointment 0.25% (Topicort)
	Fluocinonide cream, gel, lotion, ointment 0.05%
	Betamethasone valerate ointment 0.1% (Luxiq)
Group 3	Triamcinolone acetonide cream, lotion, ointment 0.05% (Kenalog)
	Flurandrenolide cream, lotion, ointment 0.05% (Cordran)
	Fluocinolone acetonide cream 0.2% (Vanos)
	Betamethasone valerate cream 0.1% (Luxiq)
Group 4	Desonide cream 0.05% (DesOwen)
	Fluocinolone acetonide cream 0.025% (Vanos)
	Hydrocortisone valerate cream 0.2% (Westcort)
	Hydrocortisone cream, ointment, lotion 2.5% (Hytone)

RED FLAGS

▶ *Anaphylaxis* may evolve rapidly from a variety of exposures, including drugs, exercise, food, insect stings, and latex; rapidly evolving symptoms may include hives, pruritus, flushing, shortness of breath, wheezing, tachycardia, difficulty swallowing, nausea, vomiting, abdominal cramping, and possible shock. Epinephrine (1:1,000) 0.3 to 0.5 mL for adults and 0.01 mL/kg for children should be administered immediately and every 20 minutes as needed, along with supportive care.

▶ *Necrotizing fasciitis* is a rapidly progressing deep infection of the subcutaneous tissue that presents as an area or rapidly enlarging erythematous, edematous plaque with a central area of necrosis, pain out of proportion to the degree of cellulitis, fever, and crepitation. It is caused by beta-hemolytic streptococcus and/or staphylococcus. Urgent hospitalization for debridement and IV antibiotics is essential to avoid excessive tissue loss or rapid multiple system failure.

▶ *Malignant melanoma* has five cardinal signs: asymmetry; border is irregular and often scalloped; color is mottled with variegated display of brown, black, gray, and/or pink; diameter is large (greater than 6.0 mm); and elevation is almost always present with subtle or obvious surface distortion, best assessed by side-lighting of the lesion.

ALLERGY

Contact Dermatitis

Description

▶ Cutaneous reaction to an external substance—either irritant or allergen—that may appear as an asymmetric distribution of red, raised, and/or inflamed rash, or rash only on exposed areas

▶ Includes metal, plant, chemical, or food substances

Etiology

▶ 80% of cases are due to universal irritants (soap, detergents, organic solvents). Irritant contact dermatitis is due to direct injury of the skin (e.g., from detergent).

▶ Allergic contact dermatitis results from previous immunosensitization; see poison ivy, oak, antimicrobials, adhesive tape, latex.

Incidence and Demographics

▶ Less common in Black people

▶ Common in all ages; age has no influence on sensitization; however, allergic contact dermatitis less common in young children

▶ Occupational sensitization a common cause of disability in industry

Risk Factors

▶ Exposure to irritant or allergen

▶ Prior sensitization to allergen

Prevention and Screening

▶ Protective clothing in presence of potential exposure

▶ Avoidance of known irritants/allergens

Assessment

History

▶ Pruritic rash in unnatural pattern on exposed skin

▶ Known exposure to irritant or allergen

▶ May include systemic symptoms of toxicity if extensive involvement

Physical Exam

▶ Morphology: erythematous papules, vesicles, or bullae on inflamed background; scaling, erythema, edema; thickened skin and weepy, encrusted lesions in chronic phase; local area hot and swollen

▶ Location/distribution: exposed skin surfaces in unnatural pattern, mimicking possible path of irritant

▶ Particular irritant or allergen may be obvious by location of symptoms

▶ Metal allergy: most common offender is nickel in jewelry and clothing

▷ Distribution: neck, wrists, waist, strap line, ear lobes

▷ Generally mild and chronic with scaling, pigmentation changes, and pruritus

▶ Plant dermatitis

▷ Distribution and arrangement: often linear pattern

▷ Most commonly caused by poison ivy, poison oak, and poison sumac

▷ Secondary signs: weeping, scaling, edema, crusting, and excoriation

Diagnostic Studies

▶ Clinical diagnosis; patch testing may be warranted for severe or recurrent episodes with unclear etiology

Differential Diagnosis

▶ Atopic dermatitis

▶ Impetigo

▶ Scabies

Management

Nonpharmacologic Treatment

▶ Remove offending irritant or allergen within 20 minutes; may require patch testing after episode is resolved.

▶ Wash potentially contacted clothing.

▶ Bathe in tepid water with soap to wash allergen/irritant off skin.

▶ Use cool compresses with astringent (Domeboro or Burow's solution) or colloidal oatmeal suspension (Aveeno) to treat pruritus.

Pharmacologic Treatment

▶ Oral antihistamines (diphenhydramine, hydroxyzine, loratadine, or cetirizine) should be used for pruritus (dose all pharmacologic interventions by weight in pediatric patients) with best time for administration before sleep because of sedating side effects.

▶ Topical antihistamines not currently recommended

▶ Topical steroids applied b.i.d.

▶ Systemic steroids for severe or extensive involvement

▷ Prednisone: Begin at 60 mg in adults and taper over 2 to 3 weeks, depending upon severity of symptoms.

▷ Medrol Dosepak considered inadequate dose for this condition

▶ Oral antibiotics for secondarily infected lesions

▶ UVA-UVB or PUVA treatments

How Long to Treat

▶ Length of treatment determined by extent of involvement and response; often 1 to 2 weeks

Special Considerations

▶ Steroids are contraindicated in pregnancy unless clinically warranted.

▶ Distribution of symptoms may help determine causative agent.

When to Consult, Refer, Hospitalize

▶ Consult with/refer to an allergist for patch testing if indicated.

▶ Hospitalization should be considered for toxic or unstable patients (infants, older adults).

Follow-Up

Expected Course
- ▶ The course is usually dictated by irritant or allergen and extent of involvement.
- ▶ Metal allergies tend to be low-level and chronic, with possible lichenification and hyperpigmentation.

Complications
- ▶ Toxicity and secondary infection

Urticaria

Description

- ▶ Represents reaction in dermis and subcutaneous tissues to various stimuli; characterized by erythematous wheals that appear on any part of the body
- ▶ The lesions may be round, oval, or form rings or arcs; often pruritic
- ▶ Acute urticaria—hives, or wheals, appear abruptly and may last 24 to 36 hours.
- ▶ Chronic urticaria—lesions persist for longer than 6 weeks.
- ▶ May occur along with angioedema or with generalized anaphylaxis

Etiology

- ▶ May be allergic or nonallergic, IgE-mediated or non-IgE–mediated hypersensitivity in which there is release of chemical mediators (histamine, prostaglandins, serotonin, kinins) from cutaneous mast cells that leads to increased vascular permeability
- ▶ Fluid extravasates from small blood vessels, causing typical lesions
- ▶ Many and varied causes—include foods, medicines, inhalants, infectious agents, physical factors (heat, cold, exercise, sunlight)

Incidence and Demographics

- ▶ Experienced by up to 20% of population at some point
- ▶ Can occur at any age; more common in children and adolescents

Risk Factors

- ▶ History of allergies, asthma, atopic diseases

Prevention and Screening

- ▶ Allergen avoidance
- ▶ Sunscreen or protective clothing if solar urticaria

Assessment

History
- ▶ Complete review of recent exposure to possible causative factors, such as medications, foods, injections, infections, inhalations, animals
- ▶ Family or personal history of previous episodes of urticaria, atopic disease

▶ Exposure to sun, cold, stress, water, exercise

▶ Chronic health problems

▶ Extent of pruritus

▶ Assess for any lip and hand swelling, shortness of breath, or signs of a more generalized reaction.

Physical Exam

▶ Mildly erythematous, blanching, flat-topped lesions with pale centers

▶ Lesions 2 mm–20 cm in diameter, scattered or coalesced, generalized or localized distribution

▶ May appear and fade within 24 hours; may reappear later

▶ Heat may intensify lesions

▶ Evaluate mucous membranes and airway

▶ Evaluate lungs for wheezing, BP for hypotension

Diagnostic Studies

▶ If fever, assess for infectious underlying cause and perform appropriate diagnostic tests as needed

Differential Diagnosis

▶ Erythema multiforme

▶ Contact dermatitis

▶ Juvenile rheumatoid arthritis

▶ Mastocytosis

▶ Pityriasis

Management

Nonpharmacologic Treatment

▶ Avoid suspected offending agent.

Pharmacologic Treatment

▶ Oral antihistamines such as diphenhydramine (Benadryl) 5 mg/kg/day in four divided doses or hydroxyzine 2 mg/kg/day in three to four divided doses

▶ Topical steroids not useful; systemic steroids are used for severe or extensive reactions

▶ Epinephrine (1:1,000) 0.01 mL/kg subcutaneously for signs of anaphylaxis; EpiPen for prophylaxis of bee sting by patient

How Long to Treat

▶ As long as needed to resolve symptoms

Special Considerations

▶ Angioedema and anaphylaxis occur by the same mechanism as urticaria.

▶ Angioedema occurs in up to 50% of children with urticaria and usually involves the face, hands, and feet.

▶ Anaphylaxis may evolve rapidly with the hives, accompanied by airway edema, pruritus, flushing, wheezing, tachycardia, difficulty swallowing, nausea, vomiting, abdominal cramping, and possible shock.

▶ A precise cause of the urticaria is often not found.

When to Consult, Refer, Hospitalize

▶ Refer to allergist or immunologist if persistent for more than 6 weeks.

▶ Immediately transfer to emergency facility if signs of anaphylaxis with emergency care en route.

Follow-Up

▶ Recheck if symptoms persist beyond 36 hours.

▶ Complications

▶ Angioedema, anaphylaxis, or secondary infection of site as a result of scratching

ECZEMATOUS CONDITIONS

Atopic Dermatitis

Description

▶ Chronic skin condition characterized by inflammation and intense itching along a typical pattern of distribution; presentation frequently varies according to the age and race of the patient; pruritus is most characteristic finding

▶ Scratch-itch-scratch cycle perpetuates and exacerbates problem.

▶ Infantile atopic dermatitis is usually erythematous and vesicular and is frustrating scratch-itch-rub cycle seen in infants, usually on the face, antecubital and/or popliteal fossae, and/or lateral legs.

▶ Childhood-type atopic dermatitis more often papular with lichenified plaques and appears as erosions and crusts as child scratches the sites.

Etiology

▶ IgE-mediated inherited dermatitis that involves abnormality in the cell-mediated immune system

▶ Often a manifestation of multisystem atopy, which includes asthma, allergic rhinitis, and atopic dermatitis

Incidence and Demographics

▶ Common condition; 66% have positive family history of atopic problems; inherited IgE-mediated hypersensitivity; frequent onset in infancy or early childhood (60% by 1 year)

▶ 12.5% of children between age of 0 and 17 years of age

▶ 75% to 85% of those with atopic dermatitis will develop allergic rhinitis; 50% of these will develop asthma

Risk Factors

▶ Positive family history of atopic problems; past medical history (PMH) of asthma, allergic rhinitis, or atopic dermatitis

▶ Dry environment; repetitive skin abrasion

▶ Emotional stress; hormonal factors (pregnancy, menses, thyroid); infections

Prevention and Screening

▶ Environmental controls

▶ Coping skills

▶ Management of pruritus

Assessment

History

▶ Pruritic rash in classic distribution

▶ PMH or family history of asthma or allergic rhinitis/dermatitis

Physical Exam

▶ Morphology: initially poorly defined erythematous patches, papules, or patches, with or without scales

▶ Develops into red, weeping, crusted patches; eventually become lichenified

▶ Distribution: extensor and exposed surfaces of infants

▶ Flexor folds: antecubital and popliteal fossae; wrists, neck, and forehead of older children and adults; upper trunk

▶ Associated findings: lichenification, excoriations, fissures and erosions, periorbital hyperpigmentation, rhinitis and/or asthma, dermatographism, keratosis pilaris, ichthyosis vulgaris, cataracts in up to 10% of patients

▶ Black people may lose pigmentation in lichenified areas

Diagnostic Studies

▶ Mainly a clinical diagnosis

▶ Increased serum IgE, eosinophilia; allergy testing

▶ Bacterial cultures to rule out *S. aureus;* viral cultures to rule out herpes simplex

Differential Diagnosis

▶ Seborrheic dermatitis

▶ Nummular eczema

▶ Psoriasis

▶ Dermatophytosis

▶ Scabies

▶ Contact dermatitis

Management

Nonpharmacologic Treatment

▶ Acute weeping lesions: humidify environment; decrease use of hot water, soap, and abrasive clothing

▶ Take long, soaking baths in warm water—pat dry; don't use abrasive towels/rubbing.

▶ Make liberal use of emollients and/or lubricating lotions after bathing; take oatmeal baths for pruritus.

▶ Relaxation techniques and behavior modification may be helpful in severe cases.

▶ Patients need to learn stress management techniques to control flare-ups as well.

Pharmacologic Treatment

▶ Use of bleach baths diluted twice weekly or more for severe cases (1/2 cup of bleach to 40 gallons of water)

▶ Oral antihistamines such as diphenhydramine (Benadryl) for pruritus

▶ Topical steroids b.i.d. sparingly, potency based on response

▶ Immunomodulators: pimecrolimus (Elidel) or tacrolimus

▶ Montelukast (Singulair): may use in children older than 2 years and adults

▶ Systemic steroids (prednisone) sometimes warranted in severe flare-ups; begin at 60 mg and taper down over 2 to 4 weeks

▶ May need oral antibiotics for secondarily infected lesions

▶ UVA-UVB and PUVA treatments for recalcitrant cases

▶ Tar preparations in those unresponsive to steroids

How Long to Treat

▶ Prednisone treatment should be limited to a 2-week tapered course.

▶ Topical preparations are used intermittently as symptoms warrant.

▶ Treat acute flares until controlled while maintaining and then continuing nonpharmacologic treatment; may require occlusive dressings at night for 2 to 6 weeks.

Special Considerations

▶ Systemic steroids are usually contraindicated in pregnancy and lactation.

▶ Geriatric patients are predisposed to atrophic skin and steroids exacerbate atrophy; use topical steroids of lower potency.

▶ *Nummular eczema* is a chronic, pruritic, inflammatory dermatitis in coin-shaped plaques of 4–5 cm; usually found on anterior aspects of the lower legs but may also appear on the trunk, hands, and fingers; pruritus is often intense.

▷ Secondary skin changes include exudative crusting, scaling, excoriation, lichenification, and post-inflammatory hyperpigmentation.

▷ Treatment is the same as for atopic dermatitis.

▶ *Dyshidrotic eczema* is an acute, chronic, or recurrent dermatosis of palms, fingers, and/or soles characterized by a sudden onset of deep pruritic rash on hands and feet, which may last for weeks.

▷   Initially clear vesicles in clusters on palms and soles; later scaling, lichenification, painful fissures

▷   Pruritus treated with wet dressings of Domeboro solution, oatmeal, high-potency corticosteroid cream b.i.d., oral antihistamines

▷   May need dermatology referral for intralesional steroid injections for small, localized involvement; systemic steroids for severe or extensive involvement; oral antibiotics for secondarily infected lesions; or possible PUVA treatments

When to Consult, Refer, Hospitalize

▶   Consult or refer patients with suboptimal response to above regimen to \ or for PUVA or UVA-UVB treatment.

Follow-Up

▶   Every 2 weeks until well-controlled

Expected course

▶   Chronic condition with subacute phases and acute flares

▶   Usually more symptomatic during winter months

Complications

▶   Secondary infection and/or cellulitis

▶   Skin atrophy, striae from overuse of topical steroids

Seborrheic Dermatitis

Description

▶   Chronic, recurrent, and sometimes pruritic inflammatory disease of skin where sebaceous glands are most active (face, scalp, body folds)

Etiology

▶   Unknown with questionable role of *Pityrosporum ovale*

Incidence and Demographics

▶   2% to 5% of population affected; males more than females

▶   Infancy ("cradle cap") and adults between 20 to 50 years

Risk Factors

▶   Family history

▶   HIV infection; zinc or niacin deficiency; Parkinson's disease

Prevention

▶   Daily cleansing of skin with soap, water, and cloth

Screening

▶   None

Assessment

History

▶ Gradual onset of greasy, scaly rash on face and scalp

▶ Possibly associated with *slight* pruritus

Physical Exam

▶ Usually see fine, dry, white, or yellow scale on erythematous base, or

▶ Dull red plaques with thick, white, or yellow, scaly, greasy lesions

▶ Morphology: yellowish-red, greasy, moist, sharply marginated lesions; 5–20 mm scaling macules and papules; in dark-skinned children, hypopigmentation may be present

▶ Distribution: scalp, eyebrow, eyelids, nasolabial folds, cheek, behind ears, intertriginous areas

▶ Secondary signs: possible inflammatory base, sticky crusting (more common on ears), fissures (more common at ear attachments to scalp)

Diagnostic Studies

▶ Diagnosis is usually made clinically.

Differential Diagnosis

▶ Psoriasis

▶ Impetigo

▶ Dermatophytosis

Management

Nonpharmacologic Treatment

▶ For infant scales: Use antiseborrheic shampoo three times per week; leave on for 5 minutes before rinsing. For stubborn infant scales, apply warm mineral or baby oil for 10 minutes before shampoo.

▶ Adolescents: Avoid cold creams and moisturizers, which may plug sebaceous glands.

▶ Remove scaling of eyelashes with baby shampoo.

Pharmacologic Treatment

▶ Shampoo frequently with selenium sulfide (Selsun or Exsel), tar (Polytar, T-Gel or Tegrin), or zinc (Head & Shoulders) shampoos.

▶ Salicylic acid may be helpful in removing crusts.

▶ Use hydrocortisone lotion for stubborn areas, and/or ketoconazole (Nizoral) cream.

▶ Treatment of face includes sulfur-based soap.

▶ Use topical steroids (1% hydrocortisone lotion with sulfur).

▶ *Do not use fluorinated steroids on the face, such as Betamethasone dipropionate 0.05% (Diprolene).*

How Long to Treat
- ▶ Chronic condition requires initial therapy until symptoms resolve, followed by maintenance therapy of ketoconazole shampoo, lotions, and/or topical steroids q.d.

Special Considerations
- ▶ Systemic steroids contraindicated in pregnancy and lactation unless clinically warranted.

When to Consult, Refer, Hospitalize
- ▶ Consult or refer for unresponsive cases.

Follow-Up
- ▶ Visits every 1 to 2 months during maintenance phase to monitor disorder and for signs of skin atrophy

Expected Course
- ▶ Chronic condition requiring initial treatment phase and maintenance therapy

Complications
- ▶ Secondary infection
- ▶ Skin atrophy, striae from chronic topical steroids

ACNE

Acne Vulgaris and Nodulocystic Acne
Description
- ▶ A polymorphic disorder of the pilosebaceous unit characterized by inflammation and a variety of lesions ranging from comedones to inflamed cysts on the face, upper torso, and back
  - ▷ Acne vulgaris consists of open and closed comedones, inflamed papules, and pustules.
  - ▷ Nodulocystic acne or acne conglobata consists of cysts, abscesses, and sinus tracts.
  - ▷ Acne fulminans is the most severe form and features suppuration of lesions; the patient may have systemic symptoms such as fever and arthritis.

Etiology
- ▶ Five factors usually involved:
  1. Excess keratin plugging of the sebaceous follicles
     - ▶ Increased androgen production during puberty; some pathologic conditions such as polycystic ovarian syndrome (POS) affect sebum production
     - ▶ Pore-blocking cosmetics and trauma from harsh scrubbing may affect keratinization and blocking of the sebaceous duct; retention of sebum, overgrowth of *Propionibacterium acnes*

2. Bacterial colonization with *Propionibacterium; P. acnes* commonly found in the pilosebaceous unit of healthy skin but proliferate in the impacted sebaceous duct

3. Sebum overproduction and increased androgenic production; disordered functioning of the pilosebaceous unit includes excessive sebum production, abnormal follicular keratinization (comedogenesis)

4. Inflammation due to distention of the hair follicle with *P. acnes* and sebum

5. Genetics

Incidence and Demographics

▶ Most common skin condition; present in 80% to 85% of all adolescents because of increased androgen production

▶ Males more than females; light-skinned more than darker-skinned

▶ May persist into the second decade of life; then more common in women

▶ Flare in perimenopausal women because of elevated unopposed adrenal androgens

Risk Factors

▶ Elevated circulating androgen hormones as described above

▶ Use of follicle-blocking cosmetics and hair spray

▶ Oral contraceptives with high progestin component; anticonvulsants; systemic or topical steroid use

▶ Genetic predisposition, male

Prevention and Screening

▶ Good daily skin hygiene, avoidance of follicle-blocking cosmetics

Assessment

History

▶ Onset associated with puberty or androgen excess

▶ May include history of use of oil-based cosmetics and/or harsh scrubbing

Physical Exam

▶ Mild to moderate acne, or acne vulgaris

▷ Presence of comedones, inflamed papules, pustules and cysts on face, upper torso and back

▶ Open comedones, or "blackheads" (follicular orifice is dilated)

▶ Closed comedones, or "whiteheads" (plug in the sebaceous duct enlarges)

▷ Inflamed papules and pustules result from the proliferation of *P. acnes*

▶ Severe acne or nodulocystic acne

▷ Cysts and nodulocystic lesions develop as plug enlarges; may result in sinus tracts forming under skin; inflamed cysts develop as abscesses

▷ Possible presence of scarring from healed lesions

Diagnostic Studies

▶ None are necessary unless the patient has acne fulminans and appears toxic, then CBC and blood cultures are appropriate; bacterial culture may be indicated to rule out folliculitis; serologic testing

Differential Diagnosis

▶ Rosacea

▶ Abscess

▶ Cutaneous manifestations of systemic lupus erythematosus (SLE)

▶ Furunculosis

▶ Tinea barbae

▶ Folliculitis

Management

Nonpharmacologic Treatment

▶ Gentle washing b.i.d. with mild soap such as Dove, Basis, or Neutrogena, or non-comedogenic cleanser

▶ Avoid oil-based cosmetics and hairsprays as these plug follicles.

▶ Avoid picking or squeezing lesions as this may lead to scarring.

Pharmacologic Treatment

▶ Acne vulgaris

  ▷ Keratolytic topical agents, including benzoyl peroxide 5% and 10% q.d. to b.i.d. or salicylic acid 0.5% to 10% in many OTC preparations

  ▷ Topical antibiotics, including erythromycin 1% to 2% gel q.d. or b.i.d. or clindamycin 1% gel or solution q.d. or b.i.d.

  ▷ Antibacterial/keratolytic agent azelaic acid (Azelex) 20% cream q.d. x 2 weeks then b.i.d.

  ▷ Topical comedolytic agent tretinoin (Retin-A) 0.025% to 0.1% cream or gel bid or adapalene (Differin) 0.1% gel q.d. to b.i.d. Reassess in 12 weeks for improvement.

  ▷ Antiandrogen therapy through oral contraceptives such as Ortho Tri-Cyclen

▶ Nodulocystic acne and widespread acne or acne resistant to other therapies

  ▷ Oral antibiotics such as erythromycin 250 mg q.d. to t.i.d.; minocycline 50 to 100 mg q.d. to b.i.d.

  ▷ Systemic isotretinoin 0.5–2 mg/kg/day in two divided doses

How Long to Treat

▶ Treatment is long-term and may continue for years. Topical agents should be started individually or with a combined keratolytic and antibiotic such as Benzamycin gel q.d. and increased to b.i.d. after 1 to 2 weeks to avoid excessive drying from these products.

▶ Start oral antibiotics b.i.d. to t.i.d. and taper over time to q.d. after improvement is achieved.

▶ Systemic isotretinoin should be used for 15 to 20 weeks; treatment may restart after 2 months off the drug.

Special Considerations

▶ Patients need to be advised that minimal response is to be expected in the first 4 to 6 weeks of therapy, and optimal response may take several months on the various regimens.

▶ Patients should be started on a single agent, with the addition of other agents as tolerated.

▶ Because all of the topical treatments can be drying, it is important to start slowly (q.d. with one agent) and increase to b.i.d., adding second and third agents one at a time.

▶ Sex: Females with polycystic ovaries or other hyperandrogenism and females with late-onset acne may benefit from the use of oral contraceptives with low androgenic activity.

▶ Race: Darker-skinned people are more likely to develop post-inflammatory hyperpigmentation. Azelaic acid cream possesses hypopigmentation properties and may be useful in limiting post-inflammatory hyperpigmentation.

▶ Most anti-acne drugs (topical and oral) cause photosensitivity reactions; sun exposure should be limited, and liberal use of oil-free sunscreen gel is advised.

▶ Pregnancy and lactation: Isotretinoin (Accutane) is a teratogen and must be avoided. **Women of childbearing age must be strongly counseled to use reliable contraception for 1 month before, during, and for 1 month following use of this drug.**

▶ Laboratory monitoring for patients on isotretinoin includes lipid panel, CBC, liver function tests (LFT), and glucose.

When to Consult, Refer, Hospitalize

▶ Referral to a dermatologist is appropriate if a suboptimal response is achieved after adequate trial on two or three of the above drugs and if isotretinoin is being considered.

Follow-Up

▶ Initial follow-up every 2 months until stable regimen established with successful control

Expected Course

▶ Long-term management often necessary for several years

Complications

▶ Excess drying of the skin from topical agents

▶ Potentially severe side effects with isotretinoin, such as pseudotumor cerebri (increased risk with tetracycline), pancreatitis, hepatotoxicity, corneal opacities, blood dyscrasias, premature epiphyseal closure; pregnancy category X

Acne Rosacea

Description

▶ Chronic acneform inflammation of central third of face

▷ Does not involve any comedones—the classic lesion of acne vulgaris

Etiology

▶ Cutaneous vascular disorder of unknown etiology with increased reaction of capillaries to heat ("flushing")

▶ Sebaceous gland hyperplasia

▶ Ocular manifestations such as conjunctivitis, blepharitis, and episcleritis occur

Incidence and Demographics

▶ Predominantly affects women in 35- to 50-year age range

▶ Severe form with rhinophyma is seen almost exclusively in men over age 40

Risk Factors

▶ Found more commonly in persons with fair skin who burn and rarely tan

▶ Positive family history of rosacea is risk factor; more common in those with migraine headaches

▶ Excessive ETOH consumption associated with flares

Prevention and Screening

▶ None

Assessment

History

▶ History of abnormal flushing of the central portion of the face after drinking hot or alcoholic beverages or eating spicy foods

Physical Exam

▶ 2 to 3 mm papular and pustular discrete and clustered lesions on central portion of face on an erythematous base; rosy coloration of nose, chin, cheeks; no comedones

▶ Dilatation of the superficial capillaries causes flushing and eventually leads to telangiectasia.

▶ Ocular symptoms such as blepharitis or keratitis may be associated.

▶ Chronic symptoms can lead to lymphatic changes causing cellulitis.

▶ Irreversible hypertrophy of the nose (rhinophyma) is a result of chronic inflammation and is seen almost exclusively in men over age 40.

Diagnostic Studies

▶ Based on clinical presentation; culture or biopsy not necessary

Differential Diagnosis

▶ Acne vulgaris

▶ Butterfly rash of SLE

▶ Cellulitis

▶ Folliculitis

Management

Nonpharmacologic Treatment

▶ Includes avoidance of triggers that cause facial flushing such as hot beverages, ETOH, highly spicy foods, exposure to sun and wind, emotional stress, and certain medications such as niacin

Pharmacologic Treatment

▶ Topical metronidazole (Metrogel) 0.75%, erythromycin 2%, or clindamycin (Cleocin T) gel b.i.d.

▶ Tetracycline 250 mg orally t.i.d. or b.i.d.

▶ Doxycycline (Vibramycin) 100 mg orally b.i.d.

▶ Minocycline (Minocin) 50–100 mg orally b.i.d.

▶ Erythromycin 250 mg orally t.i.d. or b.i.d.

How Long to Treat

▶ Long-term initially at b.i.d. or t.i.d. dosing, tapering down to q.d. maintenance dosing

▶ If no improvement with above regimens, a trial of trimethoprim-sulfamethoxazole (TMP-SMX), oral metronidazole (Flagyl), dapsone, or isotretinoin may be considered.

Special Considerations

▶ Pregnant and lactating women, use erythromycin

▶ Menopausal women who are experiencing flushing associated with hormonal fluctuations may benefit from hormone replacement therapy (HRT) or clonidine (Catapres) if HRT is contraindicated.

When to Consult, Refer, Hospitalize

▶ If response is suboptimal, refer to dermatologist.

Follow-Up

▶ 2 to 4 weeks initially; once patient responds to therapy, self-management appropriate with family nurse practitioner follow-up visits annually

Expected Course

▶ Initial response usually within 3 weeks, maximum response by 9 weeks

Complications

▶ Rhinophyma as described above; may require surgical debulking

Hidradenitis Suppurativa

Description

▶ Chronic suppurative disease of the apocrine gland region of the axillae, anogenital region, breasts, and scalp with development of sinus tracts and scarring

Etiology

▶ Unknown; may be genetic predisposition toward occlusion of the follicular orifice leading to retention of secretions, nodular formation, abscesses, draining sinuses, and eventual scarring

Incidence and Demographics

▶ Race: all, but with more extensive involvement in Black people

▶ Age: puberty to climacteric

▶ Sex: more commonly found in axillae in females, in anogenital region in males

Risk Factors

▶ Family history

▶ Nodulocystic acne

▶ Obesity

▶ Apocrine duct obstruction (antiperspirant use)

Prevention and Screening

▶ Management of obesity

▶ Avoidance of antiperspirants in people who have had previous problems with them

Assessment

History

▶ Recurrent painful lesions with suppuration in the axillae and/or anogenital area

Physical Exam

▶ Abscess of axillae and/or anogenital region, erythematous nodules

▶ Seropurulent/purulent drainage from single or multiple openings on skin

▶ Hypertrophic scarring, keloid and sinus tract formation

▶ Dilated open comedones, often double comedones which are characteristic

▶ Lymphedema possible

Diagnostic Studies

▶ Cultures not usually indicated because multiple pathogens colonize

Differential Diagnosis

▶ Furuncle or carbuncle

▶ Cat-scratch disease

▶ Ruptured inclusion cyst

▶ Lymphadenitis

In Anogenital Involvement

▶ Sinus tracts and fistulas associated with ulcerative colitis and enteritis

▶ Lymphogranuloma venereum

Management

Nonpharmacologic Treatment

▶ Local heat; keep the area clean and dry

▶ Weight loss; avoidance of antiperspirants

Surgical Treatment

▶ Initially incision and drainage acute abscesses

▶ Excision of nodules or marsupialization of sinuses in chronic cases

▶ Complete excision of axillae or involved anogenital area to the fascia with split skin grafting for extensive, chronic disease

Pharmacologic Treatment

▶ Oral antibiotics until resolution (may takes weeks). Examples include:

▷ Erythromycin 250–500 mg q.i.d.

▷ Minocycline (Minocin) 100 mg b.i.d.

▷ Tetracycline 250–500 mg b.i.d.

▷ Doxycycline 50–100 mg b.i.d.

▶ Intralesional triamcinolone (5 mg/mL) diluted with lidocaine injected into wall of lesion, followed by incision and drainage

▶ Oral prednisone taper (70 mg q.d. initially, tapered over 14 days)

▶ Oral isotretinoin 0.5–2 mg/kg/day in two divided doses

How Long to Treat

▶ Chronic and recurrent disease: Treat episodic flares with oral antibiotics; steroids as above.

▶ For frequent flares or extensive involvement, continuous antibiotics are indicated pending surgical intervention.

Special Considerations

▶ Erythromycin is recommended for pregnant women.

When to Consult, Refer, Hospitalize

▶ Referral to a surgeon is indicated for extensive and/or chronic involvement.

Follow-Up

▶ Weekly during flare

Expected Course
- ▶ Usually recurrent flares, but may be resolution after surgery
- ▶ Often spontaneous remission toward end of third decade of life

Complications
- ▶ Fistulas to urethra, bladder, and/or rectum
- ▶ Anemia of chronic disease

PAPULOSQUAMOUS ERUPTIONS

Pityriasis Rosea

Description
- ▶ Common, maculopapular, red scaly, sometimes pruritic rash appearing on trunk and proximal extremities; self-limiting with spontaneous remission

Etiology
- ▶ Unclear but most likely viral

Incidence and Demographics
- ▶ More common in spring and fall months and in temperate climates
- ▶ Age 10 to 35 years; 50% more common in women; young adults most commonly affected

Risk Factors
- ▶ Sharing a household with an affected person

Prevention and Screening
- ▶ None

Assessment

History
- ▶ Single, large herald patch appearing most commonly on trunk, followed in 1 to 2 weeks by generalized exanthem; mild to moderate pruritus
- ▶ No systemic symptoms but may be preceded by viral-like illness

Physical Exam
- ▶ Initial lesion is "herald patch": 2 to 6 cm, round, scaly plaque, usually on trunk
- ▶ Generalized fine, oval, 3 to 7 mm papules and plaques with fine "collarette" scale
- ▶ Distribution on trunk, often in Christmas tree pattern, following skin lines

Diagnostic Studies
- ▶ None; clinical diagnosis; may do KOH scraping to rule out tinea

Differential Diagnosis

▶ Drug eruptions

▶ Secondary syphilis

▶ Guttate psoriasis

▶ Tinea corporis

▶ Tinea versicolor

▶ Seborrheic dermatitis

▶ Erythema migrans

Management

Nonpharmacologic Treatment

▶ UV or natural sunlight exposure

Pharmacologic Treatment

▶ None usually necessary, but may use oral antihistamines or topical corticosteroids to relieve pruritus

How Long to Treat

▶ Spontaneous remission in 6 to 8 weeks

Special Considerations

▶ None

When to Consult, Refer, Hospitalize

▶ No need

Follow-Up

▶ For patient reassurance or when diagnosis is in question

▶ Complications rare but may be post-inflammatory hypo- or hyperpigmentation

FUNGAL AND YEAST INFECTIONS

Fungal (Dermatophyte) Infections

Description

▶ Persistent superficial fungal infection of the keratinized layer of the skin, including the stratum corneum (epidermomycosis), nails (onychomycosis), and hair (trichomycosis)

▶ Infections named by body part involved or, in the case of tinea versicolor, for the multicolored appearance

Etiology

▶ Caused by several dermatophytes with regional predominance

▶ Three common dermatophytes in the United States: *Microsporum, Trichophyton,* and *Epidermophyton*

▶ Can be spread by direct contact with an active lesion on an animal or another human; with fomites such as clothing, linens, or gym mats; or, rarely, from the soil

Incidence and Demographics

▶ Affects all ages, races, genders; Black adults believed to have lower incidence

▶ More common in tropical climates, warmer months in temperate climates

▶ More common in immunocompromised, including when secondary to prolonged use of topical steroids, with greater risk of intractable infection

Risk Factors

▶ Heat and humidity

▶ Obesity

▶ Immunocompromised: decreases host resistance to fungal infection

▶ Diabetes

Prevention and Screening

▶ Climate control as appropriate: air conditioning; loose, cotton clothing

▶ Management of obesity

▶ Air drying or using an electric hair dryer to completely dry intertriginous areas

▶ Complete drying of athletic shoes between wearings

▶ Frequently changing shoes, white cotton socks during day; wearing sandals

▶ No sharing of combs, brushes, or hair ornaments

▶ Avoid occlusive ornaments: acrylic nails; synthetic jewelry, belts, shoes

Assessment

History

▶ Known exposure to others with tinea or high-risk population

▶ Mild to moderately pruritic localized "rash" or isolated lesion

Physical Exam

▶ Presentation differs based on location of lesion: tinea corporis (scalp), tinea manus (hand), tinea facialis (face); exposed areas, commonly known as ringworm

　▷ Scaling erythematous plaque ranging from less than 1 cm up to 20 cm

　▷ Varying shapes: annular (round), arciform, or polycyclic

　▷ With or without pustules/vesicles

　▷ Usually has an elevated, sharp border with central clearing

　▷ Color is erythematous or hyperpigmented

　▷ Tinea manuum may be bilateral (50%), may occur with tinea pedis or tinea cruris

▷ May be confused with granuloma annulare, which is similar in appearance but is a self-limiting condition of the hands, feet, elbows, and knees

▶ Tinea cruris (groin), commonly known as jock itch

▷ Similar but usually arciform or polycyclic and duller red in coloring

▷ Often coexists with tinea pedis; infection transferred from feet to groin

▷ Maceration common in intertriginous areas

▶ Tinea pedis (foot), commonly known as athlete's foot

▷ Erythema, maceration between toes

▷ Diffuse desquamation with superficial white scales and possible bulla formation

▷ Hyperkeratosis of soles

▷ Painful fissuring/cracking along lateral borders of the soles and toe webs

▷ Usually bilateral foot involvement

▶ Tinea versicolor (trunk and neck)

▷ Superficial *Pityrosporum orbiculare* yeast that colonizes all human skin

▷ Clinically significant only in some persons

▷ Hypo- or hyperpigmented nummular macules

▷ Discrete, scattered, or confluent patches

▷ Usually asymptomatic but may be mildly pruritic

▶ Trichomycosis (hair): tinea capitis (head) and tinea barbae (beard)

▷ Involves dermatophyte invasion of the hair follicle by *trichophyton* dermatophytes

▷ Inflammation of the hair follicle, alopecia

▷ Painful, boggy, suppurative nodules with crusting/scabs

▶ Onychomycosis (nail): tinea unguium

▷ Nails become white, brown, yellow, or black; thicken and surface becomes roughened; eventually separate from nail bed

Diagnostic Studies

▶ Wood's lamp: Tinea capitis fluoresces green.

▷ Tinea versicolor fluoresces faint yellow-green scales.

▷ Tinea cruris does not fluoresce, but Wood's lamp exam can differentiate erythrasma, a bacterial infection that fluoresces coral-red.

▶ KOH mount: Skin scrapings placed on a slide in 10% to 30% KOH solution with a cover slip, viewed under a microscope after warming for 30 to 60 seconds, will demonstrate mycelia and hyphae.

▷ Tinea versicolor appears as long hyphae and few buds ("spaghetti and meatballs").

▶ Fungal cultures can identify a fungus but usually take weeks to grow.

  ▷ Indicated only when an infection is resistant to treatment

Differential Diagnosis

Based on location of lesions; includes many scaling skin disorders such as

▶ Psoriasis

▶ Erythrasma

▶ Candidiasis

▶ Contact dermatitis

▶ Seborrhea

▶ Dyshidrotic eczema

▶ Atopic dermatitis

▶ Lichen simplex chronicus

▶ Lichen planus

▶ Pityriasis rubra pilari

▶ Pityriasis rosea

▶ Erythema migrans

▶ Polymorphic light eruption

▶ Phototoxic drug eruption

▶ SLE

▶ Beard folliculitis

▶ Scabies

▶ Impetigo

▶ Ecthyma

Management

Nonpharmacologic Treatment

▶ Treat chronic, immunocompromising conditions.

▶ Follow preventive measures described above.

Pharmacologic Treatment

▶ Initial treatment with topical antifungal preparations such as clotrimazole 1% (Lotrimin), ketoconazole 2% (Nizoral), terbinafine 1% (Lamisil); apply to affected area, including a 2-cm peripheral border, and rub in b.i.d.

▶ Topical selenium sulfide 2.5% shampoo to skin for 30 minutes, then wash off for tinea versicolor; repeat 2 weeks later

▶ Use systemic antifungal agents for widespread, recurrent, or resistant infections, as well as onychomycosis.

▶ Apply ciclopirox (Penlac) 8% topical solution (nail lacquer) to nail and 5 mm of surrounding skin daily (remove with alcohol weekly) for up to 48 weeks for onychomycosis.

▶ Dosage

▶ Griseofulvin 250 to 500 mg b.i.d. (children more than 30 lbs: 5 mg/lb of body wt/day), adults 250–500 mg daily

▷ Ketoconazole (Nizoral) 200 mg q.d.(children older than 2 years: single dose of 3.3 to 6.6 mg/kg)

▷ Terbinafine (Lamisil) 250 mg q.d. (not indicated in children)

▷ Itraconazole (Sporanox) 200 mg q.d. (may use pulsing dose of 200 mg b.i.d. x 1 week, no meds x 3 weeks then repeat; not indicated in children)

How Long to Treat

▶ Resolution is slow, and treatment length depends on the location of the dermatophytosis; all take several weeks.

▷ Tinea capitis and tinea barbae: 4 to 6 weeks

▷ Tinea corporis, tinea manuum, tinea facialis: 4 to 6 weeks

▷ Tinea cruris: 2 to 4 weeks

▷ Tinea versicolor: 4 to 6 weeks

▷ Tinea pedis: 4 to 12 weeks

▷ Tinea unguium: 8 to 12 months

Special Considerations

▶ Side effects from systemic antifungal agents include hepatotoxicity and lowering of serum testosterone. LFTs should be evaluated before starting oral agents and q 4 to 6 weeks thereafter.

▶ Most antifungals are pregnancy category C; terbinafine is category B.

▶ Breastfeeding is not recommended with antifungal use.

When to Consult, Refer, Hospitalize

▶ Refer to a dermatologist for extensive involvement or unresponsive infection.

▶ Consider hospitalization for immunosuppressed patients with extensive disease.

Follow-Up

▶ Q 4 weeks for reevaluation and LFTs

Expected Course

▶ Relapse is common.

Complications

▶ Loss of hair, nails

Candidiasis (Moniliasis)

Description

▶ Yeast-like superficial fungus that causes pruritic rash on moist cutaneous and mucosal sites in vulnerable persons when local immunity is interrupted

Etiology

▶ *Candida* species (*Candida albicans* [most common], *Candida glabrata, Candida tropicalis*) that are normal inhabitants of mucosal surfaces and intestinal tracts of healthy persons

▶ Infection occurs when local or systemic immunity of host disrupted

Incidence

▶ All ages, both sexes equally, and all races can be affected.

▶ In babies, most commonly in the diaper region

Prevention and Screening

▶ None

Risk Factors

▶ Predisposing factors that alter immunity; immunocompromised states: HIV and chronic debilitation

▶ Chemotherapy or broad-spectrum antibiotic therapy; diabetes or poly endocrinopathies

▶ Maceration from repeated immersion in water, skin folds

▶ Occlusive clothing that traps moisture such as diapers or rubber boots; diapers' plastic outer covering

▶ Hyperhidrosis (excessive sweating); obesity with redundant skin folds

▶ Corticosteroid use

▶ Pregnancy and oral contraceptives

Assessment

History

▶ Pruritic and/or burning sensation and rash in characteristic locations such as intertriginous areas, anogenital region, and redundant skin folds

▶ Painful or sensitive white, "stuck on" lesions of the oral mucosa with decreased taste and odynophagia ("thrush")

▶ White curd-like vaginal discharge usually associated with pruritus, external dysuria, and dyspareunia (vulvovaginitis)

▶ Painful fissuring of the foreskin of uncircumcised males with dysuria

▶ Painful, inflamed nail folds, discolored nails, and a creamy discharge (paronychial candidiasis)

▶ Painful, congested ear canal with moist exudate (otitis externa)

Physical Exam

▶ Bright red, smooth macules

▶ Maceration is typical of all intertriginous infections

▶ Scaling elevated border

▶ "Satellite" lesions: similar macules outside main lesion

▶ Oral and vaginal candidiasis: white, stuck on but removable plaques on inflamed mucosa

▶ Balanoposthitis: flattened pustules, edema, erosions, fissuring on erythematous surface of penis

▶ Candida otitis externa: edematous ear canal with macerated appearance and moist, white, scaly exudate

Diagnostic Studies

▶ 5% KOH preparation under microscope demonstrates buds and pseudohyphae in clusters.

▶ Cultures may be done to identify specific species but *usually* are not done because it takes 1 to 2 weeks for results.

Differential Diagnosis

Oral Candidiasis

▶ Hairy leukoplakia

▶ Pernicious anemia

▶ Geographic tongue

▶ Bite irritation

Genital Candidiasis

▶ Bacterial vaginosis

▶ Lichen planus

▶ Condyloma acuminatum

▶ Scabies

▶ Inverse pattern psoriasis

▶ Erythrasma

Intertriginous Areas

▶ Eczema

▶ Atopic dermatitis

▶ Contact dermatitis

▶ Dermatophytosis

Paronychial Candidiasis

▶ Herpetic whitlow

▶ S. *aureus* paronychia

Management

Nonpharmacologic Treatment

▶ Management of underlying predisposing factors such as obesity, diabetes

▶ Air exposure of affected areas, such as diaper region in infants

▶ Careful drying of intertriginous areas and redundant skin folds

▶ Wear cotton undergarments; avoid tight, synthetic clothing

Pharmacologic Treatment

▶ Oral (thrush)

  ▷ Nystatin (Mycostatin) oral suspension 4–6 mL (adults), 2 mL (children), swish and swallow q.i.d.

  ▷ Clotrimazole 10 mg troches 3–5x/day (3 years and older), dissolve in mouth

  ▷ Systemic ketoconazole (Nizoral) 200 mg p.o. q.d. to b.i.d. (adults; usually not recommended in children), fluconazole (Diflucan) 100 mg p.o. q.d. to b.i.d. (adults; check manufacturer literature for children), itraconazole (Sporanox) 100 mg p.o. q.d. (adults; not recommended for children)

  ▷ Amphotericin B 3/mg/kg/day IV for resistant cases in immunocompromised hosts

▶ Intertriginous and anogenital infections

  ▷ Castellani paint x 1 (Phenol Topical)

▶ Topical antifungal: clotrimazole 1% cream, miconazole (Monistat) 2% cream, ketoconazole (Nizoral) 2% cream, econazole (Spectozole) 1% cream, terconazole (Terazol) 0.4 or 0.8% cream, terbinafine (Lamisil) 1% cream or solution bid, tolnaftate (Tinactin) 1% cream, solution, powder applied bid

  ▷ Nystatin cream or ointment applied b.i.d. to t.i.d. to diaper area in infants

  ▷ Oral antifungal treatment as described above may be necessary in extensive or recurrent infections or when host immunity is suppressed.

  ▷ Oral fluconazole (Diflucan 150 mg) x 1 has been successful in treatment of vaginal candidiasis (see Chapter 13).

How Long to Treat

▶ Oral candidiasis: 10 to 14 days

▶ Intertriginous and anogenital candidiasis: 1 to several weeks, depending on extent of the infection and the immune status of the host

▶ Paronychial candidiasis: 2 to 4 weeks

Special Considerations

▶ Immunosuppressed patients are subject to extensive and recurrent infections and may require a daily maintenance dose to limit recurrences.

When to Consult, Refer, Hospitalize

▶ Immunosuppressed patients with extensive or severe candidiasis, particularly oral/esophageal candidiasis, may require hospitalization or home IV infusion therapy of amphotericin B and nutrition supplementation.

Follow-Up

▶ Patients should be seen in 2 to 4 weeks and p.r.n. to evaluate progress.

Expected Course

▶ Resolution can be expected in patients without immunosuppression, but predisposing factors such as obesity and poorly controlled diabetes mellitus may make recurrences common.

Complications

▶ Secondary infection of excoriated lesions

▶ Weight loss secondary to odynophagia with esophagitis

BACTERIAL INFECTIONS OF SKIN

Cellulitis

Description

▶ Acute bacterial infection of the dermis and subcutaneous tissues; spreads in rapid, diffuse manner

▶ Erysipelas is type of cellulitis, usually of the face, caused by beta-hemolytic streptococci and accompanied by fever and malaise

Etiology

▶ Usually caused by beta-hemolytic streptococci and *Staphylococcus aureus*; may also be caused by *Haemophilus influenzae* in children, *Pseudomonas aeruginosa* from hot tubs, and *Pasteurella* from animal bite wounds, especially cats

▶ Occurs when break in skin allows bacteria to enter, most commonly in children younger than 3 years and older adults

Incidence and Demographics

▶ Common in all age groups

Risk Factors

▶ Breaks in the skin from lacerations, abrasions, excoriations; underlying dermatosis; previous cellulitis

▶ Diabetes mellitus; hematologic malignancies

▶ IV drug use; immunocompromised; chronic lymphedema (after mastectomy or coronary artery grafting)

Prevention and Screening

▶ Discourage scratching; maintain short, clean nails

▶ Meticulous diabetic foot care

Assessment

History

▶ May be unaware of original break in skin

▶ Possible history of fungal infection or dermatitis of the affected area

▶ Possible fever, malaise, anorexia, pain increased with weight-bearing

▶ Possible airway occlusive symptoms if cellulitis involves the face (erysipelas)

Physical Exam

▶ Puncture wound, fissure, or laceration may be visible.

▶ Erythematous plaque that is edematous, hot, and tender with sharply defined, ir-regular border

▶ Vesicles, bullae, abscesses may be seen within the plaque.

▶ Possible erythematous streaking (lymphangitis)

▶ Regional lymphadenopathy

▶ Toxic signs may be present, especially if involved area is large or if patient is immu-nocompromised or a child.

▶ *Necrotizing fasciitis,* deep infection of subcutaneous tissue, appears as a large erythematous plaque with a central area of necrosis; beta-hemolytic streptococcus is usually the invading organism; staphylococcus may or may not be involved. Refer immediately to diminish tissue loss or death.

Diagnostic Studies

▶ Culture lesion; blood cultures (false negatives in about 75% of the cases)

▶ In facial cellulitis, culture of cerebrospinal fluid

▶ Bone scan if lesion on heel or hand to rule out osteomyelitis

▶ CBC, WBC, and sedimentation rate indicated if patient appears toxic

Differential Diagnosis

▶ Deep vein thrombosis or thrombophlebitis

▶ Early contact dermatitis

▶ Giant urticaria

▶ Fixed drug eruption

▶ Necrotizing fasculitis

▶ Swelling over septic joint

▶ Erythema migrans

▶ Early herpes zoster

Management

Nonpharmacologic Treatment

▶ Rest, immobilization, and elevation of the involved extremity (bed rest if leg is involved)

▶ Application of hot, moist compresses x 20 to 30 minutes q.i.d.

Pharmacologic Treatment

▶ Oral antibiotics that cover Gram-positive organisms:

▷ Dicloxacillin (Dycill) 250–500 mg q.i.d. x 5 to 10 days (children: 12.5–25 mg/kg/day q.i.d. x 10 days)

▷ Erythromycin 250–500 mg x 5 to 10 days (children: 30–50 mg/kg/day q.i.d. x 10 days)

▷ Cephalexin (Keflex) 250–500 mg q.i.d. x 5 to 10 days (children: 25–50 mg/kg/day q.i.d. x 10 days)

▶ For human bites, amoxicillin/clavulanate (Augmentin) 875/125 mg b.i.d. (adults; see manufacturer recommendations for children)

▶ Ceftriaxone (Rocephin) 250 mg to 1 g IM q.d. (same in children)

▶ Ceftriaxone (Rocephin) 1 g IV q.d. for more severe infections (same in children)

▶ NSAIDs p.r.n. for analgesia, fever treatment, and to decrease inflammation

How Long to Treat

▶ 5 to 10 days, depending on extent of involvement

Special Considerations

▶ Young children, immunocompromised patients, and patients with synthetic heart valves are at greater risk of toxicity and may warrant hospitalization.

▶ Medical management of predisposing conditions such as diabetes, IV drug use, malignancies, or chronic lymphedema will augment the treatment of cellulitis.

When to Consult, Refer, Hospitalize

▶ Hospitalize if toxic symptoms, facial cellulitis, or debridement necessary.

▶ Refer to surgeon or infectious disease specialist if the patient is not responding to therapy.

Follow-Up

▶ The erythematous plaque should be outlined with an indelible pen on initial assessment, and the patient should return daily for the first few days to monitor progression or regression of the involved area.

Expected Course

▶ Resolution is expected in 5 to 10 days

Complications

▶ Toxicity or septicemia

▶ Patients with diabetes may lose leg following severe cellulitis.

▶ Lymphedema may result from recurrent erysipelas.

Impetigo

Description

▶ Primary or secondary superficial bacterial infection of the skin leading to nonbullous or bullous impetigo or to ecthyma, a deeper infection involving the dermis

▶ Characteristic skin lesion is honey-colored crust

▶ Characterized by its autoinoculable nature

Etiology

▶ *S. aureus*, group A beta-hemolytic streptococci, or mixed bacteria

▶ Organism gains access through breaks in integrity of skin caused by trauma, scratching, scaling, or inflammation

▶ Secondarily infected preexisting dermatitis is "impetiginization"

Incidence and Demographics

▶ Accounts for 10% of all skin problems in general outpatient pediatrics

▶ More prevalent in urban areas with poverty and overcrowding

▶ More common in young children ages 2 to 7 years

Risk Factors

▶ Young age; may be endemic in day care centers or schools; contact sports

▶ Poor hygiene, crowded living conditions

Prevention and Screening

▶ Good hygiene, including keeping children's nails cut short

Assessment

History

▶ Rash that may or may not be pruritic that has been present for days to weeks

▶ Possible history of underlying dermatitis (atopic, contact)

▶ Possible exposure to household members or school/sports exposure

Physical Exam

▶ Lesions can appear on skin in which integrity has been disturbed.

▶ Commonly found on face, torso, and extremities

▶ Nonbullous: small vesicles, pustules that rupture causing erosion and superficial honey-colored crusting, often caused by *Streptococcus pyogenes;* regional lymphadenopathy present with fever

▶ Bullous: large, transparent flaccid vesicle or bullae containing clear yellow fluid on erythematous base; rupture easily and often caused by *S. aureus*; rupture leaves a rim surrounding a moist shallow ulcer; often found in clothing-covered areas

Diagnostic Studies

▶ Diagnosis primarily clinical; cultures may be warranted if diagnosis is in doubt or if lesions fail to respond to an appropriate course of antibiotics

▶ Possible Gram stain

▶ May want to perform serology for anti-DNAse beta to look for prior strep infection

Differential Diagnosis

▶ Excoriations

▶ Perioral dermatitis

▶ Seborrheic dermatitis

▶ Contact dermatitis

▶ Herpes simplex or zoster

▶ Dermatophytosis

▶ Scabies

▶ Stasis or atherosclerotic ulcers

▶ Varicella

▶ Staphylococcal scalded skin syndrome

▶ MRSA

Management

Nonpharmacologic Treatment

▶ Wash area with soap to remove crusts prior to applying topical antibiotic

▶ Wash all linens, wash cloths, etc., separately from other clothing

▶ Meticulous handwashing

Pharmacologic Treatment

▶ Mupirocin (Bactroban) 2% t.i.d. ointment topically to lesions (if limited) x 7 to 10 days

▶ Beta-lactamase–resistant oral antibiotics such as Augmentin if widespread lesions (larger than 0.3) or if topical treatment undesired

▶ Penicillin VK 250–500 mg q.i.d. x 10 days (children: 30–60 mg/kg/day q.i.d. x 10 days)

▷ Erythromycin 250–500 mg q.i.d. x 10 days (children: 30–50 mg/kg/day q.i.d. x 10 days)

▷ Dicloxacillin 500 mg q.i.d. x 10 days (children: 12.5–25 mg/kg/day q.i.d. x 10 days)

▶ If Pen VK or erythromycin is the drug of choice, cultures are warranted to ensure sensitivity to *S. aureus.*

▶ If culture demonstrates methicillin-resistant S. aureus, vancomycin (Vancocin) or SMP/TMZ is an alternative depending upon resistance within the community.

How Long to Treat

▶ 10-day treatment usually adequate; if patient not responding to initial course, cultures should be done to demonstrate antibiotic sensitivity

Special Considerations

▶ Penicillin VK or erythromycin are drugs of choice in pregnant and lactating women.

When to Consult, Refer, Hospitalize

▶ Hospitalization is warranted in toxic-appearing patient.

Follow-Up

Expected Course

▶ Generally resolved with 10-day course of antibiotics

▶ Patients should be instructed to return sooner if symptoms do not appear to be resolving or if condition appears to be spreading.

Complications

▶ With nontreatment or noncompliance with medication regimen, infection may progress to lymphangitis, cellulitis, erysipelas, bacteremia, or septicemia.

▶ GAS complications include guttate psoriasis, scarlet fever, glomerulonephritis.

▶ Scarring often occurs after healing of ecthyma.

Folliculitis, Furuncle, and Carbuncle

Description

▶ Folliculitis: local inflammation of hair follicles by infection or irritation; usually self-limiting

▶ Furuncle (boil or abscess): infection deep in a hair follicle

▷ Furunculosis: several discrete furuncles

▶ Carbuncle: deeper abscess, involves subcutaneous tissue, arising in several contiguous hair follicles, interconnected by sinus tracts; may have several pustular openings onto skin; may be associated with systemic symptoms of fever and malaise

Etiology

▶ Usually *S. aureus*, rarely other bacteria; hot tub folliculitis caused by *P. aeruginosa*

▶ Most common in hairy areas exposed to friction, pressure, and moisture

Incidence and Demographics

▶ Age: more common in children, adolescents, and young adults

Risk Factors

▶ Chronic staphylococcus carrier state (nares, axillae, anogenital, intestine)

▶ Obesity, poor hygiene, injection of drugs

▶ Metabolic abnormalities (chronic granulomatosis, high serum IgE), diabetes mellitus, HIV

Prevention and Screening

▶ Good hygiene, improvement in underlying factors such as diabetes and obesity

Assessment

History

▶ Folliculitis appears as single or multiple small pustules with possible mild erythema.

▶ Furuncle and carbuncles present as painful, warm, erythematous lesions with central pustulation developing over days.

▶ Carbuncles are sometimes accompanied by systemic symptoms of fever and malaise.

▶ History of predisposing factors or prior boils

Physical Exam

▶ Furuncle: firm, tender nodule with a central necrotic plug; nodule becomes fluctuant below the necrotic plug, usually with a pustule over the plug

▶ Carbuncle: several adjacent, coalescing furuncles with multiple, loculated abscesses, draining pustules, and necrotic plugs

▶ Vital signs may indicate fever and tachycardia.

▶ Local lymphadenopathy

Diagnostic Studies

▶ Laboratory studies are usually not indicated.

▶ Gram staining usually demonstrates Gram-positive cocci with multiple neutrophils.

▶ Culture and sensitivity may be done to confirm *S. aureus* or identify methicillin-resistant *S. aureus* or other bacteria that may be resistant to treatment.

▶ Blood cultures are indicated if the patient remains febrile or appears toxic.

Differential Diagnosis

▶ Ruptured epidermal or pilar cyst

▶ Hidradenitis suppurativa

▶ MRSA

▶ Necrotizing HSV

Management

Nonpharmacologic Treatment

▶ Warm, moist compresses or sitz baths x 10 minutes q. 2 to 3 hours (usually all that is necessary for folliculitis)

▶ Incision and drainage required for furuncle and carbuncle if large or pointing (pustule looks "ripe"); sterile packing is often necessary to allow the incision to continue to drain

▶ Washing daily with antibacterial soap; clean razors and personal items; change towels daily

Pharmacologic Treatment

▶ Topical antibiotics are usually not effective.

▶ Mupirocin ointment (Bactroban) t.i.d. to nares is helpful in eliminating chronic *S. aureus* carrier state, or applied after shower to prevent recurrence.

▶ Systemic antibiotics are usually indicated for multiple furuncles and carbuncles, marked inflammation, or immunocompromised.

 ▷ Dicloxacillin 250–500 mg q.i.d.; children: 12.5–50 mg/kg/day in divided doses

 ▷ Cephalexin (Keflex) 250–500 mg q.i.d.; children: 25–50 mg/kg/day in divided doses

 ▷ Amoxicillin and clavulanic acid (Augmentin) 250–500 mg; children: 20–40 mg/kg/day in divided doses

 ▷ EES 400 mg t.i.d.; children: 30–50 mg/kg/day in divided doses

 ▷ Clarithromycin (Biaxin) 250–500 mg b.i.d.

 ▷ Azithromycin (Zithromax) 250 mg q.d.

 ▷ Clindamycin (Cleocin) 150–300 mg q.i.d.

▶ Methicillin-resistant *S. aureus* (MRSA)

 ▷ Minocycline (Minocin) 100 mg b.i.d. (adults); 4 mg/kg initially, then 2 mg/kg b.i.d. (children older than 8 years)

 ▷ Trimethoprim-sulfamethiazole DS b.i.d.; 8 mg/kg/day based on trimethoprim divided b.i.d. (children older than 2 months)

 ▷ Ciprofloxacin (Cipro) 500 mg b.i.d. (18 and older only)

 ▷ Rifampin (Rifadin) may be added to one of the above antibiotics.

 ▷ Vancomycin IV for severe infections

How Long to Treat

▶ 7 to 10 days

Special Considerations

▶ Erythromycin should be used in pregnant or lactating women.

When to Consult, Refer, Hospitalize

▶ Consult with physician if a large furuncle or carbuncle requires incision and drainage.

▶ Referral to general surgeon is indicated for extensive abscess involvement or recurrence.

Follow-Up

▶ Daily follow-up initially to monitor response and to remove packing from surgical site

Complications

▶ Bacteremia and possible seeding of heart valves, joints, spine, long bones, and viscera

▶ Cavernous venous thromboses and meningitis

VIRAL SKIN INFECTIONS

Herpes Simplex Virus (HSV)

Description

▶ Recurrent viral mucocutaneous infection spread by skin-to-skin, skin-to-mucosa, or mucosa-to-skin contact; only known to affect humans

▶ Sites of involvement include the vermillion border of the lips, buccal mucosa, gingiva, cheeks, distal tips of fingers (herpetic whitlow), anogenital region.

▶ Genital HSV infection is a sexually transmitted disease.

▶ Requires break in normal skin integrity for initial cutaneous infection; asymptomatic until provoked

Etiology

▶ Herpes simplex virus type 1 and type 2—HSV replicates within epithelial cells, lyses them, and then produces a thin-walled vesicle.

▶ HSV type 2 is usually associated with genital lesions.

▶ The virus migrates within several hours along sensory neurons to nerve root ganglia, where it then resides in a latent state.

▶ Viral reactivation occurs during periods of physical or emotional stress, although the exact mechanism of stimulating reactivation is unclear.

▶ When reactivated, it migrates back to the skin along sensory nerves, producing typical lesions.

Incidence and Demographics

▶ Most often affects young adults, but can affect any age

Risk Factors

▶ Intimate skin-to-skin or skin-to–mucous membrane contact with an infected person during stages of viral shedding; virus not stable at room temperature and therefore unlikely to spread through fomites or aerosol

▶ Contagious during the prodromal and vesicular stages

▶ Sun exposure to face; viral upper respiratory infection

▶ Altered hormonal status (menstruation)

▶ Immune status alteration (HIV, malignancy, chemotherapy, systemic corticosteroids, irradiation)

Prevention and Screening

▶ Safe sex practices; avoidance of close contact while symptomatic

Assessment

History

▶ May not be aware of contact with infected person (incubation period 2 to 20 days; average 6 days)

▶ Initial or primary outbreak may range from very minor to severe, with grouped vesicles at the site of exposure

▶ Commonly associated with regional lymphadenopathy, malaise, muscle pain, headaches, and possible fever

▶ In childhood, most often presents as acute gingivostomatitis with multiple shallow, painful ulcers; fever; hyper-salivation; and lymphadenopathy

▶ Recurrences preceded by prodromal tingling or aching at site of previous lesions; may be less severe, no systemic symptoms

Physical Exam

▶ Thin-roof, grouped vesicles on erythematous bases, often at border of lips, penis, labia, buttocks

▶ Vesicles burst, shallow ulcer exposed with crusting and ulcerations, then crust and dry over 1 week

▶ Regional lymphadenopathy, malaise, muscle pain, headaches, and possible fever

Diagnostic Studies

▶ Tzanck smear microscopic exam (Wright's or Giemsa's stain) would demonstrate giant, multinucleated epidermal cells

▶ Herpes culture or DNA probe of exudate from pierced vesicle or scraping from crusted ulcer (may get false-negative results from crusted lesions or after the initial 24 to 48 hours of an outbreak when viral shedding has slowed or ceased)

▶ Little clinical value from HSV serology

Differential Diagnosis

▶ Aphthous stomatitis

▶ Herpangina

▶ Chancroid

▶ Syphilis

▶ Pyoderma

▶ Trauma

▶ Hand, foot, and mouth disease

▶ Impetigo

▶ Herpes zoster

▶ Erythema multiform

Management

Nonpharmacologic Treatment

▶ Sitz baths, cool compresses, Burow's solution for comfort

▶ Safe sex practices of limited value; condoms do not reduce risk of transmission as viral shedding occurs along a wide area of the groin/perineal region

▶ Sunscreen may prevent outbreaks in infected people.

Pharmacologic Treatment

▶ Oral antivirals usually not indicated for adults unless infection is genital (see Chapter 13 for genital herpes treatment)

▶ Acyclovir (Zovirax) 15 mg/kg per day divided in five doses x 7 days in children with gingivostomatitis; for adults, 200 mg 5 times daily or 800 mg t.i.d. or valacyclovir 1,000 mg b.i.d. or famciclovir 250 mg t.i.d.

▶ Topical 5% acyclovir q.2.h. (only approved indication is for treatment of initial outbreak in immunocompromised patients) x 5 days

▶ Penciclovir (Denavir) cream q.2.h. x 4 days (indicated for treatment of recurrent orolabial herpes; only been shown to reduce average attack from 5 to 4.5 days)

▶ Prophylactic acyclovir 400 mg b.i.d.; valacyclovir 500 mg q.d. or famciclovir 125–250 mg b.i.d. when risk of triggers high (UV light exposure, dental or oral surgery)

Special Considerations

▶ Treatment of an initial outbreak of herpes genitalis during pregnancy is recommended because the risk to the fetus of complications from a severe and prolonged outbreak outweighs the risk of complications from medications.

▶ Patients with frequent outbreaks should be evaluated for other STDs, including HIV.

▶ HIV+ patients with CD4 less than 50 should be on prophylactic oral therapy; topical therapies are not effective.

When to Consult, Refer, Hospitalize

▶ Consult with a physician if hospitalization required for IV therapy if patient is immunocompromised with widespread disease.

Follow-Up

▶ Routine follow-up not necessary unless severe

Expected Course

▶ Usual resolution of symptoms within 2 weeks for first occurrence, 5 to 7 days for recurrences

▶ Recurrences less frequent with passage of time

Complications

▶ Secondary infection of lesions

▶ Post-inflammatory hyperpigmentation

▶ Erythema multiforme

Herpes Zoster

Description

▶ "Shingles"; acute, painful, unilateral, localized vesicular cutaneous infection in a dermatomal pattern

Etiology

▶ Varicella zoster virus (VZV), usually contracted in childhood as chickenpox

▶ Lies dormant in a nerve ganglion; reactivation of virus causes eruption along course of the nerve; cause of reactivation unclear

Incidence and Demographics

▶ Occurs most often in persons over 50; fewer than 10% of cases occur under age 20

Risk Factors

▶ Immunosuppression, advanced age; previous infection with varicella

▶ Trauma to the sensory ganglia

Prevention and Screening

▶ Varicella vaccine now included in routine childhood immunization schedule; may prevent development of herpes zoster in later life

▶ Varicella vaccine (Zostavax) later in life when anti-VZV antibodies are declining; may be effective in preventing development of herpes zoster; older than 50 years of age, ACIP recommends use in patients older than 60 years of age even if have had shingles in remote past. Vaccine decreases risk of developing shingles by 51%.

Assessment

History

▶ Pain (piercing, stabbing, boring), paresthesias (tingling, burning, itching), and allodynia (heightened sensitivity to mild stimuli) along neuronal pathway preceding eruption by 3 to 5 days; may mimic internal pathology

▶ Generalized malaise, fever, and headache in about 5%

Physical Exam

▶ Initially, grouped vesicles along a unilateral dermatomal pathway, followed by bullae within 2 days (more than one contiguous dermatome may be involved but noncontiguous dermatome involvement rare)

▶ By day 4, vesicles become pustules, followed by crusting in 7 to 10 days.

▶ Lesions occur on an erythematous, edematous cutaneous base.

Diagnostic Studies

▶ Can be made clinically

▶ Tzanck smear, serum VZV antibodies, viral culture

Differential Diagnosis

▶ Herpes simplex

▶ Contact dermatitis

▶ Erysipelas

▶ Bullous impetigo

▶ Poison ivy or oak

▶ Necrotizing fasciitis

Management

Nonpharmacologic Treatment

▶ Moist dressings (water, normal saline, or Burow's solution) may decrease pain.

Pharmacologic Treatment

▶ Acyclovir (Zovirax) 800 mg 5 times daily

▶ Valacyclovir (Valtrex) 1,000 mg t.i.d.

▶ Famciclovir (Famvir) 500 mg t.i.d.

▶ IV acyclovir 10 mg/kg t.i.d.

▶ IV foscarnet (Foscavir) for acyclovir-resistant strains

▶ Pain management with narcotic pain medications or NSAIDs

How Long to Treat

▶ 7 to 10 days

Special Considerations

▶ Most common risk factor is decreasing immunity, putting those with advancing age and immunocompromised conditions most at risk

When to Consult, Refer, Hospitalize

▶ Disseminated infection may require hospitalization or in-home IV therapy.

▶ Patients with corneal involvement require ophthalmology evaluation.

Follow-Up

▶ Follow-up in 2 weeks to ensure the infection is resolving

Expected course

▶ Initial course generally resolved in 2 to 3 weeks

Complications

▶ Postherpetic neuralgia

▶ Local hemorrhage, gangrene, or secondary infection

▶ Systemic meningoencephalitis, cerebral vascular syndrome, cranial nerve syndromes (ophthalmic, trigeminal, facial, and auditory), peripheral motor weakness

Human Papillomavirus/Verruca/Warts

Description

▶ Discrete, benign, epithelial hyperplasia on skin and mucous membranes

▷ Vulgaris: common wart, no particular location

▷ Plantaris: plantar wart, plantar surface of foot; plana: flat wart

Etiology

▶ Infection caused by human papillomaviruses, DNA viruses of which at least 70 types have been described; incubation period of 1 to 6 months; 65% spontaneous resolution in 12 to 24 months, but some persist for years

▶ Many varieties identified; specific morphology and predilection for different anatomical sites

▶ Most benign; subtypes that infect cervix known to have oncogenic potential; also sexually transmitted

Incidence and Demographics

▶ Occurs in all ages and races, most frequently seen in 10% of school-age children and 5% of adults

▶ Immunocompromised people at greater risk for clinically widespread disease

Risk Factors

▶ Skin-to-skin contact

▶ Household contact

▶ HIV+

Prevention and Screening

▶ Education about contagious nature of virus and avoidance of contact

Assessment

History

▶ Painless skin lesion present from days to months, possibly with known exposure (incubation period 2 to 9 months)

▶ Plantar warts generally painful with weight-bearing

▶ May bleed if disrupted by shaving or scratching

▶ May be mildly pruritic, especially if secondarily infected

Physical Exam

▶ Verruca vulgaris or "common warts": firm, hyperkeratotic 1 to 10 mm papules with surface cleft

▷ Usually flesh-colored and discrete

▷ May be vegetative

▷ Characteristic black puncta, or "dish-brown dots," are thrombosed capillary loops, best seen with hand lens; may only be apparent after paring callused surface

▷ Common on hands, fingers, and knees (sites of trauma), pressure points on feet

▶ Verruca plantaris or "plantar warts": flesh-colored, rough, hyperkeratotic papules or plaques (possible mosaic configuration) with black puncta on plantar surface of feet

▶ Verruca plana or "flat warts": small, skin-colored, flat-topped ("mesa-like") 1 to 5 mm papules

▷ Usually round or oval

▷ Always discrete and closely set multiple lesions that sometimes appear in a linear configuration (autoinoculation from scratching)

▷ Found on face, hands, or shins

Diagnostic Studies

▶ Clinical with black puncta pathognomonic; suspicious lesions should be sent for pathology evaluation

Differential Diagnosis

▶ Molluscum contagiosum

▶ Seborrheic keratosis

▶ Actinic keratosis

▶ Clavus or callus of feet

▶ Condylomata lata

▶ Squamous cell carcinoma

▶ Imbedded foreign body

Management

Nonpharmacologic Treatment

▶ Warts of the hand: laser surgery, electrodesiccation, cryotherapy (liquid nitrogen)

▶ Apply opaque ("duct") tape to verruca plantaris or planus, change weekly (shown to be as effective as other treatments)

Pharmacologic Treatment

▶ Verruca vulgaris: keratolytic agents (salicylic or lactic acids); OTC salicylic acid (Compound W, Duoplant) preparations applied nightly; soak in warm water 10 minutes, dry and "sand" lesion with emery board before applying product; cover with Band-Aid or tape to increase effectiveness; apply daily

▶ Verruca plantaris: same as with vulgaris, except use higher potency product

▶ Verruca planus: retinoic acid A or salicylic acid applied daily

▶ Anogenital warts: podophyllin topical application every 1 to 2 weeks; bi- or trichloro-acetic acid topical application every 1 to 2 weeks; imiquimod 5%

▶ Systemic H-2 blockers such as cimetidine (Tagamet) or ranitidine (Zantac) b.i.d. for persistent warts in children along vermillion border of lip or eyelid, very extensive, or treatment is painful

How Long to Treat

▶ 4 to 12 weeks

Special Considerations

▶ Podophyllin is contraindicated in pregnant and lactating women.

▶ *Molluscum contagiosum* is another cutaneous viral infection (poxvirus) with characteristic pearly white papules 1 to 2 mm in size with umbilicated center.

　▷ Spontaneous regression occurs in 6 months unless immunocompromised.

　▷ Widespread involvement in the immunocompromised requires treatment as above.

When to Consult, Refer, Hospitalize

▶ Consult with dermatology for inadequate resolution with above regimens.

Follow-Up

▶ Treatment in office as indicated

Expected Course

▶ 50% to 60% spontaneously regress within 2 years.

▶ 65% of patients have recurrences regardless of treatment.

Complications

▶ Scarring, post-inflammatory hyperpigmentation

▶ Prevention: gardisil vaccine ages 9 to 18 for boys and girls

PARASITIC INFESTATIONS AND BITES

Scabies

Description

▶ Infestation by scabies mite, spread by direct contact; leads to generalized pruritus, a hypersensitivity reaction to the scabies excretions

Etiology

▶ *Sarcoptes scabiei* that thrive and multiply only on human skin; spread by human-to-human contact; may live up to 2 days on clothing and bed linens

▶ Sensitization to *S. scabiei* must occur before developing the generalized pruritus associated with an infestation. For people with an initial infestation, sensitization takes about 10 days; subsequent infestations progress to the pruritic stage much more quickly.

Incidence and Demographics

▶ Common in young children under the age of 5 through direct contact; in young adults, usually through sexual contact; in older adults and infirm in residential facilities; worldwide distribution

▶ Epidemics occur in cycles; incubation 4 to 6 weeks

Risk Factors

▶ Institutional living

▶ Immunocompromised status

Prevention and Screening

▶ Prompt treatment and washing of linens, etc.

Assessment

History

▶ Usually can give history of close contacts with similar symptoms

▶ Severe generalized pruritus sparing head and neck, with initial infestation about 1 month after exposure; with reinfestation, pruritus begins immediately

▶ Pruritus and scratching often interfere with sleep

Physical Exam

▶ Characteristic scattered vesicles, burrows, or nodules: gray or skin-colored ridge, serpiginous or straight, 2 mm to a few cm in length; with excoriations

▶ Common distribution: axillae, anogenital region, wrists, hands (webs of fingers), waist, and flexor surfaces of elbows

▶ May develop generalized erythroderma; may also develop lichen simplex chronicus

▶ Eczematous dermatitis common in atopic persons

▶ Post-inflammatory hyperpigmentation may occur; secondary infections to denuded sites common

▶ Crusted vesicles or burrows after infestation of several months

Diagnostic Studies

▶ Serum eosinophilia

▶ Microscopic identification by placing a drop of mineral oil over a burrow and scraping burrow with a blade; mites, eggs, or fecal droppings can be identified on slide.

Differential Diagnosis

▶ Drug eruption dermatitis

▶ Atopic or contact dermatitis

▶ Pityriasis rosea

▶ Herpetiform dermatitis

▶ Pediculosis dermatitis

- ▶ Insect bites
- ▶ Impetigo
- ▶ Delusions of parasitosis
- ▶ Metabolic pruritus

Management

Nonpharmacologic Treatment

- ▶ Wash all bedding and clothing in washing machine with hot soapy water and hot dry cycle at time of treatment; seal nonwashable clothing and articles in a plastic bag for 1 week.
- ▶ Lubricants may help reduce itching.

Pharmacologic Treatment

- ▶ Relies on pharmacologic treatment for eradication of mites and their eggs, and of pruritus
- ▶ Lindane 1% cream overnight (8 to 12 hours) x 1; avoid in children and pregnant women
- ▶ Permethrin (Elimite) 5% cream overnight (8 to 14 hours) x 1 (can be used on infants from 2 months and older and by pregnant women)
- ▶ Tapered course of systemic steroids starting at 70–80 mg q.d. and tapering by 5 mg q.d. often necessary to treat widespread pruritus
- ▶ Topical steroids bid to severely pruritic areas
- ▶ Systemic antihistamines such as diphenhydramine (Benadryl) 25–50 mg q. 4 to 6 hours for pruritus

How Long to Treat

- ▶ One-time treatment with lindane or permethrin may be effective, but a repeat treatment in 14 days is often necessary to eliminate infestation.
- ▶ Systemic steroids are generally tapered over 10 to 14 days.
- ▶ Systemic antihistamines are used on an as-needed basis.

Special Considerations

- ▶ Lindane is contraindicated if pregnant, lactating, or child under 2 years of age.
- ▶ Lindane is known to cause seizures if used just after a bath or in patients with extensive dermatitis.
- ▶ Lindane-resistant cases may occur; try permethrin.

When to Consult, Refer, Hospitalize

- ▶ Refer to dermatologist when resolution is not achieved with above regimens.

Follow-Up

- ▶ Patients should be brought back in 1 to 2 weeks, then at weekly intervals if there is extensive dermatitis.

Expected Course
- ▶ Mites may be eradicated with one or two treatments, but the generalized pruritus may persist for several weeks because it is a hypersensitivity reaction to the mite.

Complications
- ▶ Secondary infection, abscesses, and/or cellulitis due to scratching

Insect Bites and Stings

Description
- ▶ Very common injury in children and all ages, caused by flying or crawling insects
- ▶ Kinds of insects include ticks, bees or wasps, fleas, and chiggers
- ▶ Two U.S. spiders are known to bite humans and are capable of producing severe reactions: brown recluse and black widow.

Etiology
- ▶ Spider venom is composed of an enzyme-spreading factor and a toxin distributed by the enzyme (not an allergic reaction); it causes toxic reaction with possible systemic symptoms.
- ▶ Many bites cause allergic reactions with local or systemic symptoms, immediate or delayed.
- ▶ Anaphylaxis is possible.
- ▶ Mosquitoes are the most common insects that afflict children and usually cause local reactions.

Incidence and Demographics
- ▶ More common in late spring or summer months
- ▶ Flea bites occur year-round.
- ▶ Spiders live in dark areas such as closets, under porches, and in woodpiles; they are most common in southern regions but can be found anywhere in the United States.

Risk Factors
- ▶ Playing or walking in grassy or wooded areas
- ▶ Wearing bright-colored clothing or perfumed products

Prevention and Screening
- ▶ Avoid infested areas.
- ▶ Apply insect repellents (containing less than 10% diethyltoluamide [DEET] or permethrin) before going outside
- ▶ Wear neutral-colored clothing.
- ▶ Avoid scented products.
- ▶ Apply permethrin to clothing.
- ▶ Wear protective clothing such as long pants and shirts.

▶ Carefully check for ticks after a hike in potentially tick-infested areas.

▶ Eliminate fleas from living areas with powders or spray.

Assessment

History

▶ Recent exposure to insect-infested areas; report of feeling a bite or sting

▶ Swelling, pain, or pruritus of affected area

▶ May be complaints of nausea, vomiting, diarrhea, headache, fever, lightheadedness, flushing, hives, dyspnea, wheezing

Physical Exam

▶ Presentation varies due to different insects and individual reaction.

▶ Mosquitoes: scattered erythematous pruritic wheals with central punctum

▶ Fleas: irregularly grouped or linear urticarial wheals or papules with central punctum

▶ Bees and wasps: redness, edema, pain, pruritus, induration

▶ Chiggers: discrete bright red papules on legs and belt line

▶ Distribution usually on exposed areas of skin, except fleas—areas where clothing is snug

▶ Spiders: swelling and erythema at site, and may develop more severe reactions in areas of fatty subcutaneous tissue; necrosis can develop in 4 hours

▶ Wheezing, hypotension, change in mental status may present in anaphylaxis

Diagnostic Studies

▶ None

Differential Diagnosis

▶ Varicella

▶ Impetigo

▶ Scabies

Management

Nonpharmacologic Treatment

▶ Cool compresses or ice; colloidal oatmeal baths

▶ Remove stinger or tick if visible

Pharmacologic Treatment

▶ Symptomatic treatment of pruritus: pramoxine (topical anesthetic), topical steroids, oral antihistamines

▶ Oral corticosteroids if more severe pruritus and swelling

▶ Tetanus prophylaxis update as needed

▶ Epinephrine and other emergency measures for anaphylactic reactions

▷ Dose of epinephrine 1:1,000 (aqueous) 0.01 mL/kg per dose administered subcutaneously;

▷ in infants/children: 0.01 mg/kg, max 0. 3 mg/dose; adults: 0.1–0.5 mg, max dose 1 mg

▶ If life-threatening systemic anaphylaxis occurs, call 911 and emergency transport; give epinephrine as above; start IV, oxygen, inhaled albuterol (Proventil) nebulizer if bronchospasm severe.

How Long to Treat

▶ Until symptoms relieved; usually 48 hours

Special Considerations

▶ Papular urticaria, a hypersensitivity reaction, may develop secondary to bites from mosquitoes, fleas, or other insects—grouped urticarial papules with a central punctum, vesicles, pustules, or bullae. This reaction usually occurs in the first decade of life, and may last for 1 to 2 years.

▶ A secondary infection may develop.

When to Consult, Refer, Hospitalize

▶ Transfer to acute care facility for anaphylactic reaction.

Follow-Up

▶ None usually necessary unless urticaria or more serious reaction

Complications

▶ Spider bites by brown recluse or black widow can cause tissue necrosis.

Pediculosis Capitis and Pubis

Description

▶ An infestation with one of the three species of parasitic lice that affect humans: *Pediculus humanus capitis, Pediculus humanus corporis*, or *Pthirus pubis,* which are wingless, blood-sucking insects

▶ Infestation of the scalp, body, or pubic hair causing mild pruritus and excoriation

Etiology

▶ Incubation period from egg to hatching, 6 to 10 days; lice mature in 2 to 3 weeks and then lay eggs

▶ Lice need to ingest blood every few hours; can survive on fomites more than 2 days

Incidence and Demographics

▶ All ages, but pediculosis capitis more common in children (estimated up to 10 million children in the United States infected annually); pediculosis pubis more common in young adults, spread through close physical or sexual contact, sharing bed linens

▶ Head lice uncommon in Black population

Risk Factors

▶ Shared hats, combs, head-to-head contact; epidemics of head lice in schools

▶ Sexual promiscuity and poor personal hygiene for pubic lice

Prevention and Screening

▶ Education of parents, children, and school personnel about modes of transmission and to avoid sharing hats, combs, etc.

▶ Educating young adults about the modes of transmission and to avoid sexual promiscuity

Assessment

History

▶ Mild pruritus of scalp and nape of neck, pubis, or axilla for days to weeks

▶ Only symptom in child may be restlessness

▶ Sexual contact with affected person; poor personal hygiene

Physical Exam

▶ Pediculosis capitis

  ▷ 2 to 5 mm mobile lice often difficult to find; usually fewer than 10 per infestation

  ▷ More commonly found are small (1.0 mm), creamy, yellowish-white nits adherent to shaft of hair as it emerges from the scalp; a few to thousands of nits may be found on one scalp

  ▷ White nits farther from the scalp indicate longer-standing infection (hair grows approximately 0.5mm/day)

  ▷ Excoriations, crusting, purulent exudate (plica polonica), eczematous dermatitis, or papular urticaria and lichen simplex chronicus along nape of neck

  ▷ Regional lymphadenopathy—may be found with long-standing infestation or extensive excoriations and crusting

▶ Pediculosis pubis

  ▷ Lice: appear as 1 to 2 mm brownish-gray adherent dots on hair in pubic region, perineum, axillae, and torso

  ▷ Nits: whitish-gray dots on hair shaft

  ▷ Papular urticaria: slate-gray or bluish-gray 0.5 to 1 cm nonblanching macules

  ▷ Excoriations, crusting, purulent exudate, regional adenopathy

Diagnostic Studies

▶ Mainly a clinical diagnosis, but may be confirmed by microscopic exam of lice, which demonstrates a 1 to 4 mm six-legged insect with a gray-white body that may be engorged with blood, or nits that are less than 0.5 mm yellowish-white eggs or, in the case of an older nit, an empty, translucent white egg

▶ Wood's lamp demonstrates pearly fluorescence of live nits

▶ Bacterial cultures confirm secondary infection and sensitivity

Differential Diagnosis

▶ Hair spray/lacquer

▶ Eczema

▶ Tinea cruris

▶ Dandruff

▶ Neurotic excoriation

▶ Impetigo

▶ Contact or seborrheic dermatitis

▶ Scabies

Management

Nonpharmacologic Treatment

▶ Vacuuming carpets and furniture; washing clothing and linens in hot water and using hot dryer; and soaking combs, brushes, and hair ornaments in rubbing alcohol are all effective means of controlling the environment to prevent spread or reinfection with lice.

▶ Hair should be combed with fine-toothed comb after treating to remove adherent nits.

▶ Wetting hair with white vinegar before combing loosens nits, facilitates removal.

▶ In resistant cases, applying oily substance such as mayonnaise, leaving on overnight, and shampooing out in morning may be effective.

▶ Children may return to day care or school on day after treatment.

▶ Seal unwashable articles in plastic bag for 10 days.

Pharmacologic Treatment

▶ Permethrin shampoo (Nix) or pyrethrin shampoo (RID), worked well into hair and scalp and left on for 10 minutes; retreat in 1 week

▶ Lindane 4% shampoo left on for 4 minutes

   ▷ Ovide lotion, 0.5% malathion in an alcohol and pine needle solution, may be used as alternative.

   ▷ Benzyl alcohol topical (Ulesfia)

▶ Secondarily infected lesions should be treated with appropriate antibiotics.

▶ Treat nits on eyebrows and eyelashes with petroleum jelly. Apply t.i.d. 8 to 10 days and comb out nits.

How Long to Treat

▶ Once, with retreatment in 1 week

Special Considerations

▶ Lindane is not recommended for pregnant and lactating women or children under 2 years.

When to Consult, Refer, Hospitalize

▶ Usually not necessary

Follow-Up

▶ Patients should be reevaluated in 1 week and re-treated if any nits or lice remain.

Expected Course

▶ Reinfection is likely if schools are not notified and other children are not evaluated and treated, or if sexual contacts or bed partners are not treated.

Complications

▶ Secondary infection, excoriated lesions

TUMORS

Basal Cell Carcinoma

Description

▶ Slow-growing carcinoma that most commonly presents as a papule or nodule that may have central umbilication, progressing to significant ulceration; no risk of metastasis, but can produce significant cosmetic deformity; most commonly seen skin cancer, arising on sun-exposed areas

Etiology

▶ Excess sun exposure, particularly in fair-skinned persons

▶ Slow-growing, common skin cancer that is result of proliferating atypical basal cells with various amounts of stroma; requires a hair follicle to develop

▶ Can become invasive if located on the face, in the ear canal, or in the posterior auricular sulcus; metastasis is rare

Incidence and Demographics

▶ Older than age 40; men more than women

▶ 400,000 cases per year

▶ Dark skin rarely affected

Risk Factors

▶ Excess sun exposure (especially sunburns in youth), fair skin with poor tanning ability

▶ Prior treatment with X-ray for facial acne

Prevention and Screening

▶ Education about risk of excess sun exposure, should start with young children

▶ Monthly skin self-exam, yearly clinical exam

Assessment

History

▶ Patients may or may not be aware of suspicious lesions

Physical Exam

▶ Waxy or "pearly" appearing firm, round, or oval papules or nodules on sun-exposed skin (80% on the face and neck); visible telangiectasia

▶ "Ulcer" or "sore" with a rolled border ("rodent bite ulcer"); central umbilication possible

▶ Crusting may be present; pink or red; pigmented lesions may be brown, blue, or black

Diagnostic Studies

▶ Biopsy demonstrating atypical basal cells

Differential Diagnosis

▶ Molluscum contagiosum

▶ Warts

▶ Cysts

▶ Scarring

▶ Other benign lesions

▶ Squamous cell carcinoma

Management

▶ Excision, cryosurgery, or electrosurgery

▶ Mohs surgery: microscopically controlled surgery for lesions in the danger zones of nasolabial folds, around eyes, in ear canal and posterior auricular sulcus

▶ Radiation therapy is alternative in areas of possible cosmetic disfigurement

How Long to Treat

▶ Retreat if reoccurs

Special Considerations

▶ Reoccurrence or development of a new lesion may occur within 5 years.

When to Consult, Refer, Hospitalize

▶ Refer all suspected skin cancer to a dermatologist or provider with experience in skin cancer assessment for biopsy.

Follow-Up

Expected Course

▶ Resolution with above therapies is the norm, but at-risk patients should be followed to monitor for new lesions.

Complications
▶ Cosmetic disfigurement

Squamous Cell Carcinoma

Description
▶ A skin malignancy that occurs on sun-exposed areas and may arise out of actinic keratoses on exposed parts in persons who burn easily; develops in the course of a few months; approximately 5% potential for metastasis; second-most common type of skin cancer
▶ Bowen's disease—carcinoma-in-situ arising on any area of skin

Etiology
▶ Skin exposure to exogenous carcinogen such as sunlight, ionizing radiation
▶ Arsenic ingestion, tobacco, human papillomavirus
▶ Malignant growth of epithelial keratinocytes developing on skin and mucous membranes

Incidence and Demographics
▶ Higher incidence in Sun Belt states
▶ Older than age 55; men more than women

Risk Factors
▶ Fair skin with poor tanning ability
▶ Sun exposure—outdoor workers and sports people
▶ Arsenic ingestion, tobacco use, radiation exposure
▶ Preexisting solar keratosis
▶ Organ transplant patients
▶ Cases around oral cavity and surrounding region and genitalia have greater risk of metastasis.

Prevention and Screening
▶ Sun precautions; monthly skin self-exam, yearly clinical exam

Assessment
History
▶ Suspicious lesion developing over months to years
▶ Most often on sun-exposed skin (face, lips, hands, and forearms)

Physical Exam
▶ Originate with small red nodule, papule, or plaque; progresses to induration
▶ Thick, adherent, keratotic scale

▶ Honey-colored exudate extruded from periphery

▶ May be eroded, crusted, ulcerated, hard, erythematous; isolated or multiple

Diagnostic Studies

▶ Biopsy demonstrating atypical squamous cells

Differential Diagnosis

▶ Basal cell carcinoma

▶ Malignant melanoma

▶ Actinic keratosis

▶ Paget's disease

▶ Other benign lesions

Management

▶ Immediate surgery or radiation depending on size, shape, and location of the tumor

▶ Strict sun precautions for rest of life; lesions 2 cm or greater prone to recur

How Long to Treat

▶ Retreat if recurs

Special Considerations

▶ Any slowly evolving isolated keratotic lesion in a high-risk patient that persists for more than 1 month is to be considered carcinoma until proven otherwise with a biopsy.

When to Consult, Refer, Hospitalize

▶ Refer all suspected skin cancer to a dermatologist or provider with experience in skin cancer assessment for biopsy.

Follow-Up

Expected Course

▶ Remission achieved in 90% of cases

▶ Monitor for reoccurrence annually and if patient reports change in any existing lesion; photographs of lesions can be kept for comparison of appearance

Complications

▶ Scarring and disfigurement

Malignant Melanoma

Description

▶ Least common but most lethal of all skin cancers; high risk of metastasis

▶ Classifications: superficial spreading melanoma (most common), nodular melanoma (poorer prognosis), lentigo maligna melanoma, acral lentiginous melanoma (Black people and dark-skinned White people), desmoplastic melanoma, and melanoma of the mucous membranes

Etiology

▶ Malignant growth of melanocytes

▶ Widely metastatic

Incidence and Demographics

▶ Only 3% of all skin cancers; accounts for two-thirds of skin cancer deaths

▶ Cases with lymph node involvement at time of diagnosis have 5-year survival rate of 30%; with distant metastasis, less than 10%

▶ More common in Sun Belt states

Risk Factors

▶ Positive family history, congenital nevi, familial dysplastic nevi syndrome

▶ Excessive sun exposure, outdoor occupation or sports

▶ Severe sunburn, particularly at an early age; fair skin

Prevention and Screening

▶ Sun exposure precautions

▶ Monthly skin self-exams and yearly clinical exams

Assessment

History

▶ New pigmented lesion or recent change in longstanding skin lesion

▶ Lesion that burns, itches, hurts, or bleeds

Physical Exam

▶ Macule, papule, or nodule

▶ Colors ranging from pink to brown, blue, or black

▶ Borders most often irregular

▶ Size from a few millimeters to centimeters

▶ The five cardinal signs of malignant melanoma are:

  ▷ A: Asymmetry

  ▷ B: Border is irregular and often scalloped.

  ▷ C: Color is mottled with variegated display of brown, black, gray, and/or pink.

  ▷ D: Diameter is large (greater than 6.0 mm).

  ▷ E: Elevation is almost always present with subtle or obvious surface distortion; best assessed by side-lighting of the lesion.

▶ Five histopathologic types:

  1. Superficial spreading malignant melanoma (most common)

  2. Nodular malignant melanoma

  3. Acral-lentiginous melanoma (palms of hands, soles of feet, nail beds)

4. Malignant melanomas of mucous membranes

5. Melanomas arising from blue or congenital nevi

Diagnostic Studies

▶ Biopsy, including margins and depth of invasion assessment

▶ Lymph node biopsy often also indicated

Differential Diagnosis

▶ Benign nevi

▶ Seborrheic keratosis

▶ Vascular skin lesions

▶ Squamous cell or basal cell carcinoma

Management

▶ Aggressive surgical management by excision with margins intact

▶ Chemotherapy for patients with high-risk melanomas, to be managed by oncology specialist

How Long to Treat

▶ To be determined by oncologist

Special Considerations

▶ People with skin phototype 1 or 2 should *never* sunbathe and should always use sunscreens with a sun protection factor (SPF) of more than 30 (see Table 5–4 for skin phototype classifications).

When to Consult, Refer, Hospitalize

▶ All suspected malignant melanomas should be referred to a dermatologist for biopsy.

Follow-Up

Expected Course

▶ Prognosis based on staging of initial lesion

▶ Monthly skin self-exam; dermatology follow-up every 6 months for suspicious lesions

TABLE 5–4.
SKIN PHOTOTYPE CLASSIFICATIONS

SKIN PHOTOTYPES		
1	Pale white	Does not tan; burns easily
2	White	Tans poorly; burns easily
3	White	Tans after initial burn
4	Light brown	Tans easily
5	Brown	Tans easily
6	Dark brown	Blackens

▶ All patients monitored annually for newly appearing and changing lesions; any lesion that is itchy or tender for more than 2 weeks should be evaluated.

Complications

▶ Lung, liver, brain, bowel metastasis

OTHER INTEGUMENTARY CONDITIONS

Alopecia Areata

Description

▶ Sudden loss of hair in discrete oval patches

▶ Severity varies; may affect eyelashes, eyebrows, body hair, and nails

▶ Alopecia areata totalis involves whole scalp; alopecia areata universalis involves all body hair

Etiology

▶ Not fully known, but most likely an autoimmune process

Incidence and Demographics

▶ Rarely occurs before age 4 years

▶ Childhood and adult cases—half occur before age 20

▶ Recurrence is common.

Risk Factors

▶ Positive family history in 20%

▶ Associated with trisomy 21, atopy, other autoimmune disorders

Prevention and Screening

▶ Screen during annual exam

▶ Prevention: none

Assessment

History

▶ Usually asymptomatic except for sudden (overnight or over a few days) loss of hair

▶ Occasionally, burning or itching of the scalp just before hair loss

Physical Exam

▶ Sudden appearance of one or more well-circumscribed patches of hair loss

▶ Scalp generally clear and unaffected, occasionally slightly inflamed

▶ Hair is easy to pull out at periphery of patches

▶ "Exclamation point hairs"—short hairs at periphery with attenuated bulb—are pathognomonic

▶ Fine nail pitting in approximately 20% of cases

Diagnostic Studies
- ▶ Usually none except to exclude other diagnoses: fungal cultures, KOH, scalp biopsy

Differential Diagnosis

- ▶ Tinea capitis
- ▶ Systemic disease, drugs, and toxins
- ▶ Trichotillomania
- ▶ Traumatic alopecia from cosmetic treatments
- ▶ Traction alopecia—tight braids, rollers
- ▶ Androgenic (male pattern hair loss)

Management

Nonpharmacologic Treatment
- ▶ Education of child and parents about disease and course
- ▶ Support groups
- ▶ Hair pieces, hats, or head coverings
- ▶ Psychological counseling

Pharmacologic Treatment
- ▶ Controversial, as spontaneous resolution often occurs, but may include topical, systemic, or intralesional steroids, or topical minoxidil or anthralin

How Long to Treat
- ▶ Monitor and reassure for regrowth in 6 to 12 months

Special Considerations

- ▶ More diffuse, nonscarring hair loss may occur due to androgen hormonal changes, postpartum factors, systemic disease, weight loss, a wide variety of drugs and toxins, thyroid disease, lupus, and congenital syndromes.
- ▶ Scarring hair loss can occur with connective tissue diseases, skin diseases, burns, radiation, congenital disorders, and tumors.
- ▶ Trichotillomania is a type of traction alopecia due to self-pulling of hair.

When to Consult, Refer, Hospitalize

- ▶ Refer to a dermatologist if diagnosis is uncertain or scarring occurs.

Follow-Up

- ▶ With routine health maintenance exams

Expected Course
- ▶ Course and prognosis is extremely variable, though there is often some resolution within 1 to 2 years.
- ▶ Hair that regrows is often hypopigmented and fine; reoccurrence may occur.

Complications

▶ Usually none

Psoriasis

Description

▶ Common benign, acute, or chronic skin disease with scaling papules and plaques in characteristic distribution

Etiology

▶ Alteration in cell kinetics of keratinocytes with shortening of cell turnover rate, resulting in increased production of epidermal cells; normal maturation of the skin cells cannot take place, keratinization develops

▶ Unknown etiology and pathophysiology with genetic link

Incidence and Demographics

▶ Age: 75% type 1 early onset (age 16 years in females, 22 years in males); 25% type 2 late onset (56 years men and women)

▶ Race: 1% to 2% of White population affected

▶ Rare in people of West African, Japanese, and Alaskan Native descent; very rare in North and South American Indians

▶ Polygenic heredity

Risk Factors

▶ Trauma (Köbner's phenomenon—lesions develop in areas of trauma)

▶ Infections (streptococcal) can lead to Guttate psoriasis

▶ Drugs: corticosteroids, lithium, interferon, beta-adrenergic blockers, and possibly alcohol can cause psoriasis drug eruptions.

▶ Stress can lead to exacerbations.

▶ Genetic predisposition

Prevention and Screening

▶ Stress management

Assessment

History

▶ Skin lesions usually with insidious onset, but may be acute

▶ Pruritus may or may not be present

▶ May be associated with acute systemic illness with fever and malaise

▶ May be associated with arthralgias/arthritis

Physical Exam

▶ Morphology: silvery-white scaling papules and plaques

▶ Distribution: usually symmetrical; involves scalp, extensor surfaces, and areas subject to trauma (Köbner's phenomenon)

▶ Associated symptoms: may involve pitting of nails, yellowing of the nail at distal end, separation of nail plate from the bed

▶ Characteristic scale attaches to skin at only one point; drop of blood where scale peels off (Auspitz sign)

▶ Variations: Guttate psoriasis (drop-like lesions), pustular psoriasis, psoriatic arthritis

Diagnostic Studies

▶ None usually needed except to rule out other conditions

▶ Rheumatoid factor is negative in psoriatic arthritis.

Differential Diagnosis

▶ Seborrheic dermatitis

▶ Tinea and candida

▶ Drug eruptions

▶ Eczema

▶ Lichen simplex chronicus

Management

Nonpharmacologic Treatment

▶ Avoid rubbing or scratching lesions.

▶ Take oatmeal baths for pruritus.

▶ Avoid excessive sun exposure.

Pharmacologic Treatment

▶ Topical fluorinated steroids with occlusive dressing (Cordran tape) for limited area

▶ Interlesional steroids

▶ Avoid general use of systemic steroids—can cause rebound flares

▶ 2% to 3% salicylic acid to peel off scales

▶ Systemic therapy: methotrexate, anthralin, oral retinoids, or hemodialysis

▶ UVB light with coal tar or psoralens; PUVA if UVB therapy fails

▶ Occlusive therapy with DuoDERM or Tegaderm for at least 7 days

▶ Calcipotriene ointment 0.005%; tazarotene gel for mild to moderate involvement

▶ May require cyclosporin or sulfasalazine

How Long to Treat

▶ Treatment duration depends on the type of psoriasis diagnosed, but primarily until flare-up subsides.

Special Considerations

▶ Von Zumbusch acute pustular psoriasis is a life-threatening problem with acute on-set. There is no known precipitating factor, and the patient may or may not have had stable plaque-like psoriasis in the past.

▶ This condition requires emergency hospitalization.

When to Consult, Refer, Hospitalize

▶ Every patient should be referred to a dermatologist for confirmation of diagnosis and assistance in developing a plan of care.

Follow-Up

▶ Routine, with laboratory monitoring if systemic medications used

Expected Course

▶ Chronic condition requiring initial treatment phase and maintenance therapy

Complications

▶ Secondary infection

Burns

Description

▶ Thermal, electrical, or chemical injury causing damage to the epidermis, dermis, and/or subcutaneous tissue

Etiology

▶ Exposure to intense heat of fire or steam or to damaging chemicals or electrical volt-age; the longer the contact with the skin, the greater the burn injury

Incidence and Demographics

▶ Approximately 1.25 million burn injuries annually in the United States

▶ Flame burns most common in adults; scald burns more common in children

▶ Scald, tar, chemical, and electrical burns more common in the workplace

Risk Factors

▶ Firefighters

▶ Unsupervised children

▶ Workplace exposure to scalding liquids (tar, steam) and chemicals or electricity

Prevention and Screening

▶ Education on fire safety and safe handling of hot liquids, chemicals, and electricity in the community and workplace

▶ Removal from source and application of cold to stop the burning process

Assessment

History

▶ Exposure to fire, chemicals, scalding liquids, or electricity

▶ Intense pain at site of exposure; third-degree burns usually painless

Physical Exam

▶ Burns are classified by extent and depth of tissue involvement, patient age, and associated illness or injury.

▶ The patient's age and health status is critical; even a minor burn on an infant or older adult patient may be fatal.

▶ Extent of involvement can be measured by using the "rule of nines":

▷ Anterior head and neck = 4.5%

▷ Posterior head and neck = 4.5%

▷ Torso and abdomen = 18%

▷ Back = 18%

▷ Anterior arms = 4.5% each

▷ Posterior arms = 4.5% each

▷ Genitalia = 1%

▷ Anterior legs = 9% each

▷ Posterior legs = 9% each

▶ Equate patient's palm size as 1% of total body size

▶ Depth of injury described as first-, second-, or third-degree burns

▷ First-degree: superficial burns involving the epidermis only; redness and blanching erythema (demonstrating capillary refill) of affected area with no initial blistering

▷ Second-degree: partial-thickness burns involve entire epidermis and variable portions of the dermis; red, moist, and edematous skin with small or large bullae

▷ Third-degree: full-thickness burn involving entire dermis and subcutaneous tissue; pale, white, tan, or charred wound that may appear dry and depressed below surrounding skin; skin may feel tight and leathery

Diagnostic Studies

▶ Immediate clinical triage is essential to allow patients to be treated in the most appropriate setting.

Differential Diagnosis

▶ Contact dermatitis

▶ Herpes zoster

▶ Atopic dermatitis

▶ Child abuse

▶ Scalded skin syndrome

Management

In office:

▶ First-degree burns (e.g., sunburn)

▶ Superficial second-degree burns of up to approximately 5% to 6% total body surface area (TBSA) that do not affect areas of function or cosmesis

▶ Selected deeper second-degree burns if not on lower extremities, hands, face, areas of function or cosmesis, or genitals and probably do not cover more than 1% to 2% TBSA

▶ Patient or family must be reliable and home situation functional

Serious burn patients:

▶ Emergency stabilization of following advanced trauma life support (ATLS) guidelines, including establishing and maintaining an airway, establishing vascular access, and instituting fluid resuscitation

Nonpharmacologic Treatment

▶ Burns involving the eye should be irrigated with water, saline, or lactated Ringer's solution.

▶ The wound should be cleaned and debrided using plain soap and water, Betadine diluted with water, or saline solution; remove any dead skin.

▶ Elevate involved extremities.

Pharmacologic Treatment

▶ Topical silver sulfadiazine (Silvadene) in 1/16-inch layer over entire surface, covered with nonabsorbent gauze (Kerlix or Telfa) and wrapped in at least a 3-inch thick non-adhesive wrap

▶ Analgesia with narcotics or NSAID as needed

▶ Tetanus prophylaxis

▶ Antibiotic coverage for secondary infection

How Long to Treat

▶ Dressing changes b.i.d. with frequent reevaluation until resolution

Special Considerations

▶ Very young, older adult, or debilitated patients are at a higher risk for hemodynamic compromise.

When to Consult, Refer, Hospitalize

▶ *Refer patients with the following characteristics to a burn center:*

▷ Deep second-degree or third-degree burns

▷ Burns of greater than 10% TBSA in patients younger than 10 years and older than 50 years

▷   Burns of greater than 20% TBSA in all other patients

▷   Burns of the face, hands, and feet; over a joint or of the perineum; or that are circumferential

▷   Burns resulting from child or adult abuse

▷   Inhalation injury, electrical burns, chemical burns

▷   Suspected toxic epidermal necrolysis syndrome

Follow-Up

▶   Within several days, to ensure proper home wound management and evaluation for signs of infection; then possibly weekly until healed

Expected Course

▶   Depends on extent and location of burn

Complications

▶   Hemodynamic compromise, multi-organ failure, sepsis

▶   Scarring

▶   Posttraumatic stress

▶   Increased photosensitivity of healed skin

CASE STUDIES

Case 1

A 15-year-old boy presents to your clinic after a camping trip with parents. Within 2 days, patient noticed a rash on his legs. Upon close examination, an erythematous linear rash was noted on both lower extremities.

PMH: asthma

Medications: montelukast 10 mg p.o. q. p.m. and albuterol inhaler p.r.n. (no more than one inhaler used every 3 months)

1. What pertinent history is it important to obtain?
2. What is the most likely diagnosis based on this history?
3. What would you expect to find on PE?
4. Is he contagious?
5. How would you treat this patient?

Case 2

A 26-year-old White man comes in with a complaint of a "funny rash" on his back and across his shoulders that has resulted in "brown and white patches." He reports that he has had this rash for 6 months and his girlfriend noticed that the rash was spreading. Seems to be more prominent when he is hot or outside.

Social history: works in an automobile factory and enjoys playing volleyball in his off time; recently joined a church volleyball league

PMH: healthy, does not smoke, drinks 2 to 3 nights per week with friends

1. What pertinent history is it important to obtain?
2. You note discrete, scattered, or confluent patches. Wood's lamp exam reveals faint yellow-green scales. What is the most likely diagnosis?
3. What laboratory tests would you order to confirm the diagnosis?
4. How would you treat this patient?

Case 3

A 5-year-old girl presents to the clinic with skin lesions that the mother reports were at first vesicular by description and have now become honey-crusted. They are in various stages of healing on her face, arms, and legs. Nothing itches at all. Has had no fever. Attends day care.

PMH: no hospitalizations, two to three bouts of otitis media per year

1. What pertinent history is it important to obtain?
2. What is the most likely diagnosis given this presentation?
3. What would you look for on PE?

4. Is she contagious?

5. What laboratory tests would you order?

6. How would you treat this patient?

CASE STUDIES DISCUSSION

Case 1

1. What pertinent history is it important to obtain?

   Any fever, systemic symptoms, any bites or other forms of exposure? Is there a history of irritant dermatitis, or other rashes? What type of allergies does patient have: environmental, food, seasonal, and/or drug?

2. What is the most likely diagnosis based on this history?

   Contact dermatitis, due to a plant such as poison ivy

3. What would you expect to find on PE?

   Eruptions along areas of skin exposure on arms and legs, possibly linear. Papules, dry scaling, and erythema. Possibly scratch marks. Later will see weeping and excoriation.

4. Is he contagious?

   No, contact dermatitis is not contagious unless clothing or other items are contaminated with oil from the plant. All clothing or shoes with oil from the plant have the potential to irritate again until oil is removed.

5. How would you treat this patient?

   Identification and removal of offending agent; relief of symptoms with colloidal oatmeal, astringent, topical corticosteroids (do not use over large areas or if infected), oral steroids if a large area is involved, antihistamines, antibiotics (for cellulitis or impetigo only)

Case 2

1. What pertinent history is it important to obtain?

   Has he used any new products? Allergies? Medications? Previous episodes of same? Any itching, scaling, flaking? Any associated symptoms of disease?

2. You note discrete, scattered, or confluent patches. Wood's lamp exam reveals faint yellow-green scales. What is the most likely diagnosis?

   Tinea versicolor

3. What laboratory tests would you order to confirm the diagnosis?

   KOH and microscope visualization

4. How would you treat this patient?

   Topical selenium sulfide 2.5% shampoo to skin for 30 minutes the wash off for tinea versicolor; repeat 2 weeks later

Case 3

1. What pertinent history is it important to obtain?

   How long have the lesions been there? Fever? Remedies tried so far? Crowded living conditions?

   In day care? Any contacts with similar? Vaccines current?

2. What is the most likely diagnosis given this presentation?

    Impetigo

3. What would you look for on PE?

    Possible poor hygiene evident in child's grooming; breakdown and secondary infection (impetiginizing) of neglected skin lesions; honey-colored fluid oozing from open lesions and others with crusted covering; bullous (large vesicle or bullae containing clear yellow fluid on erythematous base); ecthyma (ulceration with thick adherent crust); possible tenderness; possible regional lymphadenopathy

4. Is she contagious?

    Yes

5. What laboratory tests would you order?

    Diagnosis is primarily clinical; cultures may be warranted if diagnosis is in doubt or if the lesions fail to respond to an appropriate course of antibiotics; possible Gram stain; cultures demonstrate *S. aureus,* group A streptococci, possible methicillin resistant *S. aureus*; if recurrent, serology for anti-DNAse beta to look for prior strep infection.

6. How would you treat this patient?

    Wash area with soap to remove crusts prior to applying topical antibiotic penicillin for streptococci, dicloxacillin for staphylococcus; erythromycin may be used if allergic to penicillin; topical mupirocin for small lesions.

REFERENCES

Arcangelo, V. P., & Peterson, A. M. (2013). *Pharmacotherapeutics for advanced practice.* Philadelphia, PA: Lippincott, Williams & Wilkins.

Berger, T. G. (2012). Skin, hair and nails. In M. A. Papadakis, S. J. McPhee, & M. W. Rabow (Eds.), *Current medical diagnosis and treatment* (52nd ed.). New York, NY: Lange Medical Books/ McGraw Hill.

DiSantostefano, J. (2011). Dermatology procedures. *Journal for Nurse Practitioners, 7*(6), 519–520.

Domino, F. J., Baldor, R. A., Golding, J., & Grimes, J. A. (2015). *The 5 minute clinical consult.* Philadelphia, PA: Lippincott, Williams & Wilkins.

Eichenfield, L. F., Boguniewicz, M., Simpson, E. L., Russell, J. J., Block, J. K., Feldman, S. R., . . . Paller, A. S. (2015). Translating atopic dermatitis management guidelines into practice for primary care providers. *Pediatrics, 136*(3), 554–565.

Facts and Comparisons. (2015). *Drug facts and comparisons 2015.* St. Louis, MO: Wolters Kluwer Health.

Gilbert, D. N., Moellering, R. C., Jr., Eliopoulus, G. M., Chambers, H. F., & Saag, M. S. (2012). *The Sanford guide to antimicrobial therapy.* Hyde Park, VT: Antimicrobial Therapy.

Goroll, A. H., & Mulley, A. G. (2014). *Primary care medicine* (7th ed.). Philadelphia, PA: Lippincott, Williams & Wilkins.

Habif, T. P., Campbell, J. L., Chapman, M. S., Dinulos, J. G., & Zug, K. A. (2011). *Skin disease: Diagnosis and treatment* (3rd ed.). Philadelphia, PA: Saunders.

Hay, W. W., Levin, M. J., Deterding, R. R., & Abzug, M. J. (2014). *Current pediatric diagnosis & treatment.* New York, NY: McGraw-Hill.

U.S. Preventive Services Task Force. (2015). *Guide to clinical preventive services.* Retrieved from http://www.ahrq.gov/professionals/clinicians-providers/guidelines-recommendations/index.html

Wolff, K., Johnson, R. A., & Saavedra, A. (2013). *Fitzpatrick's color atlas and synopsis of clinical dermatology* (7th ed.). New York, NY: McGraw-Hill.

Woo, T. M., & Wynne, A. L. (2011). *Pharmacotherapeutics for nurse practitioner prescribers* (3rd ed.). Philadelphia, PA: F. A. Davis Co.

CHAPTER 6

EYE, EAR, NOSE, AND THROAT DISORDERS

Dawn Bucher, DNP, FNP-BC

GENERAL APPROACH

▶ Assessing visual acuity is the single most important test in evaluating eye complaints in primary care.

▶ The most important approach is to obtain a good history of illness and make a correct diagnosis.

▶ With the emergence of increasingly resistant organisms, it is imperative to be more judicious in prescribing antibiotics for upper respiratory infections, sinusitis, and acute otitis media.

▶ Proper equipment, including a hermetically sealed otoscope with a pneumatic attachment, is critical to performing a proper physical exam.

RED FLAGS

Eyes

▶ Sudden acute onset of vision loss—immediate referral to emergency care is needed

▶ Herpetic keratitis—use topical steroid eye preparations cautiously as it may increase intraocular pressure! Use caution, because herpetic keratitis may present similarly to viral conjunctivitis.

▶ Chemical burns—irrigate immediately and copiously before evaluation.

▶ History suggestive of ocular foreign body with no visible findings—refer to ophthalmology. Many eye problems require evaluation and management by a specialist. See Table 6–1 for signs and symptoms that should be referred immediately to an ophthalmologist.

TABLE 6–1.
RED FLAG SIGNS AND SYMPTOMS OF VISION-THREATENING DISORDERS

SYMPTOMS	SIGNS
Blurred vision that does *not* clear with blinking	Ciliary flush
	Corneal damage (opacities, trauma)
Acute loss or decreased vision	Abnormal pupils
Halos around sources of lights	Increased intraocular pressure
Flashing lights	Shallow anterior chamber
Sudden floating spots or sensation of "cobwebs" across field of vision	Proptosis (forward displacement of the eye globe within the orbit of the eye)
Photophobia	
Periocular headache	Severe green-yellow discharge, eye erythema, chemosis, and lid edema
Ocular pain	
Nystagmus	Absent red reflex

▶ *Acute angle closure glaucoma* results in permanent vision loss if not treated *immediately.*

▶ *Retinoblastoma* (malignant tumor of retina) may present as white pupils (leukocoria), esotropia, exotropia, or anisocoria; refer to ophthalmologist for prompt evaluation.

▶ Contact lens wearers are at higher risk for corneal damage.

Ears

▶ *Complications of ear infections:* Otitis media or externa with spreading infection, mastoid tenderness, lymphadenopathy, and neurologic abnormalities are *urgent for referral.*

▶ Suspected *perforated tympanic membrane* is a contraindication for removal of cerumen impaction by irrigation; refer to a specialist.

Nose and Sinuses

▶ Important, serious findings pointing to complications of sinusitis include external facial swelling, erythema, or cellulitis over an involved sinus (periorbital or forehead); vision changes such as diplopia; difficulty moving eyes (extraocular movements [EOMs]); proptosis; and any abnormal neurologic signs. *Urgent for referral.*

Throat

▶ *Epiglottal spasm:* In cases of suspected epiglottitis, attempting to examine the oral cavity or insert a tongue blade for visualization of the pharynx can result in acute airway obstruction and potential asphyxiation.

▶ Consider *peritonsillar abscess* when the patient with severe tonsillitis (usually more pronounced unilaterally) appears toxic with fever, trismus, "hot potato" voice, palatal bulge, and uvula deviation.

DISORDERS OF THE EYES

Blepharitis

Description

- ▶ Inflammatory disease process of the eyelid(s)
- ▶ Anterior blepharitis involves the eyelashes and follicles; usually subdivided into staphylococcal and seborrheic types
- ▶ Posterior blepharitis involves meibomian gland orifices; is more common than anterior blepharitis

Etiology

- ▶ Seborrheic: sebaceous gland dysfunction with accelerated shedding of skin cells
- ▶ Staphylococcal: super infection of Zeis glands of lid margin and meibomian glands posterior to lashes with *Staphylococcus aureus*; usually part of mixed blepharitis
- ▶ Meibomian gland dysfunction: obstruction and inflammation of the gland; associated with acne rosacea, acne vulgaris, and oral retinoid therapy

Incidence and Demographics

- ▶ One of the most common eye disorders in adults; not common in children
- ▶ Males and females affected equally
- ▶ Mixed (seborrheic and infectious) blepharitis most common type

Risk Factors

- ▶ History of skin problems: seborrheic dermatitis, contact dermatitis, acne rosacea, dry eye syndrome
- ▶ Poor hygiene, including improper cleaning of the face using old or contaminated eye makeup; contact lens use
- ▶ Immunocompromise due to chemotherapy, diabetes, or HIV

Prevention and Screening

- ▶ Maintenance of long-term regimen of lid hygiene can decrease risk of recurrence.

Assessment

History

- ▶ Unilateral or bilateral eye irritation, itching, erythema of the lids, or changes in the eyelashes
- ▶ Common complaints: burning, watering, gritty sensation, crusting and mattering of the lashes and medial canthus, red lids, red eyes, photophobia, and impaired vision
- ▶ Symptoms worse upon awakening (typically in the morning)
- ▶ Additional complaints of purulent drainage if infection has developed (conjunctivitis, stye)
- ▶ History of recurrent stye, acne, rosacea, or eczema

Physical Exam
- ▶ All types: eyelid erythema, inflammation, change in eyelash pattern (broken, missing, misdirected)
- ▶ Seborrheic type: dandruff-like flaking, scaling, waxy surface of lid margin
- ▶ Infectious: purulent discharge, concurrent papules or pustules, punctate ulcerations
- ▶ Mixed: all signs listed above
- ▶ Chronic: thickening of lid with or without above concurrent symptoms
- ▶ Conjunctiva may be infected.
- ▶ Visual acuity unaffected; exam of cornea and pupil normal

Diagnostic Studies
- ▶ Rarely, a culture of secretions may be indicated if treatment failure with usual antibiotics

Differential Diagnosis
- ▶ Chalazion, hordeolum, conjunctivitis, and keratitis may result from blepharitis.
- ▶ Sebaceous cell carcinoma of eyelid: initial presentation similar to blepharitis (usually unilateral), styes, and chalazion; consider if no response to treatments after 1 month.

Management
Nonpharmacologic Treatment
- ▶ Warm, moist compresses q.i.d. x 15 minutes to soften encrustations
- ▶ Gentle lid massage with circular motion following warm compress application
- ▶ Daily lid hygiene using dilute tear-free shampoo with warm, damp cotton tip (cotton swab or ball)
- ▶ Discontinue use of contact lens or eye makeup while symptomatic or being treated
- ▶ Maintenance: long-term regimen of lid hygiene helps prevent outbreaks of more symptomatic disease.

Pharmacologic Treatment
- ▶ Topical ophthalmic antibiotics: choice of bacitracin, sodium sulfacetamide, erythromycin, ofloxacin (Ocuflox) depending on sensitivities, allergies; frequency and duration of treatment guided by severity
- ▶ Severe cases: consider oral antibiotic use—choice of doxycycline 100 mg/d or tetracycline 1,000 mg/d in divided doses, tapered after clinical improvement (2–4 weeks) to doxycycline 50 mg/d or tetracycline 250–500 mg/d. For pregnant women or children consider erythromycin or azithromycin (500 mg on day 1, followed by 250 mg days 2–5)
- ▶ Short-term topical corticosteroids for acute eyelid or ocular surface inflammation may be useful. Should be evaluated by ophthalmologist prior to use and 2 weeks after use.

Special Considerations
- ▶ A herpes simplex infection of the eyelid may appear very similar to staphylococcus blepharitis but has acute onset.

When to Consult, Refer, Hospitalize

▶ Refer to ophthalmologist if treatment fails or if concurrent or additional symptoms develop, requiring surgical treatment (meibomian gland drainage or extraction)

Follow-Up

Expected Course

▶ Alleviate chronic inflammatory symptoms with lid hygiene.

▶ Infectious component should resolve with treatment as above.

Complications

▶ Spread of infection to conjunctiva, cornea, or both

▶ Scarring of eyelid margin

Nasolacrimal Duct Obstruction

Description

▶ Dacryostenosis: "blocked tear ducts" with tear drainage cut off between lacrimal sac and nose

▶ Most common cause of persistent tearing and ocular discharge in children

Etiology

▶ Blockage caused by residual epithelial membranes; canalization of the nasolacrimal duct is incomplete

▶ Generally not completely occluded

Incidence and Demographics

▶ Occurs in up to 6% of newborns; however, 20% of healthy infants may have symptoms sometime during the first year of life.

Risk Factors

▶ None known

Prevention and Screening

▶ No known prevention

Assessment

History

▶ Parent reports chronic or intermittent tearing and debris on eyelashes (mattering) from one or both eyes

▶ Redness of the conjunctiva is not typical; mild redness of lower lid may be present from chronic rubbing of eyes.

Physical Exam

▶ Note presence of watery or mucus discharge; may be purulent if infected; eyes look wet, tearing over lid; increase in size of tear meniscus; palpation of lacrimal sac may cause reflux of tears or mucoid discharge

▶ Maceration of eyelids from excessive tearing; crusting on lashes

Diagnostic Studies

▶ None indicated; diagnosis based on history and physical exam; if area is infected, may perform culture and sensitivity

▶ May perform fluorescein study (dye disappearance test)

Differential Diagnosis

▶ Congenital glaucoma

▶ Entropion

▶ Conjunctivitis

▶ Corneal abrasion or foreign body

▶ Blepharitis

▶ Uveitis

▶ Dacryocystocele

Management

Nonpharmacologic Treatment

▶ Observe for up to 6–7 months if asymptomatic other than watery eyes.

▶ Lacrimal sac (Crigler) massage: Apply moderate pressure downward on lacrimal sac to expel buildup 2–3 times per day until symptoms resolve.

▶ Lacrimal duct probing and irrigation: should be performed by an ophthalmologist, usually if unresolved by 12 months of age; may be done sooner if recurrent infections or lid irritation

▶ Nasolacrimal duct (NLD) intubation or balloon dacryocystoplasty have been used in treatment failure and in children >12 months of age

Pharmacologic Treatment

▶ Treat secondary infections with topical antibiotics (tobramycin, moxifloxacin, gentamicin, erythromycin, sulfacetamide, or fluoroquinolones); short course, 3–5 days.

How Long to Treat

▶ Depends on response

Special Considerations

▶ None

When to Consult, Refer, Hospitalize

▶ Reevaluate at 6–7 months; refer to ophthalmologist if patient remains symptomatic; signs and symptoms of dacryocystitis or dacryocystocele; or signs of amblyopia or anisometropia.

Follow-Up

Expected course

▶ 90% of cases will resolve spontaneously by 6 months of age.

Complications

▶ Acute or chronic dacryocystitis

▶ Secondary infection of conjunctivae or eyelids due to excessive drainage

Hordeolum (Stye) and Chalazion

Description

▶ Inflammatory disorders of the lubricating glands of the eyelids and eyelashes

▷ Hordeolum (stye): acute inflammation or infection of the eyelid margin involving the sebaceous gland of an eyelash or meibomian gland

▷ Chalazion: chronic inflammation that develops when a Zeis or meibomian gland becomes obstructed

Etiology

▶ Obstructed glands (Zeis, Moll, or meibomian) cause inflammatory papule, pustule, or granulomatous papule

▶ Hordeolum: 90%–95% caused by infection with *S. aureus*

▶ Chalazion: chronic granuloma from obstructed Zeis or meibomian gland; may also result from a chronic hordeolum

Incidence and Demographics

▶ Predominant age: none, seen in all ages

▶ Predominant sex: male = female

Risk Factors

▶ Poor eyelid hygiene

▶ Previous hordeolum

▶ Wearing contact lenses

▶ Applying makeup

▶ Blepharitis and rosacea

Prevention and Screening

▶ Eyelid hygiene

Assessment

History
- ▶ Patient complains of a sudden onset of localized tenderness, swelling, or redness of the eyelid.
- ▶ Foreign body sensation
- ▶ History of prior episodes

Physical Exam
- ▶ Localized or generalized inflammation or erythema of the eyelid
- ▶ Erythematous papule or pustule may be visible on outer or conjunctival aspect of eyelid.
- ▶ Possible ulceration at base of lash follicle where infectious head has ruptured.
- ▶ Conjunctiva may be infected.
- ▶ Visual acuity unaffected; exam of cornea and pupil normal

Diagnostic Studies
- ▶ Usually none indicated; culture of eyelid margins usually not necessary

Differential Diagnosis

- ▶ Sebaceous cell carcinoma (rare)
- ▶ Trauma
- ▶ Blepharitis
- ▶ Dacryocystitis
- ▶ Periorbital cellulitis

Management

Nonpharmacologic Treatment
- ▶ Warm compresses for 15 minutes 4 times per day
- ▶ Daily lid hygiene until resolved (see section on blepharitis)
- ▶ Educate patient not to squeeze or express hordeolum.

Pharmacologic Treatment
- ▶ Ophthalmic antibiotics on eyelid margin: erythromycin ointment (Ilotycin) up to 6 times daily for 7–10 days
- ▶ Artificial tears for underlying dry eyes
- ▶ Oral dicloxacillin or cephalexin for 2 weeks if refractory to topical antibiotics

How Long to Treat
- ▶ Lid hygiene and warm compresses continued until resolution
- ▶ Antibiotic ointment for 7–10 days

Special Considerations

▶ None

When to Consult, Refer, Hospitalize

▶ Refer nonresponding conditions to an ophthalmologist for excision and drainage or curettage.

▶ Though rare, the initial presentation of cancer is similar to blepharitis, styes, and chalazion; consider if no response to treatment after 1 month and refer to ophthalmology.

Follow-Up

Expected Course

▶ Usually resolves with good hygiene and warm compresses

▶ May be recurrent or develop in clusters that do not heal well; consider diabetes mellitus

▶ If no improvement, assess need for surgical treatment

Complications

▶ Cellulitis of the eyelid

Strabismus

Description

▶ Abnormal ocular alignment; commonly referred to as "crossed eyes"

▶ Can occur in one or both eyes, and in any direction

▶ Described as "esotropia" when eyes are crossed inward (nasal deviation); "exotropia" when eyes are crossed outward (temporal deviation); "hypertropia" or "hypotropia" when the eyes deviate upward or downward, regardless of which eye is fixated.

▶ Uncorrected, may result in amblyopia (loss or lack of development of central vision in one eye). When eyes are misaligned, the brain will receive two images instead of the normal one; the brain manages this by "shutting down" or not processing one of the images. Left untreated, this eventually becomes permanent, leading to loss of depth perception. Children do not outgrow strabismus.

Etiology

▶ Unknown cause in most children

▶ May be congenital or acquired (disease-induced); may be caused by diseases including cranial nerve palsies, orbital mass, orbital fractures, Graves's ophthalmopathy, retinoblastoma, neurologic disorders such as cerebral palsy, and certain genetic conditions

▶ May be paralytic (paralysis of one or more ocular muscles) or nonparalytic (unequal muscle tone)

▶ Viral infections can affect cranial nerves, causing development of strabismus; in case of viral illness, strabismus may resolve spontaneously.

▶ Results from an inability of the visual cortex to use the eyes together, or a disorder of the cranial nerves (III, IV, or VI) or the extraocular muscles

▶ An intermittent phoria—esophoria or exophoria—is common in the first 6 months of life. It may be noted by parents particularly when infant is tired; may report that child's eyes are "crossed" for a few seconds to minutes. Phorias resolve spontaneously by 6 months of life and do not require referral before that time.

Incidence and Demographics

▶ Genetic: Parents with strabismus have a 12%–17% chance of having a child with strabismus.

▶ Occurs in approximately 4% of children

Risk Factors

▶ Family history of strabismus

▶ Prematurity

▶ Low birth weight with history of retinopathy of prematurity or neurologic complications

▶ Any other disease that causes vision loss may also cause strabismus.

Prevention and Screening

▶ Alignment of eyes should be assessed on all well child check-ups; visual acuity should be assessed in routine exams as soon as children are capable of using eye charts (sooner if indicated).

Assessment

History

▶ Parent reports that the child's eyes "don't move together," "are crossed"

▶ Developmental/birth history

▶ Family history of strabismus or other eye disorders

▶ History of trauma, other medical problems, or exposure to toxins or medications

▶ Onset of deviation (early infancy); duration and severity of deviation; whether deviation is constant or intermittent and what exacerbates the deviation (fatigue, positions of gaze)

Physical Exam

▶ Assess general health, developmental level, neurologic status, and the presence of a head tilt.

▶ Assess visual acuity and function, pupillary reactivity, and eyelid position.

▶ Extraocular movements (EOMs): Six cardinal positions of gaze (CN III, IV, and VI) would detect primarily a paralytic strabismus, but in each position, the corneal light reflex can be used to assess for nonparalytic strabismus.

▶ Corneal light reflex (Hirschberg): demonstrates a nonparalytic tropia

▶ Cover test: No movement is detected if the patient has normal ocular alignment. Strabismus is present if the eye that is not occluded shifts to refixate.

▶ Cover/uncover test: The patient stares at a fixed point. A cover is placed over one eye for a few seconds and then is rapidly removed. The eye that was under the cover is carefully observed for movement or deviation; if detected, latent strabismus is present.

▶ Brückner test: The provider stands about 20 inches from the child in a darkened room, looks at both eyes through the ophthalmoscope, and notes symmetry of red reflexes bilaterally.

▶ Note presence of nystagmus or other involuntary eye movements.

▶ Perform a funduscopic exam; note fullness of red reflex.

Diagnostic Studies

▶ Neuroimaging studies (visual evoked response, electroretinogram, and electrooculography) may be indicated but are rarely required for routine strabismus.

▷ Consider in children with craniofacial malformations, neurologic abnormalities, trauma, or acute onset of paralytic or restrictive strabismus

▶ CAT scan and MRI studies of the orbits and head may be helpful to exclude an intracranial mass (bleed or tumor) if onset is acute or if associated with trauma, craniofacial abnormalities, or neurologic disease.

Differential Diagnosis

▶ Pseudostrabismus

▶ Amblyopia

▶ Ocular instability of infancy

▶ Cranial nerve palsies

▶ CNS or orbital tumor

▶ Orbital fractures

▶ Graves' opthalmopathy

Management

Nonpharmacologic Treatment

▶ Treatment should be started as soon as a diagnosis is made.

▶ Management depends on the cause.

▶ Goal of treatments is to improve ocular alignment and binocularity.

▶ Any child in whom strabismus is suspected must be evaluated and treated by a pediatric ophthalmologist.

▶ Use of optical devices (prisms and glasses). Eyeglasses may be sufficient to induce binocular function and correct refractive errors.

▶ Surgery on the eye muscles is successful up to 80% of the time; some patients (20%–25%) may require a second surgery.

▶ The unaffected eye may be patched, alone or before glasses or surgery, to prevent amblyopia.

▶ Visual training exercises may be useful.

Pharmacologic Treatment

▶ Topical miotic drops to manipulate accommodation (atropine 1% daily or on weekends) may be helpful in some forms of esotropia. This is done only by the ophthalmologist.

▶ Botulinum toxin A (Botox) injection: produces a dose-dependent duration of paralysis to the extraocular muscle. Two or more injections are usually necessary for lasting effects.

Special Considerations

▶ None

When to Consult, Refer, Hospitalize

▶ Constant strabismus at any age

▶ Corneal light reflex test or cover test abnormality

▶ Persistent esodeviations after 4 months of age

▶ Asymmetry of pupil with Brückner test

▶ Any deviation change

▶ Parental concern of ocular alignment

▶ Refer to an ophthalmologist *as soon as strabismus is observed*, especially in infancy; in an infant <1 year, amblyopia can occur with as little as 1 week of abnormal visual input.

Follow-Up

Expected Course

▶ Depends on type and treatment modality employed; once alignment is achieved, patients followed by ophthalmologist every 3–6 months (depending on age and type of strabismus)

▶ Decompensation and reappearance may occur in up to 40% of patients in adulthood.

Complications

▶ Amblyopia, diplopia (in acquired strabismus in patients ≥3 years of age),

▶ Secondary contracture of the extraocular muscles, limiting extraocular mobility and binocular visual fields

▶ Secondary contracture develops over a course of weeks to months if strabismus is not treated

▶ Adverse psychosocial and vocational consequences

Retinoblastoma

Description

▶ Rare malignant tumor originating from the retina; most common intraocular tumor of childhood; can be unilateral (70%) or bilateral (30%)

Etiology

▶ Genetic mutations of nerve cells in the retina; originates in retinoblasts following loss, mutation, deletion, or rearrangement of retinoblastoma gene on chromosome 13

▶ Hereditary retinoblastoma is autosomal dominant and tends to affect both eyes.

▶ Unaffected parents who have one child with retinoblastoma have a 4%–7% risk of having a subsequent child with the disease.

Incidence and Demographics

▶ Occurs in 1:15,000 to 1:16,600 live births in the United States and Northern Europe

▶ Ninety percent of all retinoblastoma cases are diagnosed by 3 years of age.

▶ Forty percent inherited; 60% noninheritable type

▶ Accounts for 3% of all childhood malignancies under age 15

Risk Factors

▶ Family history of retinoblastoma or retinomas (nonmalignant)

Prevention and Screening

▶ None known; genetic testing can identify individuals with the retinoblastoma mutation only about 5% of the time (not helpful)

▶ Red reflex checks at all well baby and well child visits

▶ Assess all children with strabismus to rule out retinoblastoma.

▶ Siblings and children of parents with retinoblastoma should have thorough ophthalmic examinations (which can be done under anesthesia) shortly after birth, every 3 months until age 3–4, and every 6 months until age 5–6.

Assessment

History

▶ Parents may note crossed eyes or outward deviation of eyes.

▶ Leukocoria may be noticed in a photograph.

▶ Pain and redness are rare; usually no complaints of visual problems because the unaffected eye maintains the vision.

▶ Note family history of malignancies, particularly of the eyes.

Physical Exam

▶ "Cat's eye reflex" (leukocoria): white pupil seen when observing the red reflex; may be unilateral or bilateral; not necessary for diagnosis

▶ Presence of strabismus, anisocoria, decreased vision, ocular inflammation, or proptosis (late finding)

Diagnostic Studies

All studies should be done by an ophthalmologist and an oncologist.

▶ Dilated indirect ophthalmoscopic examination performed under anesthesia

▶ Aqueous cytology (rarely used as it can increase risk of extraocular spread of retino-blastoma), CT scan of the head and orbits

▶ MRI to confirm presence of an intraocular mass

▶ Ocular ultrasonography

Differential Diagnosis

▶ Retinopathy of prematurity

▶ Coats's disease

▶ Hypopyon

▶ Iritis

▶ Uveitis

▶ Toxoplasmosis, other ocular infections

▶ Strabismus

Management

▶ By ophthalmology and oncology; treatment will depend on extent of disease and may include intravenous chemotherapy, radiation, radioactive plaques (I-125 brachy-therapy), cryotherapy, laser photoablation, and surgery (enucleation)

▶ Fractionated external beam radiation therapy (EBRT): reserved for eyes with residual or recurrent retinoblastoma following a complete course of intravenous chemo-therapy. EBRT is associated with fatal bony and soft tissue secondary malignant neoplasms.

When to Consult, Refer, Hospitalize

▶ All children with retinoblastoma are referred immediately to ophthalmology.

Follow-Up

▶ Frequently by ophthalmology; every 3 months for a year; if stable then can be ta-pered to every 4 months and then every 6 months, and then annually

▶ Long-term by multidisciplinary team

▶ Future evaluations for:

▷ Contralateral eye developing retinoblastoma (in about 15%)

▷ Metastasis: occurs before 5 years

▷ Second malignancies; may include osteosarcoma (most common), bladder, breast, lung cancer, and melanoma; occurs in about 10% of children

Expected course

▶ 94% overall 5-year survival rate in the United States

▶ Development of metastatic disease usually seen within 1 year of diagnosis

▶ Poor prognosis for children with metastatic disease

▶ Vision salvageable in large percentage of children diagnosed at early stages

Complications

▶ Increase risk of cancer returning in eye and other areas

▶ Death

▶ Blindness

Conjunctivitis

Description

▶ Acute inflammation of the palpebral and/or bulbar conjunctival layer of the eyes

▶ Commonly referred to as "pink eye" or "red eye"; may be bilateral or unilateral

▶ Conjunctivitis in first month of life is most commonly caused by infections passed through vaginal delivery; known as ophthalmia neonatorum.

Etiology

▶ Many causative organisms; *Chlamydia trachomatis* and *Neisseria gonorrhoeae* most common in newborns

▶ Viral: adenoviruses (most common), herpes zoster, herpes simplex virus (HSV) type 1 and type 2, enterovirus

▶ Bacterial: *S. aureus* (common in adults), *Streptococcus pneumoniae* (common in children), *Haemophilus influenzae*, *C. trachomatis*, *N. gonorrheae*, *Neisseria meningitidis*

▶ Allergic: allergic rhinitis ("hay fever"), seasonal allergies, atopy, contact blepharitis, nonspecific

▶ Irritative: topical medications, wind, dry eye, contact lens solutions, UV light exposure, smoke

▶ Autoimmune: Sjögren's syndrome, Wegener's granulomatosis, pemphigoid

▶ Rare: fungal, parasitic, rickettsial, tuberculosis, syphilis, Kawasaki disease, gout, Graves' disease, sarcoidosis, psoriasis, Stevens-Johnson syndrome, Reiter syndrome

Incidence and Demographics

▶ Common eye disorder in all ages

▶ Pediatric: viral, bacterial

▶ Adult: viral, bacterial, allergic

▶ Increased incidence in the fall because of higher incidence of viral infections and exposure to seasonal allergens

Risk Factors

▶ History of contact with infected people

▶ Contact lenses: especially wearing lenses overnight

▶ Sexually transmitted disease contact: gonococcal, *Chlamydial*, syphilis, or herpes

▶ Exposure to infectious agents, chemical agents, wind, extreme temperatures, allergens

Prevention and Screening

▶ Avoid known allergens, irritants, and others with conjunctivitis.

▶ Frequent handwashing and good hygiene to reduce risk of transmission

▶ Provide gonorrhea prophylaxis for newborns: 1% silver nitrate, 0.5% erythromycin, or 1% tetracycline ointment.

Assessment

History (see Table 6–2)

▶ Irritated eyes with redness, mild pain, or itching in one or both eyes, or spread from one to the other

▶ Gritty, scratching or burning sensation, sensation of fullness around the eyes, itching, and photophobia

▶ Watery or purulent drainage, crusting on eyelashes upon awakening

▶ Visual complaints limited to complaints of blurry vision that clears with blinking

▶ Assess for associated symptoms that may indicate systemic disease, such as rash, lesions, joint pain, fever, genitourinary complaints, constitutional symptoms.

Physical Exam

▶ Must document visual acuity

▶ Pupillary reaction and EOMs intact

▶ Edema of eyelids and matted eyelashes

▶ Red eye, conjunctival injection

▶ Foreign body sensation

▶ *Note:* ciliary flush, corneal changes, pupil abnormalities, and photophobia are not associated with simple conjunctivitis; must rule out keratitis, iritis, or other serious conditions through urgent referral (see Box 6–1)

Diagnostic Studies

▶ Conjunctival scrapings for microscopic examination and culture are recommended for all cases; mandatory for purulent, membranous, or pseudomembranous

▶ May consider fluorescein staining to assess for epithelial integrity (keratitis, ulcer)

▶ Enzyme immunoassays for *Chlamydia* organisms if suspected as etiology

Differential Diagnosis

▶ Acute uveitis

▶ Foreign body/corneal ulcers

▶ Acute glaucoma

▶ Scleritis, episcleritis

▶ Blepharitis

▶ Pingueculitis

▶ Keratitis

TABLE 6–2.
DIFFERENTIATING CHARACTERISTICS OF CONJUNCTIVITIS

CAUSE	SYMPTOMS
Bacterial	Often starts in one eye, spreads to both
	Occasionally associated with sore throat or fever
	Mild pruritus
	Moderate tearing
	Generalized hyperemia
	Profuse exudate (flaky and amorphous; copious and eyelids "stuck together")
	Preauricular adenopathy uncommon
	Stained scrapings/exudates: bacteria or polymorphonuclear cells (PMNs)
	Conjuntival chemosis/edema
	If patient wears contact lenses, rule out microbial keratitis
N. gonorrhea	Copious amounts of purulent discharge
	Chemosis/conjunctival/lid edema
Chlamydia	Mild pruritus
	Moderate tearing
	Hyperemia generalized
	Profuse exudates: copious and eyelids "stuck together"
	Preauricular lymphadenopathy common with inclusion conjunctivitis
	Stained scrapings/exudates: PMNs, plasma cells, inclusion bodies
	Never associated with sore throat or fever
	Genitourinary symptoms may be evident
	Photophobia (indicator of advanced infection)
Viral	Minimal pruritus
	Profuse tearing
	Generalized hyperemia
	Minimal exudate
	Preauricular lymphadenopathy common
	Stained scrapings/exudates: monocytes
	Occasionally associated with sore throat and fever
	Herpetic type may be associated with cold sores, burning sensation; rarely—itching
Allergic	Severe itchy eyes
	Moderate tearing (stringy discharge; usually bilateral)
	Generalized hyperemia
	Minimal exudates
	Preauricular lymphadenopathy: not present
	Stained scraping/exudates: eosinophils
	Never associated with sore throat or fever
	+/– associated allergy type symptoms (rhinitis, sneezing)
	Seasonal or dander allergies
	Chemosis/conjunctival/eyelid edema
	"Cobblestone" appearance of conjunctival edema

Management

Nonpharmacologic Treatment

- ▶ Apply cool moist compresses: up to 4x/day, to ease irritation and itch
- ▶ Replacing eye makeup, especially mascara
- ▶ Patient should avoid wearing contact lenses until conjunctivitis resolves and consider replacement with new lenses.
- ▶ Educate patient on proper use of eye drops.
- ▶ Patient should avoid irritants (smoke, wind, sun).

Pharmacologic Treatment

- ▶ Allergic and atopic:
  - ▷ Ketotifen (Zaditor, Alaway) 0.25%, 1 drop b.i.d.
  - ▷ Cromolyn (Opticrom) 4% q.i.d.
  - ▷ Epinastine (Elestat) 0.05% b.i.d.
  - ▷ Ketorolac (Acular) 0.1%, 1 drop q.i.d.
  - ▷ Emedastine 0.05%, 1 drop q.i.d.
  - ▷ Azelastine (Optivar) 0.05% 1 drop b.i.d.
  - ▷ Olopatadine (Patanol) 0.1%, 1 drop b.i.d. or 0.2%, 1 drop daily
  - ▷ Oral nonsedating antihistamines: cetirizine (Zyrtec), fexofenadine (Allegra), for nasal and urticarial symptoms
  - ▷ Oral antihistamine (diphenhydramine) in severe cases
- ▶ Bacterial (nonsexually transmitted infection [STI]): self-limited (5–7 days); treatment optional (consider cost versus bacterial resistance-production)
  - ▷ Trimethoprim/polymyxin (Polytrim) ophthalmic 1 to 2 drops q.i.d. x 7 days
  - ▷ Erythromycin (Ilotycin) ophthalmic ointment ½ inch b.i.d./q.i.d. x 5 days
  - ▷ Sulfacetamide sodium (Bleph-10) 2 drops q 4 hrs while awake x 5 days
  - ▷ Tobramycin 3% (Tobrex) ophthalmic drops q 4 hrs; ointment q 8 hrs
- ▶ Bacterial (gonococcal)
  - ▷ Gonococcal: hospitalize and treat with systemic ceftriaxone (Rocephin) 25–50 mg/kg/d IV or IM, or cefotaxime (Claforan) 25–50 mg/kg/d IV or IM q 12h x 7 days; if no corneal lesions, ceftriaxone 1 g IM x1 and topical bacitracin ophthalmic ointment ½ inch q.i.d. x 7 days
  - ▷ Chlamydial:
    - ▶ Adults—doxycycline (Vibramycin) 100 mg p.o. b.i.d. x 3 weeks; children— erythromycin 50 mg/kg/d p.o. ÷ 4 doses x 14 days
  - ▷ Neonates: erythromycin ethylsuccinate 30mg/kg/d q 6 hrs p.o. x 14 days
    - ▶ If other bacteria suspected, base treatment on culture and sensitivity results

- Viral (nonherpetic):
  - ▷ Artificial tears for symptomatic relief
  - ▷ Vasoconstrictor/antihistamine (naphazoline/pheniramine) q.i.d. for severe itching
  - ▷ May consider topical antibiotics (see above)
- Viral (herpetic): Refer to ophthalmologist for treatment.

How Long to Treat

- Length of treatment determined by etiology and responsiveness to treatment
- If not resolved in 5–7 days, consider alternate diagnosis/ophthalmologic consultation
- Refer to ophthalmologist if condition is worse in 24 hours.

Special Considerations

- Geriatric: suspect autoimmune, systemic, or irritative conditions
- Pregnancy or lactation: Do not use doxycycline.
- Day care regulations may require a child to be treated with a topical antibiotic despite lack of evidence.

When to Consult, Refer, Hospitalize

- Hospitalization for hyperacute bacterial conjunctivitis requiring IV antibiotics or for penetrating ocular trauma
- Immediate referral to ophthalmologist if severe pain, ciliary flush, changed visual acuity, abnormal eye exam, contact lens–related bacterial conjunctivitis, or signs of herpetic etiology
- Referral to ophthalmologist symptoms worsen within 24 hours

Follow-Up

Expected Course

- Bacterial conjunctivitis: 2–5 days with treatment, 5–7 days without treatment
- Viral conjunctivitis: 5–14 days
- Herpes simplex: 2–3 weeks

Complications

- Potential for spread of infection to surrounding areas (blepharitis, keratitis, iritis)
- Corneal ulcers or perforation (gonococcal infection)
- Scars on cornea, lids, with eyelids or lashes misdirected
- Hypopyon

Iritis/Uveitis/Keratitis

Description

- Iritis: inflammation of the iris

▶ Keratitis: corneal inflammation or infection that is potentially vision-threatening; result of infection or direct irritation

▶ Uveitis: acute intraocular inflammation of one or more of the components of uveal tract (iris, ciliary body, choroids, and retina)

   ▷ Anterior uveitis: inflammation of the iris (iritis) or iris and ciliary body (iridocyclitis); ~ 90% of patients with uveitis

   ▷ Intermediate uveitis: inflammation of structures posterior to the lens (pars planitis or peripheral uveitis)

   ▷ Posterior uveitis: inflammation of the choroid (choroiditis), retina (chorioretinitis) or vitreous near the optic nerve and macula

▶ Panuveitis: all components affected

   ▷ May be acute or chronic

Etiology

▶ Uveitis (caused by trauma, infections, inflammation, or, rarely, neoplasms); isolated eye disease (lens-induced uveitis, trauma, pars planitis, acute retinal necrosis); masquerade syndromes (ocular lymphoma, leukemia, retinoblastoma); idiopathic (~25%)

▶ Cause differs by location

▶ Anterior uveitis (iritis): trauma is common; 50% of nontraumatic causes are idopathic; 20% are caused by seronegative spondyloarthropathies (ankylosing spondylitis, reactive arthritis, psoriatic arthritis, inflammatory bowel disease); 10% are caused by juvenile ideopathic arthritis. Less common infections include herpes, syphilis, and tuberculosis.

▶ Intermediate: most are idiopathic

▶ Posterior: toxoplasmosis is the most common, followed by idiopathic

▶ Panuveitis: idiopathic (22% to 45%) and sarcoidosis (14% to 28%). Unilateral panuveitis is often endophthalmitis (endogenous or related to trauma or surgery). Bilateral panuveitis can be caused by sarcoidosis or syphilis.

▶ Keratitis: frequently associated with trauma, history of HSV, bacterial infections, or contact lens wear

Incidence and Demographics

▶ Noninfectious uveitis accounts for 10% of legal blindness in the United States.

▶ Eighty percent of uveitis cases seen in children are caused by juvenile rheumatoid arthritis.

▶ Affects all ages

▶ Affects males more than females (2.5:1) in HLA-B27 anterior uveitis, otherwise affects males the same as females

▶ Iritis is 4 times more prevalent than posterior uveitis.

Risk Factors

▶ Immunocompromised status

BOX 6–1.

CHARACTERISTICS OF KERATITIS/IRITIS/UVEITIS

	Definition	Causes	Exam Findings	Plan
Keratitis	Corneal inflammation or infection that is potentially vision-threatening; due to infection or direct irritation	Trauma, contact lens use and refractive corneal surgery are common causes of bacterial keratitis; herpes simplex virus types 1 and 2 or varicella zoster virus	Ciliary injection often with constricted pupils, watery or purulent discharge, photophobia, possible corneal clouding or lesions, vision loss depending on the location, extraocular herpetic rash	Refer to ophthalmology
Iritis/Uveitis	Inflammation of the uveal tract, including the iris and the ciliary body (anterior) and/or choroid (posterior)	Often associated with immunologic disorders; infection with TB, syphilis, cytomegalovirus (CMV), toxoplasmosis, herpes, Lyme disease; may be idiopathic	Deep eye pain, ciliary flush, photophobia, redness, tearing, decreased vision, 360-degree perilimbal injection	Refer to ophthalmology; consider HLA-B27, ANA, PPD, Lyme serology, RPR if severe or recurrent

▶ Autoimmune and inflammatory systemic conditions (Behcet's disease and ankylosing spondylitis, associated with the gene for human leukocyte antigen [HLA] B51/B5 and B27 respectively)

▶ Contact lenses

▶ HSV history or close contact with an HSV-infected person

Prevention and Screening

▶ High-risk groups: screened routinely by ophthalmology

▶ Contact precautions with active HSV lesions; varicella vaccination

Assessment

History

▶ Determine history of autoimmune diseases, sexually transmitted diseases, tuberculosis, AIDS.

▶ Note decreased visual acuity.

▶ Usually unilateral eye pain, redness, tearing, photophobia, and decreased vision; 360-degree perilimbal injection

▶ History of eye trauma, an associated systemic disease, or risk factors for infection

▶ Anterior uveitis: acute onset of deep eye pain, redness, photophobia, visual loss

▶ Intermediate uveitis and posterior uveitis: insidious onset; presents with altered vision or floaters; typically no pain, redness, tearing, or photophobia

▶ Keratitis: history of varicella or herpes simplex infection; prodromal period of fever, malaise, headache, and eye pain before eruptions or lesions may be common; acute onset of eye pain, headache, photophobia, tearing, ocular redness, decreased or blurred vision

Physical Exam

▶ Slit-lamp exam and indirect ophthalmoscopy are necessary for precise diagnosis.

▶ Assess visual acuity and extraocular movement; perform funduscopic exam.

▶ Anterior (iritis): tenderness to palpation, diffuse redness with perilimbal erythema; constricted pupil; frequently unilateral

▶ Iritis: opacities or haziness on the cornea and within the aqueous (may hinder funduscopic exam). If visualized, funduscopic findings may include keratic precipitates ("mutton fat"), nodules on the iris, hypopyon, macular changes (lesions, edema), and optic neuropathy (rare).

▶ Posterior uveitis: Funduscopic findings will vary with the offending organism; commonly bilateral.

▶ Keratitis: diffuse redness with ciliary injection, often with constricted pupil; eye discharge; and pain, photophobia, and vision loss depending on the location of ulceration; typically unilateral

Diagnostic Studies

▶ Usually unnecessary, but may need studies to determine whether an undiagnosed underlying cause exists

▶ Slit-lamp exam, dilated fundus exam, and intraocular pressure measurements by ophthalmologist

Differential Diagnosis

See Table 6–3

▶ Conjunctivitis

▶ Acute angle-closure glaucoma

▶ Retinal detachment

▶ Intraocular tumors

▶ Scleritis/episcleritis

▶ CNS lymphoma

Management

Nonpharmacologic Treatment

▶ Educate patient on proper method for instilling eye drops.

▶ Instruct patient to wear dark glasses if photophobia is a problem.

▶ Avoid all contact with nonimmune people

TABLE 6–3.
SELECTED DIFFERENTIAL DIAGNOSES OF THE RED EYE

	CONJUNCTIVITIS	SCLERITIS	UVEITIS/IRITIS	KERATITIS	CLOSED-ANGLE GLAUCOMA
Eye pain	No	Severe, boring	Sometimes	Usually	Yes
Redness	Diffuse; not associated with perilimbal erythema	Segmental or diffuse; dark red, purple, or blue	360-degree perilimbal (worse at limbus)	Diffuse, ciliary injection	Diffuse, scleral
Discharge	Usually	No	No	Maybe	No
Photophobia	No	Yes	Yes, if anterior	Yes	Yes
Pupils	Normal	Normal	Constricted	Normal to constricted	Mild dilation, less responsive
Cornea	Clear	Clear	Clear to hazy	Hazy	Usually hazy
Vision loss	No	Sometimes	Sometimes	Possibly, depends on location	Yes
Associated findings	Upper respiratory infection, allergy, exposure	Systemic disease	Systemic disease, idopathic	Contact lenses, HSV or varicella, rosacea	Causes headaches, nausea, vomiting, GI symptoms

Reference: "Diagnosis and Management of Red Eye in Primary Care," by H. Cronau, R. R. Kankanala, & T. Mauger, 2010, *American Family Physician, 81*(2), pp. 137–144.

▶ Avoid contact lenses during treatment period

▶ Cool compresses

Pharmacologic Treatment (Under Management of an Ophthalmologist)

▶ Identify and treat any infections

▶ Artificial tears; oral pain medications

▶ Corticosteroids with or without cycloplegics

▶ Antimicrobials, systemic immunosuppression, chemotherapy,

▶ Anti-inflammatory therapy, treatment of underlying cause

When to Consult, Refer, Hospitalize

▶ Refer all patients immediately with red eye and vision loss to an ophthalmologist.

▶ Iritis and viral keratitis: urgent referral

▶ Bacterial keratitis: emergent referral

Follow-Up

Expected Course

▶ Uveitis/iritis: variable depending on underlying disease and tolerance to medications; need to evaluate other associated systemic disease

▶ Viral keratitis: patients monitored with slit-lamp exam every 1–2 days until improvement, then every 3–4 days until epithelial defect improves, and then weekly until antiviral drops have been completed

Complications

▶ Loss of vision

▶ Cycloplegia: paralysis of ciliary muscle

▶ Cataract formation

▶ Glaucoma

▶ Recurrence of viral infection

Glaucoma

Description

▶ An optic neuropathy that leads to progressive, irreversible vision loss; frequently associated with increased intraocular pressure (IOP)

▶ Second leading cause of blindness

▶ Many different types—two main types are open-angle and angle-closure glaucoma

▷ Open-angle: most common form in the United States (90% of all cases); optic neuropathy with progressive peripheral visual field loss followed by central field loss usually (not always) in the presence of elevated IOP; can be primary or chronic

▷ Angle-closure glaucoma: narrowing or closure of the anterior chamber angle resulting in aqueous humor drainage leading to elevated IOP and damage to the optic nerve; also known as acute or narrow-angle glaucoma

Etiology

See Table 6–4

Incidence and Demographics

See Table 6–4

Risk Factors

See Table 6–4

Prevention and Screening

▶ Screening eye exam starting at age 40 biannually; sooner if high risk

▶ IOP screening after age 65 (per U.S. Preventive Services Task Force; controversial)

▶ Prophylactic laser treatment to second eye for prevention of damage

Assessment

History

▶ Variable presentation depending on type; see Table 6–4

▶ Thorough history to identify precipitating events, other medical problems, medications

Physical Exam

▶ Findings are presented in Table 6–4 below as they correlate to the classifications of glaucoma.

▶ Screening exams include visual acuity, peripheral vision by confrontation, inspection of outer eye and sclera, pupillary response, and funduscopic exam to assess optic cup-to-disc ratio.

▶ Further examination by a specialist is required to assess with slit lamp.

Diagnostic Studies (Performed by Ophthalmologist)

▶ Tonometry: intraocular pressure measurement; IOP normal range is 10–20 mmHg; >20 indicates need for further specialist evaluation

▶ Ophthalmoscopy: shape and color of optic nerve

▶ Perimetry: complete examination of field of vision

▶ Gonioscopy: angle in the eyes where iris meets cornea

▶ Pachymetry: thickness of the cornea

Differential Diagnosis

See Table 6–4

Management

Nonpharmacologic Treatment

▶ Open-angle glaucoma: argon laser trabeculoplasty; trabeculectomy (filtering surgery); shunt surgery, canaloplasty

▶ Angle-closure glaucoma: laser peripheral iridotomy after medical stabilization; surgical peripheral iridectomy if laser is not possible, cataract surgery with anterior lens implant

▶ Patient education: avoidance of certain medications (over-the-counter decongestants, motion sickness medications, adrenergic agents, antipsychotics, antidepressants, and anticholinergic agents) to prevent angle-closure attack; medication counseling and administration; instruction to seek emergency medical attention if there are changes in visual acuity, blurred vision, eye pain, or headache

Pharmacologic Treatment

▶ Open-angle glaucoma: ophthalmic and oral maintenance medications to reduce IOP

  ▷ Decrease aqueous formation (timolol [Timoptic] 0.5%, acetazolamide [Diamox] 250 mg, or brimonidine tartrate 0.1%).

  ▷ Increase aqueous outflow (pilocarpine [Isopto Carpine] 1–4%).

  ▷ Enhance uveoscleral outflow (latanoprost [Xalatan] 0.005%).

TABLE 6–4.
CHARACTERISTICS OF OPEN-ANGLE GLAUCOMA AND ANGLE-CLOSURE GLAUCOMA

	OPEN-ANGLE GLAUCOMA	ANGLE-CLOSURE GLAUCOMA
Etiology	Slow clogging of the drainage canals, resulting in increase in IOP Develops slowly and is a lifelong condition Wide-open angle between the iris and cornea	Blocked drainage canals (anatomically predisposed, mass, or hemorrhage), resulting in sudden increase in IOP Develops suddenly Demands immediate medical attention Closed or narrow angle between the iris and cornea
Incidence/ Demographics	Usually >40 years Increases with age Male = female European and African descent > Asian descent 44 million people affected worldwide	Age >40–50 years Female > male Inuit and Asian > African and European Most common form worldwide, but only 10% in the U.S. 20 million people affected worldwide (75% Asian)
Risk Factors	Increased IOP Myopia Diabetes mellitus African American Older age Hypothyroidism Hypertension Diabetes Cardiovascular disease Family history Prolonged use of corticosteroids	Hyperopia (farsightedness) Age >40–50 years old Shallow anterior chamber Female Family history Asian or Inuit descent Medications: antihistamines, adrenergic agents, antipsychotics, antidepressants, anticholinergic agents Emotional stress or sudden papillary dilation
Symptoms	Painless, slowly progressive visual loss; central visual acuity remains unaffected until late in disease	Severe unilateral ocular pain, blurred vision, lacrimation, photophobia, halos around lights/objects, frontal ipsilateral headaches, nausea and vomiting
Physical Exam	Detected incidentally during comprehensive ophthalmic examination Normal (8–20 mmHg) or increased IOP (>20 mmHg) Increased cup-to-disc ratio Normal pupil	Elevated IOP (40–80 mm Hg) Corneal and lid edema, conjunctival hyperemia, ciliary flush Fixed, mid-dilated pupil Pain with eye movement Shallow anterior chamber
Differential Diagnosis	Normal tension glaucoma Optic nerve pits Anterior ischemic optic neuropathy Compressive lesions of optic nerve or chiasm Posthemorrhagic (shock optic neuropathy)	Acute orbital compartment syndrome Traumatic hyphema Conjunctivitis, episcleritis Corneal abrasion Herpes zoster ophthalmicus Iritis and uveitis Glaucoma, malignant/neovascular Orbital/periorbital infection Lens-induced angle closure

Adapted from *The 5 Minute Clinical Consult 2015* (23rd ed.), by F. J. Domino, 2015, Philadelphia, PA: Lippincott, Williams & Wilkins.

▶ Angle-closure glaucoma: goal is to prevent or reverse angle closure, control IOP, and prevent damage to optic nerve

   ▷ Beta-adrenergic blockers: 0.5% timolol maleate

   ▷ Alpha-adrenergic agonists: 1% apraclonidine (Iopidine)

   ▷ Prostaglandin analogs: latanoprost

   ▷ Miotics: 2% pilocarpine

   ▷ Carbonic anhydrase inhibitors: acetazolamide

   ▷ Systemic hyperosmotic agents: mannitol (Osmitrol)

How Long to Treat

▶ Medical management is ongoing.

Special Considerations

▶ Medications must be used with caution in patients who are on diuretics or who have renal failure, asthma, chronic obstructive pulmonary disease (COPD), heart failure, cirrhosis, diabetes, or acidosis.

When to Consult, Refer, Hospitalize

▶ Angle-closure glaucoma: requires immediate initiation of medication and referral to an ophthalmologist for surgical treatment

▶ Open-angle glaucoma: requires consult/referral to an ophthalmologist for examination and monitoring of the condition

Follow-Up

▶ Angle-closure glaucoma: postsurgical, chronic monitoring post-acute attack per ophthalmologist

▶ Open-angle glaucoma: every 3–6 months as directed by ophthalmologist

Expected Course

▶ Varies greatly depending on severity, duration, early/late diagnosis

▶ If treated surgically and in a timely manner, recurrence of acute attack is rare

▶ Medical management of open-angle glaucoma may prevent visual loss if initiated early and treated adequately.

Complications

▶ Loss of visual fields and visual acuity leading to blindness if untreated

▶ Cornea damage: chronic edema, fibrosis, vascularization, or cataracts

▶ Atrophy of the iris, malignant glaucoma, central retinal vein occlusion

Cataract

Description

▶ Progressive, painless clouding (opacity or discoloration) of the lens of the eye, resulting in localized or generalized partial or total blindness

▶ Leading cause of blindness worldwide

Etiology

▶ Age related or senile (90% of the cause)

▶ Congenital (intrauterine infections, inborn errors of metabolism)

▶ Ocular trauma, infectious or inflammatory conditions (uveitis/scleritis)

▶ Secondary to systemic disease (diabetes, thyroid, parathyroid, sarcoid, myotonic dystrophy, atopic dermatitis)

▶ Systemic or inhaled corticosteroids

▶ Physical (radiation or infrared heat) exposure

▶ Protein (crystallins) changes in the normally transparent lens, causing opacity and scattering of light

Incidence and Demographics

▶ Leading cause of treatable blindness in the world

▶ Approximately 30 million blind people worldwide; 50% because of cataracts

▶ Cataracts present in 50% of those ages 65–74 and 70% of those age >75 years

▶ Predominant sex: variable, some believe females > males

Risk Factors

▶ Aging

▶ Cigarette smoking

▶ Ultraviolet B sunlight exposure

▶ Diabetes, metabolic syndrome

▶ Prolonged high-dose steroids

▶ Positive family history

▶ Poor lifestyle habits (malnutrition and physical inactivity)

▶ Alcohol consumption

Prevention and Screening

▶ No definite measures to prevent cataract formation

▶ Theoretical measures to slow the process include using glasses with ultraviolet protection in sunny conditions; antioxidants such as vitamins C or E; avoiding tobacco products; controlling diabetes; care with high-dose, long-term steroid use.

▶ Screening for cataracts is part of every routine annual eye exam after age 40–50.

Assessment

History

- ▶ Painless, progressive decline in vision that is highly variable among individuals
- ▶ Typically bilateral, although often asymmetrical
- ▶ Complaints of problems with night driving, reading road signs, or fine print; near-sightedness occurs before opacity
- ▶ Symptoms associated with worsening vision related to falls, injuries, or accidents
- ▶ Non–aging-related cataracts have several etiologies; history must be thorough.

Physical Exam

- ▶ Comprehensive eye exam: visual acuity testing will establish baseline; follow-up visits to track changes
- ▶ Funduscopic exam reveals altered red reflex (dark spots or generally diminished) and clouding of the lens; at highly advanced stage, pupil will appear white or leukocoria will be evident in congenital cataracts
- ▶ All other aspects of the outer eye exam are unremarkable.
- ▶ Dilated funduscopic exam may detect other age-related changes that also affect vision (macular degeneration, diabetic or hypertensive retinopathies).

Diagnostic Studies

- ▶ Visual quality assessment by ophthalmologist: glare test, contrast sensitivity, and retinal or macular function assessment

Differential Diagnosis

- ▶ Corneal scarring/edema
- ▶ Lens opacities
- ▶ Tumor
- ▶ Retinal scar
- ▶ Retinal detachment
- ▶ Macular degeneration

Management

Nonpharmacologic Treatment

- ▶ Vision correction with corrective lenses in early stages or after surgery for some patients
- ▶ Surgery necessary when cataract markedly decreases visual acuity (i.e., cataract extraction and artificial lens implant)
- ▶ Wear eye protection from UV light

Pharmacologic Treatment

- ▶ No drugs will halt the progression of the aging process in the eye.
- ▶ Postoperatively, topical antibiotic and ophthalmic steroids under direction of ophthalmologist

Special Considerations

▶ The presence of other diseases (e.g., macular degeneration, diabetic or hypertensive retinopathy) influences the decision to perform corrective surgery.

▶ Make surgeon aware if patient is taking an alpha-1 antagonist (tamsulin, doxazosin, terazosin, or alfuzosin) before surgery because of the increased risk of intraoperative floppy iris syndrome.

▶ If possible, patients on anticoagulants may need to be temporarily discontinued for 1–2 weeks before surgery.

When to Consult, Refer, Hospitalize

▶ All patients with cataracts should be referred to an ophthalmologist for eye assessment, management, and treatment.

Follow-Up

Expected Course

▶ Surgical extraction with lens implant improves vision in the absence of other diseases in 95% of the cases

▶ Ophthalmologists follow-up postoperatively: day 1, then 1 week, and then 1 month. Change in prescriptive glasses is determined 1–3 months after surgery

Complications

▶ Vary widely: delay in visual recovery, protracted visual discomfort, blindness, to loss of eye

▶ Retinal detachment, glaucoma, hemorrhage, infection postoperatively, lens malposition/dislocation, cystoid macular edema, endophthalmitis

OCULAR TRAUMA

Subconjunctival Hemorrhage (SCH)

Description

▶ Bleeding beneath the conjunctiva from small vessels

Etiology

▶ May occur spontaneously or by trauma

▶ Improper contact lens placement/cleaning

▶ Valsalva maneuvers (sneezing, coughing, vomiting, straining)

▶ Hypertension: most common cause in patients >60 years of age

▶ Atherosclerotic disease, diabetes, bleeding factors (thrombocytopenia, elevated prothrombin time)

▶ Rupture of conjunctival blood vessel causes bright red, sharply delineated area surrounded by normal-appearing conjunctiva.

Risk Factors

▶ Age

▶ Contact lens wearer

▶ Systemic diseases

▶ Bleeding disorders

▶ Recent cataract surgery

Prevention and Screening

▶ Correct cleaning and maintenance of contact lenses

▶ Protective eyewear in sports/hobbies

▶ Control of systemic diseases (atherosclerosis, hypertension, diabetes)

▶ Control of prothrombin time in patients on warfarin therapy

Assessment

History

▶ Generally asymptomatic

▶ Report of sudden appearance of blood in the eye

▶ Obtain history of trauma, contact lens usage, cataract surgery, and comprehensive past medical history.

▶ Sometimes noticed upon awakening

▶ No reports of pain, blurred vision, or other related symptoms

Physical Exam

▶ Normal-appearing external eye; PERRLA (pupils equal, round, reactive to light and accommodation) and normal funduscopic exam and visual acuity; no discharge or exudates present with SCH

▶ Blood noted under part or the entire conjunctiva; usually unilateral but may be bilateral

▶ Evaluate BP

Diagnostic Studies

▶ Usually none if suspected

▶ Fluorescein stain if foreign body is expected

▶ Work up for bleeding disorder if repeated episodes

Differential Diagnosis

▶ Foreign body

▶ Hyphema

▶ Penetrating trauma

▶ Acute-angle glaucoma

▶ Conjunctivitis

▶ Iritis

Management

Nonpharmacologic Treatment

▶ Self-limiting—no treatment required. Warm compresses and eye lubricants may be useful.

▶ Control blood pressure, blood glucose, international normalized ratio; use of protective eyewear as indicated

Pharmacologic Treatment

▶ None indicated unless there are associated infectious findings (conjunctivitis)

Special Considerations

▶ May be seen in hypertension and in neonates or their mothers as a result of labor and delivery

When to Consult, Refer, Hospitalize

▶ Refer to ophthalmologist if suspicious or associated with history of blunt trauma, patient complains of decreased visual acuity or disturbances, or no resolution of SCH within 2 weeks.

▶ Refer to hematologist if recurrent to rule out bleeding disorders.

Follow-Up

Expected course

▶ Hemorrhages resorb in 1–2 weeks.

Hyphema

Description

▶ Hemorrhage (gross visible blood) into the anterior chamber of the eye

▶ Frequently accompanies penetrating eye injuries

▶ Can result in permanent vision loss

Etiology

▶ Blunt or penetrating injury to eye such as from a rock, paintballs, BB gun pellet, dart, stick, fists, belt, elastic bungee cords, air bag deployment, or baseball; or from a fall

▶ Child abuse

▶ Traumatic eye injury during sports

▶ Intraocular surgery

▶ Spontaneous (uncommon): secondary to neovascularization (e.g., diabetes mellitus, ischemia, cicatrix formation), ocular neoplasms (e.g., retinoblastoma), coagulation disorders, uveitis, and vascular anomalies

Incidence

▶ Approximately 12 injuries/100,000 population

▶ Males 3–5 times > females

▶ Approximately 70% occur in children, with peak incidence between 10–20 years of age

Risk Factors

▶ Blunt trauma to the eye, especially penetrating type

▶ Anticoagulant therapy

▶ Hemophilia

▶ Sickle cell anemia

Prevention and Screening

▶ Use of protective eyewear in high-risk situations

▶ Maintenance and control of hematologic disorders

Assessment

History

▶ Obtain details regarding precipitating event (recent eye trauma).

▶ Eye pain usually is present from trauma or increased intraocular pressure.

▶ Decreased vision

▶ Nausea and vomiting may accompany injury.

▶ Patient or family history of hemophilia, blood disorders (including sickle-cell disease); medications (especially those that would affect clotting such as aspirin, NSAIDs, and herbal preparations such as ginkgo biloba)

▶ History of sickle-cell disease or trait increases risk of rebleeding and the development of complications; usually needs more aggressive management.

▶ Children, especially young children, often are somnolent; needs to be differentiated from decreased level of consciousness associated with a head injury.

Physical Exam

▶ Open globe must be ruled out prior to any examination procedure that causes pressure to the eyeball (eyelid retraction, IOP measurement).

▶ Comprehensive eye exam (inspection of eyelids, lashes, lacrimal ducts, and cornea; extraocular movement, and visual fields by confrontation)

▶ Decrease visual acuity, photophobia

▶ Eye pain with papillary constriction to bright light (direct and consensual)

▶ Blood in the anterior chamber is visible to varying degrees, from partial filling seen as a visible fluid level line to a completely filled chamber. (Bleeds are graded according to the amount of blood in the anterior chamber, with grade 4 being the worst—entire chamber filled. Incidence of complications increases with higher grades.)

▶ Damage to adjacent structures or abnormal IOP

- ▶ May have increased ocular pressure (32%), may occur several days after injury
- ▶ Obtain a neurological exam if patient is somnolent.
- ▶ Assess for other signs of bleeding (e.g., bruising).
- ▶ Direct ophthalmoscopy is useful for closer visualization of anterior structures and lens.
- ▶ Funduscopic examination may be difficult because of miosis (pupillary constriction) and photophobia, or with a large hyphema
- ▶ Fluorescein examination should be deferred if the ruptured globe is highly suspected or evident.

Diagnostic Studies

- ▶ Clotting times (PT, PTT, INR), CBC with differential if indicated
- ▶ Possible sickle cell prep (African, Hispanic, or Mediterranean descent)
- ▶ Orbital CAT scan without contrast as indicated (globe rupture, intraocular foreign body)
- ▶ Cranial CAT scan may be needed in other facial/head trauma.

Differential Diagnosis

- ▶ Globe trauma
- ▶ Eye contusion
- ▶ Systemic disease
- ▶ Melanoma
- ▶ Retinoblastoma
- ▶ Medication induced anticoagulation

Management

Nonpharmacologic Treatment

- ▶ Apply bilateral eye patches to limit additional injury or blinking during transport to an emergency facility or ophthalmologist (put no pressure on the globe); eye shield to affected eye should be worn at all times until the hyphema resolves or for at least one week to avoid further injury to the affected eye.
- ▶ Keep the patient in an upright position during transfer.
- ▶ Limit activity: no TV viewing or reading; head elevation. Some experts recommend patient remain ambulatory versus bed rest for 5–7 days.
- ▶ If severe or developing complications, surgery may be done to evacuate blood.
- ▶ The goal is to prevent secondary hemorrhage and intraocular hypertension.
- ▶ Monitor intraocular pressure daily.

Pharmacologic Treatment

- ▶ Acetaminophen with or without codeine may be used as needed for pain.
- ▶ Avoid NSAIDs and aspirin.

▶ Other topical or oral agents may be used to suppress aqueous flow and decrease intraocular pressure or inflammation.

Special Considerations

▶ Aspirin products, miotics, and mydriatics should not be used.

▶ Sedation may be needed to ensure complete rest, especially in children.

When to Consult, Refer, Hospitalize

▶ Immediate referral to emergency facility, hospital, or ophthalmologist

▶ Greater than 50% affected require intervention by an ophthalmologist

▶ Outpatient management is acceptable if compliant with treatment plan

▶ If at home, must follow-up daily to check intraocular pressure and for rebleeds

Follow-Up

Expected course

▶ Variable, dependent on severity; ophthalmologist may manage patient at home or as inpatient

▶ Followed by ophthalmologist daily for 5 or more days

▶ Blood usually reabsorbs in 5–10 days (if no rebleeding)

Complications

▶ Decreased visual acuity

▶ Recurrent bleeding (~25%): most common time is ≥5 days postinjury; increases risk of complications

▶ Retinal detachment or ocular rupture

▶ Permanent corneal staining (from the hemorrhage) and subsequent haziness

▶ Glaucoma (immediately or later in life)

▶ Optic atrophy

Corneal Abrasion

Description

▶ Defect in the epithelial layer of the cornea caused by mechanical trauma to the surface of eye

Etiology

▶ Traumatic: fingernails, paws, paper or cardboard, branches, etc. (64% of cases)

▶ Foreign body: rust, wood, glass, plastic, fiberglass, etc.

▶ Contact lens related: removal of an over-worn, improperly fitting, or improperly cleaned contact lens (12% of cases)

▶ Spontaneous (recurrent erosions): occurs with no immediate injury or foreign body; seen in previous traumatic eye abrasions or eyes that have an underlying defect in the corneal epithelium

Incidence and Demographics

▶ Common in all ages; more males treated for corneal abrasion than females

Risk Factors

▶ Contact lens wear

▶ Foreign body in eye

▶ Any abrasive injury

▶ Lack of protective eyewear

▶ Contact sports

▶ Blepharitis

▶ Dry eye syndrome

▶ Entropion

▶ Autoimmune disorders

▶ Chronic corneal exposure (Bell's palsy, exophthalmos)

▶ Chronic topical steroid use or abuse of topical anesthetics

▶ Recent eye surgery

▶ Flash burn (welding burn)

Prevention and Screening

▶ Use of eye protection during high-risk activities

▶ Proper contact lens handling

▶ Use of artificial tears

▶ Lenses to block UV rays (welding helmets)

Assessment

History

▶ Complaints of excruciating eye pain, inability to open eye, photophobia, tearing, foreign body sensation, blurred vision, or conjunctival injection

▶ Usually unilateral

▶ History of contact lens use, dry eyes, trauma from foreign body or chemical burn

▶ History of connective tissue disorder

Physical Exam

▶ Conjunctival injection, photophobia, increased lacrimation on affected side, blepharospasm

▶ Altered integrity of normally smooth cornea seen as irregular light reflex; actual abrasion may be visible with the naked eye or only upon fluorescein staining.

▶ Visual acuity may be decreased if abrasion is centrally located, pupils are reactive, and funduscopic exam is normal.

▶ Invert upper eyelid to assess for foreign body.

Diagnostic Studies

▶ Fluorescein staining will reveal epithelial disruption on the cornea.

▶ Slit-lamp exam by ophthalmologist may be required to determine corneal penetration.

Differential Diagnosis

▶ Foreign body

▶ Unilateral iritis

▶ Keratitis

▶ Acute or chronic glaucoma

▶ Herpes simplex or zoster

▶ Corneal ulcer

▶ Scleritis

Management

Nonpharmacologic Treatment

▶ Irrigation with normal saline to flush any nonpenetrating particles or foreign body after applying topical anesthetic (proparacaine or tetracaine)

▶ Patching of eye no longer recommended

▶ Avoid wearing contact lenses until abrasion healed and patient pain free.

Pharmacologic Treatment

▶ Topical antibiotic ointment or solution to prevent infection: oflaxacin, ciprofloxacin, sulfacetamide 10%, erythromycin, gentamicin or polymyxin B/trimethoprim; continue until eye pain resolves

▶ Topical NSAIDs: help relieve pain; use with caution, may cause corneal melting and perforation

▶ Analgesics for pain (systemic)

▶ Never treat with topical steroids; may delay healing

▶ Tetanus booster if indicated

How Long to Treat

▶ Topical antibiotics for 3–5 days or until eye pain is resolved

Special Considerations

▶ Topical analgesics are used for evaluation of the eye in a clinic setting only and should not be prescribed for pain management at home.

▶ Advise patients of the risk of severe complications and need for follow-up next day.

When to Consult, Refer, Hospitalize

▶ Referral to an ophthalmologist if injury is extensive, signs of infection, severe ocular pain not explained by apparent pathology, or no improvement in 24 hours

Follow-Up

▶ Contact lens wearers: reevaluate daily with slit-lamp exam

▶ Minor abrasions: reevaluated only if they become more painful

▶ Large abrasions (>4 mm): reevaluate in 24 hours

Expected Course

▶ Variable depending on severity; simple corneal abrasion resolves in 24–48 hours

Complications

▶ Recurrence

▶ Scarring of the cornea

▶ Corneal perforation

▶ Infection, ulceration

▶ Loss of vision

Ocular Foreign Body

Description

▶ Abnormal substance (foreign body) on the epithelium of the eye surface such as dust, dirt, metal, glass, or organic material

Etiology

▶ Accidental trauma

▶ Foreign body becomes lodged in the corneal epithelium or stroma

▶ Disruption in the epithelial integrity of the cornea causes symptoms

▶ If foreign body penetrates further than the epithelial surface, ophthalmologist referral is indicated.

Incidence and Demographics

▶ Commonly occurring condition

▶ Males > females

Risk Factors

▶ Lack of or improper use of protective eyewear during at-risk activities

▶ Living or playing in dusty or sandy environment (e.g., desert, beach)

Prevention and Screening

▶ Use of protective eyewear in appropriate or at-risk situations

Assessment

History
- ▶ Patients may complain of pain, foreign body sensation, photophobia, tearing, red eye.
- ▶ Determine event, timing, and place of injury; some projectiles puncture the eye and become lodged in the deeper layers, leaving only a relatively minor injury apparent. If history suggests this, immediate referral is advised.

Physical Exam
- ▶ Comprehensive eye exam. Include visual acuity, inspection of the outer eye, and both the outer and inner aspect of the upper and lower eyelids; check pupillary response and EOMs; and do funduscopic examination.
- ▶ Evert the eyelids for visualization of inner aspect of the eyelids.
- ▶ Findings may include a quiet eye (no tearing, discharge, injection, or edema), dark specks on the iris, "rust ring" at site of entry of steel or iron projectile, diffuse injection, or abrasion or tear of the epithelial layer.

Diagnostic Studies
- ▶ Fluorescein staining detects defects on the epithelial lining of the conjunctiva and cornea.
- ▶ Slit-lamp exam to assess inner eye thoroughly if no foreign body found

Differential Diagnosis

- ▶ Corneal abrasion
- ▶ Infection
- ▶ Herpetic ulcer
- ▶ Keratitis, bacterial
- ▶ Foreign body, intraocular
- ▶ Keratitis, fungal

Management

Nonpharmacologic Treatment
- ▶ Goal is to relieve pain, avoid infection, and prevent permanent loss of function.
- ▶ Irrigate eye with normal saline solution for 10 minutes or more.
- ▶ After application of eye anesthetic drops (proparacaine HCL [e.g., Ophthaine]), foreign bodies that are superficial may be dislodged with irrigation alone, or gentle touch with a moistened cotton-tipped applicator. Evert the eyelid to remove foreign bodies under eyelids.
- ▶ *Note:* Use moistened cotton-tipped applicator *only* if object is not embedded.
- ▶ Application of patch to injured eye is no longer recommended.

Pharmacologic Treatment
- ▶ Topical ophthalmic anesthetic is reserved for examination *only*, not treatment.

▶ Topical antibiotics are applied for prophylaxis until the epithelial defect heals; see corneal abrasion for list of pharmacologic treatment

▶ Provide a tetanus booster if indicated.

Diagnostic Studies

▶ Fluorescein staining will detect a concurrent corneal abrasion.

▶ A slit-lamp exam may be necessary to assess for intraocular penetration of foreign body.

How Long to Treat

▶ Depends on extent of injury; patient seen by ophthalmologist for follow-up if necessary

Special Considerations

▶ Do not prescribe ophthalmic anesthetics for home pain control; use systemic analgesics (acetaminophen with codeine p.r.n.).

When to Consult, Refer, Hospitalize

▶ Urgent referral to an ophthalmologist if a corneal foreign body cannot be removed, or if there is suspicion of corneal infection or penetrating injury

▶ Presence of a rust ring requires referral to ophthalmologist for treatment.

▶ Patients with a suspected intraocular foreign body must be referred emergently to an ophthalmologist.

Follow-Up

Expected Course

▶ Depends on type of foreign body and severity of the injury

Complications

▶ Penetration of foreign body

▶ Infection, corneal abrasion, tissue necrosis

▶ Glaucoma secondary to intraocular inflammation, cataract formation

PROBLEMS OF THE EARS

Hearing Loss

Description

▶ Diminished or absent sense of hearing with inability to detect or comprehend sound or speech

▶ Can be partial, complete, unilateral, or bilateral

▶ Categorized as either conductive or sensorineural or both

Etiology

▶ *Conductive hearing loss (CHL):* dysfunction of the external or middle ear; decreased hearing by air conduction

  ▷ Common causes in adults include: cerumen impaction, otosclerosis, cholesteatoma, and tympanic membrane perforation secondary to chronic otitis media

  ▷ Common causes in children: otitis media and related conditions such as middle ear effusion and eustachian tube dysfunction

  ▷ Often correctable with medical therapy, surgical therapy, or both

▶ *Sensorineural hearing loss (SNHL):* deterioration of the cochlea (inner ear) or eighth cranial nerve or both; decreased hearing through bone conduction; can be congenital or acquired and hereditary or nonhereditary; affects older adults (~90%) more than children (<10%)

  ▷ There are many different causes of SNHL. Presbycusis the most common, followed by noise-induced hearing loss. Other causes include: pharmacologic toxicity (aminoglycosides, loop diuretics, antimalarials, salicylates), trauma (head injury, noise, barotraumas, irradiation), infections (otitis media, CMV, syphilis, labyrinthitis), and other disorders (multiple sclerosis, migraine, sickle-cell disease, blood dyscrasia, polyarteritis nodosa, HIV, meningioma).

  ▷ Presbycusis: the most common cause of SNHL is due to the aging process; nonpathological, high-frequency hearing loss, etiology unknown.

  ▷ SNHL usually is not correctable with medical or surgical therapy; however, it may be preventable or stable.

▶ *Mixed:* both air and bone conduction impaired

Incidence and Demographics

▶ Is the third most common chronic condition in older Americans after hypertension and arthritis

▶ Twenty-eight million Americans have some degree of hearing loss

▶ Affects between 25% and 40% of patients over the age of 65

▶ All ages are affected; males = females

▶ Affects approximately 1.4 million children (<18 years)

▶ 1 of every 1,000 newborns in the United States is completely deaf; >3 million children have hearing loss

▶ Congenital hearing loss affects newborns approximately 1–3 cases per 1,000; >60% are genetic causes and occur before speech development.

▶ Otosclerosis is the most common cause of conductive, slowly progressive hearing loss in people aged 30–40 years; caused by bone dyscrasias; can be unilateral or bilateral.

Risk Factors

► Conductive:
  ▷ Chronic sinusitis; allergy
  ▷ Cigarette smoking
  ▷ Sleep apnea with CPAP use
  ▷ Eustachian tube dysfunction
  ▷ Neuromuscular disease
  ▷ Family history/heredity
  ▷ Prematurity and low birth weight
  ▷ Adenoid hypertrophy; nasopharyngeal mass

► Sensorineural:
  ▷ Aging/older age
  ▷ Loud noise/acoustic trauma
  ▷ Dizziness/vertigo
  ▷ Medications (aminoglycosides, loop diuretics, quinine, aspirin, chemotherapeutic agents)
  ▷ Bacterial meningitis
  ▷ Head trauma
  ▷ Infectious diseases (chickenpox, measles, encephalitis, influenza, mumps)
  ▷ Neoplasm, bone disorders, immune disorders, neurologic disorders, and vascular and hematologic disorders

Prevention and Screening

► Mandatory newborn screening; NICU screening before discharge
► Audiologic testing after major intracranial infection (meningitis)
► Routine screening after age 65 (U.S. Preventive Services Task Force, 2007)
► Limiting noise exposure—using hearing protection
► Avoiding ear canal instrumentation (e.g., cotton swabs, hairpins)
► Limiting ototoxic medications
► Vaccination for *Haemophilus influenzae* type b meningitis and for measles, mumps, and rubella (MMR)

Assessment

See Table 6–5

Diagnostic Studies

► Tympanometry: assessing tympanic membrane (TM) mobility and middle ear's ability to receive sound waves

TABLE 6–5.
CHARACTERISTICS OF HEARING LOSS

	CONDUCTIVE (CDHL)	SENSORINEURAL (SNHL)	PRESBYCUSIS (SNHL)
Etiology	Congenital Impaction with wax or foreign body Infection Perforated TM Trauma Tissue overgrowth: otosclerosis, cholesteatoma Tumor	Prolonged exposure to loud noises Ototoxic substances Inner ear infections Ménière's disease Metabolic diseases: diabetes, myxedema, thyroid Infectious: syphilis, viral Trauma: temporal bone injury or fracture Autoimmune disease	Aging process Multifactorial Associated with smoking Systemic disease Ototoxic drugs
Pattern of Loss	Decreased low tones, vowels; may have 60–70 dB deficit	Decreased high-frequency pitch, consonant discrimination, and background noise	Gradual loss of all tones; begins with highs then progresses to lows
History	Unilateral loss With or without tinnitus	Unilateral or bilateral Hears better in quiet room Associated with tinnitus and dizziness Sudden loss (assess for acoustic neuroma)	Presents bilaterally Develops tinnitus, sensitivity to loud and high pitches Reduced hearing sensitivity and speech understanding in noisy environments
Exam	Speaks softly Variable findings: normal, foreign body, wax impaction, edema, obstruction, fluid behind TM; stiff, retracted or bulging TM Rinne: BC > AC in affected ear Weber test—lateralizes to affected ear	Speaks loudly Exam normal Rinne: AC > BC bilaterally Weber test lateralizes to unaffected ear	Speaks loudly Exam normal Whisper voice test difficult Nonspecific Weber or Rinne findings Otoscopy (rule out conductive hearing loss)

▶ Antinuclear antibody and sedimentation rate to screen for autoimmune disease if indicated

▶ Audiometry evaluation for all chronic hearing loss and for acute hearing loss of unknown etiology

▶ Vestibular testing if tinnitus or vertigo is involved

▶ CAT if tumors/bony lesions are suspected

▶ MRI if acoustic neuroma is suspected

Differential Diagnosis

▶ Presbycusis

▶ Infectious, vascular, metabolic, problems

▶ Ménière's disease

▶ Acoustic neuromas

▶ Ototoxicity (aspirin, quinine, aminoglycosides)

▶ Viral labyrinthitis

▶ Conductive problems: obstruction of canal, TM impairment, otosclerosis, cholesteatoma, cochlear damage

Management

Nonpharmacologic Treatment

▶ Depends on etiology; remove obstructing wax or foreign body (ceruminolytics, such
as Debrox, and irrigation), treat underlying infections, discontinue ototoxic medications, surgical treatment (e.g., cochlear implants, tympanostomy and tube placement, tympanoplasty, mastoidectomy, stapedectomy/stapedotomy, canaloplasty),
hearing aids, adaptive measures (lip-reading, sign language)

Pharmacologic Treatment

▶ Antibiotics if indicated

▶ Steroid therapy may be indicated for sudden sensorineural loss of unknown etiology

How Long to Treat

▶ Variable depending on underlying cause

Special Considerations

▶ Sign language interpreters should be considered in the primary care office for communication with patients with hearing impairments.

▶ Otosclerosis can worsen during pregnancy.

▶ Loss of communication produces emotional stress and is a physical risk for older
adults.

When to Consult, Refer, Hospitalize

▶ Emergent referral for SNHL with sudden acute hearing loss

▶ Otolaryngologist for hearing loss of unknown etiology

▶ Audiology if hearing loss is suspected; also provides hearing aid options and
maintenance

▶ Genetics if congenital syndrome or familial hearing loss is suspected

▶ Speech therapist if speech delay or speech impediment is present

▶ Endocrinology if associated endocrine disorders are suspected

▶ Neurotology and neurosurgery if intracranial lesions are suspected or intracranial
complication of middle ear disease

Follow-Up

Expected Course
- ▶ Presbycusis and sensorineural loss is usually permanent and may be progressive.
- ▶ Temporary hearing alterations are reversible when related to minor problems such as congestion, otitis, cerumen, or foreign body obstruction that is responsive to treatment.

Complications
- ▶ Potential for serious sequelae with cholesteatoma, including balance problems, facial nerve paralysis, meningitis, brain abscess
- ▶ Neurologic abnormalities, perforations, cholesteatoma, tinnitus, vertigo, deafness

Impacted Cerumen

Description
- ▶ Obstruction of the external auditory canal due to accumulation of cerumen (ear wax), a naturally occurring lubricant that serves as a protective lining of the canal

Etiology
- ▶ Excessive production of ear wax beyond what can be cleared by natural mechanisms
- ▶ Manipulation of canal (e.g., introduction of cotton-tipped applicator) that pushes cerumen deeper into canal, resulting in a buildup that is beyond the ability of the natural process of clearing

Incidence and Demographics
- ▶ Farmers and industrial workers around grains, powders, and textiles; greater incidence among older adults

Risk Factors
- ▶ Ear hygiene practices that compact cerumen in ear canal (i.e., cotton swabs)
- ▶ Age, occupation (wearing headphones, ear plugs), use of hearing aids

Prevention and Screening
- ▶ Gentle cleaning of external opening with washcloth without entering canal itself may be helpful.
- ▶ Avoid pushing cerumen further into external canal.

Assessment

History
- ▶ Decreased or partial hearing loss
- ▶ Feeling of fullness or pressure, itching
- ▶ Dizziness/tinnitus
- ▶ Pain if pushed against tympanic membrane

Physical Exam
- ▶ Dark brown wax, may be moist or dry
- ▶ Partial or complete obstruction of ear canal
- ▶ Visualization of canal and TM may be partially or completely blocked by the wax

Differential Diagnosis
- ▶ Foreign body in canal
- ▶ Otitis media
- ▶ Otitis externa

Management

Nonpharmacologic Treatment
- ▶ Removal of the cerumen can be achieved by use of a curette, or by irrigation with body-temperature water to dislodge and rinse it out of canal
- ▶ Contraindications for irrigation: tympanostomy tube, perforated tympanic membrane, previous or current history of otitis media, severe otitis externa, organic foreign body (e.g., legumes swell in contact with water)

Pharmacologic Treatment
- ▶ Soften hardened cerumen by instilling 3 drops of hydrogen peroxide and water (1:1), 1–2 drops of baby oil or ceruminolytic solvents (Debrox) for 10–30 minutes before irrigation.

How Long to Treat
- ▶ May require ongoing maintenance indefinitely

Special Considerations
- ▶ Provide education about proper ear hygiene.

When to Consult, Refer, Hospitalize
- ▶ Referral to a specialist is required if the affected ear is the only ear with intact hearing, there is suspected perforation of the TM, or coexisting problems of the ear are present, such as severe infection, unexplained hearing loss, or hearing loss that did not clear with treatment of the impaction.

Follow-Up

Expected Course
- ▶ Acute impaction is generally resolved completely following treatment.
- ▶ Ongoing potential for repeated impaction is minimized by maintenance.

Complications
- ▶ Pain, bleeding, TM perforation

Otitis Externa (OE)

Description

▶ Inflammation or infection of the external auditory canal

▶ Commonly called "swimmer's ear"

Etiology

▶ Traumatized external auditory canal (as with a cotton-tipped swab)

▶ Bacterial infection (90%): *Pseudomonas aeruginosa* (67%), *Staphylococcus aureus*, *Streptococcus pyogenes*

▶ Fungal infection (10%): *Aspergillus* (90%) or *Candida* infection

▶ Eczematous conditions: seborrheic dermatitis, atopic dermatitis, psoriasis, neurodermatitis

Incidence and Demographics

▶ Unknown; higher in summer months and in warm, wet climates

▶ All ages

▶ Males = females

Risk Factors

▶ Trauma to external ear canal

▶ Swimming

▶ Hot, humid weather

▶ Hearing aid use

▶ Eczema

▶ Advanced age, diabetes, AIDS, debilitating disease, leukopenia, malnutrition for necrotizing OE

Prevention and Screening

▶ Avoiding prolonged exposure to moisture

▶ Using preventive antiseptics (2% acetic acid solution [OTC] 1–2 drops) after swimming or bathing and/or blow-dryer on cool setting and hold several inches away from ear

▶ Treating predisposing skin conditions

▶ Eliminating self-inflicted trauma to canal with cotton swabs

▶ Diagnosing and treat underlying system conditions

▶ Using earplugs when swimming

Assessment

History

▶ Reports of itching, plugging of ear, ear pain, and discharge from ear

Physical Exam

▶ Ear canal is red, containing purulent discharge and debris

▶ Pain on manipulation of pinnae

▶ Possible periauricular adenitis

▶ Possible eczema of pinna

▶ May have cranial nerve VII, IX-XII involvement (extremely rare)

▶ TM normal or dull

▶ Indicators of advanced infection or necrotizing malignant otitis externa: ulcerations, facial nerve palsy, mastoid tenderness, cellulitis, fever, chills, malaise; requires *immediate referral.*

Diagnostic Studies

▶ For general uncomplicated otitis externa, no diagnostic studies are indicated.

▶ Resistant infections may warrant gram stain and culture of canal discharge.

▶ An erythrocyte sedimentation rate (ESR) will be significantly increased in malignant otitis externa.

Differential Diagnosis

▶ Idiopathic ear pain

▶ Otitis media with perforation

▶ Hearing loss

▶ Wisdom tooth eruption

▶ Basal cell or squamous cell carcinoma

▶ Mastoiditis

▶ Temporomandibular joint (TMJ) problems

▶ Cranial nerve (VII, IX-XII) palsy with necrotizing OE

Management

Nonpharmacologic Treatment

▶ Removal of debris for enhancing examination by cleansing using a curette or cotton-tipped swab with 1:1 hydrogen peroxide/water solution. (*Note*: Do not irrigate.)

▶ Placement of a wick or gauze strip in canals with greatly narrowed lumen to draw in otic drops

▶ Application of local heat (water bottle, warm pack) to outer ear for pain relief

▶ Avoidance of swimming with active infection

Pharmacologic Treatment

▶ OTC pain management (acetaminophen, NSAIDs); may need opioids

▶ First-line topical otic antibiotic: ofloxacin (Floxin), polymyxin B sulfate/neomycin sulfate/hydrocortisone (Cortisporin); acetic acid (VosoL HC) to fight infection in combination with a corticosteroid to decrease inflammation

- Second-line topical otic antibiotics: betamehasone 0.05% solution; azole antifungals for fungal otitis externa

- Topical acidifying agent such as acetic acid to inhibit growth of bacteria and fungi (Vosol)

- Oral antibiotics in combination with topical otic antibiotics indicated only if associated otitis media or cellulitis of outer ear is present

How Long to Treat
- Usually 5–7 days

- Complicated case or malignant otitis externa requires prolonged therapy (6–8 weeks).

Special Considerations

- Necrotizing malignant otitis externa is typically found in those who are older than age 65, diagnosed with diabetes, or immunocompromised and requires *immediate specialist referral*.

When to Consult, Refer, Hospitalize

- Referral to a specialist is indicated for those who do not respond to treatment or with severe infections, systemic involvement, cellulitis, or malignant external otitis.

- Hospitalization is required for necrotizing otitis media requiring parenteral antipseudomonal antibiotics.

Follow-Up

Expected Course
- Forty-eight hours after therapy to assess improvement

- Simple cases will resolve with treatment; however, reoccurrence or chronic problems will require ongoing monitoring and prophylactic measures (earplugs, acetic acid 2% after bathing or swimming).

Complications
- Mastoiditis, malignant external otitis, cellulitis, chondritis

Otitis Media
Description

- Acute otitis media (AOM): moderate to severe bulging of the tympanic membrane (TM) or new onset of otorrhea not due to acute otitis externa with acute signs of illness or signs and symptoms of middle ear inflammation, often associated with recent viral upper respiratory infection.

- Otitis media with effusion (OME) also called "serous otitis media": presence of middle ear effusion in the absence of acute signs of infection; in children, may follow AOM; in adults, associated with Eustachian tube (ET) dysfunction

Etiology

▶ Acute otitis media:

▷ Typically follows viral upper respiratory infection, causing ET dysfunction

▷ Involved bacterial organisms include *Streptococcus pneumonia* (20–35%), *H. influenza* (20%–30%), *Moraxella catarrhalis* (15%), Group A β-hemolytic *Streptococcus* (3%), *S. aureus* (12%)

▶ Viral: involves respiratory syncytial virus (RSV), parainfluenza, influenza, enteroviruses, adenovirus, human metapneumovirus; 15–44% of AOM

▶ Otitis media with effusion:

▷ Residual fluid in middle ear following acute otitis media

▷ Eustachian tube dysfunction: The typically short, narrow, flexible, and horizontal ET found in children predisposes them to accumulation of nasopharyngeal secretions in the ET and middle ear. Supine bottle feeding and sucking may also contribute to reflux of fluid from the nasopharynx.

Incidence and Demographics

▶ AOM: predominant age: 6–24 months; declines >7 years; rare in adults; male > female; increased incidence in the fall and winter months

▶ OME: Nearly 90% of children aged 6 months to 4 years have had at least one episode.

Risk Factors

▶ Premature birth

▶ Bottle feeding while supine

▶ Routine day care attendance

▶ Frequent pacifier use after 6 months of age

▶ Smoking in household

▶ Male gender

▶ Native American/Inuit ethnicity

▶ Low socioeconomic status

▶ Family history of recurrent otitis

▶ Underlying ear, nose, or throat disease (adenoid hypertrophy, cleft palate, allergic rhinitis, Down syndrome)

Prevention and Screening

▶ Breastfeeding for >6 months is protective.

▶ Avoiding supine bottle feeding, passive smoke, and pacifiers >6 months may be helpful.

▶ Pneumococcal vaccination: reduces AOM cases by 6–28%

▶ Influenza vaccination: reduces AOM by ~30% in children >2 years of age

Assessment

History

▶ Acute otitis media

▷ Rapid onset

▷ Symptoms: otalgia, ear pulling, fever, irritability, otorrhea, sleeplessness, hearing loss, balance problems, anorexia, vomiting, diarrhea

▷ Fever common but not universal

▷ Patient may report extreme pain that is suddenly relieved with popping sensation, indicative of ruptured tympanic membrane

▷ Proceeds or accompanies symptoms of upper respiratory infection

▶ Otitis media with effusion

▷ Symptoms variable, from none to severe with pain, vertigo, and ataxia

▷ Patient typically complains of a sense of fullness in the ear and decreased hearing; popping or crackling sounds in the ear with yawning, chewing, swallowing, or blowing nose

▷ Is transient in most children and may not be diagnosed

▷ May report recent history of upper respiratory infection, allergy symptoms, or airplane travel

Physical Exam

▶ Acute otitis media

▷ Fever

▷ Decreased TM mobility; eardrum bulging, opaque, often yellowish or inflamed; eardrum may be red

▷ Presence of air/fluid behind TM

▷ Redness alone does not indicate AOM.

▷ Otorrhea if perforated TM

▷ Bullae on the TM are indicative of *M. pneumoniae*.

▷ May be preauricular or have cervical lymph node tenderness and enlargement

▷ An entirely normal exam warrants further examination of related structures for conditions that may present with referred ear pain (e.g., TMJ dysfunction, sinusitis, cranial nerve abnormalities, dentition problems, nasopharyngeal carcinoma).

▶ Otitis media with effusion

▷ TM often dull but not bulging; blunting of landmarks and diffuse light reflex

▷ Presence of air/fluid level

▷ Pneumatic otoscopy: decreased mobility of TM

▷ Weber test is positive to affected ear

Diagnostic Studies

▶ Pneumatic otoscopy

▶ Tympanometry to confirm tympanic membrane mobility

▶ Audiometry when hearing loss persists > 3 months or at any time that language delay, significant hearing loss, or learning problems are suspected

▶ No routine testing is indicated, although CBC may be done if complicated or systemic infection is suspected

Differential Diagnosis

▶ Otitis externa

▶ Tympanosclerosis

▶ Otitis-conjunctivitis syndrome

▶ Redness because of crying

▶ Referred pain from jaw, teeth, or throat

▶ Bullous myringitis

▶ Trauma

▶ Nasopharyngeal carcinoma

Management

Nonpharmacologic Treatment

▶ Observation

▶ Valsalva maneuver or chewing gum to facilitate opening of Eustachian tubes for draining middle ear

Pharmacologic Treatment

▶ Acute otitis media

▷ Disagreement exists regarding the usefulness of antibiotic treatment, because most cases are self-resolving.

▷ American Academy of Pediatrics/American Academy of Family Physicians (AAP/

▷) guidelines:

▶ Less than 6 months of age: antibacterial therapy recommended regardless of degree of diagnostic certainty

▶ Children >6 months: antibacterial therapy is recommended when the diagnosis of AOM is certain and illness is severe

▶ Observation for 48–72 hours is an option when the diagnosis is certain but illness is mild, and in patients with uncertain diagnosis

▷ If antibiotic therapy is used: penicillins, cephalosporins, macrolides, sulfonamides (see Table 6–6)

TABLE 6–6.
ANTIBIOTICS FOR ACUTE OTITIS MEDIA

DRUG/BRAND NAME	ADULT DOSAGE	PEDIATRIC DOSAGE
Amoxicillin (Amoxil, Trimox, Wymox)	500 mg t.i.d., 3.5 g/day	80–90 mg/kg in 2–3 divided doses b.i.d x 5–7 days in children >2 years and 10 days for children <2 years
Amoxicillin-clavulanate (Augmentin) Augmentin XR Augmentin is also available in chewable tablets and suspension in a variety of dose ranges.	875 mg q 12 h (based on amoxicillin component) 2 tabs q 12 h	90 mg/kg in 6.4 mg/kg/day divided doses b.i.d.
Azithromycin (Zithromax)	250 mg (2) to start, then 1 q.d. x 4 days	10 mg/kg/day on day 1, then 5 mg/kg/day on days 2–5
Cefaclor (Ceclor)	250–500 mg q 8 h	40 mg/kg/day in 3 divided doses
Cefdinir (Omnicef)	300 mg q 12 h (for 5 days in adults)	14 mg/kg/day in 1 dose or 2 divided doses (for 5 days in children >2 years old)
Cefixime (Suprax)	400 mg q.d.	8 mg/kg/day once a day
Cefpodoxime (Vantin)	200 mg q 12 h for 5 days	10 mg/kg/day in 2 divided doses for 5 days
Cefprozil (Cefzil)	250–500 mg q 12 h	30 mg/kg/day in 2 divided doses
Ceftibuten (Cedax)	400 mg q.d.	9 mg/kg/day once a day
Ceftriaxone (Rocephin)	1 g q12h IM or IV	50 mg/kg IM x 1–3 days
Cefuroxime axetil (Ceftin)	250–500 mg b.i.d.	30 mg/kg/day in 2 divided doses
Clarithromycin (Biaxin)	500 mg q 12 h	15 mg/kg/day in 2 divided doses
Erythromycin-sulfisoxazole (Pediazole)	Not indicated	50 mg/kg in 3 or 4 divided doses (based on erythromycin component)
Loracarbef (Lorabid)	200 mg q 12 h	30 mg/kg in 2 divided doses
Trimethoprim-sulfamethoxazole (Septra, Bactrim)	1 double-strength tablet q 12 h (160 mg trim. + 800 mg sulfa)	8 mg/kg trim + 40 mg/kg sulfa in 2 divided doses x 10 days. Do not use if group A streptococcus is suspected.
Trimethoprim (Trimpex, Proloprim)	Not indicated	10 mg/kg in 2 divided doses

▷ CDC guidelines for antibiotic therapy:

► First-line therapy: amoxicillin 80–90 mg/kg/day, in divided doses; 5–7 day treatment for children >2 years old with no complications and 10-day course for children <2 years old; adult dose: 500 mg p.o. t.i.d.

► Consider use of a cephalosporin (cefdinir, cefpodoxime, cefuroxime), azithromycin, clarithromycin, or sulfamethoxazole-trimethoprim in the event of penicillin allergy.

▷ When choosing an antibiotic, consider risk of infection with resistant strains of bacteria.

▷ For clinically defined treatment failures after 3 days of therapy, an alternative agent should be selected after considering risk of infection with resistant strains. Choose a drug effective against drug-resistant *S. pneumoniae* (DRSP) and beta-lactamase–producing pathogens, such as oral amoxicillin-clavulanate (Augmentin XR), cefuroxime axetil (Ceftin), or intramuscular ceftriaxone (Rocephin) x 3 days.

▷ Pain management with OTC preparations such as acetaminophen or NSAIDs; codeine additionally if needed; warm compresses over affected ear

▷ Decongestants for the associated congestion of the nose or sinuses. (*Note*: Does not affect otitis media, but provides symptom relief for congestion.)

▷ Antihistamines *only* if patient has allergies with increased watery secretions

► Otitis media with effusion

▷ Antibiotic therapy is not routinely indicated for serous otitis media.

▷ AAP/AFPP recommends watchful waiting for 3 months

How Long to Treat

► Antibiotic therapy is generally for 7–10 days with the exception of azithromycin (Zithromax), cefpodoxime (Vantin), and cefdinir (Omnicef), which are given for 5 days.

Special Considerations

► Accurate diagnosis is essential to avoid overuse of antibiotics.

► Airplane travel in patients with ET dysfunction may cause painful barotraumas, bleeding into TM, or TM perforation. Chewing gum or food (or sucking of pacifier or bottle in infants) may help equalize pressure.

When to Consult, Refer, Hospitalize

► Refer to ENT specialist for surgery in recurrent AOM if >3 episodes in 6 months, >4 episodes in 12 months with at least one occurring the the past 6 months, or AOM episodes occur while patient is on chemoprophylaxis.

► Complications of severe infection such as mastoiditis or cholesteatoma

► Refer to ENT specialist for chronic middle ear effusion.

► Referral to ENT specialist for OME is individualized: if bilateral OME >3 months, unilateral OME >6 months, hearing loss >25 dB, or for high-risk individuals any time.

▶ If a child is at risk for speech, language, or learning problems

▶ Refer to ENT specialist for perforation of the TM, nonresponsive to treatment within 48–72 hours, or a hearing loss of 20 dB or more post-treatment.

Follow-Up

Expected Course

▶ Simple cases are resolved in 7–10 days for AOM and should be reevaluated after treatment is completed to monitor resolution of middle ear effusion.

▶ Middle ear effusion commonly persists after course of treatment for acute otitis media.

▶ Recheck can be made in 2–8 weeks depending on reliability of patient/parent.

▶ Follow-up in 48–72 hours in children who fail to improve on antibiotic therapy.

Complications

▶ Permanent conductive hearing loss, pain, balance disturbance, and tinnitus

▶ Speech and language disabilities can occur with OME.

▶ Perforation of tympanic membrane, facial nerve paralysis, otitic hydrocephalus

▶ Cholesteatoma, tympanosclerosis

▶ Advanced infection (acute mastoiditis, meningitis, epidural abscess)

▶ Atrophy and scarring of eardrum, chronic perforation and otorrhea, cholesteatoma, and permanent hearing loss are possible in recurrent AOM and OME.

PROBLEMS OF NOSE/SINUSES

Rhinitis

Description

▶ Inflammation of the nasal mucous membranes, accompanied by itchy eyes, nose, and palate, postnasal drip, cough, irritability, fatigue, and edema of mucosa; may be allergic, nonallergic (vasomotor rhinitis), or infectious

Etiology

▶ *Allergic rhinitis* is an IgE-mediated hypersensitivity reaction, most commonly related to inhaled seasonal pollen allergens (tree, grass, weeds) and perennial allergens of dust mites, pet dander, cockroaches, molds, indoor pollutants, and cigarette smoke.

▶ *Infectious rhinitis (common cold)* is most commonly due to the rhinovirus, as well as coronavirus, influenza, parainfluenza, and adenoviruses, or, less commonly, bacteria.

▶ *Nonallergic or vasomotor rhinitis* etiologies are not well understood but are thought to be autonomic responses that result in dilation of the nasal submucosal vessels. Influencing or triggering factors include temperature/humidity change, odors, selected drugs, emotional response, and body positions such as lying down.

▶ *Other causes*: The perennial form of nonallergic rhinitis is associated with atrophy of the nasal bones and nasal lining in the geriatric population; nasal polyps, benign overgrowths of the nasal mucous membrane, and connective tissue disorders; abuse of nasal decongestants oxymetazoline (Afrin) with rebound edema of the nose after continuous use; and transient rhinitis associated with pregnancy due to hormonal influences in women or foreign body in children.

Incidence and Demographics

▶ Increased incidence since the industrial revolution

▶ Affects 1 in 5 Americans

▶ Forty-four to 87% of patients have mixed rhinitis (allergic and nonallergic).

▶ Infectious: common in all ages, especially children

Risk Factors

▶ Family history of atopy

▶ Higher socioeconomic status

▶ Tobacco smoke

▶ Other allergies (asthma)

▶ Pets in house; cockroaches in home

▶ Genetics (80% have family history of allergic conditions)

Prevention and Screening

▶ Avoid environmental allergens.

▶ Frequent handwashing to reduce risk of infection

▶ Environmental control measures indoors: frequent vacuuming with particulate filters, air cleaners (HEPA filters), mattress and pillow encasements, removal of carpeting, air conditioner, dehumidifier to reduce indoor humidity (<50%), closing doors and windows during allergy season

Assessment

See Table 6–7

Diagnostic Studies

▶ Based on history and physical

▶ Skin testing for allergies

▶ Nasal smear for eosinophils

▶ Serum IgE levels (test has limited value)

▶ CBC if infectious process

▶ Rapid flu test if influenza is suspected

Differential Diagnosis

▶ URI

▶ Foreign body

▶ Hormonal: oral contraceptives or pregnancy

▶ Sinusitis

TABLE 6–7.
COMPARISON OF RHINITIS PRESENTATIONS

	ALLERGIC RHINITIS	INFECTIOUS RHINITIS (COLD)	VASOMOTOR RHINITIS	ATROPHIC RHINITIS
Onset	Age 8–11	Anytime	Adulthood	Older adulthood
Common Primary Symptoms	Nasal congestion, sneezing, itchy nose, clear rhinorrhea	Congestion or obstruction, sneezing, scratchy sore throat, nasal crusting, cloudy or colored drainage	Abrupt onset congestion and pronounced rhinorrhea and postnasal drip, sneezing	Nasal congestion, thick postnasal drip, frequent clearing of throat, bad smell in nose
Associated Symptoms	Cough, sore throat, itching and puffy eyes, headache	Cough, hoarseness, malaise, headache, fever >100°F, may c/o facial or sinus tenderness	Watery eyes	May have nasal discomfort
Physical Exam Findings	Nasal mucosa pale and boggy, blue-gray nasal mucosa Enlarged turbinates Clear, watery discharge Postnasal discharge "Allergic shiners" Transverse nasal crease Nasal salute Mouth-breathing	Edema and hyperemia of mucous membranes, throat erythema without edema, rhinorrhea (clear, yellow or green), postnasal drainage, dull TMs, lungs clear, cervical lymph nodes tender and enlarged	Turbinates pale and edematous, rhinorrhea No other findings	Nasal mucosa dry, smooth, and shiny Studded with crust Foul odor may be present Nonedematous Airway patent No other findings

▶ Nasal polyps or overgrowths

▶ Adenoid hypertrophy

▶ Otitis media

▶ Endocrine disease (hypothyroidism)

Management

Nonpharmacologic Treatment

▶ General measures for all types: hydration, humidification (except for allergic), intranasal irrigation with saline solutions

▶ Avoidance of known triggers

Pharmacologic Treatment

▶ Topical antihistamine azelastine HCL 0.1% (Astelin), olopatadine (Patanase)

▶ Oral antihistamines:

▷ 1st-generation products such as diphenhydramine (Benadryl) cause sedation and may impair performance; use with caution

▷ 2nd-generation nonsedating: fexofenadine (Allegra), loratadine (Claritin), cetirizine (Zyrtec) are preferred for regular use

▶ Intranasal glucocorticoids: first generation—beclomethasone (Beconase AQ), flunisolide (Nasarel), budesonide (Rhinocort Aqua, trimacinolone (Nasacort). Second generation—fluticasone propionate (Flonase), mometasone furoate (Nasonex), fluti-casone furoate (Veramyst), ciclesonide (Ominaris or Zetonna). Refer to packaging for age-appropriate usage and dosage.

▶ Oral decongestants cause vasoconstriction, decrease blood supply to the nasal mucosa, decrease mucosal edema; can be used with antihistamines; numerous preparations available

▶ Cromolyn sodium

▶ Antileukotriene agent: montelukast (Singulair)

▶ Ipratropium bromide (Atrovent) for profuse rhinorrhea

▶ OTC nasal decongestant sprays: phenylephrine, oxymetazoline, xylometazoline, naphazoline: not recommended as monotherapy in chronic rhinitis because rebound congestion may occur

▶ Systemic glucocorticoids: short course may be indicated in severe cases; do not use repeatedly or for prolonged periods of time

▶ Allergen immunotherapy: subcutaneously or sublingual tablets available; series of injections with specific allergens, once or twice weekly; should be initiated only by a trained specialist

▶ Specific recommendations for each disorder:

▷ Allergic rhinitis: intranasal steroids first; oral antihistamines may be added, also topical antihistamine (Astelin) and mast cell stabilizer (NasalCrom); if patient has concomitant allergic eye symptoms, treat also with ocular antihistamine, mast cell stabilizer, or both; leukotriene antagonist (montelukast) used as adjunct, not monotherapy

▷ Infectious rhinitis: acetaminophen or NSAIDs for pain or fever; topical or oral decongestants; inhaled or topical anticholinergics, antihistamines

▷ Atrophic rhinitis: guaifenesin (Naldecon Senior EX syrup) for stimulation of mucus, or intranasal saline solution spray

How Long to Treat

▶ Infectious rhinitis: for symptom relief only

▶ Allergic rhinitis: usually daily throughout allergy season

▶ Nonallergic rhinitis: daily may be needed to prevent symptoms

Special Considerations

▶ Use medications (especially decongestants and antihistamines) with caution in the older adult population; medications commonly produce adverse reactions or may interact with other medications that older adults take routinely.

▶ Use OTC decongestants with caution in patients with diabetes, hypertension, or glaucoma.

When to Consult, Refer, Hospitalize

▶ Referral to an allergist for allergen immunotherapy for allergic rhinitis that is not easily managed by medications or avoidance of known allergens

▶ Referral to ENT for those with complications, nasal polyps or growths, or symptoms unmanageable with above-described treatments

Follow-Up

▶ Routine generally 2–4 weeks after initiation of treatment for allergic and nonallergic rhinitis

▶ If infectious rhinitis has not resolved in 10 days

Expected Course

▶ Viral rhinitis usually resolves within 7–10 days.

▶ Allergic, vasomotor, and atrophic rhinitis are ongoing problems that are managed, not cured.

Complications

▶ Rhinitis medicamentosa (rebound)

▶ Worsening of related pulmonary conditions (e.g., COPD, asthma)

▶ Spread of infection: otitis media, acute sinusitis, pneumonia, bronchitis

▶ Nasopharyngeal lymphoid hyperplasia

▶ Epistaxis

▶ Sleep disturbance

Epistaxis

Description

▶ Hemorrhage from the nostrils, nasopharynx, or nasal cavity (anterior or posterior); "nosebleed"

▶ May be a symptom of an underlying problem

Etiology

▶ Primarily idiopathic, but may have many other causes; <10% related to neoplasm or coagulopathy

▶ Trauma: nose picking, foreign body, septal perforation, sinus fracture, abuse of inhaled recreational drugs (cocaine)

▶ Localized inflammation or irritation: infection, irritant inhalation, topical steroid use, septal deviation, low humidity

▶ Vascular abnormalities such as aging sclerotic vessels, arteriovenous malformations

▶ Hypertension (bleeding worsened by but not caused by hypertension)

▶ Coagulation problems from diseases such as von Willebrand disease, leukemias, blood dyscrasias, platelet dysfunction; medications such as warfarin (Coumadin), clopidogrel (Plavix), NSAIDs; or aspirin, alcoholism

▶ Neoplasm: rare, but consider in persistent unilateral cases

Incidence and Demographics

▶ Common in the United States

▶ Estimated lifetime incidence ~60%

▶ Bimodal: peaks in children up to age 15 and in adults >50

▶ Rare in children under age 2

Risk Factors

▶ All of the concomitant or precipitating problems listed under Etiology

Prevention and Screening

▶ Adequate moisturizing of the mucous membranes (humidifier, saline nasal spray); keeping nails clipped short and away from nose

▶ Petroleum jelly or antibiotic ointment applied to the anterior nasal septum

▶ Control of underlying nasal and systemic problems

▶ Protective athletic equipment, safety precautions to prevent trauma

▶ Avoid trauma and irritants

Assessment

History

▶ Patients may present with actively bleeding nose or may consult for episodes that were resolved with self-care.

▶ Ascertain precipitating events; from which nostril blood first appeared; associated symptoms, including nausea and vomiting, URI indications.

▶ Inquire about trauma (including nose picking), previous episodes, comorbid conditions, current medications (including over-the-counter and supplements).

Physical Exam

▶ Inspect for site of bleed; note localized or diffuse mucosal irritation, bleeding from 1 or 2 nostrils, venous or arterial source (Table 6–8); obtain vital signs, do complete ENT exam.

Diagnostic Studies

▶ Only recurrent or severe cases warrant extensive evaluation with head radiograph or CAT scan.

▶ CBC, platelet count, prothrombin time (PT) for recurrent or intractable cases

TABLE 6–8.
CHARACTERISTICS OF NASAL BLEEDING SITES

	ANTERIOR EPISTAXIS	POSTERIOR EPISTAXIS
Presentation	Typically unilateral	Unilateral or bilateral
Timing	Lasts between a few to 30 minutes, in isolation or recurrently	Intermittent
Source of Bleed	Typically venous from Kiesselbach's plexus	Typically arterial from posterior nasopharynx
	90% are located here	More common location in older adults
Other	Usually less severe, easier to treat	Can result in significant hemorrhage
	More common in young patients	May have nausea or coffee-ground emesis

▶ PT/partial thromboplastin time (PTT) if patient is on warfarin or other medications affecting coagulation

▶ Cross-match when appropriate

▶ Toxicology screen when illicit drug use is suspected

Differential Diagnosis

▶ Drug-related as an anticoagulant side effect or from abuse (nasal cocaine inhalation)

▶ Symptom of one of the etiologic agents identified above

▶ Localized, isolated, benign event

Management

Nonpharmacologic Treatment

▶ For simple (anterior) nosebleeds, application of direct pinching-type pressure just below the bridge of the nose for 5–20 minutes will stop the bleeding; can be taught to the patient for self-care in the event of recurrence of a simple nosebleed. Keep the patient in an upright position and apply ice packs over the bridge of the nose.

▶ If not responsive to above measures, most anterior venous bleeds can be controlled by placing a cotton ball moistened with 1:1,000 epinephrine *or* vasoconstrictor nose drops (e.g., phenylephrine) just inside the nares and then applying pressure for 5–10 minutes. Some practitioners may also initiate cauterization with silver nitrate sticks or chemical cautery with chromic acid beads to the site of the bleeding.

▶ For maintenance of nasal hygiene and to avoid recurrence, apply petroleum jelly (Vaseline) to nares routinely for lubrication. Use humidifiers, cut fingernails, and avoid picking.

▶ For arterial (posterior) bleeds or epistaxis not responding to above acute treatment, immediate referral to an ER or ENT specialist for further treatment procedures, which may include cauterization via silver nitrate stick, bead of chromic acid, or 25% trichloroacetic acid or electrocautery or thermal cautery followed by packing with ribbons of gauze impregnated with petroleum jelly, nasal tampons, or balloon inflation compression.

Pharmacologic Treatment
- ▶ Vasoconstrictors and topical anesthetics for bleeding cessation and analgesia
  - ▷ Cocaine 4%, phenylephrine 0.25%, epinephrine 1:1,000, lidocaine laryngeal spray, lidocaine jelly 2%, lidocaine solution 4%, viscous lidocaine 2%
- ▶ Treatment of underlying disorders

How Long to Treat
- ▶ Episodic for the actual bleeding incident
- ▶ Ongoing monitoring and treatment as indicated for the associated underlying disorders

Special Considerations
- ▶ Pediatrics: more likely anterior, idiopathic, and recurrent
- ▶ Older adults: more likely to be posterior bleed

When to Consult, Refer, Hospitalize
- ▶ Posterior bleeding: frequently requires otolaryngology consultation
- ▶ Intractable bleeding: may require endoscopic laser or electrocauterization or angiography with arteriolar embolization; therefore, immediate referral to an emergency facility or ENT
- ▶ Recurrent epistaxis: refer to an ENT specialist

Follow-Up

Expected Course
- ▶ Excellent prognosis for isolated, idiopathic epistaxis
- ▶ Variable outcome depending on underlying cause

Complications
- ▶ Septal perforation from cauterization therapy
- ▶ Toxic shock syndrome with packing
- ▶ Arrhythmias triggered by packing
- ▶ Pressure-induced tissue necrosis of nasal mucosa

Sinusitis

Description
- ▶ Symptomatic inflammation of the nasal cavity and paranasal sinuses, categorized as acute, recurrent, subacute, or chronic
  - ▷ *Acute*: an infection of one or more paranasal sinuses of <4 weeks' duration; considered recurrent if >3 acute episodes per year
  - ▷ Subacute: ongoing symptoms of purulent nasal discharge and inflammation of the sinuses for 4–12 weeks

▷ Chronic: prolonged inflammation of the sinuses with or without associated infection >12 weeks; irreversible damage to the mucosa is possible

Etiology

▶ Viral: vast majority of cases (rhinovirus, influenza A and B, parainfluenza virus, respiratory syncytial, adenovirus, coronavirus, enterovirus)

▶ Bacterial: ore likely if symptoms worsen after 5–7 days or do not improve >10 days (*S. pneumonia*, *H. influenzae*, *M. catarrhalis*); often overdiagnosed, leading to overuse of antibiotics and an increase antibiotic resistance

▶ Fungal: seen in immunocompromised hosts (uncontrolled diabetes, neutropenia, use of corticosteroids) or nosocomial infection

Incidence and Demographics

▶ Highest in early fall through early spring

▶ Affects 31 million Americans each year

▶ About 2% of viral rhinosinusitis episodes have bacterial superinfections.

Risk Factors

▶ Viral URI

▶ Allergic rhinitis

▶ Asthma

▶ Cigarette smoking

▶ Dental infections and procedures

▶ Anatomic variations: tonsillar and adenoid hypertrophy, turbinate hypertrophy, nasal polyps, deviated septum, cleft palate

▶ Immunodeficiency (HIV)

▶ Cystic fibrosis

Prevention and Screening

▶ Handwashing to prevent transmission of viral infection

Assessment

History

▶ Major challenge is to distinguish between viral and bacterial disease

▶ Predictive symptoms of bacterial infection: worsening symptoms >5–7 days after initial improvement; persistent symptoms for >10 days; persistent purulent nasal discharge; unilateral upper tooth or facial pain; unilateral maxillary sinus tenderness; fever

▶ Other associated symptoms: headache, nasal congestion, retro-orbital pain, otalgia, hyposomia, halitosis, chronic cough worse at night

Physical Exam
- ▶ Complete HEENT (head, eyes, ears, nose, throat) and pulmonary exam, with typical findings in the case of acute sinusitis:
  - ▷ Fever
  - ▷ Edema and erythema of nasal mucosa
  - ▷ Purulent discharge
  - ▷ Tenderness to palpation over sinus(es)
- ▶ Chronic sinusitis merits a more detailed examination for underlying risk factors
- ▶ *Note*: Important serious findings include external facial swelling, erythema, or cellulitis over an involved sinus (periorbital or forehead); vision changes such as diplopia; difficulty moving eyes (EOMs); proptosis; and any abnormal neurologic signs. *These are all indicative of serious complications requiring urgent referral and treatment.*

Diagnostic Studies
- ▶ Diagnostic tests are not routinely recommended; no diagnostic test can differentiate between viral and bacterial rhinosinusitis.
- ▶ Lab: none indicated in routine evaluations; transillumination of sinuses may confirm fluid in sinuses (helpful if asymmetric; not helpful if symmetric)
- ▶ Imaging: value of imaging studies is limited; they do not distinguish between viral and bacterial etiology
- ▶ Limited coronal CAT scan can be useful in recurrent infection or failure to respond to medical therapy

Differential Diagnosis
- ▶ Dental disease
- ▶ Nasopharyngeal tumor
- ▶ Wegener's syndrome
- ▶ HIV infection
- ▶ Immotile cilia syndrome
- ▶ Kartagener syndrome
- ▶ Headache, tension or migraine
- ▶ Trauma, foreign body
- ▶ Cystic fibrosis
- ▶ Granuloma

Management

Nonpharmacologic Treatment
- ▶ Hydration
- ▶ Steam inhalation 20–30 minutes t.i.d.
- ▶ Saline irrigation (neti pot) or nose drops
- ▶ Sleeping with head of bed elevated

- ▶ Avoiding exposure to cigarette smoke or fumes
- ▶ Avoiding caffeine and alcohol
- ▶ Warm facial packs

Pharmacologic Treatment

- ▶ Analgesics: acetaminophen, aspirin, NSAIDs, acetaminophen with codeine (severe cases)
- ▶ Decongestants: pseudoephedrine HCl, phenylephrine nasal spray (limit use), oxymetazoline nasal spray (Afrin; limited to 3-day use)
- ▶ Antibiotics: indicated only when findings suggest bacterial infection (symptoms that persist >10 days or worsen in 5–7 days)
- ▶ First-line antibiotics:
  - ▷ Amoxicillin: 1 g t.i.d. (adults) and 80–90 mg/kg/day divided q 8 h (children)
  - ▷ Trimethoprim-sulfamethoxazole (TMP/SMX): 160/800 mg q 12 h (adults) and 8–12 mg/kg/day of trimethoprim component divided q 12 h (children)
  - ▷ Doxycycline: 100 mg p.o. b.i.d. (adults only)
- ▶ Second-line antibiotics: use if no response to first-line therapy after 72 hours or if patient has had antibiotics within the past 4–6 weeks
  - ▷ Amoxicillin-clavulanate: 875/125 mg q 12 h (adults) and 30 mg/kg/day of amoxicillin component divided b.i.d. (children)
  - ▷ Augmentin XR b.i.d. in adults and Augmentin ES-600 in children (for beta-lactam and penicillin-binding protein resistance)
- ▶ Other second-line antibiotics: cefpodoxime, cefuroxime axetil, azithromycin, clarithromycin, levofloxacin (Levaquin). See specific dosages in Table 6–6 as for otitis media.
- ▶ If lack of response after 3 weeks of antibiotics, consider CAT scan, ENT referral
- ▶ Oral antihistamines: loratadine, fexofenadine, cetirizine, desloratadine (Clarinex) or levocetirizine (Xyzal), diphenhydramine
- ▶ Leukotriene inhibitors: montelukast, zafirlukast (Accolate), especially in patients with asthma
- ▶ Nasal steroids: fluticasone. Refer to Rhinitis section for a list of intranasal glucocorticoids.

How Long to Treat

- ▶ Recommendations are not consistent; however, a 10–14-day course is typical for acute sinusitis.
- ▶ Chronic sinusitis should be treated until the patient is well for 7 days.

Special Considerations

▶ Avoid prolonged use of topical decongestants to prevent rebound congestion and dependence.

▶ Resist the urge and patient demand to treat viral URIs with antibiotics.

▶ Pregnancy: avoid clarithromycin and levofloxacin as they may cause fetotoxicity; other safer alternatives available

When to Consult, Refer, Hospitalize

▶ Complications or failure of treatment

Follow-Up

Expected Course

▶ Improvement of symptoms within 72 hours and resolution of sinusitis within 10–14 days

▶ Follow-up if no improvement after 72 hours or no resolution after 10 days of antibiotic use

Complications

▶ Serious complications are rare: brain abscess, meningitis, osteomyelitis, orbital cellulitis, cavernous sinus thrombosis, subdural empyema

PROBLEMS OF THE PHARYNX

Pharyngitis/Tonsillitis

Description

▶ Inflammation of the pharynx commonly caused by acute viral infection; infection by Group A beta-hemolytic streptococci is of greatest concern, because of the potential preventable rheumatic sequelae (scarlet fever, rheumatic fever, glomerulonephritis)

Etiology

▶ Spread by person-to-person contact via droplets of oral, respiratory, and nasal secretions

▶ Viral infection accounts for 90% of pharyngitis.

▶ Viral agents include: rhinovirus, adenovirus, parainfluenza, coxsackie, echovirus, herpes simplex virus, Epstein-Barr, cytomegalovirus

▶ Most common bacterial agents: Group A B-hemolytic streptococci, *N. gonorrhoeae*, *Corynebacterium diphtheriae*, *H. influenzae*, *M. catarrhalis*, Groups C and G *Streptococcus* (rarely)

▶ Infectious mononucleosis: Epstein-Barr virus; affects adolescents most frequently

▶ Chronic causes: more likely noninfectious; irritation from postnasal discharge of chronic allergic rhinitis or reflux; referred pain, chemical irritation, or smoking; neoplasms and vasculitides

Incidence and Demographics

▶ Commonly occurring illness; approximately 30 million cases per year estimated

▶ Group A *Streptococcus* is the most common bacterial cause, ~15%–30% of cases in children and 5%–10% of cases in adults

▶ Rheumatic fever is rare in the United States; greatest incidence is in children ages 5–18 years

Risk Factors

▶ Epidemics of Group A beta-hemolytic streptococcal disease

▶ Age (the young are most susceptible)

▶ Family history

▶ Communal living (dormitories, barracks)

▶ Immunosuppression; diabetes mellitus

▶ Recent illness; fatigue

▶ Excess alcohol consumption, smoking, receptive oral sex

Prevention and Screening

▶ Frequent handwashing, especially in situations of contact with infected people

▶ Avoiding contact with infected people

Assessment

History

▶ Complaint of sore throat, cough, hoarseness, lower respiratory symptoms, fever, anorexia, chills, malaise, headache; contacts with similar symptoms or diagnosed infection are common

Physical Exam

▶ Enlarged tonsils, pharyngeal erythema, tonsillar exudates, soft palate petechiae, cervical adenopathy, fever >102.5° F

▶ Scarlet fever rash: streptococcal pharyngitis

▶ Gray pseudomembrane found in diphtheria and, occasionally, mononucleosis

▶ Erythematous-based clear vesicles are found in herpes stomatitis.

▶ Conjunctivitis is found with adenovirus infections.

Diagnostic Studies

▶ Diagnostic testing is done only in patients with history of fever, tonsillar exudates, and tender anterior cervical adenopathy without presence of cough.

▶ Rapid strep antigen screen: 50%–80% sensitivity; >95% specificity; do not culture if positive

▶ Throat culture remains the "gold standard" for diagnosis of Group A beta-hemolytic streptococcus.

▶ If a negative rapid strep screen is found in a patient with a high probability of streptococcus, culture to confirm.

TABLE 6–9.
CHARACTERISTICS OF PHARYNGITIS BY ETIOLOGY

	SYMPTOMS	EXAM FINDINGS
VIRAL		
Coxsackie and others	Sore throat, malaise, fever, headache	Small oral vesicles, ulcers on posterior pharynx, tonsils, buccal mucus
Epstein-Barr	Above + fatigue	Exudative tonsillitis, palatial petechiae, posterior cervical adenopathy; possible maculopapular rash
Primary HIV	Above + myalgia, photophobia lasting a few days to 2 weeks	Posterior cervical lymphadenopathy Similar to Epstein-Barr with rash
BACTERIAL		
Group A strep	Sore throat, fever, odynophagia (primarily) Abdominal pain, vomiting, headache	Fever > 101° F Erythema and white or yellow exudate of tonsils and/or pharynx Anterior cervical lymphadenopathy Absence of other URI symptoms/signs generally but not always
Scarlet fever	Abrupt-onset fever, pharyngitis, headache	Sandpaper-like fine, erythematous rash on trunk and extremities (absent on face) that blanches on pressure Appears within 24–48 hours, lasts 4–10 days
Rheumatic fever	Symptoms develop 1–6 months after strep infection	Various manifestations: heart murmur, polyarthritis, rash (see Chapter 4, Infectious Diseases)
STI		
Chlamydia or Gonorrhea	Chronic sore throat History of oral sex or sexual abuse	Exudative, erythematous pharynx Anterior cervical lymphadenopathy
Mycoplasma	Same as strep	Same as strep
FUNGAL		
Candida albicans	History of antibiotic use, immunosuppression, use of inhaled corticosteroids	Thin, diffuse, or patchy white plaques on red base on mucous membranes, pharynx, tongue
Peritonsillar abscess	Unilateral throat and ear pain Dysphagia, dysphonia, drooling, trismus (difficulty opening mouth because of pain and inflammation)	Erythema and swelling of soft palate Uvula and soft palate edema such that it may appear the uvula "points" toward side of abscess Exquisitely tender, palpable, fluctuant abscess on tonsil Similarly tender, enlarged anterior cervical lymph nodes

▶ Culture of the pathogen may help identify causative organism; however, may not be cost-effective or influence outcome.

▶ Mono spot is indicated for suspicion of mononucleosis.

▶ CBC with differential reveals increased WBC if bacterial, decreased if viral (not routinely done)

▶ If indicated, culture for gonorrhea and/or *Chlamydia* infection.

▶ Potassium hydroxide (KOH) wet mount reveals pseudohyphae and budding spores in candidiasis.

Differential Diagnosis

▶ Strep "carrier state"

▶ Etiologic agents identified above

▶ Epiglottitis

▶ Thyroiditis

▶ Peritonsillar abscess (rare)

▶ Postnasal drip related to rhinitis or sinusitis

Management

▶ Goal: identify and treat Group A beta-hemolytic streptococcal pharyngitis to decrease risk of acute rheumatic fever

Nonpharmacologic Treatment

▶ Symptomatic treatment includes: force fluids, salt water gargles, OTC analgesics (acetaminophen, NSAIDs if no contraindications), throat lozenges, cool-mist humidifier

▶ Rest is advisable with pharyngitis associated with mononucleosis.

▶ *Note*: Peritonsillar abscess requires urgent referral to otolaryngologist for possible IV antibiotics, incision, and drainage; tonsillectomy may be recommended as definitive treatment after the acute episode resolves.

Pharmacologic Treatment

▶ First-line therapy:

▷ Penicillin V (Pen-Vee K) 250 mg t.i.d (<27 kg) or 500 mg b.i.d. or t.i.d. (>27 kg) is the drug of choice for *Streptococcus*; children: 25–50 mg/kg/day, divided b.i.d–q.i.d all for 10 days *or*

▷ Amoxicillin 50mg/kg/day once daily x 10 days (use with caution, because EBV infection may induce rash)

▶ If allergic to penicillin:

▷ Erythromycin (E-mycin 500 mg b.i.d. x 10 days); children: 30–50 mg/kg/day, divided t.i.d.–q.i.d.; *or*

▷ Cephalexin (Keflex) 250 mg p.o. t.i.d. adults and 30 mg/kg/d b.i.d. x 10 days for children

▶ Second-line therapy: first-generation cephalosporins, azithromycin, clarithromycin

▶ Intramuscular penicillin G benzathine (single dose) for patients who are unable to complete the full 10-day dose or for those who are at increased risk for rheumatic fever

▶ Eradication of carrier state:

▷ Clindamycin 20 mg/kg/day in 3 divided doses x 10 days (most effective)

▷ Cephalexin 25–50 mg/kg/day b.i.d. x 10 days

▷ Penicillin + rifampin: use above penicillin doses + rifampin 20 mg/kg/day b.i.d. for final 4 days

▷ Consider repeat throat culture after treatment to document eradication of Group A strep

▷ Asymptomatic carriers: generally no treatment indicated

▶ For *Chlamydial* or mycoplasmal infections, which, when present, are usually accompanied by lower respiratory tract symptoms: children—erythromycin 30–50 mg/kg b.i.d. x 10 days; adults—doxycycline 100 mg b.i.d. x 10 days or azithromycin 500 mg for 1 day followed by 250 mg for 4 days

▶ For gonococcal pharyngitis: ceftriaxone 125–250 mg IM (consider treatment for *Chlamydia* as well)

▶ For candidiasis pharyngitis: nystatin (Mycostatin) 100,000 U/ml oral suspension 4–6 mL q.i.d.

How Long to Treat

▶ Patients being treated with penicillin should complete the full 10 days of oral antibiotic. Five-day therapy is acceptable with cefpodoxime, cefdinir, or azithromycin.

Special Considerations

▶ Patient must complete full course of antibiotic for strep regardless of symptom response

▶ Household and close personal contacts of the patient with strep are treated only if symptomatic.

▶ Children may return to school once afebrile and on antibiotic for at least 24 hours.

▶ Advise those diagnosed with mononucleosis to avoid contact sports for 4 weeks to avoid possible splenic rupture.

When to Consult, Refer, Hospitalize

▶ Any patient with peritonsillar or retropharyngeal abscess requires urgent referral.

▶ Patients with symptoms or edema affecting the ability to breathe or swallow (e.g., inability to swallow their own saliva) require immediate transfer to hospital.

Follow-Up

▶ No follow-up necessary unless not resolving

Expected Course

▶ Strep pharyngitis typically lasts for 5–7 days, with fever peaking at second to third day; will spontaneously resolve, but early treatment of strep pharyngitis decreases symptomatic period by ½–2 days and decreases risk of rheumatic complications.

▶ Viral pharyngitis will resolve spontaneously.

▶ Symptoms of rheumatic complications develop in weeks to months following resolution of pharyngitis.

Complications

▶ Otitis media, mastoiditis, septicemia, rhinitis, sinusitis, pneumonia

▶ Rheumatic fever

▶ Poststreptococcal glomerulonephritis, peritonsillar abscess, systemic infection

Epiglottis

Description

▶ Rapid development of inflammation and edema of the supraglottic structures, epiglottis, vallecula, aryepiglottic folds, and arytenoids leading to narrowed airway and respiratory compromise

▶ *Note:* **An acute and sudden onset of a potentially life-threatening illness**

Etiology

▶ Infectious etiology:

▷ Bacterial: *H. influenzae* type b (HiB), *S. pyogenes, S. pneumoniae, S. aureus, Haemophilus parainfluenzae, Escherichia coli,* and many more

▷ Fungal (*Candida* spp.)

▷ Viral: herpes simplex type 1, varicella zoster, parainfluenza type 3, influenza B, Epstein-Barr

▶ Traumatic (caustic ingestion, thermal injury, foreign body ingestion)

▶ Allergic reactions

Incidence and Demographics

▶ Has decreased dramatically since the introduction of HiB vaccine

▶ Predominant age shifting to older children (median age, 7 years) and adults

▶ Predominant sex: male > female (1.8:1)

Risk Factors

▶ Absence of immunization against HiB vaccine

▶ Immunocompromise

▶ Associated with comorbid conditions (hypertension, diabetes mellitus, substance abuse)

Prevention and Screening

▶ Immunization with *H. influenzae* type B vaccine, although not 100% affective; available only for children up to age 5

▶ Rifampin 20 mg/kg/day x 4 days (max daily dose 600 mg) for close contacts (may be carriers) of invasive HiB

Assessment

History

▶ Sudden onset of severe pain with swallowing *or* already unable to swallow own saliva by time of examination

▶ Fever, toxic appearing, respiratory distress (stridor, tachypnea, anxiety, refusal to lie down, and labored breathing)

▶ Dysphagia, refusal to eat, drooling, sore throat, anterior neck pain

▶ Muffled "hot potato" voice/cry (vs. hoarseness in croup)

▶ Minimal cough (vs. barking cough in croup); usually no precipitating URI (vs. positive history in croup)

▶ In adults, presentation more indolent (sore throat and odynophagia are predominant symptoms)

▶ PMH including immunization history and current medications

Physical Exam

▶ Toxic appearance/shock

▶ Marked restlessness, irritability, and anxiety

▶ Airway obstruction resulting in respiratory distress

▶ Marked substernal and subcostal retractions and labored breathing indicate impending respiratory failure

▶ Stridor softer and less prominent than in croup

▶ Anterior neck exam may reveal tender adenopathy.

▶ Classic posturing of sitting up and leaning forward, tongue hanging out, often holding something (a cup) to spit their saliva out as they cannot swallow it without severe pain

▶ Cyanosis indicates poor prognosis.

▶ *Note*: Examination of the pharynx should be carried out *only* with equipment and personnel in place for emergency intubation or tracheotomy for airway maintenance. Insertion of a tongue blade into the oral cavity may precipitate laryngeal spasm and acute airway obstruction.

Diagnostic Studies

▶ Blood and epiglottis cultures (obtained under the same conditions as examination described above)

▶ Blood cultures are positive in 75%–90% of children.

▶ CBC positive for leukocytosis with left shift

▶ HiB antigen test in serum/urine is useful in children with previous antibiotic treatment.

   ▷ Lateral neck X-ray is consistent with enlarged edematous epiglottitis (the thumbprint sign), but contraindicated because of the risk of sudden complete airway obstruction. If obtained, ensure adequate staff in case complete airway obstruction occurs.

   ▷ Chest X-ray for screening of pneumonia (25% occurrence rate) and placement of endotracheal tube

Differential Diagnosis

▶ Viral croup

▶ Acute angioneurotic edema

▶ Foreign body aspiration

▶ Peritonsillar abscess

▶ Retropharyngeal abscess

▶ Diphtheria in unimmunized patients

▶ Lingual tonsillitis

▶ Sepsis

▶ Uvulitis

▶ Angioedema

Management

▶ Immediately arrange for monitoring, IV, and maintenance of secure airway with appropriate personnel and equipment and transport to an emergency setting or hospital with ICU.

▶ Monitor vital signs, oxygen saturation, and be alert for potential abrupt deterioration.

▶ Begin IV antibiotics.

▶ Monitor patient in the ICU

▶ Two goals: maintain airway and administer antimicrobial agents

Special Considerations

▶ Incidence decreasing in children since use of HiB vaccine

When to Consult, Refer, Hospitalize

▶ All patients with epiglottitis require immediate transport to the hospital.

Follow-Up

Expected Course

▶ With prompt and appropriate treatment, morbidity and mortality rates are low.

▶ Airway management measures are usually discontinued within 24–48 hours of treatment.

▶ Immunization recommended

Complications

▶ Pneumonia, meningitis, cervical adenitis, septic arthritis, cellulitis

▶ Progression of infection to deep neck tissue

▶ Epiglottic abscess

▶ Septic shock

▶ Pneumothorax

▶ Death from airway obstruction (asphyxia)

PROBLEMS OF THE MOUTH

Oral Candidiasis (Thrush)

Description

▶ Fungal infection of the oral mucous membranes

Etiology

▶ *Candida albicans* is part of the normal flora of the oral cavity that causes overt infection when there is a reduction in the competitive oral microflora.

Incidence and Demographics

▶ Essentially a disease of infants; in adults it may be a sign of immunosuppression

▶ Common with immunodeficiency, persons with obesity, diabetes, hyperhidrosis

Risk Factors

▶ Most common cause in infants and children is long-term use of broad-spectrum antibiotics

▶ May also arise in the immunosuppressed patient (HIV)

▶ Conditions that cause decrease in the host resistance—stress, diabetes, malnutrition, prematurity, use of inhaled corticosteroids (ICS)

▶ Denture wear

Prevention and Screening

▶ Judicious use of antibiotics

▶ Patient should rinse mouth after inhaled steroid use.

▶ Dentures should be cleaned appropriately and fit well.

▶ Control of diabetes, weight loss, decrease in stress, proper nutrition

Assessment

History

▶ White coating in the mouth

▶ Decreased sucking or appetite because of discomfort, sore throat

▶ Ask about recent antibiotic use

Physical Exam

▶ White, raised, distinct patches in the mouth, particularly the tongue, buccal mucosa, and hard palate, which rubs off easily, leaving an underlying red, raw surface

▶ Membrane consists of an almost pure colony of fungus

▶ Immunocomprimised hosts: oral lesions are white, raised, nontender, distinct patches; red, slightly raised patches; thick, dark-brownish coating; deep fissures

▶ Angular chelitis: infection in corners of the mouth

Diagnostic Studies

▶ KOH preparation for microscopy of plaque can be made but is not necessary

▶ Culture for rare types of fungal/yeast infections or alternative infection if first-line treatment fails

Differential Diagnosis

▶ Exudative pharyngitis

▶ Hairy leukoplakia (adults), does not rub off

▶ Lichen planus

▶ Geographic tongue

▶ Herpes simplex erythema multiforme

▶ Pemphigus

▶ Baby formula or breast milk

Management

Nonpharmacologic Treatment

▶ Determine and treat underlying cause (e.g., antibiotic use, immune problem).

▶ Boil pacifiers and bottle nipples; assess mother's breasts/nipples for *Candida* infections.

▶ Disinfect dentures.

Pharmacologic Treatment

▶ First-line therapy:

▷ Clotrimazole (Mycelex) troches 10 mg (suck on for 20 minutes) 5x day for 7–14 days

▷ Nystatin pastilles: 200,000 U each, q.i.d. for 7–14 days

▷ Denture wearers: nystatin ointment 100,000 U/g on fitting surfaces of denture and corners of mouth for 3 weeks; remove dentures at night; clean 2x/week with diluted (1:20) bleach or soaking solution containing benzoic acid, 0.12% chlorhexidine gluconate, or alkalize proteases

▷ Moderate to severe disease: fluconazole (Diflucan) 100–200 mg (3 mg/kg) daily x 7–14 days or itraconazole (Sporanox) solution or capsules

▶ Second-line therapy:

▷ Nystatin oral suspension (100,000 U/ml: Infants: 0.5 mL in each cheek q.i.d x 10 days; children; 5–10 mL q.i.d x 10 days; adults: swish and swallow 5–10 mL q.i.d. x 14 days; prophylaxis—same dosages x 2–5 days

▷ Fluconazole 100 mg daily for 7–14 days (load immunocompromised patient with 200 mg)

▷ Itraconazole (Sporanox) suspension: 200 mg (20 mL) daily; swish and swallow for 7–14 days; capsules 200 mg daily with food for 2–4 weeks

▷ Miconazole (Daktarin) oral gel (20 mg/mL) q.i.d., swish and swallow

▷ Amphotericin B (Fungizone) oral suspension (100 mg/mL), 1 mL q.i.d. daily, swish and swallow; use between meals

▷ Ketoconazole (Nizoral): 200–400 mg p.o. daily for 14–21 days

▶ Probiotics: *Lactobacillus* and *Bifidobacterium* may be beneficial

How Long to Treat

▶ Usually 7–14 days or continue until 2 days after disappearance of infection

Special Considerations

▶ Miconazole is usually the drug of choice in pregnancy.

▶ Use caution when prescribing oral agents because of possible severe allergic or adverse reactrions (renal failure or hepatoxicity) may occur.

When to Consult, Refer, Hospitalize

▶ Consult with physician or infectious disease specialist for immunocompromised patient, esophageal infection, or failure to resolve as expected.

Follow-Up

Expected Course

▶ Resolves in 1–2 weeks depending on severity and host immune status

Complications

▶ Feeding problems, weight loss

▶ Immunocompromised hosts: complications depend on severity of immunosuppression

Gingivostomatitis

Description

▶ Inflammation of the mucosal lining of the oral cavity that may involve the gingiva, mouth, cheeks, lip, tongue, and floor or roof of mouth that leads to painful sores.

Etiology

▶ Many oral lesions are caused by viruses

▶ Children:

  ▷ Primary herpetic lesions

  ▷ Hand-foot-mouth disease (HFMD)

  ▷ Herpangina

  ▷ Angular stomatitis

  ▷ Aphthous stomatits (peak onset age 10–19 years)

▶ Teenagers and adults:

  ▷ Vincent stomatitis (trench mouth)

  ▷ Behcet disease

  ▷ Nicotinic stomatitis

  ▷ Chronic ulcerative stomatitis

▶ Smoking

▶ Food hypersensitivity (citrus, nuts, coffee, chocolate, potatoes, cheeses, figs, gluten)

▶ Nutritional deficiencies: vitamin B_6, vitamin B_{12}, folic acid, vitamin C, iron deficiencies

▶ Malnutrition

▶ Hormonal, bacterial, traumatic, uremic; ill-fitting dentures; chemotherapy or radiation

▶ Allergic or toxic drug reactions

Incidence and Demographics

See Table 6-10

Risk Factors

▶ Poor oral hygiene or oral trauma

▶ Dietary deficiencies and malnutrition

▶ Chronic systemic disease (celiac disease, Crohn's disease, Behçet syndrome, HIV, reactive arthritis)

▶ Medications (NSAIDs, β-blockers, angiotensin-converting enzyme inhibitors [ACEIs])

▶ Vitamin deficiencies (zinc, iron, B_{12}, folate)

▶ Food and chemical sensitivities

▶ Immune deficiencies

▶ Poor denture fit/quality

▶ Smoking

▶ Cancer therapies

▶ Crowded living conditions, day care

▶ Sunlight exposure

▶ Stress

Prevention and Screening

▶ Avoiding causative factors

▶ Good oral hygiene

▶ Good nutrition

▶ Avoiding/discontinuing smoking

▶ Properly fitting dentures

▶ Avoiding contact with infected individuals

▶ UV protection

▶ Decrease stress

▶ Proper nutrition

▶ Frequent handwashing, avoidance of scratching

Assessment

History and Physical Exam

▶ Patient will complain of burning sensation, intolerance to temperature, and irritating foods. Diagnosis depends on etiology:

▷ Varies from minimal to severe pain

▷ Fever, malaise, headaches

▶ Physical exam should include comprehensive oral examination along with cervical, submandibular, and submental lymph node evaluation. See Table 6–10.

TABLE 6–10.
DIFFERENTIATING CHARACTERISTICS OF COMMON GINGIVOSTOMATITIS

COMMON GINGIVOSTOMATITIS	DESCRIPTION

Herpes simplex ("cold sores")	• Viral: herpes simplex-1 (90%) and HSV-2 (10%)
	• Affects: all ages; acquired in childhood (6 months–5 years of age)
	• Contagious—transmitted through infectious saliva
	• Can occur anytime and are recurrent
	• Lesion location: buccal mucosa, anterior tonsillar pillars, inner lips, tongue, and gingiva; spares posterior pharynx
	• History and Physical Exam:
	  o Poor oral intake, drooling
	  o Fever + irritability precede development of lesions
	  o Swollen, erythematous friable lesions, then vesicles that break down and become gray ulcers that bleed
	  o Tender cervical adenopathy
	  o Associated symptoms (common in primary disease): fever, headache, malaise, abdominal pain, and myalgia

Hand, foot, and mouth disease (HFMD)	• Viral: Coxsackie A16 and Enterovirus A7 are the most common
	• Affects children <5 years of age; more common in infants and toddlers
	• Highly contagious through aerosolized droplets and/or oral secretions through fecal-oral route, or contact with skin lesions
	• Seasonal: spring and summer
	• Lesion location: any area of mucosa including hands and feet; spares posterior pharynx; most common on tongue and buccal mucosa
	• H & P:
	  o Low-grade fever (2–3 days), decreased appetite, malaise, vague abdominal pain, mouth or throat pain, and mild URI, evolving to lesions
	  o Painful oral lesions rupture to form ulcers
	  o Usually not pruritic
	  o Cervical or submandibular adenopathy may be present.
	  o Associated symptoms: cutaneous lesions on palms of hands, soles of feet, and buttocks; may cause CNS symptoms

CONTINUED

COMMON GINGIVOSTOMATITIS	DESCRIPTION
Herpangina	• Viral: Coxsackie Group A 16 most common
	• Affects: all ages; common in children 3–10 years of age
	• Highly contagious through aerosolized droplets and/or oral secretions through fecal-oral route, or contact with skin lesions
	• Seasonal: summer and early fall
	• Lesion location: tonsils and soft palate; spares anterior pharynx
	• H & P:
	o Painful vesicles, fever, sore throat, difficulty swallowing, and dysphagia; gray, pinhead-sized vesicles rupture and form large, fibrin-covered ulcers
	o Associated symptoms: headache, vomiting, and abdominal pain may occur
Aphthous ulcers ("canker sores")	• Etiology unknown; stress, systemic disease, medications, oral trauma, etc.
	• Affects any age; common in ages 10–19 years
	• Not contagious
	• Not seasonal: can occur anytime
	• Lesion location: labial and buccal mucosa, ventral tongue; spares gingiva and hard palate
	• H & P:
	o Burning sensation, hurts to eat and swallow, especially foods and drinks with a high acid content
	o Obtain history of GI symptoms, genital ulcers, HIV risk factors, and joint pain
	o Recurring, 1 or more ulcers covered by a painful oral lesions appear as localized, round-to-oval ulcers with grayish base

Diagnostic Studies

▶ Viral cultures and polymerase chain reaction (PCR) testing can be done but are not usually necessary

▶ Consider:

   ▷ Tzanck test (HSV), does not differentiate HSV1 from HSV2

   ▷ Serologic test for syphilis

   ▷ CBC, cultures to determine secondary infection

   ▷ Ferritin, B_{12}, folate,

   ▷ Erythrocyte sedimentation rate (ESR)

   ▷ KOH

   ▷ Skin biopsy

   ▷ HIV testing

Differential Diagnosis

▶ Etiologies mentioned above

▶ Pharyngitis/tonsillitis

▶ Oral trauma

▶ Syphilis

▶ Squamous cell carcinoma

▶ Stevens-Johnson syndrome

▶ Scarlet fever

▶ Burning mouth syndrome

Management

▶ Treatment depends on causative factors.

Nonpharmacologic Treatment

▶ Palliative and supportive, because many cases are self-limiting

▶ Fluids, popsicles may be beneficial; gargle/swish with mild mouthwash or 1:1 hydrogen peroxide and water; maintain good oral hygiene; stop smoking; refit dentures; avoid specific allergens; replace vitamin deficiencies

▶ Avoid salty, acidic, or sharp foods

Pharmacologic Treatment

▶ Acetaminophen or ibuprofen for analgesia; narcotics may be necessary

▶ "Miracle mouth rinses": swish, gargle, and spit out (viscous lidocaine 2%, Maalox, and diphenhydramine is one formulation used)

▶ 2% viscous lidocaine (Xylocaine); swish and spit for local discomfort (generally not recommended because of risk of swallowing and associated seizures)

▶ Liquid diphenhydramine by mouth or swish and spit, for allergic reactions

▶ Oral anesthetics, but can be harmful and result in self-injury when children chew on anesthetized lips

▶ Antibiotics for gangrenous stomatitis (penicillin and metronidazole IV recommended)

▶ Topical valacyclovir (Valtrex) or penciclovir (Deavir); docosanol (Abreva; sold OTC) is often used in treatment of recurrent oral herpes to decrease the duration of HSV shedding, but has minimal effect on symptoms

  ▷ Consider oral acyclovir: primary herpatic stomatitis in children—5 mg/kg divided 5x/day x 7 days; adults—400 mg t.i.d. x 7–10 days

  ▷ Recurrence: acyclovir 400 mg p.o. t.i.d. x 5 days or 800 mg b.i.d. x 5 days or 800 mg t.i.d. x 2 days or famciclovir (Famvir) 250 mg t.i.d. x 5 days

  ▷ Suppression: use 400 mg b.i.d. daily

▶ Sucralfate (Carafate) suspension 1 tsp; swishing in mouth or placing on ulcers q.i.d. may be helpful

► Possible corticosteroids in severe cases

► Severe cases may require parenteral fluids and antiviral therapy, particularly in children and immunocompromised patients.

How Long to Treat

► Continue symptomatic treatment until resolution; depends on etiology

► Lesions to be followed until resolved; if they fail to resolve, continuously recur, or appear suspicious, biopsy may be needed.

Special Considerations

► Herpetic (primary), hand-foot-mouth disease, herpangina, and traumatic ulcers are common causes in pediatric population

► Ill-fitting dentures, nutritional deficiencies seen in older adult population

► HSV is always present in dormant state and can reactivate.

When to Consult, Refer, Hospitalize

► If dehydration is caused by decreased fluid intake or immunocompromised state, patient may require hospitalization for IV fluids or IV acyclovir therapy.

Follow-Up

► Follow-up visit in 3–7 days if case is severe

► Extensive/primary cases should be rechecked in 1 week

► Monitor for secondary bacterial infections

Expected Course

► Most cases are self-limiting and resolve in 7–14 days.

► Consider long-term suppression therapy (HSV).

Complications

► Usually none

► Recurrent scarifying stomatitis may result in intraoral scarring with restriction of oral mobility.

► Behcet disease may result in vision loss, pneumonia, colitis, vasculitis, or encephalitis.

► Herpetic stomatitis may be complicated by ocular or CNS involvement; herpes pneumonia.

PROBLEMS OF THE NECK

Cervical Adenitis

Description

► Inflammation of one or more cervical lymph nodes; most common cause is infection

► Most common site is submandibular and anterior cervical

► Also called "cervical lymphadenitis"

Etiology

▶ Infection: local (dental caries or periodontal disease, URI, otitis media, pharyngitis, stomatitis) or systemic infection

  ▷ Viral (most common cause in children): Epstein-Barr (EBV), cytomegalovirus (CMV), varicella zoster, HIV, herpes simplex (HSV), adenovirus, rhinovirus, enterovirus,

  ▷ Bacterial: β-hemolytic streptococcal (70%), staphylococci (20%); methicillin-resistant *Staphylococcus aureus* (MRSA) must also be considered

  ▷ Other infections: Cat-scratch disease (*Bartonella henselae*), atypical mycobacteria, toxoplasmosis

▶ Malignant neoplasms (80% of isolated solitary neck masses in adults >S40 years of age)

▶ Manifestation of systemic autoimmune diseases such as lupus, rheumatoid arthritis, and sarcoidosis

▶ Rarely due to trauma

▶ Easily mistaken for goiter or thyroid nodule or parotitis

Incidence and Demographics

▶ More commonly found in children

▶ About 55% of healthy children in all age groups have palpable cervical nodes that are not associated with acute infection or systemic illness

▶ Can occur at any age

Risk Factors

▶ Infection

▶ Systemic disease

▶ Cat scratch

▶ Tobacco and alcohol use (associated with squamous cell carcinoma and 80% of cervical lymphatic tumors)

Prevention and Screening

▶ Avoid use of tobacco and abuse of alcohol.

▶ Maintain general health with strategies such as adequate nutrition, exercise, and rest

▶ Avoid contact with those known to have contagious viral infections.

▶ Good handwashing hygiene

Assessment

History

▶ History of recent or current infection

▶ Duration and mode of onset of node enlargement, any tenderness, warmth, or change in size

▶ Pain with eating suggests parotid gland involvement.

▶ Patient with malignancy—describes lymphadenitis as being present for an undetermined time (gradual enlargement) and becoming larger, nontender, and firm

▶ Fever, sore throat, ear pain, toothache, rash, unexplained weight loss, night sweats, irritability, cough, and wheezing

▶ Exposure to cats (cat-scratch disease)

Physical Exam

▶ A thorough examination of the teeth, gingiva, oropharynx, and ears is required, assessing for indicators of infection.

▶ All lymph nodes should be assessed to differentiate between an isolated and localized adenitis versus the generalized, diffuse lymphadenopathy associated with systemic disease.

▶ Assess whether the node(s) are soft, firm, hard; assess for matting, adherence to skin or to deeper tissues; fluctuant

▶ Physical findings vary depending upon the etiology.

▶ Infection-related lymphadenitis is typically found in the anterior cervical chain and the submandibular nodes. These are soft, tender, and warm, and may reveal erythema of the overlying skin. The size of enlargement is variable (2–6 cm) and is usually bilateral.

▶ Malignancy-related lymphadenitis is often found in the supraclavicular area with a firm texture that is fixed to the skin and underlying tissue. Exam may reveal one or several enlarged nodes along the anterior cervical chain. Lesions may be found in the oral cavity, nose (e.g., unilateral obstruction), or pharynx.

▶ Examination should carefully differentiate among other structures (thyroid, parotid, or salivary glands).

Diagnostic Studies

▶ Suspected infectious lymphadenitis may be diagnosed clinically.

▶ Tests to consider in the workup include:

▷ Rapid group A streptococcal test and culture

▷ CBC with differential

▷ TB skin testing

▷ Rapid mononucleosis test

▷ Serologic testing for EBV, CBV, toxoplasmosis, *Bartonella henslae*, HIV, and fungi

▷ Chest X-ray

▷ Large fluctuant nodes are aspirated for culture and sensitivity if unresponsive to therapy or worsening.

▷ Node biopsy if there is no improvement or malignancy is suspected

▷ CAT scan, ultrasound, or MRI can be done to differentiate among solid, fluctuant, or cystic mass.

▶ Refer to a specialist if the patient is over age 40.

Differential Diagnosis

▶ Malignancy

▶ Localized infection

▶ Lymphatic malformation

▶ Thyroid enlargement

▶ Cat-scratch disease

▶ Parotid or salivary gland inflammation

Management

Nonpharmacologic Treatment

▶ For localized infection, warm compresses for 15 minutes q.i.d.

▶ Good handwashing and washing cat scratches/bites with warm soapy water

Pharmacologic Treatment

▶ OTC analgesics such as NSAIDs or acetaminophen for fever or pain

▶ Most cases of cervical lymphadenopathy or lymphadenitis do not require specific therapy, because they often represent reactive enlargement or viral infection.

▶ Suppurative cases can be treated for suspected bacterial infections and should cover *S. aureus* and *S. pyogenes*. Immunocompromised patients should always be treated with antibiotics.

   ▷ First-line therapy: amoxicillin plus clavulanic acid, 30–40 mg/kg/day divided b.i.d. (500 mg t.i.d for adults) or clindamycin (30–40 mg/kg/day divided t.i.d/q.i.d. for 10 to 14 days

   ▷ Failure to improve in 36 to 48 hours should prompt reassessment of diagnosis and therapy.

   ▷ Second-line therapy: erythromycin 10 mg/kg/dose q.i.d., cephalexin 10–20 mg/kg/dose q.i.d. or (500 mg b.i.d. for adult), dicloxacillin (Dynapen) 25 mg/kg/day

▶ For atypical mycobacteria and atypical tuberculosis:

   ▷ Surgical excision is the treatment of choice for nontuberculous mycobacterial lymphadenitis.

▶ For cat-scratch disease:

   ▷ Usually a self-limiting disorder requiring no specific treatment

   ▷ Controlled studies have not shown antibiotics to affect course, but they can be used.

      ▶ Azithromycin x 5 days

      ▶ Rifampin 5–10 mg/kg/dose q 12–24 hours or

      ▶ TMP-SMX (Bactrim) 5 mg of TMP/kg/dose b.i.d.

      ▶ Ciprofloxacin (Cipro) 500 mg b.i.d. (not recommended for children under 18)

      ▶ Erythromycin, clarithromycin, doxycycline, and gentamicin are other agents used.

How Long to Treat

▶ Antibiotic therapy should be continued for 1–2 weeks.

Special Considerations

▶ Have a high index of suspicion for malignancy in patients who abuse alcohol or tobacco, or who present with weight loss and night sweats.

▶ In patients with risk factors, screen for HIV infection.

When to Consult, Refer, Hospitalize

▶ Follow-up in clinic if symptoms do not resolve 48–72 hours after treatment is initiated.

▶ Refer immediately to an emergency facility if the patient has difficulty swallowing or breathing.

▶ Refer to surgeon or ENT specialist for excision biopsy if malignancy is suspected (nodes that are matted, hard, or painless without source of regional infection).

Follow-Up

Expected Course

▶ Benign lymphadenitis will resolve over time, sometimes within days of treatment, other times over the course of 2–3 weeks with or without treatment; if not resolved after 4 weeks, refer to ENT as biopsy may be indicated.

Complications

▶ Localized infection that spreads hematologically with sepsis

▶ Obstruction of airway from extending edema and inflammation

▶ Malignancy and death

CASE STUDIES

Case 1

A 16-year-old female presents with a "severe cold" x 4–5 days.

> **HPI**: Was previously well. Until last week, she had a cold, which is persisting without much improvement. Patient's mother is very concerned that she needs antibiotics; claims that previous providers had always used them to treat her daughter's head colds. Patient feels feverish, has dry cough, runny nose, mostly clear drainage with some yellow mucus in the mornings, scratchy sore throat, and ears "popping." Tried ibuprofen cold and sinus product with benefit.

> **PMH**: Is in general good health, single, and sexually active with boyfriend x 2 months. Denies food, drug, or environmental allergies, smokes 5 cigarettes per day.

> **Medications**: Oral contraceptive; took amoxicillin 500 mg b.i.d. yesterday—left over from a prescription she was given 2 months ago for "sinusitis."

> 1.   What additional history do you need?
>
> 2.   What are the risk factors for possible diagnoses?

> **Exam**: Temp is 99.0°F, thin-appearing White female, in no acute distress, looks mildly ill. Voice quality "nasal." Posterior oropharynx has mild erythema, no lesions or exudate, tonsils not enlarged, neck supple with no lymphadenopathy, ear canals and TMs clear bilaterally. Nasal turbinates mildly erythematous and edematous, watery discharge. Heart: RRR at 88 BPM, lungs clear.

> 3.   What diagnostic tests would you order?
>
> 4.   What is your differential diagnosis?
>
> 5.   What treatment plan will you carry out?

Case 2

A 22-year-old female college student presents with sore throat and earache.

> **HPI**: Sore throat began 3 days ago, was seen at student health center 2 days ago and treated with penicillin V potassium 250 mg q.i.d. Sore throat worse last night and patient especially complained of severe right ear pain. Notes fever and chills, but did not take temperature; overall, feels very tired and achy. Hurts to swallow, only drinking liquids. Lives in the dormitory. Denies problems with SOB, chest pain, rash, joint pains, nausea, vomiting, or diarrhea.

> **PMH**: Healthy, denies any preexisting medical problems.

> **Medications**: Pen V K, ibuprofen p.r.n. for fever and pain x 3 days, last dose 4 hours ago

Exam: Young Asian female, looks ill. Temp 102.3°F, sinuses nontender, nasal mucosa clear. Ear canals and TMs negative. Throat 4+ erythema on posterior wall, white-yellow purulent exudate on right tonsillar area. Positive trismus, palatal bulge on the right. Neck positive for anterior cervical lymphadenopathy, tender, soft, and mobile. Chest clear. Heart: RRR at 110 BPM.

1. What are the most likely possibilities for a differential diagnosis?
2. What information in the history is the most significant?
3. What physical examination components are especially useful for this presentation?
4. Are the findings from the history and physical adequate to make the diagnosis?
5. What diagnostic studies will rule in or out any of the possibilities?
6. What treatment plan will you carry out?

Case 3

A 6-year-old boy presents with severe right ear pain.

HPI: Child was well until this morning, when he awoke at 6 a.m. crying with right ear pain. Mother noted that he felt very hot, did not take temp. Gave children's acetaminophen and he slept a little. Mother later noted drainage from the ear on his pillow.

PMH: Frequent otitis media as an infant/toddler, which he seemed to "grow out of"; never required long-term antibiotics or ventilation tubes; last otitis media was about 2 years ago.

Exam: Young Black male, looks moderately ill. Temp 101.2°F orally, right ear canal has whitish crust and is moist, no erythema or edema, tragus nontender with manipulation. TM red and bulging, small perforation present. Oropharynx clear, nose clear, neck supple, no lymphadenopathy. Heart: RRR 110, respirations 32, lungs clear.

1. What additional history is important?
2. What is the differential diagnosis?
3. What historical and physical exam features support the differential?
4. What are the risk factors for otitis media?
5. How will you treat this child?

CASE STUDIES DISCUSSION

Case 1

1. What additional history do you need?

    Details on history of frequent head colds (review the symptoms and signs, number of episodes in past few years, how treated, whether the episodes resolved). Any change in environment (dusty or damp, pets)? Has she ever had allergy tests or radiographic sinus imaging or endoscopy? Does she have asthma or allergic symptoms? Any symptoms/signs of systemic disease (diabetes)? Any intranasal (or other) drug use? ETOH? OTC nasal decongestants? Does she use condoms? Assess her STI risk.

2. What are the risk factors for possible diagnoses?

    Cigarettes predispose to allergic rhinitis and sinusitis. Allergic rhinitis predisposes to sinusitis. Oral contraceptives may cause vasomotor rhinitis. Oral sex and new partner may cause gonococcal pharyngitis, risk for HIV, and immunosuppression.

3. What diagnostic tests would you order?

    Probably none at this time unless the history and physical exam suggests HIV risk or other systemic disease (diabetes, anemia)

4. What is your differential diagnosis?

    Infectious rhinitis, probably viral; allergic rhinitis; acute bacterial sinusitis; vasomotor rhinitis

5. What treatment plan will you carry out?

    Patient/family education on various types of rhinitis/sinusitis and what treatment is appropriate in this case versus indiscriminate use of antibiotics; also prevention measures and maintenance care. Suggest saline lavage q.i.d., intranasal corticosteroid spray, nonsedating antihistamine, OTC oral decongestants, infection prevention, and allergy control in her environment.

Case 2

1. What are the most likely possibilities for a differential diagnosis?

    Peritonsillar abscess, streptococcal tonsillitis, infectious mononucleosis, antibiotic noncompliance, acute otitis media, antibiotic-resistant infection

2. What information in the history is the most significant?

    Failure to improve on antibiotics; symptoms worse with ear pain, which may be referred from pharynx

3. What physical examination components are especially useful for this presentation?

    Fever, erythematous posterior pharynx with exudative tonsil, trismus, palatal bulge, tender lymphadenopathy, negative ear findings

4. Are the findings from the history and physical adequate to make the diagnosis, and what diagnostic studies will rule in or out any of the possibilities?

The history and physical are very revealing for peritonsillar abscess; however, CBC with differential, mono screen test, quick streptococcal screen, throat culture, and possibly blood cultures will help define her diagnosis.

5.   What treatment plan will you carry out?

Start parenteral antibiotics (ceftriaxone is a good choice) and consult with ENT specialist for urgent evaluation and possible admission. If urgent referral to ENT is not possible, make arrangements for her to be seen at the nearest emergency department for evaluation and treatment.

Case 3

1.   What additional history is important?

Any recent URI? Cigarette smoke exposure? Is the child in day care? Any siblings? Recent swimming? Has he ever had otitis externa or TM rupture? Has he ever put anything in his ear?

2.   What is the differential diagnosis?

Acute otitis media with perforation, acute otitis externa, foreign body

3.   What historical and physical exam features support the differential?

The external auditory canal is without erythema or edema, no tragal tenderness, so otitis externa is ruled out; the red, bulging TM with a perforation and acute illness supports acute otitis media; the whitish crust in the ear canal is from the perforation of the tympanic membrane with extrusion of exudate.

4.   What are the risk factors for otitis media?

Male, day care, Eustachian tube dysfunction, secondhand cigarette smoke exposure

5.   How will you treat this child?

Amoxicillin 80–90 mg/kg/day in divided doses; or ofloxacin (Floxin) otic 5 gtts b.i.d.; acetaminophen or ibuprofen for pain and fever; follow-up in 2 weeks but instructed to return if not improving in 48–72 hours

REFERENCES

Alliman, K. J., Smiddy W. E., Banta, J., Qureshi, Y. Miller, D. M., & Schiffman, J. C. (2009). Ocular trauma and visual outcome secondary to paintball projectiles. *American Journal of Ophthalmology*, 147(2), 239-242.e1.

American Academy of Pediatrics. (2004). Managing otitis media with effusion. *Pediatrics*, 113(5), 1412–1429.

American Academy of Pediatrics. (2006). *Red book: 2006 Report of the Committee on Infectious Diseases* (26th ed.). Elk Grove Village, IL: Author.

Baskin, D. E., Reddy, A. K., Chu, Y. I., & Coats, D. K. (2008). The timing of antibiotic administration in the management of infant dacryocystitis. *Journal of American Association for Pediatric Ophthalmology and Strabismus, 12*(5), 456–459.

Behrman, R., & Kliegman, R. (2007). *Nelson's textbook of pediatrics* (17th ed.). Philadelphia, PA: W.B. Saunders.

Broaddus, E., Topham, A., & Singh, A. D. (2009). Incidence of retinoblastoma in the USA: 1975–2004. *British Journal of Ophthalmology, 93*(1), 21–23.

Calder, L. A., Balasubramanian, S., & Fergusson, D. (2005). Topical nonsteroidal anti-inflammatory drugs for corneal abrasions: Meta-analysis of randomized trials. *Academic Emergency Medicine, 12*(5), 467–473.

Cronau, H., Kankanala, R. R., & Mauger, T. (2010). Diagnosis and management of red eye in primary care. *American Family Physician, 81*(2), 137–144.

Domino, F. J. (2015). *The 5-minute clinical consult 2015* (23rd ed.). Philadelphia, PA: Lippincott, Williams & Wilkins.

Dykewicz, M. S., & Hamilos, D. L. (2010). Rhinitis and sinusitis. *Journal of Allergy and Clinical Immunology, 125*(2), S103–S115.

Edmunds, M .W., & Mayhew, M. S. (2004). *Pharmacology for the primary care provider* (2nd ed.). St. Louis, MO: Mosby.

Ferri, F. F. (2008). *Ferri's clinical advisor*. St. Louis, MO: Mosby.

Gilbert, D. N., Moellering, R. C., Eliopoulos, G. M., & Sande, M.A. (2008). *The Sanford guide to antimicrobial therapy* (37th ed.). Hyde Park, VT: Antimicrobial Therapy, Inc.

Goroll, A. H., & Mulley, A. G. (2006). *Primary care medicine* (4th ed.). Philadelphia, PA: Lippincott, Williams & Wilkins.

Hay, W. W., Levin, M. J., Deterding, R. R., & Abzug, M. J. (2014). *CURRENT diagnosis & treatment: Pediatrics* (22nd ed.). New York, NY: McGraw-Hill Education.

Henderson, M. C., Tierney Jr., L. M., & Smetana, G.W. (2012). *The patient history: An evidence-based approach to differential diagnosis* (2nd ed.) New York, NY: McGraw-Hill Companies.

Humair, J. P., Revaz, S. A., Bovier, P., & Stalder, H. (2006). Management of acute pharyngitis in adults: Reliability of rapid streptococcal tests and clinical findings. *Archives of Internal Medicine, 166*(6), 640–644.

Kleigman, R. M., Marcdante, K. J., Jensen, H. B., & Behrman, R. E. (2006). *Nelson essentials of pediatrics* (5th ed.). Philadelphia, PA: Saunders.

Lalwani, A. K. (2012). *CURRENT diagnosis & treatment in otolaryngology: Head & neck surgery*, (3rd ed.) New York, NY: McGraw-Hill Companies.

Lieverthal, A. S., Carroll, A. E., Chonmaitree, T., Ganiats, T. G., Hoberman, A., Jackson M. A., Tunkel, D. E. (2013). The diagnosis and management of acute otitis media. *Pediatrics, 131(3),* e964–e999.

McPhee, S. J., Papadakis, M. A., & Tierney, L. M. (2008). *Current medical diagnosis and treatment* (44th ed.). Norwalk, CT: Appleton and Lange.

Pizzo, P. A., & Poplack, D. G. (2011). Retinoblastoma. *Principles and practice of pediatric oncology* (6th ed.). Philadelphia, PA: Lippincott Williams & Wilkins.

Repka, M. X., Chandler, D. L., Beck, R. W., Crouch, E. R. 3rd, Donahue, S., Holmes, J. M. … Wallace, D. K. (2008). Primary treatment of nasolacrimal duct obstruction with probing in children younger than 4 years. *Ophthalmology, 115*(3), 577–584.

Riordan-Eva, P., & Cunningham Jr., E.T. (2011). *Vaughan & Asbury's general ophthalmology* (18th ed.). New York, NY: McGraw-Hill Companies.

Schwartz, M. W. (2008). *The 5-minute pediatric consult.* Philadelphia: Lippincott, Williams & Wilkins.

Stahl, S. M. (2006). *Essential psychopharmacology: The prescriber's guide.* New York: Cambridge University Press.

Taylor, R. (2007). *Manual of family medicine* (2nd ed.). Philadelphia, PA: Lippincott, Williams & Wilkins.

Tham, Y. C., Li, X., Wong, T. Y., Quigley, H. A., Aung, T., & Cheng, C. (2014). Global prevalence of glaucoma and projections of glaucoma burden through 2040: A systemic review and meta-analysis. *Ophthalmology, 121*(11), 2081–2090.

Tierney, L. M., McPhee, S. J., & Papadakis, A. (2008). *Current medical diagnosis and treatment* (44th ed.). Norwalk, CT: Appleton & Lange.

Tintinalli, J. E., Stapczynski, J. S., Ma, O. J., Cline, D. M., Cydulka, R. K., & Meckler, G. D. (2011). *Tintinalli's emergency medicine: A comprehensive study guide* (7th ed.). New York, NY: McGraw-Hill.

Usatine, R.P., Smith, M.A., Chumley, H.S., & Mayeaux Jr., E.J. (2013). *The color atlas of family medicine* (2nd ed.). New York, NY: McGraw-Hill Companies

Walton, W., VonHagen, S., Grigorian, R., & Zarbin, M. (2002). Management of traumatic hyphema. *Survey of Ophthalmology, 47*(4), 297–334.

Williams, C., Northstone, K., Howard, M., Harvey, I., Harrad, R. A., & Sparrow, J. M. (2008). Prevalence and risk factors for common vision problems in children: Data from the ALSPAC study. *British Journal of Ophthalmology, 92*(7), 959–964.

CHAPTER 7

RESPIRATORY DISORDERS
Dawn Bucher, DNP, FNP-BC

GENERAL APPROACH

Note: Some respiratory infections can be found in Chapter 4, "Infectious Diseases."

▶ Through careful history and physical examination, determine the etiology of the problem: infectious (bacterial, viral, or other), allergic, occupational, environmental, or congenital defect.

▶ Most respiratory infections are viral. Treat empirically with antibiotics only if the patient has a secondary bacterial infection, underlying respiratory condition, or prolonged symptoms.

▶ Determine whether symptoms are acute or chronic to guide management.

▶ For dyspnea, determine patient's position at onset of symptoms, relationship to activity, and any factors that improve or exacerbate symptoms.

▶ Assess rate, depth, rhythm, work of breathing, and symmetry of chest movement. Rate is a critical indicator of respiratory status, especially in children (see Table 7–1).

▶ Obtain smoking history and smoking exposure.

▶ Is cough productive or nonproductive? Note color, amount, and consistency of sputum.

▶ Note nature of cough: paroxysmal, continuous, or staccato.

▶ Assess exercise tolerance and activity level.

▶ In infants, assess ability to take bottle or nurse.

▶ Antitussives should not be given in conditions in which retention of respiratory secretions may be harmful.

▶ Encourage patients to stay well-hydrated.

TABLE 7–1.
NORMAL RESPIRATORY RATES (COUNTED FOR 1 MINUTE AT REST)

	PRETERM	BIRTH–1 YEAR	1–3 YEARS	3–6 YEARS	6–12 YEARS	12–18 YEARS	ADULTS	ADULTS >65 YEARS OLD
Normal rate (breaths/ minute)	40–70	30–60	20–30	20–25	18–30	12–18	16–20	12–30

▶ Assess lung status with pulmonary function testing and spirometry (this can usually be obtained beginning at age 5).

▶ Patients with cardiovascular disease, peripheral vascular disease, hyperthyroidism, diabetes mellitus, urinary retention, prostatic hypertrophy, hypertension, and increased intraocular pressure should avoid decongestants.

▶ In pediatric patients, assess appetite; fluid intake (hydration status); change in sleep pattern; activity in home, school, and day care environment; and immunization history.

RED FLAGS

Post-tussive emesis and signs and symptoms of respiratory distress should be quickly evaluated, treated with oxygen and bronchodilators if appropriate, or referred to an emergency department.

▶ *Community-acquired pneumonia*—consider hospitalization in:

▷ Adult patients over age 50 with history of comorbid conditions, altered mental status, leukopenia (less than 4,000), leukocytosis (greater than 30,000), tachycardia, tachypnea, systolic blood pressure less than 90 mm HG, and temperature 35°C (95°F) or lower or 40°C (104°F) or higher

▷ Pediatric patients appearing toxic, who have immunodeficiencies or cardiac or pulmonary disease, or are in respiratory distress or dehydrated

▶ *Hemoptysis*: Older patients, smokers, and those who do not respond to treatment for infection have a high index of suspicion for lung cancer. Obtain chest radiograph and refer for bronchoscopy and further workup.

▶ *Asthma*: Acute exacerbation may present as diminished breath sounds without audible wheezing, but a patient may be in severe respiratory distress. Begin treatment, monitor closely, and be on the alert to transfer to an emergency facility.

ACUTE CONDITIONS

Acute Bronchitis

Description

▶ Self-limited inflammation of the bronchi due to upper airway infection associated with cough lasting more than 5 days with or without mucus production. Causes injury to epithelial surfaces causing increased mucous production and thickening bronchiole wall. Most common cause of antibiotic abuse.

Etiology

▶ Viruses most common (95% of cases): rhinovirus, coronavirus, adenovirus, influenza A and B, parainfluenza virus, respiratory syncytial virus (RSV), coxsackie virus

▶ Bacterial infections: *Bordetella pertussis* (second leading cause); *Haemophilus influenzae* and *Streptococcus pneumoniae* (more common in smokers and patients with COPD); *Chlamydia pneumoniae*, *Mycobacterium tuberculosis*, and *Moraxella catarrhalis* are other causes

▶ Possible fungal infections

▶ Chemical irritants

Incidence and Demographics

▶ Affects all ages: Severity and frequency increases with cigarette smoking and preexisting pulmonary disease.

Risk Factors

▶ Infants

▶ Older adults

▶ Air pollutants/environmental changes

▶ Smoking/secondhand-smoke

▶ Chronic bronchopulmonary diseases/chronic sinusitis/bronchopulmonary allergy

▶ Tracheostomy

▶ Immunosuppression: immunoglobulin deficiency, HIV infection, alcoholism

▶ GERD

▶ Environmental changes; hypertrophied tonsils and adenoids in children

Prevention and Screening

▶ Avoid smoking and secondhand smoke.

▶ Control underlying risk factors (asthma, sinusitis, GERD).

▶ Avoid exposure, especially in day care.

▶ Get pneumovax and influenza immunizations.

Assessment

History

▶ Persistent cough lasting more than 5 days (typically 1 to 3 weeks) with purulent-appearing sputum production

▶ Mild dyspnea, bronchospasm, wheeze, fever, and fatigue may be present; smoking status of patient or household members; infectious illness of household members; past medical history of respiratory diseases

▶ Acute bronchitis due to pertussis causes a paroxysmal "whooping" cough.

Physical Exam

▶ Afebrile or low-grade temperature less than 101°F (38°C)

▶ Tachypnea

▶ Pharynx injected

▶ Respiratory wheezes or rhonchi; rales should not be present

▶ No physical findings of lower airway congestion or consolidation. In children, upper airway congestion may be heard in the lungs; to differentiate, listen to breathing, then compare to auscultation sounds.

Diagnostic Studies

▶ Diagnosis generally based on clinical presentation

▶ Chest X-ray to exclude pneumonia for patients with severe respiratory symptoms and temperature over 38°C (100.4°F), pulse over 100/min, respiratory rate over 24, and abnormal lung exam

▶ CBC and sputum culture: not generally performed unless uncertain of diagnosis

▶ Influenza titers during seasonal peaks

▶ Nasopharyngeal culture and PCR if necessary to exclude pertussis

▶ PPD if at risk for tuberculosis

▶ Pulmonary function tests (PFT) if asthma or obstructive disease suspected (seldom needed during acute phases)

▶ Pulse oximetry if available

▶ Arterial blood gases: hypoxemia (rarely)

Differential Diagnosis

▶ Pneumonia

▶ Asthma

▶ Upper respiratory infection/sinusitis/PND

▶ Influenza

▶ Aspiration

▶ Retained foreign body

▶ Inhalation injury

▶ Allergies

▶ Cystic fibrosis

▶ Tuberculosis

▶ Chronic bronchitis

▶ Respiratory tract anomalies

▶ Gastroesophageal reflux

▶ Congestive heart failure

▶ Bronchogenic tumors

Management

Nonpharmacologic Treatment

▶ Rest, adequate hydration, steam inhalations, vaporizers, smoking cessation or avoid smoke, treat associated illnesses

Pharmacologic Treatment

▶ Antibiotic treatment not generally recommended unless treatable pathogen has been indentified or significant comorbidities present; most cases are viral.

▷ Amoxicillin 500 mg every 8 hours or trimethoprim-sulfamethoxazole DS (Bactrim DS) every 12 hours for routine infection

▷ Clarithomycin (Biaxin) 500 mg every 12 hours or azithromycin (Zithromax) Z-pack for penicillin allergy or *Mycoplasma* infection

▷ Doxycycline 100 mg/day x 10 day if *Moraxella*, *Chlamydia*, or *Mycoplasma* suspected; do not use during pregnancy or in children

▷ Quinolone for more serious infections or other antibiotic failure, or in older adults or patients with multiple comorbidities; do not use during pregnancy or in children

▷ Macrolide for pertussis

▷ For children with cystic fibrosis and comorbidity of chronic lung disease and persistent cough (longer than 10 days), consider antibiotic therapy.

▶ Consider antivirals if influenza suspected: amantadine (Symmetrel), rimantadine (Flumadine), oseltamivir (Tamiflu), or zanamivir (Relenza); start within 24 to 48 hours of symptom onset for demonstrable clinical benefit.

▶ Avoid antihistamines; they dry out secretions.

▶ Decongestants if accompanied by sinus condition

▶ Antipyretic analgesics: aspirin (avoid in children), acetaminophen, ibuprofen

▶ Cough suppressants for troublesome cough (not with COPD); guaifenesin with codeine or dextromethorphan

▶ Mucolytic agents not recommended

▶ Inhaled beta-agonist (albuterol) or in combination with steroids for cough with bronchospasm

▶ Consider steroids for bronchospasm

▶ Cough and cold preparations should not be used in children under age 6.

How Long to Treat

▶ If uncomplicated, generally self-limiting, recovery 7 to 14 days

▶ Cough may linger for several weeks.

▶ In children, if recurrent, need to consider other diagnoses (asthma)

Special Considerations

▶ Geriatrics: Monitor closely for complications such as pneumonia.

▶ Other: Symptoms and duration may be worse in smokers.

▶ Adults with pertussis may transmit it to unimmunized children.

When to Consult, Refer, Hospitalize

▶ Outpatient treatment unless an older adult or complicated by severe underlying disease

▶ Refer if hypoxia, severe bronchospasm present, or exacerbation of underlying disease

▶ Refer to pulmonologist or asthma specialist for further evaluation if no improvement in 4 to 6 weeks or if more severe symptoms.

Follow-Up

▶ If no improvement or symptoms worsen after 72 hours

Expected Course

▶ Generally symptoms resolve in 7 to 14 days, but cough may persist for 3 to 4 weeks.

Complications

▶ Secondary bacterial infection, pneumonia, bronchiectasis, hemoptysis, acute respiratory failure, chronic cough

Bronchiolitis

Description

▶ Acute inflammation and obstruction of small airways and reactive airways, generally affecting infants and young children

▶ Leading cause of illness and hospitalization in infants and children

Etiology

▶ 70% to 85% caused by respiratory syncytial virus (RSV), followed by rhinovirus

▶ Other causes: parainfluenza virus, adenovirus, influenza virus, *Mycoplasma pneumonia*, and *Chlamydiaphila pneumonia*

Incidence and Demographics

▶ 21% in North America

▶ 18.8% of all pediatric hospitalizations in children under 2 years of age

▶ Predominant age: newborn–2 years (peak age less than 6 months)

▶ Predominant sex: male more than female

▶ Seasonal occurrence, more common winter, early spring,and often occurs in epidemics

Risk Factors

▶ Prematurity (gestational age less than 37 weeks)

▶ Age less than 12 weeks

▶ Smoking exposure

▶ Low birth weight

- ▶ Immunodeficiency
- ▶ Formula feeding (not breastfed)
- ▶ Contact with infected person (primary mode of transmission)
- ▶ Children in day care environment
- ▶ Heart-lung transplant patient (immune compromise)
- ▶ History of bronchopulmonary dysplasia, congenital heart disease, neurologic disease
- ▶ Adults: exposure to toxic fumes, connective tissue disease (respiratory epithelial damage)

Prevention and Screening

- ▶ Handwashing
- ▶ Contact isolation of infected babies
- ▶ Contact with infants to a minimum for people with colds
- ▶ Palivizumab (Synagis) administered monthly (October through May), 15 mg/kg IM in high-risk patients
  - ▷ 32 to 35 week gestation and younger than 3 months old at start of RSV season with at least one risk factor: either attending day care or with a sibling younger than 5 years old at home
  - ▷ 28 to 32 weeks gestation and younger than 6 months old
  - ▷ Less than 28 weeks gestation and younger than 12 months old
  - ▷ Moderately severe bronchopulmonary dysplasia and up to 2 years of age
  - ▷ Hemodynamically significant congenital heart disease (until age 6 months)
  - ▷ Once begun, continue through end of season, regardless of age attained
- ▶ RSV immunoglobulin can also be used in at-risk patients; monthly infusions of 750 mg/kg, October through May
  - ▷ Influenza vaccine for children 6 to 59 months of age and their household contacts

Assessment

History

- ▶ Exposure to upper respiratory infection
- ▶ 1 to 3 days history of upper respiratory symptoms (nasal discharge, congestion, and mild cough)
- ▶ Diminished appetite, irritability, noisy breathing, cough, grunting, vomiting
- ▶ Afebrile or low-grade temperature present
- ▶ Apnea or cyanosis (apnea maybe only symptom in very young infants), respiratory distress

Physical Exam

- ▶ Afebrile or low-grade fever
- ▶ Nasal congestion with thick, purulent secretions; nasal flaring; rhinorrhea; pharyngitis; conjunctivitis; otitis may be present

▶ Cough; tachypnea; retractions

▶ Hyperresonance

▶ Wheezing; prolonged expiratory phase; fine crackles (wheezing may not be audible if airways profoundly narrowed)

▶ Tachycardia and/or mild hypoxemia

▶ Signs of dehydration: depressed fontanels, tacky mucous membranes, crying without tears

▶ Cyanosis of oral mucosa and nail beds

▶ Hepatosplenomegaly (due to hyperinflated lungs)

Diagnostic Studies

▶ Usually diagnosed by clinical presentation

▶ Pulse oximetry to monitor respiratory status (less than 94% significant)

▶ Laboratory studies and radiographics usually are not necessary for diagnosis; however, they may be useful to evaluate complications and other comorbid infections.

▶ Chest radiography: increased AP diameter, flattened diaphragm, air trapping, patchy infiltrates, focal atelectasis (right upper lobe common), peribronchial cuffing

▶ CBC with differential

▶ Urine specific gravity to monitor hydration

▶ Nasopharyngeal washings for RSV enzyme immunoassay (rapid results) and culture (usually not necessary during RSV season, but may be useful)

▶ Consider sweat test for chronic reoccurrence to exclude cystic fibrosis.

Differential Diagnosis

▶ Pneumonia

▶ Aspiration

▶ Foreign body

▶ Vascular rings asthma

▶ Croup

▶ Gastroesophageal reflux (GERD)

▶ Cystic fibrosis

▶ Pertussis

▶ Heart failure

Management

Goal: supportive to prevent hypoxia and dehydration

Nonpharmacologic Treatment

▶ In uncomplicated cases, frequent offerings of clear fluids or diluted milk; frequent suctioning of secretions, with saline and a bulb syringe

▶ Cool, humidified oxygen if hypoxemic

Pharmacologic Treatment

▶ Humidified oxygen if needed for pulse oximetry less than 94% on room air

▶ Nebulized albuterol (0.15 mg/kg) in 2 cc of saline every 20 minutes for 1 hour with continual reevaluation; refer if no response or respiratory distress apparent after treatments

▶ Racemic epinephrine may reduce wheezing, reduce tachypnea.

▶ Oral dexamethasone (1 mg/kg loading dose, then 0.6 mg/kg b.i.d. x 5 days)

▶ Nebulized dexamethasone (2–4 mg in 3 ml NS) may be beneficial

▶ Antibiotics only if secondary bacterial infection present

How Long to Treat

▶ Depends on age, severity of illness, associated high-risk conditions, and causative agent

▶ Inhaled bronchodilators should be continued only if there is a documented clinical response and then given every 4 to 6 hours; discontinue once signs and symptoms of respiratory distress improve.

▶ Most infants show marked improvement in 3 to 5 days in respiratory status; however, wheezing may persist for weeks.

▶ If patient is receiving home care, follow daily by telephone for 2 to 4 days; patient may need frequent office visits.

Special Considerations

▶ Glucocorticoids are not routinely recommended in the treatment of previously healthy infants hospitalized with the first episode of bronchiolitis but may be beneficial to those with chronic lung diseases and those with recurrent episodes of wheezing suggestive of asthma.

▶ Bronchiolitis can be associated with apnea in children younger than 6 weeks of age.

When to Consult, Refer, Hospitalize

▶ Respiratory rate over 45/min with repiratory distress or apnea

▶ Hypoxia (pulse oximetry less than 94%)

▶ Ill or toxic appearance, dehydration

▶ Underlying heart, respiratory condition, or immune suppression

Follow-Up

Expected Course

▶ Most children who do not require hospitalization recover by 28 days.

Complications

▶ Bacterial superinfection

▶ Bronchiolitis obliterans

▶ Apnea

▶ Respiratory failure

▶ Death

▶ Increased incidence of development of reactive airway disease (asthma)

Croup (Laryngotracheobronchitis)

Description

▶ Acute inflammatory disease of larynx and subglottic airway, with characteristic "barking" cough, inspiratory stridor, and hoarseness. Is the most common cause of upper-airway obstruction or stridor in children.

Etiology

▶ Parainfluenza the most common organism in all age groups (75% of cases)

▶ Respiratory syncytial virus (infants)

▶ *M. pneumoniae* and influenza virus (children over 5 years)

▶ Paramyxovirus, adenovirus, rhinovirus, enteroviruses, reovirus, measles virus (were vaccination not common)

▶ Viral infection causes inflammation, edema of subglottic space

Incidence and Demographics

▶ Most prevalent in late fall and winter, but can occur any time of the year

▶ Most common in children 7 months to 3 years of age, with peak at 2 years; rare among those older than 6 years

▶ Male-to-female ratio is 1.5:1.

Risk Factors

▶ History of croup

▶ Recurrent upper respiratory infections

Prevention and Screening

▶ No specific prevention measures except proper handwashing and other measures aimed at decreasing transmission of respiratory viruses

Assessment

History

▶ Acute onset of "seal-like" barky cough, inspiratory stridor, and chest-wall indrawing

▶ History of 2 to 3 days of nonspecific prodromal syndrome (low-grade fever, coryza, and rhinorrhea)

▶ Cough is worse at night; symptoms often resolve en route to the hospital as the child is exposed to cool night air.

▶ Symptoms progress rapidly (upper airway obstruction after fewer than 12 hours of onset)

▶ Changes in activity level, alertness, fluid intake, or voiding patterns

▶ Underlying abnormalities of the upper airway

▶ History of neuromuscular disorders

▶ Inquire about *H. influenzae* immunization status.

Physical Exam

See Table 7–2

▶ Signs and symptoms are variable, depending upon age, degree of airway obstruction, hydration status, and level of fatigue.

▶ Level of consciousness, irritability, lethargy, stuggling

▶ Work of breathing: labored, tachypnea, nasal flaring, retractions, prolonged expiratory phase

▶ Inspiratory stridor or stridor at rest; wheezing; short sentences; hoarseness

▶ Breath sounds may be diminished from airway narrowing, crackles, or rhonchi.

▶ "Barking" cough is characteristic.

▶ Tympanic membranes, throat, and sinus may be involved.

▶ Low-grade or moderate fever

▶ Tachycardia caused by fever, respiratory distress, hypovolemia

Diagnostic Studies

▶ Diagnosis usually made on clinical presentation without testing.

▶ Minimize laboratory testing, imaging, procedures as it may agitate child and worsen tachypnea.

▶ Pulse oximetry (often normal)

▶ WBCs may be low, normal, or elevated.

▶ Anteroposterior and lateral X-ray of neck shows funnel-shaped subglottic region with normal epiglottis: "steeple," "hour glass," or "pencil point" sign (present in 40% to 60% of children).

▶ CT scan may be more sensitive for defining cause for obstruction in difficult cases.

Differential Diagnosis

▶ Epiglottitis

▶ Foreign body aspiration

▶ Subglottic stenosis

▶ Bacterial tracheitis

▶ Trauma

▶ Simple URI

▶ Asthma

▶ Airway anomalies

▶ Anaphylaxis

TABLE 7-2.
DIFFERENTIATING CROUP FROM OTHER ILLNESSES

	LARYNGO-TRACHEITIS	SPASMODIC CROUP	EPIGLOTTITIS	FOREIGN BODY	BACTERIAL TRACHEITIS
Age	6 mo–3 yr	3 mo–3 yr	2–6 yr	6 mo–2 or 3 yr	6 mo – 8 yr
Etiology	Parainfluenza, RSV, mycoplasma, adenovirus	Noninfectious form with sudden resolution. May be postviral, allergic, GERD, or psychogenic.	H. influenzae type B, other bacteria or viruses	Small objects, food, toys	S. aureus, M. catarrhalis, H. influenzae; often polymicrobial
Onset	Gradual progressing over 12 to 48 hrs	Sudden, at night; short duration, sudden cessation, recurrent	Rapid	Sudden with choking	Slow onset, rapid deterioration
Retractions	Yes, with severe obstruction	Uncommon	Yes	Variable	Yes
Voice	Normal	Hoarse	Muffled, drooling	Variable	Usually normal
Position	Normal	Normal	Tripod-sitting, leaning forward, anxious	Variable	Variable, usually normal
Barking Cough	Yes: "seal-like"	Yes: "seal-like"	No	Possible if object lodged in esophagus	Yes: "brassy"
Fever	Yes	No	Yes	No	Yes

▶ Peritonsillar abscess

▶ Spasmodic croup

Management

Nonpharmacologic Treatment

▶ Mild cases can be managed at home.

▶ Deliver humidified air by cool mist vaporizer or steam-filled bathroom.

▶ Take outside into cool night air.

▶ Keep patient quiet; crying may exacerbate symptoms.

Pharmacologic Treatment

▶ Cornerstone: immediate nebulized epinephrine and dexamethasone

▶ Racemic epinephrine: 0.05 mL/kg/dose (max 0.5 mL) of 2.25% solution nebulized in normal saline total volume 3mL

▶ L-epinephrine: 0.5 mL/kg/dose (max 5 mL) of a 1:1,000 dilution; onset in 1 to 5 minutes, duration 2 hours; repeat as necessary if side effects tolerated; observe child for 3 to 4 hours

▶ Corticosteroids:

▷ Dexamethasone (Decadron) 0.15–0.6 mg/kg; single dose IM/IV/PO have equal efficacy

▷ Other steroids: betamethasone and prednisolone can be used, but not as good as dexamethasone

▷ Nebulized bedesonide can also be effective.

▶ Antibiotics not indicated; subsequent bacterial infection possible, but uncommon.

▶ Oxygen as needed

▶ Amantadine for influenza A: 100 mg p.o. b.i.d. for 3 to 5 days

▶ Probiotics may decrease incidence of upper respiratory tract infections.

How Long to Treat

▶ Length of treatment is based on clinical response.

▶ Concern about a rebound phenomenon from racemic epinephrine exists; patients who are clinically stable can safely be discharged if 4 hours have elapsed since the last dose of racemic epinephrine and systemic corticosteroids have been given as long as patient has reliable caretakers and good access to medical services.

Special Considerations

▶ Close monitoring of disease progression, stridor, respiratory rate, pulse oximetry, hydration status, and mental status are critical.

▶ Must exclude epiglottitis; watch for preferred sitting position (tripod position with hands extended), drooling, and muffled voice.

▶ When examining, do not place supine or use tongue blade to examine throat until epiglottis excluded.

When to Consult, Refer, Hospitalize

▶ Admit patients who do not respond to therapy or have recurrent stridor at rest after epinephrine wears off.

▶ Admission also indicated for those with hypoxia, pneumonia, congestive heart disease.

Follow-Up

Expected Course

▶ Symptoms may worsen over the first 3 days, so parents/guardian should be advised to return to clinic for increasing stridor or respiratory distress.

▶ For children with moderately severe croup who are discharged, phone contact or clinic follow-up is warranted in 8 to 24 hours.

▶ Up to one-third of patients will have a recurrence.

▶ Usually full recovery without lasting effects

Complications

▶ Rare

▶ Subglottic stenosis in intubated patients

▶ Bacterial tracheitis

▶ Cardiopulmonary arrest

▶ Pneumonia

Persistent Cough

Description

▶ Productive or nonproductive cough—subacute cough lasting 3 to 8 weeks; chronic cough persists longer than 8 weeks; in children, chronic cough is defined as cough longer than 4 weeks duration

▶ Chronic cough affects respiration, sleep, and social function.

Etiology

▶ Multiple etiologies; most related to bronchial irritation

▶ Coughing helps defend against pathogens and clear the tracheobronchial tree of foreign particles, noxious aerosols, and mucous.

▶ Etiology of persistent cough may not be readily apparent, due to the wide variety of infectious, mechanical, and physiologic causes (see Table 7–3).

Incidence and Demographics

▶ Common and frequent presenting complaint in all age groups

▶ Occurs in males and females equally

Risk Factors

▶ Cigarette smoking or exposure

TABLE 7–3.
MOST COMMON ETIOLOGY OF CHRONIC COUGH BY AGE

INFANTS	TODDLER/ PRESCHOOL	SCHOOL-AGE/ ADOLESCENT	ADULTS
Infection	*Infection*	*Infections*	Smoking, passive smoke
Viral (RSV, adenovirus, influenza, parainfluenza)	Viral (RSV, adenovirus, influenza, parainfluenza)	Viral	Postnasal drip from sinusitis, allergic rhinitis
Bordetella pertussis	*B. pertussis*	M. pneumoniae	GERD
Chlamydia trachomatis	*M. pneumoniae*	M. tuberculosis	Asthma
M. tuberculosis	*M. tuberculosis*		R\
		Other	Chronic bronchitis
Congenital Anomalies	*Other*	Asthma	Bronchiectasis
Cleft palate	Foreign body	Sinusitis, postnasal drip	Pneumonia
Tracheo-esophageal fistula	Asthma	Irritants, smoking	Drug-induced (ACE inhibitors)
Tracheobronchomalacia	Cystic fibrosis	Allergic rhinitis	Irritants
Vascular ring	Irritants, passive smoke	Cystic fibrosis	Foreign body
	Immunodeficiency	Ciliary dyskinesia	Tuberculosis
Other	Ciliary dyskinesia	Psychogenic (habit)	Lung malignancy
Cystic fibrosis	GERD		Psychogenic factors
Irritants, passive smoke	Sinusitis, postnasal drip		Congestive heart failure (CHF)
Asthma	Immunodeficiency		Sleep apnea
Foreign body			Interstitial lung disease
Neurologic impairment			*B. pertussis*
GERD			Nonasthmatic eosinophilic bronchitis
Immunodeficiency			

- ▶ Occupational exposure
- ▶ Allergens
- ▶ Pulmonary diseases

Prevention and Screening

- ▶ Smoking cessation
- ▶ Removing respiratory irritants
- ▶ Therapeutic lifestyle changes

Assessment

History

- ▶ Characteristics and timing of cough: onset and duration
    - ▷ Cough at night suggests sinusitis with postnasal drainage, asthma, CHF
    - ▷ Paroxysmal coughing longer than 14 days: pertussis, cystic fibrosis
    - ▷ Cough at school, not at home/on weekend: psychogenic, consider allergy (e.g., mold in building)

▶ Productive or nonproductive cough (presence or absence of sputum production not used as sole basis for treatment)

▶ Productive: bronchitis, cystic fibrosis, tuberculosis, infection (mucopurulent), pneumococcal pneumonia (rust-colored), asthma (thick, tenacious, clear)

▶ Frequent respiratory infections: cystic fibrosis

▶ In children, poor weight gain, delayed milestones: cystic fibrosis, immunodeficiency

▶ Foul-smelling, steatorrheic bowel movements: cystic fibrosis

▶ Family history of cystic fibrosis (genetic disorder, primarily in White children)

▶ Exercise-induced cough associated with asthma, bronchiectasis, or cardiac disease

▶ Associated symptoms: fatigue, weight loss, night sweats, fever, indigestion, rhinitis, epistaxis, hemoptysis (consider cancer, tuberculosis, foreign body obstruction, cystic fibrosis, HIV, sinusitis, or GERD)

▶ Precipitating factors: exercise, cold temperatures, laughing; seasonal irritants may indicate asthma

▶ Past medical history may be significant for bronchitis, pneumonia, asthma, allergy; choking episodes or heartburn: gastroesophageal reflux

▶ Family members ill: infection; family history of atopy/asthma

▶ Smokers: lung tumor, emphysema, chronic bronchitis

▶ Medication history: ACE inhibitors or beta blockers

Physical Exam

▶ Appearance/nutritional status

▶ Nasal discharge, throat clearing, and mucous or mucopurulent drainage in posterior pharynx: postnasal drip rhinitis, sinusitis

▶ Respiratory rate, evidence of distress, wheezing, adventitious sounds: asthma, cystic fibrosis, foreign body, bronchitis, pneumonia, tuberculosis

▶ Tracheal shift suggests mediastinal mass or foreign body

▶ Observe for clubbing: lung malignancy, cardiac source, COPD

▶ In children, evaluate height and weight, and plot on growth curve.

Diagnostic Studies

▶ Tuberculosis skin testing: PPD

▶ Chest X-ray for cough in smokers, cough longer than 8 weeks in nonsmokers, patients with hemoptysis, and in children and those over 40 years of age

▶ Sinus imaging for suspected acute or chronic sinusitis (paranasal sinuses only in children 18 months to 6 years) not necessary.

▶ Pulmonary function testing for asthma

▶ Methacholine bronchoprovocation testing may be positive in absence of clinical findings of asthma.

▶ Barium swallow/esophageal pH monitoring for suspected GERD

▶ CBC with differential; if infection is suspected

► Wright and gram stains, culture of sputum for productive cough

► Bronchoscopy/endoscopy (particularly useful in children from birth to 18 months)

► Sweat test for suspected cystic fibrosis

► Allergen testing if needed

► Echocardiogram for suspected cardiac etiology

► Sleep study for suspected sleep apnea

Differential Diagnosis

See Table 7–3 above.

Management

It is important to determine the underlying disorder causing the cough and treat accordingly. While determining cause, consider the following to manage.

Nonpharmacologic Treatment

► Eliminate irritant exposure (smoke, occupational agents); discontinue ACE inhibitors or beta blockers; increase humidification.

► Therapeutic lifestyle changes for GERD (e.g., stop smoking, avoid reflux-inducing foods, small frequent meals, avoid eating 2 to 3 hours before lying down, elevate head of bed)

► Warm fluids, hard candy (for adults), or nasal drops; bulb syringe suction in infants and children

Pharmacologic Treatment

► Nasal steroids, antihistamines, antacids, bronchiodilators, inhaled corticosteroids, PPIs, antibiotics are some treatments used for cause of specific cough.

► Initial empiric treatment: oral antihistamine/decongestant therapy with first-generation antihistamine or nasal steroid spray

► Ipratropium bromide therapy for chronic bronchitis

► Central-acting antitussive drugs (dextromethorphan or narcotics) are recommended for short-term symptomatic relief of nonproductive cough. Use with caution; these should not be given in conditions in which retention of respiratory secretions may be harmful; may reserve for nighttime use only. American Academy of Pediatrics (AAP) does not recommend for pediatric use.

　▷ Dextromethorphan: patients older than 12 years: 10–20 mg p.o. q. 4 hrs; patients 6 to 12 years: 5–10 mg p.o. q. 4 hrs (use with caution as pediatric recommendations are not available)

　▷ Narcotics: codeine 15–30 mg p.o. q. 6 hrs; hydrocodone (Vicodin) 5 mg p.o. q. 6 hrs; hydrocodone (Tussionex Pennkinetic) 10 mg (5ml) p.o. q. 12 hrs in patients older than 12 years

► Narcotic cough suppressants recommended for cough associated with lung cancer.

► Peripherally acting antitussive: benzonatate (Tessalon Perles) 100–200 mg p.o. t.i.d. for patients older than 10 years

▶ Amiloride 0.625 mg/kg/day may improve cough clearance of sputum in patients with cystic fibrosis.

How Long to Treat

▶ May take weeks to months for cough to resolve; resolution depends on treatment of underlying cause of cough

Special Considerations

▶ Geriatrics: Use decreased dose of antihistamines in allergy; observe and use caution with first-generation antihistamine because of increased sedation.

▶ Pediatrics: Avoid OTC cough and cold medicines (antitussives, expectorants, nasal decongestants, antihistamines, or combinations) in children younger than 2 years of age.

When to Consult, Refer, Hospitalize

▶ Refer undiagnosed patients with risk factors to specialist.

▶ Consult with pulmonologist for signs of respiratory distress or unresponsive to treatment.

Follow-Up

Expected Course

▶ Depends on patient status; patients with negative workup; follow every 1 to 3 months if cough continues

Complications

▶ Cardiovascular: arrhythmias, syncope

▶ Stress urinary incontinence

▶ Abdominal and intercostals muscle strain

▶ GI: emesis, hemorrhage, herniation

▶ Neurologic: dizziness, headache, seizures

▶ Respiratory: pneumothorax, laryngeal or tracheobronchial trauma

▶ Skin: petechiae, purpura, disruption of surgical wounds

▶ Medication side effects

▶ Other: negative impact on quality of life

Hemoptysis

Description

▶ Expectoration of gross blood or blood-stained sputum originating from lungs or bronchial tubes is a symptom of underlying disease or pulmonary injury.

▶ Classifications: nonmassive (blood loss less than 200 mL/day) or massive (more than 200 mL/day)

▶ Pseudohemoptysis: blood expectorated from the upper respiratory tract or upper gastrointestinal tract

Etiology

▶ Most common cause: acute and chronic bronchitis, pneumonia, tuberculosis (TB), and lung cancer

▶ Inflammation of tracheobronchial mucosa due to minor erosion from bronchiectasis, sarcoidosis, Wegner's granulomatosis, lupus pneumonitis

▶ Bronchovascular fistula

▶ Injury to pulmonary vasculature due to lung abscess, aspergillomas, or pulmonary emboli causing pulmonary infarction; trauma; foreign body

▶ Increase pulmonary capillary pressure due to pulmonary edema, mitral stenosis, AV malformations, or granuloma formation

▶ Bleeding disorders or anticoagulant therapy

▶ Nonpulmonary sources: nose or gastrointestinal tract

▶ Cryptogenic hemoptysis: negative workup; etiology unknown in 30% to 40% of patients, 90% resolve in 6 months

▶ Major cause in children: lower respiratory tract infection followed by foreign body aspiration (younger than 4 years of age), bronchiectasis (secondary to cystic fibrosis). Primary pulmonary tuberculosis or blunt-force trauma, although rare, should also be considered.

Risk Factors

▶ Crack cocaine inhalation, tobacco use

Prevention and Screening

▶ Avoid smoking tobacco and crack cocaine use.

Assessment

History

▶ Identify patients at risk for conditions noted above.

▶ Smoking and travel history

▶ Onset and duration of symptoms; amount, frequency, and characteristics of sputum; is there white or purulent phlegm mixed with blood?

▶ Determine if nonpulmonary source of bleeding: vomiting, expectoration from nasopharynx, anticoagulant drug use, substance use, chest trauma

▶ Associated symptoms: weight loss, night sweats, dyspnea, fever, fatigue, bruising, hematuria, rash, joint pain or swelling

▶ TB exposure, dates of last TB test and chest X-ray

▶ Past cardiac, pulmonary, hematological, or immunological history

▶ Environmental exposure, asbestos

▶ Family history of respiratory, cardiac, or hematologic disease

Physical Exam

▶ Fever and tachypnea, tachycardia, cyanosis, fatigue, diaphoresis

▶ Nail clubbing: indicates severe disorder such as lung abscess, tumor, bronchiectasis

▶ Skin: bruising, rash, palpable purpura

▶ Ears, nasal, pharyngeal exam to determine bleeding source

▶ Jugular venous distention and ankle edema: heart failure

▶ Chest exam for pulmonary and cardiac findings: wheezing, diffuse crackles, use of accessory muscles, heart murmur

▶ Lymphadenopathy: TB, carcinoma, sarcoidosis

▶ Extremities: peripheral edema, joint effusions or periarticular warmth

Diagnostic Studies

▶ Directed by history and physical findings

▶ Tuberculin skin test (PPD), unless positive in the past

▶ Chest X-ray

▶ CBC with differential and platelets

▶ Gram stain of sputum: infection; acid-fast stain: TB

▶ Sputum cytologic exam: malignancy

▶ Renal function, urinalysis, liver function tests, brain natriuretic peptide (BNP)

▶ Serologic testing: antinuclear antibodies, antineutrophil cytoplasmic antibodies, anti-glomerular basement membrane antibodies, anticardiolipin antibodies

▶ Coagulation studies: PT, PTT, bleeding time if bleeding present in more than one site

▶ Bronchoscopy for patients at risk of cancer, TB

▶ High-resolution chest CT: complementary to bronchoscopy (test of choice for suspected small peripheral malignancies)

▶ Ventilation-perfusion scan/angiography: pulmonary embolism

Differential Diagnosis

▶ See Etiology.

▶ Must differentiate from epistaxis, hematemesis, and bleeding from nasopharyngeal sources

Management

Goal: bleeding cessation, aspiration, prevention, and treat underlying cause; initial step is to manage ABCs (airway, breathing, circulation)

Nonpharmacologic Treatment

▶ Surgical interventions: flexible bronchoscopy; angiography for embolization if indicated

Pharmacologic Treatment

▶ Treat underlying illness or infection; refer to specific conditions in text.

Special Considerations

▶ In older adult smoker, think lung cancer until proven otherwise.

When to Consult, Refer, Hospitalize

▶ Refer patients at high risk for malignancy to pulmonologist or if bronchoscopy is indicated.

▶ Refer if blood persists more than 2 to 3 days after treatment initiated for respiratory infection.

▶ Hospitalization for patient with massive hemoptysis or unstable condition

Follow-Up

Expected Course

▶ Mild streaking due to infection should resolve in 2 to 3 days; with true hemoptysis, patient should follow-up in 12 to 48 hours.

Complications

▶ Massive hemoptysis is life-threatening.

Pneumonia

Description

▶ An acute inflammation of the lungs caused by infection

▶ Etiology, presentation, risk factors, management, and prognosis differ depending on if the infection is acquired in the community, hospital, or other healthcare facility.

▶ Community-acquired pneumonia (CAP): Lower-respiratory tract infection not acquired in a hospital, long-term care facility, or during other recent contact with the healthcare system; is acquired in the community setting—described as "typical" pneumonia when caused by bacteria; "atypical" when caused by *Chlamydia, Mycoplasma*, or viruses

▶ Healthcare-associated pneumonia (HCAP): Lung infection that develops at least 48 hours after hospital admission, in a long-term care facility or any recent contact with healthcare facility

▶ Other forms of pneumonia not discussed in this chapter include: aspiration pneumonia, pneumonia in immuncompromised patient, *Pneumocystis jirovecii* pneumonia

Etiology

Community-Acquired Pneumonia

Infants and Children

▶ Birth to 20 days: *E. coli*, group B streptococci, *Listeria monocytogenes*

▶ 3 weeks to 3 months: *Chlamydia trachomatis, S. pneumoniae*

▶ 4 months to 18 years:

▷ Typical: *S. pneumoniae*

▷ Atypical: *C. pneumoniae, M. pneumoniae*

Adults

▶ Typical: *S. pneumoniae, H. influenzae, Staphylococcus aureus*, Group A *Streptococcus, Moraxella catarrhalis*

▶ Atypical: *Legionella* species, *Mycoplasma pneumoniae, Chlamydophila pneumoniae*

▶ While bacterial causes are the most common, viral, fungal, and chemical aspiration all contribute.

Healthcare Associated-Acquried Pneumonia

▶ Enteric gram-negative bacilli (*Enterobacter, Klebsiella pneumoniae, Escherichia coli, Serratia marcescens, Proteus,* and *Acinetobacter*), *Pseudomonas aeruginosa,* methicillin-sensitive *Staphylococcus aureus,* and methicillin-resistant *S. aureus* (MRSA) most common

Incidence and Demographics

▶ Common and increasing in both groups

▶ CAP: Eighth leading cause of death in the United States, 5 to 11 cases per 1,000 people; increased incidence in winter months

Risk Factors

▶ CAP: Age older than 65; pulmonary, cardiac, liver, renal disease; preceding influenza; alcohol abuse; tobacco abuse; immunosuppression; HIV/AIDS; chronic corticosteroid use

▶ HCAP: mechanical ventilation; ICU admission; aspiration risks: swallowing dysfunction, supine positioning, tracheal intubation, tracheostomy; oropharyngeal microbial colonization; elevated gastric pH; immunosuppression; hyperglycemia/poor glycemic control

Prevention and Screening

▶ Good handwashing

▶ Routine PCV-13 vaccination to all children 2 to 59 months of age: given at 2, 4, 6, and 12 to 15 months of age

▶ PCV-13 is recommended for those older than 65 years of age, followed by a dose of 23-valent pneumococcal polysaccharide (PPSV23) vaccine 6 to 12 months later.

▶ 23-valent pneumococcal polysaccharide vaccination:

▷ Older than 65 years of age; second dose if patient received first dose 5 years prior and was younger than 65 years of age

▷ Age 19 to 64 with history of chronic cardiovascular disease, chronic pulmonary disease including asthma, diabetes mellitus, chronic liver disease, alcoholism, cochlear implants, CSF leaks, tobacco use or live-in long-term care facilities. Revaccination not recommended if younger than 65 years of age.

▷ Age 19 to 64 with history of immunosuppression: second dose recommended if more than 5 years elapsed since first dose

▶ Influenza and pertussis vaccines

▶ RSV prophylaxis in high-risk children younger than 2 years

▶ Avoid invasive mechanical ventilation

▶ Infection control measures

- ▶ Elevate head of bed
- ▶ Subglotic suctioning
- ▶ Oral/pharyngeal decontamination
- ▶ Maintain gastric acidity
- ▶ Treat comorbidities
- ▶ Avoid smoking

Assessment

History

See Table 7–4

- ▶ Onset either abrupt, insidious, or current or recent stay at healthcare-related facility
- ▶ Recent or concurrent URI, fever, cough (productive or nonproductive), dyspnea, chills, sweats, rigors, fatigue, malaise, myalgias, chest discomfort, headache, anorexia, abdominal pain; pleuritic chest pain; patients generally feel unwell
- ▶ Pediatrics: atypical pneumonia: slowly progressive; malaise, low-grade fever, sore throat, and cough developing over 3 to 5 days
- ▶ Older adults: often present with weakness and mental status change
- ▶ History of chronic obstructive pulmonary disease or human immunodeficiency virus infection
- ▶ Occupation, animal exposures, and sexual history helpful to identify specific infectious agent
- ▶ Recent travel history (within 2 weeks) may help identify *Legionella* pneumonia (seen on cruise ships and hotel stays).
- ▶ Influenza suggested with typical symptoms during peak influenza season
- ▶ ICU admission, mechanical ventilation, or aspiration history

TABLE 7–4.
HOW TO DIFFERENTIATE BETWEEN TYPICAL AND ATYPICAL PNEUMONIA

CHARACTERISTIC	TYPICAL PNEUMONIA	ATYPICAL PNEUMONIA
Onset	Often sudden	Usually gradual
Myalgias/headaches	Not prominent	Often prominent
Fever/shaking chills	Common	Rare
Appearance	Quite ill	Mild to moderately ill
Cough	Productive	Nonproductive paroxysms
Pleuritic pain	Common	Rare
Lung exam	Dullness, with signs of consolidation	Often minimal abnormal findings
Chest X-ray (CXR)	Localized findings correlate with examination	Involvement in excess of examination findings
Leukocyte count	>15,000/mm³	<15,000/mm³

Physical Exam

▶ Fever higher than 100.4°F (38°C), tachypnea, tachycardia

▶ Lungs: rales, rhonchi, egophony, increased tactile femitius, bronchial breath sounds, dullness to percussion, asymmetric breath sounds, use of accessory muscles, nasal flaring

▶ **Red flag**: respirations in 2 to 6 months old higher than 50; 7 to 35 months old higher than 40; over 35 months old higher than 35

▶ Abdominal tenderness

▶ Cardiac evaluation is normal unless underlying disease

▶ Signs of dehydration

▶ Assess mental status

▶ Increased respiratory secreations and leukocytosis also seen in HCAP

Diagnostic Studies

▶ Chest X-ray: infiltrates confirmed

▶ Routine laboratory testing usually unnecessary to establish an etiology in outpatients with CAP

▶ Suctioned or expectorated sputum gram stain

▶ Nasopharyngeal washings for RSV enzyme immunoassay (children)

▶ CBC, two sets of blood cultures (usually reserved for hospitalized patients), CRP, procalcinonin levels, CMP

▶ WBC elevated (may be low in older adults or immunocompromised patients)

▶ *Legionella* urine antigen test if *Legionella* suspected

▶ Bronchoalveolar lavage or protected specimen brush with quantitative cultures

▶ Serial chest X-rays or chest CT scanning if healthcare-associated pneumonia

Differential Diagnosis

▶ Pulmonary edema

▶ Asthma exacerbation

▶ Atelectasis

▶ Acute bronchitis

▶ Bronchiolitis

▶ Bronchiectasis

▶ COPD

▶ Foreign body aspiration

▶ Fungal pneumonia

▶ Lung abscess

▶ Respiratory failure

▶ Viral pneumonia

▶ *Pneumocystis jiroveci* pneumonia

▶ Pulmonary tuberculosis

▶ Lung cancer

Management

Nonpharmacologic Treatment

▶ Hydration, high humidity

▶ Monitoring of respiratory status, rest

▶ Smoking cessation, avoidance of secondhand smoke

▶ Chest physiotherapy for bacterial pneumonia

▶ Oxygen, if needed

▶ Semiupright or upright positioning

▶ Noninvasive ventilation using continuous positive airway pressure (CPAP) or bilevel positive airway pressure (BiPAP) with endotracheal intubation

▶ Incentive spirometry to help prevent postoperative pneumonia

Pharmacologic Treatment

▶ Empiric treatment often necessary because often not able to identify pathogen

▶ Adult CAP outpatient:

　▷ Previously healthy, no antibiotics in past 3 months

　　▶ Macrolide:

　　　▷ Azithromycin (Zithromax): over 12 years old: 500 mg (two 250 mg tablets) initially, then 250 mg (one tablet) q.d. x 4 days or 500 mg p.o. daily x 3 days; or

　　　▷ Clarithromycin (Biaxin): adults: 500 mg (one tablet) b.i.d. x 5 days; clarithromycin XL: two 500 mg tablets (1000 mg) once daily p.o. x 5 days or erythromycin (Erythrocin) 500 mg b.i.d. p.o. x 10 days (not generally used due to side effects); or

　　　▷ Tetracycline: Doxycycline 100 mg p.o. b.i.d. x 10 days

　▷ Comorbidities, immunosuppressed, antibiotic use in past 3 months:

　　▶ Fluoroquinolone: levofloxacin 750 mg p.o. q.d. x 5 days; moxifloxacin 400 mg p.o. q.d. x 10 days; gemifloxacin 320 mg p.o. q.d. x 5 days

　　▶ B-Lactam (amoxicillin 1 g p.o. t.i.d.; amoxicillin-clavulanate 2 g p.o. b.i.d.) plus macrolide or clarithromycin or clarithromycin XL or erythromycin

▶ Pediatric outpatient (more than 3 months):

　▷ Antibiotic treatment in preschool-age children not routinely recommended, as viral pathogens are more common.

　▷ For typical bacterial pneumonia: amoxicillin 90 mg/kg/d p.o. b.i.d. (max 4 g/d); amoxicillin-clavulanate 90 mg/kg/d p.o. b.i.d. (max 4 g/d); levofloxacin 16–20 mg/kg/d (ages 6 months to 5 years) and 8–10 mg/kg/d (over 5 years old) max 750 mg/d

▷ For atypical bacterial pneumonia: azithromycin 10 mg/kg p.o. on day 1, then 5 mg/kg/d on days 2 through 5; clarithromycin 15 mg/kg/d p.o. b.i.d. (max 1 g/d); erythromycin 40 mg/kg/d p.o. daily

▶ CAP, inpatient (non-ICU): IV antibiotic initially, then switch to oral after clinical improvement

▷ Cefotaxime, ceftraxone, or ampicillin-sulbactam plus macrolide (clarithromycin or erythromycin) x 14 days

▷ Gatifloxacin or levofloxacin x 14 days

▶ For pseudomonas CAP:

▷ Piperacillin/tazobactam (Zosyn), cefepime, imipenem/cilastatin (Primaxin), meropenem (Merrem) or doripenem (Doribax) plus either ciprofloxacin (Cipro) or levofloxacin (Levaquin); or

▷ Piperacillin/tazobactam (Zosyn), cefepime, imipenem/cilastatin (Primaxin), meropenem (Merrem) or doripenem (Doribax) plus an aminoglycoside and azithromycin; or

▷ Piperacillin/tazobactam (Zosyn), cefepime, imipenem/cilastatin (Primaxin), meropenem (Merrem) or doripenem (Doribax) plus aminoglycoside and an antipneumococcal respiratory fluoroquinolone

▶ HCAP: antipseudomonal beta-lactams, antipseudomonal fluoroquinolones, aminogly-cosides, vancomycin, or linezolid are used

▶ Viral pneumonia

▷ Bronchodilator if wheezing present

▷ Consider amantadine (Symmetrel) or rimantadine (Flumadine) 100 mg p.o. b.i.d. for influenza A

▶ Antitussives

▷ Generally cough should not be suppressed and antitussives should be avoided; however, in patients with severe chest discomfort and persistent cough, may consider use of nonnarcotic or low-dose narcotic antitussive for night use only; see the section on Persistent Cough.

How Long to Treat

▶ For mild to moderate CAP: short course antimicrobial agents are sufficient in treatment.

▶ Patients should be afebrile for 48 hours and clinically stable before therapy is discontinued.

▶ Some symptoms (cough, fatigue, and dyspnea) may be present for 2 to 4 weeks. Infiltrates on CXR may last up to 30 days.

▶ Most patients improve within 2 weeks. Older adults or very sick patients may need longer treatment.

Special Considerations

▶ Drug resistance: Suspect drug-resistant *S. pneumonia* in communities with increased prevalence. Risk factors include younger than 2 year of age or older than 65 years, betalactam or macrolide treatment within the past 3 to 6 months, alcoholism, medical comorbidities, immunosuppression, and exposure to day care.

When to Consult, Refer, Hospitalize

▶ Consider hospitalization for adult patients over age 65, with history of comorbid conditions, altered mental status, leucopenia (less than 4,000), leukocytosis (more than 30,000), tachycardia, tachypnea, systolic blood pressure less than 90 mmHG, and temperature lower than 35°C (95°F) or higher than 40°C (104°F).

▶ Consider hospitalization in pediatric patients that are less than 3 to 6 months; look toxic; have immunodeficiencies, cardiac, or pulmonary disease; are in respiratory distress; or are dehydrated.

▶ Consider chest CT scan if patient fails to improve on current management.

▶ Consult specialist if there is little improvement or deteriotation after 48 to 72 hours of therapy.

Follow-Up

▶ 24-hour follow-up contact for patients moderately to severely ill, and 72 hours after beginning antimicrobials for reevaluation

▶ For patients who are improving, routine follow-up in 2 to 3 weeks

▶ Patients older than 40 years and all smokers, follow-up CXR in 4 to 8 weeks to rule out underlying bronchogenic carcinoma, which may present as pneumonia

▶ In children with recurrent pneumonia, repeat CXR in 4 to 6 weeks

Expected Course

▶ Dependent upon pathogen, patient response, comorbidities, and complications

Complications

▶ Necrotizing pneumonia, respiratory failure, empyema, abscesses, cavitation, bronchopleural fistula, sepsis

Primary Lung Malignancies

Description

▶ Cancer that forms in tissues of the lung, usually in the cells lining air passages

▶ There are three broad categories:

▷ Non–small cell lung cancer (NSCLC): over 85% of all lung cancers; includes adenocarcinoma, squamous cell carcinoma, large cell

  ▶ Adenocarcinoma: most common in United States and in nonsmokers; about 40% of NSCLC, metastasizes early, poor prognosis

  ▶ Squamous cell carcinoma: less than 25% of NSCLC, dose-related effect with smoking, slower growing

▶ Large cell carcinoma: about 10% of NSCLC, poor prognosis

▷ Small cell lung cancer (SCLC), also known as *oat cell carcinoma*: 10% to 15% of all lung cancers; centrally located; early metastases; aggressive

▷ Lung carcinoid tumor (also called *lung neuroendocrine* tumors): 5% of lung cancers, most of these tumors grow slowly and rarely spread

▶ Other: mesothelioma, sarcoma

▶ Most metastasize to lymph nodes (pulmonary, mediastinal), then liver, adrenal, bone, kidney, brain

Etiology

▶ Cigarette smoking, most important cause in both men and women in the United States

▶ Other causes: secondhand smoke, ionizing radiation (radon gas, therapeutic radiation), asbestos exposure, heavy metals (nickel, chromium), industrial carcinogens

▶ Possible causes: lung scarring, air pollution, genetic factors

▶ Carcinogen causes chromosomal damage, abnormal cell growth, leads to malignancy

▶ Besides direct damage to the airways, lung cancers cause complications through direct extension, metastasis, and paraneoplastic syndromes such as syndrome of inappropriate antidiuretic hormone (SIADH).

Incidence and Demographics

▶ Lung cancer is the leading cause of cancer death for both men and women.

▶ Approximately 221,200 new cases of lung cancer in the United States (2015 estimate)

▶ 1.6 million deaths worldwide in 2012

▶ Predominant sex: men more than women

▶ Predominant age: over 40 years; peak at 70 years

Risk Factors

▶ Smoking (cigarette, pipe, cigars)

▶ Secondhand smoke

▶ Radon

▶ Environmental and occupational exposures: asbestos exposure, air pollution, ionizing radiation, mutagenic gases (halogen ethers, mustard gas, aromatic hydrocarbons), metals (inorganic arsenic, chromium, nickel)

▶ Lung scarring from tuberculosis

▶ Radiation therapy to the breast or chest

Prevention and Screening

▶ Aggressive smoking-cessation counseling and therapy (20% to 30% risk reduction occurs within 5 years of cessation)

▶ Avoid supplemental B-carotene and vitamin E in smokers

▶ Avoid hormone replacement therapy in postmenopausal smokers or former smokers

▶ Avoid industrial exposures

▶ Screening controversial: annual low-dose CT of chest annually compared to CXR alone until age 74, decreased lung cancer mortality but did not increase life expectancy

Assessment

History

▶ May be asymptomatic for most of course

▶ Pulmonary: cough (new or change in chronic cough), wheezing and stridor, dyspnea, hemoptysis, pneumonitis (fever and productive cough)

▶ Constitutional: malaise, bone pain (metastatic disease), fatigue, weight loss, anorexia, fever, anemia, clubbing of digits

▶ Other: chest pain (dull, pleuritic), shoulder/arm pain (Pancoast tumors), dysphagia, plethora (redness of face or neck), hoarseness, Horner syndrome, neurologic abnormalities (headaches, syncope, weakness, cognitive impairment), pericardial temponade (pericardial invasion)

Physical Exam

▶ General: pain, performance status, weight loss

▶ HEENT: Horner syndrome, dysphonia, stridor, sclera icterus

▶ Neck: supraclavicular/cervical lymph nodes, mass

▶ Lungs: effusion, wheezing, airway obstruction, pleural effusion

▶ Abdomen/groin: hepatomegaly or lymphadenopathy

▶ Extremities: signs of hypertrophic pulmonary osteoarthropathy, DVT

▶ Neurologic: exclude cognitive and focal motor defects

Diagnostic Studies

▶ Initial lab tests: CBC, BUN, serum creatinine, liver function tests, LDH, electrolytes (hypercalemia: paraneoplastic syndrome; hyponatremia: SIADH), sputum cytology

▶ Chest radiographs: most important initial diagnostic test in predicting whether lung cancer is potential cause of chronic cough (compare with old films); possible findings: nodule or mass, persistent infiltrate, atelectasis, mediastinal widening, hilar enlargement, pleural effusion

▶ CT scan of chest (with IV contrast): nodule or mass, lymphadenopathy, and for cancer staging

▶ Fine needle aspiration (FNA) biopsy

▶ Other test to evaluate for metastatic disease and staging:

▷ Brain MRI: necrotic or bleeding lesions

▷ Abdomen: hepatic, adrenal, renal masses

▷ PET scan: to determine metastasis

▷ Bone scan: advanced disease or bone pain

▶ Fiberoptic bronchoscopy when the chest radiograph suggests that a tumor or an inflammatory pulmonary parenchymal process is present

Management

▶ Treatment options for patients are determined by histology, stage, general health, and comorbidities of the patient.

▶ Chemotherapy is the mainstay of treatment for SCLC and advanced NSCLC.

▶ Adjuvant chemotherapy following surgery is used in patients with fully resected stage II-III NSCLC.

▶ Radiation is used in some unresectable diseases in combination with chemotherapy.

Nonpharmacologic Treatment

▶ Palliative therapy includes general care of the patient, with particular attention to pain control, symptom control, maintenance of adequate nutrition/hydration, and psychological support.

▶ Acupuncture has been found effective in the management of chemotherapy-associated nausea and vomiting, and in controlling pain associated with surgery.

▶ Oxygen may be necessary in some patients experiencing dyspnea.

Pharmacologic Treatment

▶ Multiple therapies are used in lung cancer treatment including surgery, chemotherapy, radiation therapy, targeted therapy, laser therapy, photodynamic therapy, cryosurgery, electorcautery, watchful waiting. For more complete information, see http://www.cancer.gov/cancertopics/types/lung.

How Long to Treat

▶ Duration of treatment depends on type and stage of cancer.

Special Considerations

▶ Discuss end-of-life care with patient and family members.

▶ Consider bisphospinates or denosumab in patients with bone metastases.

When to Consult, Refer, Hospitalize

▶ Any patient with suspected lung malignancy should be referred to a pulmonologist for evaluation, with subsequent referral to a thoracic surgeon and/or oncologist for treatment.

Follow-Up

Expected Course

▶ Depends on clinical history: postoperative visits every 3 to 6 months with physical exam and CXR

▶ Follow-up CT scans as indictated

▶ Overall 5-year survival rate for all types and stages is 17.4% (NSCLC: 17%; SCLC: 6%); patients with SCLC rarely live 5 years (4%)

Complications
- ▶ Development of metastatic disease (brain, bones, adrenals, and liver)
- ▶ Local recurrence of disease
- ▶ Postoperative complications
- ▶ Side effects of chemotherapy and radiation

Tuberculosis (TB)

Description
- ▶ Contagious bacterial infection (*Mycobacterium tuberculosis*) that involves the lungs, but may spread to other organs (skin, kidneys, bones, genitourinary, meninges, peritoneum, and heart)
- ▶ Classified as active (disease from initial infection) or latent (asymptomatic with positive PPD, negative chest X-ray, noninfectious)

Etiology
- ▶ Caused by *Mycobacterium tuberculosis* (*M. tuberculosis*) when inhaling aerosolized droplets from a cough or sneeze of an infected person
- ▶ Reactivation may occur years later and symptoms of active disease appear
- ▶ Structure of the bacterium *M. tuberculosis* makes it relatively resistant to destruction by macrophages and drugs; it multiplies slowly and may lay dormant for long period of time.

Incidence and Demographics
- ▶ 33% of world's population are infected with TB.
- ▶ TB is the leading killer of people who are HIV infected.
- ▶ 9 million people diagnosed worldwide in 2013 and 1.5 million TB-related deaths
- ▶ TB death rate worldwide dropped 69% between 1992 and 2013.
- ▶ TB incidence for 2013: U.S. 3.0 case/100,000 persons
- ▶ In 2013, 65% of reported TB cases in the United States occurred among foreign-born persons (13 times higher than U.S.-born persons)
- ▶ In the United States, highest rates are in people of Asian, Native Hawaiian and other Pacific Islander, African American, Native American, and Hispanic descent.

Risk Factors
- ▶ HIV infection is the strongest known risk factor.
- ▶ For infection:
  - ▷ Homeless, minority, residents and employees in institutionalized settings, close contact with infected persons, people from high-risk countries (Asia, Africa, Latin America), healthcare workers, travel to high-risk areas, medically underserved areas, low income, substance abuse

▶ For development of disease once infected:

▷ HIV, lymphoma, silicosis, diabetes mellitus, chronic renal failure, cancer of head/neck/lung, children younger than 5 years of age, malnutrition, systemic corticosteroids, immunosuppressive drugs, IV drug abuse, alcohol abuse, cigarette smokers, less than 2 years since infection with *M. tuberculosis*, history of gastrectomy or jejuna bypass, less than 90% ideal body weight, conversion from negative to positive tuberculin skin test (PPD) or interferon-gamma release assay (IGRA) within previous 2 years

Prevention and Screening

▶ Treat latent infection and report to health department; test and treat all close contacts

▶ Tuberculin skin tests (TST): Mantoux (PPD) is standard test, establishes exposure to TB; see Table 7–5 for PPD interpretation

▶ A whole-blood interferon gamma assay (IGRAs) (e.g., QuantiFERON-TB Gold test or QFT-G test)

▶ The Centers for Disease Control and Prevention (CDC) recommend that the QFT-G test can be used in all circumstances in which the TST is currently used. Compared with the TST, the QFT-G test is less subject to reader bias and error, can be accomplished after a single patient visit, and may not be as likely to be positive following the BCG vaccine.

▶ A positive TST or IGRA result only indicates if someone has been infected with *M. tuberculosis*. These tests cannot identify if a person has TB disease.

▶ Practice appropriate infection control procedures in the workplace. The Bacillus Calmette-Guerin (BCG) vaccine: Consider use in United States for children with negative PPD and HIV tests with unavoidable high risk and for healthcare workers at high risk for drug-resistant infection; used in countries with endemic TB; may cause persistent positive PPD.

Assessment

History

▶ Assess for history of TB, exposure to TB, or treatment for active or latent disease.

▶ Assess HIV status and other risk factors.

▶ Often a person with latent TB infection doesn't feel sick, is asymptomatic, cannot spread TB to others, and is at risk of developing TB disease.

▶ TB disease: Patient will feel sick, usually will have one or more symptoms, and may spread TB bacteria to others.

▶ General symptoms of TB disease: chills, night sweats, weight loss, appetite loss, fatigue, malaise

▶ Symptoms of pulmonary TB disease: cough lasting 3 or more weeks, chest pain, hemoptysis

▶ Symptoms of extrapulmonary TB disease depend on part of body affected:

▷ Back pain: TB of spine

▷ Hematuria: TB of kidneys

▷ Lymphadenapathy: TB of lymph nodes

▶ Children are usually asymptomatic at initial infection; symptoms may occur 1 to 6 months later.

▶ Extrapulmonary TB symptoms depend on site affected.

Physical Exam

▶ Often entirely normal

▶ Specific findings vary based on system involved

▶ May find weight loss, adenopathy, apical rales/crackles on lung exam

▶ Evaluate for extrapulmonary TB

▶ HIV testing and counseling should be regularly offered to all patients during a physical examination.

Diagnostic Studies

▶ PPD to assess exposure (see Table 7–5); 5 U (0.1 mL) intradermal injection into volar forearm; measure induration at 48 to 72 hours; repeat second test in 1 to 3 weeks after initial test for persons with no recent PPD, age older than 55, nursing home resident, prison inmate, healthcare worker, or interferon-gamma release assays (IGRAs)

▶ Chest X-ray: infiltrate in middle and lower lobes in primary TB; fibronodular upper lobe infiltrate in reactivation of disease; see small, homogenous infiltrates, cavitation, hilar, and paratracheal lymph node enlargement

TABLE 7–5.
GUIDELINES FOR DETERMINING A POSITIVE TUBERCULIN SKIN TEST AND NEED FOR PREVENTIVE TREATMENT

INDURATION >5 MM	INDURATION >10 MM	INDURATION >15 MM
HIV-positive people	Recent immigrants (<5 years) from high-prevalence countries	All persons with no known risk factors for TB
Fibrotic changes on CXR consistent with old TB	IV drug users	
Patients with organ transplants, other immunosuppressed patients (e.g., receiving the equivalent of >15 mg/d of prednisone for >1 month)	Residents and employees of high-risk congregate settings: prisons, jails, nursing homes and other healthcare facilities; residential facilities for AIDS patients; and homeless shelters	
Recent contact of a person with TB disease	Mycobacteriology laboratory personnel	
	Preexisting medical conditions: weight loss >10% below ideal body weight, diabetes mellitus, gastrectomy, jejuneal bypass, silicosis, chronic renal failure, malignancy	
	Any child <4 years; infants, children, and adolescents exposed to adults in high-risk categories	

Adapted from *Tuberculin skin testing for tuberculosis,* by the Centers for Disease Control and Prevention, 2012. Retrieved from http://www.cdc.gov/tb/publications/factsheets/testing/skintesting.htm.

▶ Three different morning sputum samples for acid-fast bacilli (AFB) stain and culture; if positive treat right away. TB is a reportable disease. Positive results must be reported within 24 hours to the state or local TB control program.

▶ Nucleic acid amplification (NAA) test identifies *M. tuberculosis* by amplifying tuberculous DNA and RNA segments found in the patient's specimen. If NAA test and AFB smears are both positive, patients are presumed to have TB disease and should begin treatment. If NAA test is negative and AFB smears are positive, patients may be infected with nontuberculous mycobacteria (NTM).

▶ Drug susceptibility testing is done when culture is found to be positive and is important because it determines which drugs can kill the tubercle bacilli, which can prevent further drug resistance.

▶ CBC with differential and platelets, creatinine, AST, ALT, bilirubin, alkaline phosphatase

▶ HIV testing; if positive, need baseline CD4 count

▶ CT chest bronchoscopy

Differential Diagnosis

▶ COPD

▶ Asthma

▶ Pneumonia

▶ Cancer

▶ Pleurisy

▶ Histoplasmosis

▶ Silicosis

▶ Interstitial lung disease

Management

Nonpharmacologic Treatment

▶ Education and counseling regarding the importance of adherence; consider use of community resources such as directly observed therapy (DOT) to ensure adherence

▶ Review transmission of disease and need for good hygiene, handwashing, secretion precautions, and no sharing of utensils, glasses, etc., for active disease.

▶ Education on the symptoms caused by adverse reactions of the TB treatment medications (no appetite, nausea, vomiting, jaundice, fever longer than 3 days, abdominal pain, neuropathy of fingers and toes, skin rash, easy bleeding, aching joints, dizziness, easy bruising, blurred or changed vision, ringing in ears, hearing loss, tingling/numbness around mouth). If symptom(s) present, stop medication and contact healthcare provider immediately.

Pharmacologic Treatment

▶ Latent TB infection: See Table 7–6. Consider modifications for HIV infection, suspected drug resistance, pregnancy, or treatment of children. Refer to www.thoracic.org and/or www.cdc.gov for further treatment recommendations for these groups. Patients should be given documentation of treatment upon completion.

TABLE 7–6.
LATENT TB INFECTION TREATMENT REGIMENS

DRUGS	DURATION	INTERVAL	MINIMUM DOSES
Isoniazid (INH)	9 months	Daily	270
		Twice weekly*	76
Isoniazid	6 months	Daily	180
		Twice weekly*	52
Isoniazid and rifapentine Not recommended for: – Children <2 years old – People with HIV/AIDS who are taking antiviral agents – People who are presumed to have been infected with INH- or RIF-resistant *M. tuberculosis* – Pregnant women or women expecting to be pregnant within the 12-week regimen	3 months	Once weekly *	12
Rifampin (RIF) – For persons who cannot tolerate INH or are exposed to INH-resistant TB – Should not be used with certain combinations of ARV therapy	4 months	Daily	120

*Use DOT

Reprinted from *Treatment for latent TB infection*, by the Centers for Disease Control and Prevention, 2015. Retrieved from http://www.cdc.gov/tb/topic/treatment/ltbi.htm.

▶ TB disease treatment regimen: See Table 7–7. DOT is required for children, institutionalized patients, risk for nonadherence, and non-daily regimens. Current recommendations can be obtained from http://www.thoracic.org and www.cdc.gov.

  ▷ TB disease must be treated for at least 6 to 9 months, 18 to 24 months or longer to treat multidrug-resistant TB (MDR TB).

  ▷ Regimens for treating TB have an initial phase of 2 months, followed by a continuation phase of either 4 or 7 months.

▶ Continuation phase: 4-month used in the large majority of patients

  ▷ 7-month recommended only for patients with cavitary pulmonary tuberculosis caused by drug-susceptible organisms and whose sputum culture obtained at the time of completion of 2 months of treatment is positive; patients whose initial phase of treatment did not include pyrazinamide (PZA); and patients being treated with once weekly INH and rifapentine and whose sputum culture obtained at the time of completion of the initial phase is positive.

  ▷ The preferred regimen for treating drug-susceptible TB disease in the continuation phase in persons not infected with HIV is daily isoniazid (INH) and rifampin (RIF) for 126 doses (18 weeks) or twice-weekly INH and RIF for 36 doses (18 weeks).

TABLE 7–7.
X BASIC TB DISEASE TREATMENT REGIMENS

PREFERRED REGIMEN	ALTERNATIVE REGIMEN	ALTERNATIVE REGIMEN
Initial phase: Daily INH (5 mg/kg), RIF (10 mg/kg), PZA (15–30 mg/kg), and ethambutol (EMB)* (15–20 mg/kg) for 56 doses (8 weeks)	Initial phase: Daily INH/RIF/PZA/EMB* for 14 doses (2 weeks), then twice weekly for 12 doses (6 weeks)	Initial phase: INH/RIF/PZA/EMB* 3 times weekly for 24 doses (8 weeks)
Continuation phase: Daily INH/RIF for 18 weeks or INH/RIF 2–3 times weekly for 18 weeks	Continuation phase: INH/RIF 2 times weekly for 36 doses (18 weeks)	Continuation phase: INH/RIF 3 times weekly for 54 doses (18 weeks)

*EMB can be discontinued if drug susceptibility studies demonstrate susceptibility to first-line drugs.

Adapted from *Treatment for TB disease*, by the Centers for Disease Control and Prevention, 2015. Retrieved from http://www.cdc.gov/tb/topic/treatment/tbdisease.htm.

> ▷ A continuation phase of once-weekly INH/rifapentine can be used for HIV-negative patients who do not have cavities on the chest film *and* who have negative acid-fast bacilli (AFB) smears at the completion of the initial phase of treatment.

▶ Treatment completion is determined by the number of doses ingested over a given period of time, not by number of weeks or months on the regimen.

▶ Drug-resistant TB should be managed by or in close consultation with an expert in the disease.

▶ DOT should always be used in treating drug-resistant TB to ensure adherence.

Special Considerations

▶ Geriatric patients often have atypical presentation of disease.

▶ INH major adverse reactions are hepatotoxicity, peripheral neuropathy (vitamin B6 daily to decrease neuropathy and CNS effects), and interactions with other drugs. Monitor closely.

▶ Pregnancy: PZA given along with INH; streptomycin contraindicated

▶ Lactation: Small doses of antituberculosis drugs are found in breast milk; however, do not discourage breastfeeding.

▶ Pharmacotherapy may cause interactions with other drugs.

▶ HIV-infected patients should be treated for 9 months.

When to Consult, Refer, Hospitalize

▶ All suspected or confirmed cases should be reported to local and state health departments.

▶ Refer all patients with active disease to specialist for treatment.

▶ Hospitalize patients if incapable of self-care, or if patient is likely to expose new susceptible persons.

▶ Some states may incarcerate noncompliant patients to ensure they take medication.

Follow-Up

Expected Course

▶ Baseline monitoring is not routinely indicated. Baseline monitoring of ALT is recommended for those persons who chronically consume alcohol, take concomitant hepatotoxic drugs, have viral hepatitis or other liver disease, and are pregnant or within 3 months postpartum, and are HIV-infected. Some experts recommend monitoring for those older than 35 years. Treatment should be interrupted and generally modified for those with ALT 3x the upper limit of normal (ULN) in the presence of hepatitis symptoms and/or jaundice, or 5x ULN in the absence of symptoms.

▶ Patients should be evaluated at least monthly during therapy for adverse reactions, adherence to regimen, and signs and symptoms of TB disease. Bacteriologic examination of patient's sputum or other specimens should be done monthly until culture results are negative.

▶ If culture is positive after 2 months of therapy, reassess drug sensitivity and intiate DOT.

▶ Typically there are few complications and there is full resolution of infection when medications are taken as prescribed for full course.

Complications

▶ Drug-induced hepatitis, particularly in patient younger than 35 years, frequent monitoring of liver function indicated; drug-induced neuropathy

▶ Treatment failure most often due to noncompliance

▶ Cavitary lesions can become secondarily infected.

▶ Drug resistance high if HIV-positive, treatment taken improperly, or from an area with high incidence of resistance

▶ Hemoptysis, pneumothorax, bronchiectasis, extensive pulmonary destruction, malignancy and chronic pulmonary aspergillosis

CHRONIC CONDITIONS

Asthma

Description

▶ Chronic, reversible inflammatory airway disease

▶ Episodes are variable and recurring with airflow obstruction, bronchial hyperresponsiveness, and underlying inflammation.

▶ Classified into four groups based on severity; see Table 7–8:

▷ Intermittent, mild persistent, moderate persistent, and severe persistent

Etiology

▶ Inflammation and bronchospasm caused by allergic and nonallergic triggers

▶ Allergy triggers:

▷ Seasonal or environmental allergens: pollens, feathers, warm-blooded pet epithelia, dust mite and cockroach excrement, molds, food additives/ preservatives such as sulfites (rare)

▶ Nonallergic triggers:

▷ Exercise-induced asthma, occurring 5 to 10 minutes following onset of strenuous activity; related to bronchial heat or water loss

▷ Occupational asthma: triggers in workplace such as fumes, dyes, and chemicals

▷ Diseases or infections such as bronchitis, gastroesophageal reflux, rhinitis/sinusitis, viral respiratory infections (especially RSV infections during infancy, rhinovirus younger than 2 years of age)

▷ Drug induced: aspirin, NSAIDs, indomethacin, beta blockers

▷ Smoke and pollutants

Incidence and Demographics

▶ Affects people of all ages

▶ More than 25 million people affected in United States; about 7 million children affected

▶ Children, females, and Black and Puerto Rican people are more likely to have asthma.

▶ People with lower annual household income and residents of the Midwest and Northeast are more likely to have asthma.

Risk Factors

▶ Environmental exposure: dust mites, cats/dogs, cockroaches, RSV, fungus/molds, secondhand smoke, air pollution, grass/trees/weed pollen

▶ Occupational exposure: formaldehyde, fragrances, fumes

▶ Genetic charactreristics: atopy, eczema, allergic rhinnitis

Prevention and Screening

▶ Avoid allergens, tobacco smoke, aspirin, and NSAIDs if sensitive.

▶ Avoid exercise in cold temperatures and during high pollution/pollen levels.

▶ Reduce exposure to triggers by use of air filters and air conditioners; removal of rugs, stuffed animals, pets, etc.

▶ Consider allergy immunotherapy when indicated.

▶ Treat upper respiratory infections, rhinitis, and gastroesophageal reflux when present.

▶ Recommend influenza vaccination annually.

▶ Carry EpiPen if at risk for anaphylaxis.

Assessment

History

▶ Characteristic symptoms: episodic wheezing (absent in severe exacerbation), chest tightness, dyspnea, chronic dry or spasmodic cough; symptoms worse at night, with exercise, exposure to cold temperatures, smoke, allergens

▶ Symptoms of emotional stress, upper respiratory infection, rhinitis/sinusitis, eczema/atopic dermatitis, nasal polyps

▶ Family history of asthma, allergies, or atopy

▶ Severity of symptoms (see Table 7–8)

Physical Exam

▶ Findings may be normal, vary with severity of attack

▶ Vital signs, with particular attention to respiratory rate

▶ General appearance: signs of respiratory distress (use of accessory muscles)

▶ Skin: atopic dermatitis/eczema

▶ Upper respiratory tract: rhinitis, nasal polyps, swollen nasal turbinates

▶ Lower respiratory tract: tachypnea, prolonged expiration phase, audible wheezing (may be absent in severe attacks due to decreased breath sounds)

Diagnostic Studies

▶ Blood test not routinely required; may find esinophilia or elevated serum IgE levels

▶ Spirometry: measures forced expiratory volume in 1 second (FEV1) and forced vital capacity (FVC) in patients younger than 5 years of age. Baseline measurements are essential for diagnosis, then periodic monitoring. See Table 7–8 regarding lung function values and severity.

▶ Bronchoprovocation testing: confirms diagnosis; used in patients with atypical presentation (normal baseline spirometry, no variable airflow limitation with spirometry or peak flow)

   ▷ Inhaled methacholine, histamine, cold dry air, or exercise challenge test induces symptoms

▶ Peak expiratory flow (PEF) used for monitoring lung status, not to confirm diagnosis.

▶ Values vary with height, age, gender. Patient determines "personal best" or average of three readings on optimal day's PEF; less than 200 mL indicates severe obstruction.

   ▷ 80% to 100% of patient's "personal best": good control, maintain treatment

   ▷ 50% to 79%: acute exacerbation, adjust treatment

   ▷ Less than 50%: severe asthma exacerbation, emergency treatment

▶ Chest X-ray: almost always normal; routinely recommended in severe asthma and in patients with co-morbid conditions and/or with atypical symptoms; shows hyperinflation in uncomplicated episodes also used to evaluate patients for complicating cardiopulmonary processes

▶ Skin testing to determine allergic triggers

TABLE 7–8.
CLASSIFYING ASTHMA SEVERITY AND INITIATING THERAPY

INITIAL VISIT: CLASSIFYING ASTHMA SEVERITY AND INITIATING THERAPY
(in patients who are not currently taking long-term control medications)

Level of severity (Columns 2–5) is determined by events listed in Column 1 for both impairment (frequency and intensity of symptoms and functional limitations) and risk (of exacerbations). Assess impairment by patient's or caregiver's recall of events during the previous 2–4 weeks; assess risk over the last year. Recommendations for initiating therapy based on level of severity are presented in the last row.

Components of Severity		Intermittent			Persistent								
					Mild			Moderate			Severe		
		Ages 0–4 years	Ages 5–11 years	Ages ≥12 years	Ages 0–4 years	Ages 5–11 years	Ages ≥12 years	Ages 0–4 years	Ages 5–11 years	Ages ≥12 years	Ages 0–4 years	Ages 5–11 years	Ages ≥12 years
Impairment	Symptoms	≤2 days/week			>2 days/week but not daily			Daily			Throughout the day		
	Nighttime awakenings	0	≤2x/month		1–2x/month	3–4x/month		3–4x/month	>1x/week	>1x/week but not nightly	>1x/week	Often 7x/week	
	SABA* use for symptom control (not to prevent EIB*)	≤2 days/week			>2 days/week but not daily and not more than once on any day			Daily			Several times per day		
	Interference with normal activity	None			Minor limitation			Some limitation			Extremely limited		
	Lung function ♦ FEV₁* (% predicted)	Not applicable	Normal FEV₁ between exacerbations >80%	Normal FEV₁ between exacerbations >80%	Not applicable	>80%	>80%	Not applicable	60–80%	60–80%	Not applicable	<60%	<60%
	♦ FEV₁/FVC*		>85%	Normal†		>80%	Normal†		75–80%	Reduced 5%†		<75%	Reduced >5%†
Risk	Asthma exacerbations requiring oral systemic corticosteroids‡	0–1/year	0–1/year		≥2 exacerb. in 6 months, or wheezing ≥4x per year lasting >1 day AND risk factors for persistent asthma	≥2/year							

Consider severity and interval since last asthma exacerbation. Frequency and severity may fluctuate over time for patients in any severity category.

Relative annual risk of exacerbations may be related to FEV₁.

Generally, more frequent and intense events indicate greater severity.

| | Recommended Step for Initiating Therapy (See "Stepwise Approach for Managing Asthma Long Term," page 7) | Step 1 | | | Step 2 | | | Step 3 | Step 3 medium-dose ICS* option | Step 3 | Step 3 | Step 3 medium-dose ICS* option or Step 4 | Step 4 or 5 |

In 2–6 weeks, depending on severity, assess level of asthma control achieved and adjust therapy as needed.

Consider short course of oral systemic corticosteroids.

The stepwise approach is meant to help, not replace, the clinical decisionmaking needed to meet individual patient needs.

For children 0–4 years old, if no clear benefit is observed in 4–6 weeks, consider adjusting therapy or alternate diagnoses.

* Abbreviations: EIB, exercise-induced bronchospasm; FEV₁, forced expiratory volume in 1 second; FVC, forced vital capacity; ICS, inhaled corticosteroid; SABA, short-acting beta₂-agonist.

† Normal FEV₁/FVC by age: 8–19 years, 85%; 20–39 years, 80%; 40–59 years, 75%; 60–80 years, 70%.

‡ Data are insufficient to link frequencies of exacerbations with different levels of asthma severity. Generally, more frequent and intense exacerbations (e.g., requiring urgent care, hospital or intensive care admission, and/or oral corticosteroids) indicate greater underlying disease severity. For treatment purposes, patients with ≥2 exacerbations may be considered to have persistent asthma, even in the absence of impairment levels consistent with persistent asthma.

Source: National Heart, Lung, and Blood Institute. (2012). *Expert panel report 3 (EPR 3): Asthma care quick reference: Diagnosing and managing asthma.* Retrieved from http://www.nhlbi.nih.gov/files/docs/guidelines/asthma_qrg.pdf.

Differential Diagnosis

All Ages

- ► Foreign body aspiration
- ► Acute infections, viral, pneumonia, bronchitis, TB
- ► GERD
- ► Aspiration
- ► AIDS
- ► Psychogenic cough
- ► Neuromuscular weakness
- ► Vocal cord dysfunction

Adults

- ► COPD
- ► CHF
- ► Pulmonary embolism
- ► Bronchogenic carcinoma
- ► Cough secondary to ACE inhibitors
- ► Alpha antitrypsin deficiency

Children

- ► Allergic rhinitis
- ► Sinusitis
- ► Bronchiolitis (RSV)
- ► Laryngotracheobronchitis (croup)
- ► Cystic fibrosis
- ► Bronchopulmonary dysplasia
- ► Tracheoesophageal fistula
- ► Congenital heart disease

Management

Goals of therapy

- ► Reduce impairment:
    - ▷ Prevent chronic and troublesome symptoms.
    - ▷ Require infrequent use of inhaled short-acting beta-2 agonists (SABA)
    - ▷ Maintain near-normal pulmonary function
    - ▷ Maintain normal activity levels
    - ▷ Meet patient and family expectations of satisfaction with asthma care

▶ Reduce risk:

▷ Prevent recurrent exacerbations and minimize ED visits/hospitalization

▷ Prevent loss of lung function or reduced lung growth in children

▷ Provide optimal pharmacotherapy with minimal or no adverse effects of therapy

Nonpharmacologic Treatment

▶ Develop written asthma action plan with patient/family

▶ Identify and avoid factors that trigger asthma; control environmental triggers

▶ Allergy skin testing to determine allergens

▶ Maintain hydration; increase fluids during exacerbation

▶ Address family, school, and/or day care issues; provide education, support, and counseling

▶ Establish a patient/provider partnership with a detailed asthma action plan

▶ Delivery of inhaled agents via "spacer" or holding chamber provides increased efficacy.

▶ Educate patients to rinse mouth out with water immediately after use of inhaler to avoid thrush

▶ No smoking

Pharmacologic Treatment

Based on age and severity (see Tables 7–8, 7–9, and 7–10)

Quick-Relief Medications ("Rescue")

▶ Short-acting beta-agonist (SABA) for quick relief of acute symptoms and prevention of exercised-induced bronchospasm

▷ Albuterol HFA (Proventil HFA, Ventolin HFA), pirbuterol (Maxair), metaproterenol (Alupent): generally two inhalations or one nebulization q4h in adults and children

▷ Levalbuterol (Xopenex HFA): children older than 4 years and adults: 2 inh every 4 to 6 hours p.r.n.

▷ or in adults and children older than 4 years: levalbuterol (Xopenex) 0.63 or 1.25 mg one nebulized solution q6–8h

▷ or especially in young children: albuterol syrup (Proventil, Ventolin) 2 mg/5 mL; children 2 to 6 years; 0.1–0.2 mg/kg tid max 2 gm/day; 6 to 14 years: 5 mL t.i.d. to q.i.d.

▶ Anticholinergic: Ipratropium (Atrovent) 1–2 inh or 1–2 unit dose neb q6h p.r.n. (adults only) in combination with SABA

▶ Systemic corticosteroids may be used:

▷ In moderate-to-severe asthma as adjunct

▷ In patients with all but the mildest of acute asthma exacerbations

▷ Prescribed for up to 7 days in adults and 3 days in children with no need for tapering

▷ In corticosteroid doses of prednisolone 1–2 mg/kg/d or equivalent; max 60 mg/day for 3 to 10 days

Long-Term Control Medications ("Controllers")

▶ Inhaled corticosteroids are the most effective long-term control therapy recommended in children and adults with persistent asthma.

▷ Beclomethasone propionate HFA (QVAR) 40–80 mcg. Adults: 40–320 mcg twice daily; children 5 to 11: 40–80 mcg twice daily; budesonide (Pulmicort) preferred in pregnancy; 90–180 mcg

▶ Adults: 360 mcg twice daily; max 720 mcg twice daily

▶ Children ages 6 to 17: 180 mcg twice daily; max 360 mcg twice daily

▷ Pulmicort respules: 0.25mg/2ml, 0.5mg/2ml, or 1mg/2ml susp; once daily or in divided doses ages 12 months to 8 years

▷ Triamcinolone acetate (Azmacort) 75 mcg/spray: adults: 4–16 puffs/day in divided doses; children 6 to 12 years of age: 2–8 puffs/day in divided doses

▷ Ciclesonide (Alvesco) 80 mcg, 160 mcg; ages 12 years and older; b.i.d.

▷ Flunisolide (Aerobid) 250 mcg/puff; adults, 2–4 inh twice daily; children ages 6 years and older, 2 inh twice daily

▷ Fluticasone propionate (Flovent HFA) 44 mcg, 110 mcg, 220 mcg; for children and adults 4 years of age and older; dose varies; Flovent diskus: 50, 100, 250 mcg; 1–2 inh twice daily

▷ Mometasone (Asmanex Twisthaler) 110, 220 mcg

▶ Adults and children 12 years old and older: 220–880 mcg

▶ Children ages 4 to 11: 110 mcg every evening

▷ Mometasone furoate HFA (Asmanes HFA): 100 or 200 mcg; 12 years of age and older; 2 puffs twice daily

▶ Inhaled long-acting beta$_2$ agonists (LABA)

▷ Salmeterol (Serevent): 50 mcg/inh, adults:1 inh q 12 hrs; children older than 4 years: (Serevent discus) 1 inh q 12 hrs

▷ Formoterol (Foradil): 12 mcg/inh, adults and children (older than 5 years): 1inh q 12 hrs

▷ Should not be used alone as maintance therapy in persistent asthma; doing so leads to increased risk of asthma-related mortality

▶ Combination medication: inhaled corticosteroid plus long-acting beta-agonist: dose depends on level of severity or control

▷ Fluticasone/salmeterol: DPI 100 mcg/50 mcg, 250 mcg/50 mcg, or 500 mcg/50 mcg; MDI 45 mcg/21 mcg, 115 mcg/21 mcg, or 230 mcg/21 mcg: 1 inh 2x/day for patients 5 years or older

▷ Budesonide/formoterol: MDI 80 mcg/4.5 mcg or 160 mcg/4.5 mcg 2 puffs 2x/day for patients 5 years or older

▷ Mometasone/formoterol: MDI 100 mcg/5 mcg, 2 inh 2x/day for patients age 12 years and older only

▶ Oral long-acting beta-agonists: albuterol extended release tabs (Volmax, Proventil Repetabs); adults: 4–8 mg q 12 hrs; children older than 12 years: 4 mg q 12 hrs; ages 6 to 11: 2 mg q12 hrs

▶ Oral systemic corticosteroids: methylprednisolone, prednisolone, or prednisone: children 0 to 11 years old: 0.25–2 mg/kg daily in single dose in a.m. or every other day p.r.n. for control; short course burst is 1–2 mg/kg/day, max 60 mg/d for 3 to 10 days. For patients older than 12 years of age: 7.5–60 mg daily in single dose in a.m. or every other day p.r.n. for control; short burst to achieve control is 40–60 mg/day as single or two divided doses for 3 to 10 days

▶ Anti-IgE Omalizumab (Xolair) subcutaneous injection for 12 years of age and older with a positive skin test reactive to perennial aerollergen and symptoms uncontrolled with inhaled corticosteroids

▶ Anti-inflammatory (noncorticosteroid): adults and children older than 2 years: cromolyn sodium (Intal) 2 inh of metered dose inhaler (MDI) 0.8 mg/inh q.i.d.; neb sol 20 mg/2 mL q.i.d.; nedocromil (Tilade) 2 inh q.i.d. (avoid in children younger than 2 years of age)

▶ Leukotriene receptor antagonists

▷ Zafirlukast (Accolate): adults (12 years and older): 20 mg b.i.d.; children age 7 to 11 years: 10 mg b.i.d.; take on empty stomach; monitor liver function

▷ Montelukast (Singulair): adults: 10 mg q.HS.; age 1 to 4 years: 4 mg q.HS.; age 6 to 14 years: 5 mg q.HS

▶ Methylxanthines: theophylline dose dependent on preparation; maintain serum levels of 12–15 mcg/L

▶ The National Heart, Lung, and Blood Institute of the National Institutes of Health has developed general guidelines for the treatment of asthma based on age group (see Tables 7-8, 7–9, and 7–10).

How Long to Treat

▶ Dependent on the severity of the attacks; goal is to gain control as quickly as possible and decrease treatment gradually to least amount of medication needed to maintain control

Special Considerations

▶ Pregnancy:

▷ Check asthma control at all prenatal visits. Asthma can improve or worsen during pregnancy; adjust medications as needed.

▷ Most ICS agents are category C, except budesonide, montelukast, and zafirlukast, which are category B.

▷ Remind patients to avoid exposure to tobacco smoke.

▷ Treating asthma with medications is safer for mother and fetus than having poorly controlled asthma.

▷ Maintaining lung function is essential for good fetal outcome.

TABLE 7–9.
ASSESSING ASTHMA CONTROL AND ADJUSTING THERAPY

FOLLOW-UP VISITS: ASSESSING ASTHMA CONTROL AND ADJUSTING THERAPY

Level of control (Columns 2–4) is based on the most severe component of impairment (symptoms and functional limitations) or risk (exacerbations). Assess impairment by patient's or caregiver's recall of events listed in Column 1 during the previous 2–4 weeks and by spirometry and/or peak flow measures. Symptom assessment for longer periods should reflect a global assessment, such as inquiring whether the patient's asthma is better or worse since the last visit. Assess risk by recall of exacerbations during the previous year and since the last visit. Recommendations for adjusting therapy based on level of control are presented in the last row.

Components of Control	Well Controlled			Not Well Controlled			Very Poorly Controlled		
	Ages 0–4 years	Ages 5–11 years	Ages ≥12 years	Ages 0–4 years	Ages 5–11 years	Ages ≥12 years	Ages 0–4 years	Ages 5–11 years	Ages ≥12 years
Impairment									
Symptoms	≤2 days/week	≤2 days/week but not more than once on each day	≤2 days/week	>2 days/week	>2 days/week or multiple times on ≤2 days/week	>2 days/week	Throughout the day	Throughout the day	Throughout the day
Nighttime awakenings	≤1x/month	≤1x/month	≤2x/month	>1x/month	≥2x/month	1–3x/week	>1x/week	≥2x/week	≥4x/week
Interference with normal activity	None	None	None	Some limitation	Some limitation	Some limitation	Extremely limited	Extremely limited	Extremely limited
SABA* use for symptom control (not to prevent EIB*)	≤2 days/week	≤2 days/week	≤2 days/week	>2 days/week	>2 days/week	>2 days/week	Several times per day	Several times per day	Several times per day
Lung function — FEV$_1$* (% predicted) or peak flow (% personal best)	Not applicable	>80%	>80%	Not applicable	60–80%	60–80%	Not applicable	<60%	<60%
— FEV$_1$/FVC*	Not applicable	>80%	Not applicable	Not applicable	75–80%	Not applicable	Not applicable	<75%	Not applicable
Validated questionnaires† — ATAQ*	Not applicable	Not applicable	0	Not applicable	Not applicable	1–2	Not applicable	Not applicable	3–4
— ACQ*			≤0.75‡			≥1.5			Not applicable
— ACT*			≥20			16–19			≤15
Risk									
Asthma exacerbations requiring oral systemic corticosteroids§	0–1/year	0–1/year	0–1/year	2–3/year	≥2/year	≥2/year	>3/year	≥2/year	≥2/year
	Consider severity and interval since last asthma exacerbation.								
Reduction in lung growth/Progressive loss of lung function	Not applicable	Evaluation requires long-term follow-up care.	Evaluation requires long-term follow-up care.	Not applicable	Evaluation requires long-term follow-up care.	Evaluation requires long-term follow-up care.	Not applicable	Evaluation requires long-term follow-up care.	Evaluation requires long-term follow-up care.
Treatment-related adverse effects	*Medication side effects can vary in intensity from none to very troublesome and worrisome. The level of intensity does not correlate to specific levels of control but should be considered in the overall assessment of risk.*								

Recommended Action for Treatment	Well Controlled	Not Well Controlled	Very Poorly Controlled
(See "Stepwise Approach for Managing Asthma Long Term," page 7) *The stepwise approach is meant to help, not replace, the clinical decisionmaking needed to meet individual patient needs.*	Maintain current step. Regular follow-up every 1–6 months. Consider step down if well controlled for at least 3 months.	Step up 1 step (0–4 yrs); Step up at least 1 step (5–11 yrs); Step up 1 step (≥12 yrs). Reevaluate in 2–6 weeks to achieve control. For children 0–4 years, if no clear benefit observed in 4–6 weeks, consider adjusting therapy or alternative diagnoses.	Consider short course of oral systemic corticosteroids. Step up 1–2 steps. Reevaluate in 2 weeks to achieve control.

Before step up in treatment: Review adherence to medication, inhaler technique, and environmental control. If alternative treatment was used, discontinue and use preferred treatment for that step. For side effects, consider alternative treatment options.

* **Abbreviations:** ACQ, Asthma Control Questionnaire©; ACT, Asthma Control Test™; ATAQ, Asthma Therapy Assessment Questionnaire©; EIB, exercise-induced bronchospasm; FVC, forced vital capacity; FEV$_1$, forced expiratory volume in 1 second; SABA, short-acting beta$_2$-agonist.
† Minimal important difference: 1.0 for the ATAQ; 0.5 for the ACQ; not determined for the ACT.
‡ ACQ values of 0.76–1.4 are indeterminate regarding well-controlled asthma.
§ Data are insufficient to link frequencies of exacerbations with different levels of asthma control. Generally, more frequent and intense exacerbations (e.g., requiring urgent care, hospital or intensive care admission, and/or oral corticosteroids) indicate poorer asthma control.

Source: National Heart, Lung, and Blood Institute. (2012). *Expert panel report 3 (EPR 3): Asthma care quick reference: Diagnosing and managing asthma.* Retrieved from http://www.nhlbi.nih.gov/files/docs/guidelines/asthma_qrg.pdf.

TABLE 7–10.
STEPWISE APPROACH FOR MANAGING ASTHMA LONG TERM

The stepwise approach tailors the selection of medication to the level of asthma severity (see page 5) or asthma control (see page 6). The stepwise approach is meant to help, not replace, the clinical decisionmaking needed to meet individual patient needs.

ASSESS CONTROL:

STEP UP IF NEEDED (first, check medication adherence, inhaler technique, environmental control, and comorbidities)

STEP DOWN IF POSSIBLE (and asthma is well controlled for at least 3 months)

		STEP 1	STEP 2	STEP 3	STEP 4	STEP 5	STEP 6
		At each step: Patient education, environmental control, and management of comorbidities					
0–4 years of age		**Intermittent Asthma**	**Persistent Asthma: Daily Medication** Consult with asthma specialist if step 3 care or higher is required. Consider consultation at step 2.				
	Preferred Treatment[†]	SABA* as needed	low-dose ICS*	medium-dose ICS*	medium-dose ICS* + either LABA* or montelukast	high-dose ICS* + either LABA* or montelukast	high-dose ICS* + either LABA* or montelukast + oral corticosteroids
	Alternative Treatment[†,‡]		cromolyn or montelukast				
		If clear benefit is not observed in 4–6 weeks, and medication technique and adherence are satisfactory, consider adjusting therapy or alternate diagnoses.					
	Quick-Relief Medication	• SABA* as needed for symptoms; intensity of treatment depends on severity of symptoms. • With viral respiratory symptoms: SABA every 4–6 hours up to 24 hours (longer with physician consult). Consider short course of oral systemic corticosteroids if asthma exacerbation is severe or patient has history of severe exacerbations. • Caution: Frequent use of SABA may indicate the need to step up treatment.					
5–11 years of age		**Intermittent Asthma**	**Persistent Asthma: Daily Medication** Consult with asthma specialist if step 4 care or higher is required. Consider consultation at step 3.				
	Preferred Treatment[†]	SABA* as needed	low-dose ICS*	low-dose ICS* + either LABA,* LTRA,* or theophylline[(b)] **OR** medium-dose ICS	medium-dose ICS* + LABA*	high-dose ICS* + LABA*	high-dose ICS* + LABA* + oral corticosteroids
	Alternative Treatment[†,‡]		cromolyn, LTRA,* or theophylline[§]		medium-dose ICS* + either LTRA* or theophylline[§]	high-dose ICS* + either LTRA* or theophylline[§]	high-dose ICS* + either LTRA* or theophylline[§] + oral corticosteroids
			Consider subcutaneous allergen immunotherapy for patients who have persistent, allergic asthma.**				
	Quick-Relief Medication	• SABA* as needed for symptoms. The intensity of treatment depends on severity of symptoms: up to 3 treatments every 20 minutes as needed. Short course of oral systemic corticosteroids may be needed. • Caution: Increasing use of SABA or use >2 days/week for symptom relief (not to prevent EIB*) generally indicates inadequate control and the need to step up treatment.					
≥12 years of age		**Intermittent Asthma**	**Persistent Asthma: Daily Medication** Consult with asthma specialist if step 4 care or higher is required. Consider consultation at step 3.				
	Preferred Treatment[†]	SABA* as needed	low-dose ICS*	low-dose ICS* + LABA* **OR** medium-dose ICS*	medium-dose ICS* + LABA*	high-dose ICS* + LABA* **AND** consider omalizumab for patients who have allergies[††]	high-dose ICS* + LABA* + oral corticosteroid[§§] **AND** consider omalizumab for patients who have allergies[††]
	Alternative Treatment[†,‡]		cromolyn, LTRA,* or theophylline[§]	low-dose ICS* + either LTRA,* theophylline,[§] or zileuton[‡]	medium-dose ICS* + either LTRA,* theophylline,[§] or zileuton[‡]		
			Consider subcutaneous allergen immunotherapy for patients who have persistent, allergic asthma.**				
	Quick-Relief Medication	• SABA* as needed for symptoms. The intensity of treatment depends on severity of symptoms: up to 3 treatments every 20 minutes as needed. Short course of oral systemic corticosteroids may be needed. • Caution: Use of SABA >2 days/week for symptom relief (not to prevent EIB*) generally indicates inadequate control and the need to step up treatment.					

* **Abbreviations:** EIB, exercise-induced bronchospasm; ICS, inhaled corticosteroid; LABA, inhaled long-acting beta₂-agonist; LTRA, leukotriene receptor antagonist; SABA, inhaled short-acting beta₂-agonist.

† Treatment options are listed in alphabetical order, if more than one.

‡ If alternative treatment is used and response is inadequate, discontinue and use preferred treatment before stepping up.

§ Theophylline is a less desirable alternative because of the need to monitor serum concentration levels.

** Based on evidence for dust mites, animal dander, and pollen; evidence is weak or lacking for molds and cockroaches. Evidence is strongest for immunotherapy with single allergens. The role of allergy in asthma is greater in children than in adults.

†† Clinicians who administer immunotherapy or omalizumab should be prepared to treat anaphylaxis that may occur.

‡‡ Zileuton is less desirable because of limited studies as adjunctive therapy and the need to monitor liver function.

§§ Before oral corticosteroids are introduced, a trial of high-dose ICS + LABA + either LTRA, theophylline, or zileuton, may be considered, although this approach has not been studied in clinical trials.

Source: National Heart, Lung, and Blood Institute. (2012). *Expert panel report 3 (EPR 3): Asthma care quick reference: Diagnosing and managing asthma.* Retrieved from http://www.nhlbi.nih.gov/files/docs/guidelines/asthma_qrg.pdf.

- For postmenopausal women using inhaled corticosteroids, consider calcium supplements (1,000–1,500 mg a day) and vitamin D (800 units a day).
- Bone mineral density testing if on long-term inhaled or oral corticosteroids to monitor osteoporosis
- Periodic ophthalmology exam if on oral corticosteroids
- Most medications are secreted in breast milk.
- Assess for ACE inhibitor use.
- Avoid ipratropium in patients with allergy to peanuts or soy; it contains soya lecithin and may precipate an allergic reaction.
- In children, monitor growth if using steroids to manage asthma.
- Withhold varicella vaccine if child receiving 2 mg/kg or more or 20 mg/day of oral prednisone.

When to Consult, Refer, Hospitalize

- When diagnosis is unclear
- Additional asthma education needed
- Specialized testing (bronchoprovocation, skin testing)
- Specialized treatments (immunotherapy, anti-IgE therapy)
- Moderate-to-severe persistent asthma in adults
- Moderate-to-persistent asthma in children
- Comorbidities: rhinitis, GERD, sinusitis, obstructive sleep apnea, COPD
- Poorly controlled asthma: frequent ED visits and hospitalizations for asthma
- Hospitalization: based on duration and severity of symptoms, severity of airflow obstruction, response to emergency department treatment, course and severity of prior exacerbations, access to medical care and medication, and adequacy of home condition

Follow-Up

Expected Course

- Follow-up depends on symptom severity, symptom control, knowledge level, social support, and other resources.
    - ▷ Every 2 to 6 weeks while gaining control
    - ▷ Every 1 to 6 months to monitor control
    - ▷ Every 3 months if step down in therapy is anticipated
- New asthmatics require frequent monitoring and patient education.
- Children need more frequent monitoring during growth spurts.
- Patients should monitor peak flow rates twice daily to establish baseline and then regularly.

▶ For acute exacerbation, follow-up in 24 hours, then 3 to 5 days, then weekly until symptoms are controlled and peak flow consistently 80% of predicted, then monthly.

▶ Monitor theophylline levels 2 weeks after initiation of therapy, then every 4 months.

Complications

▶ Atelectasis, pneumonia, air leak syndromes (pneumomediastinum, pneumothorax), medication-specific side effects/interactions, respiratory failure, death (approximately 50% of asthma deaths occur in adults older than 65 years)

Chronic Obstructive Pulmonary Disease (COPD)

Description

Chronic progressive disease that is common and preventable, characterized by airflow limitation that is not fully reversible, with inflammatory responses in the airways and lungs from noxious irritants

▶ Includes chronic bronchitis, emphysema, and—in some cases—asthma

▷ Chronic bronchitis: presence of increased mucus production and recurrent cough most days for at least 3 months of a year, for 2 consecutive years, without other underlying disease to explain the cough

▷ Emphysema: destruction of interalveolar septa within the distal or terminal bronchiole involving both airways and lung parenchyma

▶ Patients with asthma whose airflow obstruction is not completely reversible are considered to have COPD. The etiology and pathogenesis of the COPD in these patients may vary from those who have chronic bronchitis or emphysema.

Etiology

▶ Cigarette and/or cannabis smoking

▶ Air pollution

▶ Antiprotease deficiency (alpha-1 antitrypsin deficiency)

▶ Occupational exposure (firefighters)

▶ Infection (bacterial or viral)

▶ Occupational pollutants (cadmium, silica)

Incidence and Demographics

▶ COPD affects more than 15 million people in the United States.

▶ Seen more in women than men

▶ Onset in middle-aged or older adults; COPD with asthma is the third leading cause of death in the United States

Risk Factors

▶ Smoking

▶ Passive smoking

▶ Cannabis use (1 joint equivalent to 2½–5 cigarettes)

▶ Severe viral pneumonia early in life

▶ Aging

▶ Alcohol consumption

▶ Airway hyperactivity

▶ Pollution: indoor or outdoor (dust, fumes, coal miners, metal molders, grain handlers)

▶ Periodontal disease

Prevention and Screening

▶ Smoking cessation and reduction of exposure to secondhand smoke

▶ Early detection through pulmonary function tests (PFTs) in high-risk groups

▶ Avoid outdoor activities when air pollutant concentrations are high.

Assessment

History

▶ Duration and characteristics of chronic cough, dyspnea, chronic sputum production

▶ Exercise/activity tolerance, dyspnea on exertion or at rest

▶ Chills/fever, weight gain/loss, edema, fatigue, angina

▶ Tobacco exposure (current smoking, pack year history, environmental tobacco exposure)

▶ Environmental/occupational history

▶ Asthma history

▶ Sleep habits (number of pillows used)

▶ Increase in sputum production or purulence along with dyspnea signals exacerbation

▶ Family history of COPD

▶ Impact on quality of life, activities of daily living, socioeconomic status

▶ Risk of exacerbations, history of previous treated events (2 or more per year)

▶ Other comorbidities: cardiovascular diseases, osteoporosis, depression, anxiety, skeletal muscle dysfunction, metabolic syndrome, and lung cancer increase morbidity and hospitalizations. Assess for and manage diseases appropriately.

Physical Exam

▶ Rarely diagnostic for COPD

▶ Early disease: normal exam or may have prolonged expiration or wheezes or forced exhalation

▶ Progression of disease: exam may show hyperinflation, decreased breath sounds, wheezes, crackles at lung bases or distant heart sounds; "barreled chest" may be present

▶ End-stage COPD: unusual positions to relieve dyspnea at rest (leaning forward with arms outstretched and weight supported on palms or elbow), use of accessory respiratory muscles of neck and shoulder girdle, pursed lip breathing, paradoxical retractions with inspiration, cyanosis, asterixis due to severe hypercapnia, enlarged tender liver, neck vein distention, yellow stains on fingers

▶ Chronic bronchitis: cyanosis, wheezing, weight gain, diminished breath sounds, distant heart sounds

▶ Emphysema: barrel chest (increased anteroposterior [AP] diameter), minimal wheezing, accessory muscles used, pursed lip breathing, cyanosis slight or absent, breath sounds diminished

▶ COPD symptoms are classified using the GOLD staging system based on degree of airflow limitation severity measured during PFTs. See Table 7–11.

▶ Comprehensive symptom assessment using validated questionnaires: COPD Assessment Test (CAT) and Clinical COPD Questionnaire (CCQ) are recommended. Medical Research Council (mMRC) scale used only to assess breathlessness.

▶ Patient's symptoms, risk of exacerbations, severity of spirometric abnormality and other comorbid conditions important to assess in the diagnosis of COPD. See Global Initiative for Chronic Obstuctive Lung Disease at: http://goldcopd.org/pocket-guide-copd-diagnosis-management-prevention-2016/, Table 3. Combined Assessment of COPD.

Diagnostic Studies

▶ PFT (spirometry): Reduced FEV1 determines severity of airflow limitation, while decreased FEV1/FVC ratio determines airflow limitation. FEV1/FVC <0.70 with use of postbronchiodilator is diagnostic for COPD

▶ Chest radiographs in emphysema: small heart, hyperinflation, possible bullous changes; flattened diaphragm; chronic bronchitis: increased bronchovascular markings and cardiomegaly

▶ Consider pulse oximetry during acute exacerbations or in those patients who may be considered for long-term oxygen therapy.

▶ Arterial blood gases (ABGs) unnecessary unless FEV1 is less than 40% of predicted, hypoxia, or hypercapnia suspected; no abnormalities in early COPD; hypoxemia in advanced chronic bronchitis; compensated respiratory acidosis with chronic respiratory failure in chronic bronchitis

▶ Alpha 1 antitrypsin level to look for deficiency if COPD occurs before 45 years of age or family history of genetic disease

▶ Increased hemoglobin/hematocrit may be present with chronic bronchitis but not with emphysema.

▶ Chest CT may show diffuse bullous changes or upper lobe predominance; is not needed for diagnosis of COPD.

Differential Diagnosis

▶ Bronchial/occupational asthma

▶ Bronchiectasis

▶ Bronchopulmonary mycosis

▶ Congestive heart failure

▶ Tuberculosis

TABLE 7–11.
CLASSIFICATION OF SEVERITY OF AIRFLOW LIMITATION IN COPD

CLASSIFICATION OF SEVERITY OF AIRFLOW LIMITATION IN COPD. (BASED ON POST-BRONCHODILATOR FEV1) IN PATIENTS WITH FEV1/FVC <0.70:		
GOLD 1	Mild	FEV1 ≥ 80% predicted
GOLD 2	Moderate	50% ≤ FEV1 < 80% predicted
GOLD 3:	Severe	30% ≤ FEV1 < 50% predicted
GOLD 4	Very Severe	FEV1 < 30% predicted

Reprinted with permission from "Global Strategy for Diagnosis, Management and Prevention of COPD", page 14, at www.goldcopd. org by Global Initiative for Chronic Obstructive Lung Disease (GOLD). Copyright 2016 by Global Initiative for Chronic Obstructive Lung Disease.

▶ Lung cancer

▶ GERD

▶ Sleep apnea

▶ Acute viral infection

▶ Normal aging of lungs

▶ Chronic pulmonary embolism

Management

Goal: relieve symptoms, improve exercise tolerance and health status, prevent disease progression, prevent and treat exacerbations, and reduce mortality

Nonpharmacologic Treatment

▶ Initiate and support smoking cessation.

▶ Reduce other risk factors: avoid exposure to colds and influenza; avoid respiratory irritants (secondhand smoke, dust, other air pollutants)

▶ Vaccinations: influenza and pneumococcal vaccines

▶ Oxygen therapy for patients with chronic hypoxemia

▶ Pulmonary rehabilitation decreases symptoms, improves quality of life, and promotes physical and emotional involvement in daily activities

▶ Maintain ideal body weight, high protein/caloric diet, and regular daily exercise; rest often.

▶ Increase fluids and humidification.

▶ Breathing exercises with manual incentive spirometer; effective cough techniques

▶ Lung reduction surgery or lung transplantation in selected cases

▶ Palliative care, end-of life care, and hospice care for advanced COPD

Pharmacologic Treatment

▶ See Table 7–12 for pharmacologic therapy for stable COPD based on GOLD recommendations

▶ Short-acting beta-agonist: levalbuterol (Xopenex) MDI (metered dose inhaler) or solution for nebulizer q 6–8 hrs; salbutamol (Albuterol) MDI, DPI (dry powder inhaler), or solution for nebulizer q 4–6 hrs.

TABLE 7–12.
PHARMACOLOGIC THERAPY FOR STABLE COPD

PATIENT GROUP	RECOMMENDED FIRST CHOICE	ALTERNATIVE CHOICE	OTHER POSSIBLE TREATMENTS**
A	SA anticholinergic p.r.n. *or* SA beta-agonist p.r.n.	LA anticholinergic *or* LA beta$_2$-agonist *or* SA beta$_2$-agonist and SA anticholinergic	Theophylline
B	LA anticholinergic *or* LA beta$_2$-agonist	LA anticholinergic and LA beta$_2$-agonist	SA beta$_2$-agonist *and/or* SA anticholinergic Theopylline
C	ICS + LA beta$_2$-agonist *or* LA anticholinergic	LA anticholinergic and LA beta$_2$-agonsit *or* LA anticholinergic and PDE-4 Inhibitor *or* LA beta$_2$-agonist and PDE-4 Inhibitor	SA beta$_2$-agonist *and/or* SA anticholinergic Theopylline
D	ICS + LA beta$_2$-agonist *and/or* LA anticholinergic	ICS + LA beta$_2$-agonist and LA anticholinergic *or* ICS + LA beta$_2$-agonist and PDE-4 inhibitor *or* LA anthicholinergic and LA beta$_2$-agonist *or* LA anticholinergic and PDE-4 inhibitor	Carbocysteine N-acetylcyteine Sa beta$_2$-agonist *and/or* SA anticholinergic Theophylline

*Medications in each box are mentioned in alphabetical order and therefore not necessarily in order of preference.

**Medications in this column can be used alone or in combination with other options in the First and Alternative Choice colums. Glossary: SA: short-acting. LA: long-acting. ICS: inhaled corticosteroid. PDE-4: phospadiesterase-4. prn: when necessary.

Reprinted with permission from "Global Strategy for Diagnosis, Management and Prevention of COPD", page 36, at www.goldcopd.org by Global Initiative for Chronic Obstructive Lung Disease (GOLD). Copyright 2016 by Global Initiative for Chronic Obstructive Lung Disease.

- Short-acting anticholinergic: ipratropium bromide (Atrovent) MDI or solution for nebulizer q 6–8 hrs.

- Long-acting beta-agonist: salmeterol (Serevent) MDI, DPI q 12 hrs; formoterol (Foradil) MDI or DPI or (Perforomist) nebulized q 12 hrs; arformoterol (Brovana) solution for nebulizer, indacaterol (Arcapta Neohaler) DPI once daily

- Long-acting anticholinergic: aclidinium bromide (Tudorza Pressair) DPI q 12 hrs; tiatropium (Spiriva) DPI q 24 hrs; umedidnium (Incruse Ellipta) DPI q 24 hrs

- Combinatation short-acting beta-agonist plus anticholinergic inhaler: fenoterol/ipratropium (Respimat) SMI or nebulized solution (Duovent) q 6–8 hrs.; salbutamol/ipratropium MDI (Combivent) or nebulized solution (DuoNeb) q 6–8 hrs.

- Combination long-acting beta-agonist pluse anticholinergic: undacaterol/gylcopyrronium (Utibron Neohaler) DPI q 12 hrs; olodaterol/tiatropium (Rispimat) SMI q 24 hrs

- Phosphodiesterase-4 inhibitor (PDE-4): roflumilast (Daliresp) 500 mcg p.o. q.d. used as maintance therapy to prevent exacerbations; decreases inflammation

- Inhaled corticosteroids: beclomethasone (QVAR), budesonide (Pulmicort) inhaler; fluticasone (Flovent); flunisolide (Aerospan); mometasone (Asmanex). For moderate or severe disease and frequent exacerbation when long-acting bronchodilators are inadequate. Increase risk of pneumonia and fractures if used long term

- Combined long-acting beta-agonist plus inhaled corticosteroids: formeterol/budesonide (Symbicort); salmeterol/flticasone (Advair); vilamerol/fluticasone (Breo Ellipta) MDI and/or DPI

- Systemic corticosteroids: Prednisone (Deltasone) 40–60 mg p.o. daily or methylprednisolone 30–40 mg/day for 5–7 days for moderate or severe COPD exacerbations. Long-term therapy is not recommended

- Methylxanthines: Aminophylline pill, syrup, or suppository. Theophylline: short-acting or long-acting pills. Up to 800 mg/d; monitor carefully; decrease dose used in renal impairment, liver dysfunction, CHF, or age older than 55 years; must monitor serum level, maintain therapeutic range. Use only if other bronchodilators are unaffordable or unavailable

- Other medications:
  - ▷ Mucolytic agent: N-acetylcyteine (Mucomyst) nebulizer solution improves secretion
  - ▷ Low-dose macrolides: decrease inflammation (clarithromycin, azithromycin, or erythromycin)
  - ▷ Antibiotics for severe exacerbation or presence of purulent sputum
    - Most common organisms: *H. influenzae, S. pneumoniae, M. catarrhalis;* may be due to viral infection, pneumonia
    - Choice of antibiotic is based on local bacterial resistance pattern
    - Trimethoprim-sulfamethoxazole (Bactrim DS): 160/800 mg q 12 h
    - Amoxicillin-clavulanate (Augmentin): 875/125 mg q 12 h or 500/125 mg t.i.d.
    - Doxycycline (Vibramycin): 100 mg b.i.d.
    - May use a fluoroquinolone such as levofloxacin (Levaquin), moxifloxacin (Avelox); azithromycin, cephalosporins

> ▶ Antibiotics not indicated in younger patients with mild symptoms and infrequent exacerbation

> ▶ Consider use in patients under 65 years old with mild–moderate impairment of lung function (FEV1 50% or more predicted value with fewer than four exacerbations per year), or patients over 65 years old with FEV1 less than 50%, more than 4 exacerbations/year, or use of antibiotic within the last 3 months

▶ Home oxygen therapy: may improve survival in hypoxemia and cor pulmonale; initiate early if oxygen level is less than 88% on room air

▶ Noninvasive positive-pressure ventilation if acute repiratory acidosis is present

▶ α1-antitrypsin if deficient: 60 mg/kg/wk to maintain level over 80 mg/dl

How Long to Treat

▶ Chronic condition requiring ongoing therapeutic treatments and monitoring

▶ Antibiotics use in COPD exacerbation is controversial. However, is recommended in patients with increase dyspnea, sputum volume, and sputum purulence or in patients requiring mechanical ventilation. Length of antibiotic therapy is usually 5-10 days.

Special Considerations

▶ Use caution with beta blockers, cough suppressants, antihistamines, or sedatives.

▶ Discuss advance directives and end-of-life decisions.

When to Consult, Refer, Hospitalize

▶ Consult: severe exacerbation, frequent hospitalizations, age younger than 40 years, rapid progression, weight loss, severe disease, comorbidities, or surgical evaluation

▶ Refer: to pulmonary rehabilitation program

▶ Hospitalize: acute decompensation (sudden development of resting dyspnea); severe underlying COPD; new physical signs (cyanosis, peripheral edema); response failure to initial medical management; frequent exacerbations; older age; insufficient home support; need for mechanical ventilation; serious comorbidities (decompensated CHF, new arrhythmias)

Follow-Up

Expected Course

▶ Routine follow-up is essential. Monitor disease progression, development of complications, comorbidities, smoking status, exacerbation history, and pharmacotherapy.

▶ Malnutrition, cor pulmonale, hypercapnia, and pulse higher than 100 indicate poor prognosis.

Complications

▶ Malnutrition, poor sleep quality, infections, secondary polycythemia

▶ Acute or chronic respiratory failure, bullous lung disease, pneumothorax, lung cancer

▶ Arrhythmias, cor pulmonale, pulmonary HTN, cardiovascular disease

▶ Osteoporosis, anxiety/depression, metabolic syndrome, diabetes

CASE STUDIES

Case 1

A 40-year-old woman, on vacation visiting family in Florida, presents to the clinic for the first time with complaints of nonproductive cough and shortness of breath with wheezing for the past 4 days. She reports having similar symptoms in the past and was prescribed an albuterol inhaler, which relieved the symptoms. Today, she reports chest tightness and difficulties catching her breath, especially with activity.

PMH: Seasonal allergic rhinitis, HTN, GERD, obese

Medications: Norethindrone/ethinyl estradiol (Loestrin), albuterol inh p.r.n., lisinopril 10 mg q.d. p.o., omeprazole (Prilosec) 20 mg q.d. p.o.

Social History: Married, has one daughter age 13 years; lives on ranch with family; has pets, livestock, and horses; is a social worker assisting immigrant population; reports tobacco use of ½ pack of cigarettes per day since she was 18.

1.   What additional history would you like to obtain?

Exam: Temp 99.6°F, pulse 88 bmp, resp 22, blood pressure 128/40 mmHg, and resting oxygen saturation of 92%. She appears to be mildly uncomfortable but is able to speak in sentences. Skin: pink, warm, dry, intact without bruising or rash. Nose: clear sinus drainage, no sinus tenderness, mild turbinate inflammation. Mouth: pink, moist mucous membranes with postnasal drainage noted in posterior pharynx. Chest: mild wheezing that is worse with forced expiration and no other adventitious sounds audible on auscultation. Heart: regular sinus rate and rhythm without murmurs, gallops, clicks.

2.   What are the possible diagnoses?
3.   What diagnostic tests would you initially order?
4.   Your working diagnosis is asthma. What is your treatment plan?
5.   On follow-up, patient is doing much better; however, her tuberculin skin test came back positive with induration greater than 10 mm. What is your course of action now?

Case 2

A 64-year-old Native American woman presents to clinic with complaints of cough for past 8 days. States she was seen in the clinic last week and has been using OTC antihistamines and cough syrup; however, the symptoms appear to be worsening. Reports feeling warm, no energy, productive cough of green sputum. Reports her blood sugars have been higher than normal (220 mg/dl) the past 3 days. She states that her four grandchildren, who live with her, were sick 2 weeks ago with URI but are fine now.

PMH: Diabetes

Medications: Metformin 1,000 mg b.i.d. p.o., lisinopril 10 mg q.d. p.o., ASA 81 mg q.d. p.o., atorvastatin (Lipitor) 10 mg q.d. p.o.

Social History: Single, lives in a two-bedroom home with four grandchildren under the age 10 years; has no running water in home; denies tobacco, alcohol, or drug use.

1. What additional history would you obtain?

Exam: Temp 102°F, pulse 110 bpm, resp 28, blood pressure 102/78, oxygen saturation is 98% on room air. Alert, appears ill, fatigued, with continuous coughing throughout exam. HEENT: unremarkable other than clear sinus drainage and mild congestion. Neck: supple without adenopathy or thyromegally. Chest: rhonchi and decreased breath sounds, bilateral dullness to bases with percussion. Heart: sinus tachycardia without murmurs. Extremities: without signs of cyanosis or edema. Remainder of her examination is normal. Laboratory results include: complete blood count (CBC) with elevated white blood cell (WBC) count of 18,000 cells/mm3, with a differential of 85% neutrophils and 20% lymphocytes; basic metabolic panel (BMP) with glucose elevated at 196 mg/dL, creatinine 1.3 mg/dL, BUN 30 mg/dL, and normal electrolytes.

2. What are the most likely differential diagnoses?
3. What other diagnostic tests would you order?
4. What is your treatment plan?
5. What are potential complications to this condition?

Case 3

A 45-year-old man presents to the clinic with complaints of sinus congestion and pain with intermittent nosebleeds for the past 4 weeks. States he has tried OTC antihistamines and saline nasal spray with some relief. However, today, he states he is just not feeling good. He reports fatigue, body aches, low-grade fever, and night sweats for the past 5 days. This morning he reports having a productive cough of white sputum tinged with nickel-sized blood clots. He also complains of pleuritic chest pains but no shortness of breath.

PMH: Unremarkable, denies cardiac or pulmonary disease

Social History: Divorced, construction worker, has smoked a pack of cigarettes per day since he was 15, occasionally consumes alcohol (six-pack of beer every month).

1. What additional history would you like to obtain?

Exam: Temp 97.4°F, pulse 88, resp 18, blood pressure 126/72, oxygen saturation is 98% on room air. He is alert, oriented, fatigued. HEENT: unremarkable other than dry blood in nares. Chest: lungs clear bilaterally without wheezing, rhonchi, rales. Heart: regular sinus rate and rhythm without murmurs, clicks, or gallops.

2. What are the most likely differential diagnoses?
3. Which initial test is most appropriate?
4. What are the major causes of hemoptysis?
5. Your working diagnosis is bronchitis. What is your treatment plan?
6. What is your diagnosis and treatment plan in a patient who expectorates a large amount of blood over a 24-hour period?

CASE STUDIES DISCUSSION

Case 1

1. What additional history would you like to obtain?

    Characteristic symptoms of asthma: episodic wheezing (absent in severe exacerbation), chest tightness, dyspnea, chronic dry or spasmodic cough; symptoms worse at night, with exercise, exposure to cold temperatures, smoke, allergens. History of emotional stress, upper respiratory infection, rhinitis/sinusitis, eczema/atopic dermatitis, heartburn, acid reflux, nasal polyps. Any family history of asthma, allergies, or atopy. Severity of symptoms

2. What are the possible diagnoses?

    COPD, CHF, Pulmonary embolism, bronchogenic carcinoma, Acute infections, viral, pneumonia, bronchitis, TB, GERD, psychogenic cough, lung cancer, AIDS, vocal cord dysfunction, neuromuscular weakness

3. What diagnostic tests would you initially order?

    Blood test not routinely required in the diagnosis of asthma. PPD to rule out tuberculosis. Spirometry: measures forced expiratory volume in 1 second (FEV1) and forced vital capacity (FVC) in patients younger than 5 years of age. Baseline measurements are essential for diagnosis, then periodic monitoring. Bronchoprovocation testing: confirms diagnosis; used in patients with atypical presentation (normal baseline spirometry, no variable airflow limitation with spirometry or peak flow). Peak expiratory flow (PEF) used for monitoring lung status, not to confirm diagnosis. Chest X-ray: almost always normal; routinely recommended in severe asthma and in patients with co-morbid conditions and/or with atypical symptoms. Skin testing to determine allergic triggers. CT scan to rule out PE may be warrented.

4. Your working diagnosis is asthma. What is your treatment plan?

    Education. Develop written asthma action plan with patient/family. Identify and avoid factors that trigger asthma; control environmental triggers. Allergy skin testing to determine allergens if needed. Maintain hydration; increase fluids during exacerbation. Establish a patient/provider partnership with a detailed asthma action plan. Educate patients to rinse mouth out with water immediately after use of inhaler to avoid thrush. Smoking cessation/No smoking. Short-acting beta-agonist (SABA) for quick relief of acute symptoms and prevention of exercised-induced bronchospasm. Anticholinergic: Ipratropium (Atrovent) 1–2 inh or 1–2 unit dose neb q6h p.r.n. (adults only) in combination with SABA is another option. Systemic corticosteroids might also be used in more moderate-to-severe symptoms as adjunct.

5. On follow-up, patient is doing much better; however, her tuberculin skin test came back positive with induration greater than 10 mm. What is your course of action now?

    Patient has latent TB. Education and counseling regarding the importance of adherence. Education on the symptoms caused by adverse reactions of the TB treatment medications (no appetite, nausea, vomiting, jaundice, fever longer than 3 days, abdominal pain, neuropathy of fingers and toes, skin rash, easy bleeding, aching joints, dizziness, easy bruising, blurred or changed vision, ringing in ears, hearing loss, tingling/numbness around mouth). If symptom(s) present, stop medication and contact healthcare provider immediately. There are four different treatment plans for latent TB: isoniazid (INH) for 9 months or 6 months duration (depending on patient's age and or health status), rifapentine (RPT) or rifampin (RIF). Treatment must be modified in the patient is a contact of an individual with drug-resistant TB disease. Consultation with a TB expert is advised if the known source of TB infection has drug-resistant TB.

Case 2

1. What additional history would you obtain?

    Onset either abrupt, insidious, or current or recent stay at health care related facility. Recent or concurrent URI, fever, cough (productive or nonproductive), dyspnea, chills, sweats, rigors, fatigue, malaise, myalgias, chest discomfort, headache, anorexia, abdominal pain; pleuritic chest pain; patients generally feel unwell. Older adults: often present with weakness and mental status change. History of chronic obstructive pulmonary disease or human immunodeficiency virus infection. Occupation, animal exposures, and sexual history helpful to identify specific infectious agent . Recent travel history (within 2 weeks) may help identify *Legionella* pneumonia (seen on cruise ships and hotel stays). Influenza suggested with typical symptoms during peak influenza season. ICU admission, mechanical ventilation, or aspiration history.

2. What are the most likely differential diagnoses?

    Pulmonary edema, asthma exacerbation, atelectasis, acute bronchitis, bronchiolitis, bronchiectasis, COPD, foreign body aspiration, fungal pneumonia, lung abscess, respiratory failure, viral pneumonia, *pneumocystis jiroveci* pneumonia, pulmonary tuberculosis, lung cancer

3. What other diagnostic tests would you order?

    Chest X-ray: infiltrates confirmed. Routine laboratory testing usually unnecessary to establish an etiology in outpatients with CAP. Suctioned or expectorated sputum gram stain. Nasopharyngeal washings for RSV enzyme immunoassay (children). CBC, two sets of blood cultures (usually reserved for hospitalized patients), CRP, procalcinonin levels, CMP. WBC elevated (may be low in older adults or immunocompromised patients). Legionella urine antigen test if *Legionella* suspected. Bronchoalveolar lavage or protected specimen brush with quantitative cultures. Serial chest X-rays or chest CT scanning if health care associated pneumonia

4. What is your treatment plan?

    Hydration, high humidity, rest, smoking cessation, avoidance of secondhand smoke, chest physiotherapy for bacterial pneumonia, oxygen if needed, semiupright or upright positioning, noninvasive ventilation using continuous positive airway pressure (CPAP) or bilevel positive airway pressure (BiPAP) with endotracheal intubation, incentive spirometry to help prevent postoperative pneumonia.

    Empiric treatment often necessary because often not able to identify pathogen. Adult CAP outpatient (previously healthy, no antibiotics in past 3 months): Macrolide: Azithromycin (Zithromax): over 12 years old: 500 mg (two 250 mg tablets) initially, then 250 mg (one tablet) q.d. x 4 days or 500 mg p.o. daily x 3 days; or Clarithromycin (Biaxin): adults: 500 mg (one tablet) b.i.d. x 5 days; clarithromycin XL: two 500 mg tablets (1000 mg) once daily p.o. x 5 days or erythromycin (Erythrocin) 500 mg b.i.d. p.o. x 10 days (not generally used due to side effects); or Tetracycline: Doxycycline 100 mg p.o. b.i.d. x 10 days

5. What are potential complications to this condition?

    Necrotizing pneumonia, respiratory failure, empyema, abscesses, cavitation, bronchopleural fistula, sepsis

Case 3

1. What additional history would you like to obtain?

   Smoking and travel history. Onset and duration of symptoms; amount, frequency, and characteristics of sputum; is there white or purulent phlegm mixed with blood? Determine if nonpulmonary source of bleeding: vomiting, expectoration from nasopharynx, anticoagulant drug use, substance use, chest trauma. Associated symptoms: weight loss, night sweats, dyspnea, fever, fatigue, bruising, hematuria, rash, joint pain or swelling. TB exposure, dates of last TB test and chest X-ray. Past cardiac, pulmonary, hematological, or immunological history. Environmental exposure, asbestos

2. What are the most likely differential diagnoses?

   Acute and chronic bronchitis, pneumonia, tuberculosis (TB), and lung cancer

3. Which initial test is most appropriate?

   Directed by history and physical findings. Tuberculin skin test (PPD), unless positive in the past. Chest X-ray. CBC with differential and platelets. Gram stain of sputum: infection; acid-fast stain: TB. Sputum cytologic exam: malignancy. Renal function, urinalysis, liver function tests, brain natriuretic peptide (BNP). Serologic testing: antinuclear antibodies, antineutrophil cytoplasmic antibodies, antiglomerular basement membrane antibodies, anticardiolipin antibodies. Coagulation studies: PT, PTT, bleeding time if bleeding present in more than one site. Bronchoscopy for patients at risk of cancer, TB. High-resolution chest CT: complementary to bronchoscopy (test of choice for suspected small peripheral malignancies). Ventilation-perfusion scan/angiography: pulmonary embolism.

4. What are the major causes of hemoptysis?

   Acute and chronic bronchitis, pneumonia, tuberculosis (TB), and lung cancer. Inflammation of tracheobronchial mucosa due to minor erosion from bronchiectasis, sarcoidosis, Wegner's granulomatosis, lupus pneumonitis. Bronchovascular fistula, injury to pulmonary vasculature due to lung abscess, aspergillomas, or pulmonary emboli causing pulmonary infarction; trauma; foreign body. Increase pulmonary capillary pressure due to pulmonary edema, mitral stenosis, AV malformations, or granuloma formation. Bleeding disorders or anticoagulant therapy. Nonpulmonary sources: nose or gastrointestinal tract. Cryptogenic hemoptysis: negative workup; etiology unknown in 30% to 40% of patients, 90% resolve in 6 months. Cocaine and tobacco use are risk factors.

5. Your working diagnosis is bronchitis. What is your treatment plan?

   Rest, adequate hydration, steam inhalations, vaporizers, smoking cessation or avoid smoke, treat associated illnesses. Antibiotic treatment not generally recommended unless treatable pathogen has been indentified or significant comorbidities present; most cases are viral. Amoxicillin or Clarithomycin (Biaxin) or Doxycycline or Quinolone for more serious infections or Macrolide for pertussis. Consider antivirals if influenza suspected.

6. What is your diagnosis and treatment plan in a patient who expectorates a large amount of blood over a 24-hour period?

   Hemoptysis. Admit to hospital for further evaluation and management for massive blood loss (200ml/day or more).

REFERENCES

American Academy of Allergy Asthma & Immunology. (2015). AAAAI allergy & asthma medication guide. Retrieved from http://www.aaaai.org/conditions-and-treatments/treatments/drug-guide/inhaled-corticosteroids.aspx

Anzueto, A. (2010). Short-course fluoroquinolone therapy in exacerbations of chronic bronchitis and COPD. *Respiratory Medicine, 104*(10), 1396–1403.

Bidwell, J. L., & Pachner, R. W. (2005). Hemoptysis: Diagnosis and management. *American Family Physician,72*(7), 1253–1260.

Bolser, D. C. (2006). Cough suppressant and pharmacologic protussive therapy: ACP evidence-based clinical practice guidelines. *Chest, 129*(Suppl. 1), 238S–249S.

Centers for Disease Control and Prevention. (2014a). *TB in children in the United States.* Retrieved from http://www.cdc.gov/tb/topic/populations/TBinChildren/default.htm

Centers for Disease Control and Prevention. (2014b). *Tuberculin skin testing for tuberculosis.* Retrieved from http://www.cdc.gov/tb/publications/factsheets/testing/skintesting.htm

Centers for Disease Control and Prevention. (2015). Trends in tuberculosis–United States, 2011. *Morbidity and Mortality Weekly Report (MMWR), 64*(10), 265–269. Retrieved from http://www.cdc.gov/mmwr/preview/mmwrhtml/mm6111a2.htm

Cherry, J. D. (2008). Croup. *New England Journal of Medicine, 358*(4), 384–391.

Crawford-Faucher, A. (2008). Levofloxacin appears safe and effective for CAP in children. *American Family Physician, 77*(6), 838–840.

Domino, F. J., Baldor, R. A., Golding, J., & Grimes, J. A. (2014). *The 5-minute clinical consult, 2015* (23rd ed.). Philadelphia, PA: Lippincott, Williams & Wilkins.

Genentech. (2015). Xolair. Retrieved from http://www.gene.com/download/pdf/xolair_prescribing.pdf

Gilbert, D. N., Moellering, R. C. Jr., Eliopoulos, G. M., Sande, M. A., & Chambers, H. F. (2008). *Sanford guide to antimicrobial therapy.* Vienna, VA: Antimicrobial Therapy.

Global Initiative for Chronic Obstructive Disease (GOLD). (2016). *At-a-glance outpatient management reference for chronic obstructive pulmonary disease (COPD).* Retrieved from http://goldcopd.org/pocket-guide-copd-diagnosis-management-prevention-2016/

Graber, M. A., Dachs, R., & Darby-Stewart, A. (2008). Fluticasone or salmeterol alone vs. combination therapy for COPD. *American Family Physician, 77*(5), 587–588.

Hall, R. G., Leff, R. D., & Gumbo, T. (2009). Treatment of active pulmonary tuberculosis in adults: Current standards and recent advances. *Pharmacotherapy, 29*(12), 1468–1481.

Hao, Q., Lu, Z., Dong, B. R., Huang, C. Q., & Wu, T. (2015). Probiotics for preventing acute upper respiratory tract infections. Cochrane Database Sys Rev, 2015; 2:CD006895. Retrieved from http://www.ncbi.nlm.nih.gov/pubmed/21901706

Hay, W.W., Levin, M. J., Deterding, R. R., & Abzug, M. J. (2014). *CURRENT diagnosis & treatment: Pediatrics* (22nd ed.). New York, NY: Lange/McGraw-Hill Education.

Llor, C., Moragas, A., Bayona, C., Morros, R., Pera, H., Plana-Ripoll, O., ... Miravitlles, M. (2013). Efficacy of anti-inflammatory or antibiotic treatment inpatients with non-complicated acute bronchitis and discoloured sputum: A randomized control trial. *BMJ, 347*, f5762. Retrieved from http://www.bmj.com/content/347/bmj.f5762.long

Mannino, D. M., & Buist, S. (2007). Global burden of COPD: Risk factors, prevalence, and future trends. *Lancet, 370*(9589), 765–773.

McPhee, S. J., Papadakis, M. A., & Tierney, L. M. (Eds.). (2008). *Current medical diagnosis and treatment* (47th ed.). New York, NY: Lange Medical Books/McGraw-Hill.

Musher, D. M., & Thorner, A. R. (2014). Community-acquired pneumonia. *New England Journal of Medicine, 371*(17), 1619–1628.

National Cancer Institute. (2015a). *Non–small cell lung cancer (PDQ) treatment – Health professionals.* Retrieved from http://www.cancer.gov/types/lung/patient/ non-small-cell-lung-treatment-pdq#section/_164

National Cancer Institute. (2015b). *Small cell lung cancer (PDQ) treatment – Health professionals.* Retrieved from http://www.cancer.gov/types/lung/patient/ small-cell-lung-treatment-pdq#section/_50

National Cancer Institute. (2015c). *SEER stat fact sheets: Lung and bronchus cancer.* Retrieved from http://seer.cancer.gov/statfacts/html/lungb.html

National Heart, Lung, and Blood Institute. (2012). *Expert panel report 3 (EPR 3): Asthma care quick reference diagnosing and managing asthma.* Retrieved from http://www.nhlbi.nih.gov/ files/docs/guidelines/asthma_qrg.pdf

National Lung Screening Trial Research Team. (2011). Reduced lung-cancer mortality with low-dose computed tomographic screening. *New England Journal of Medicine, 365*(5), 395–409.

Petruzella, F. D., Gorelick, M. H., & Marc, H. (2010). Current therapies in bronchiolitis. *Pediatric Emergency Care, 26*(4), 302–307.

Pickering, L. K. (2012). *Red book: 2012 report of the committee on infectious disease* (29th ed.). Elk Grove Village, IL: American Academy of Pediatrics.

Qaseem, A., Wilt, T. J., Weinberger, S. E., Hanania, N. A., Criner, G., van der Molen, T., . . . European Respiratory Society. (2011). Diagnosis and management of stable chronic obstructive pulmonary disease: A clinical practice guideline update from the American College of Physicians, American College of Chest Physicians, American Thoracic Society, and European Respiratory Society. *Annals of Internal Medicine, 155*(3), 179–191.

Rodriguez-Molinero, A., Narvaiza, L., Ruiz, J., & Galvez-Barron, C. (2013). Normal respiratory rate and peripheral blood oxygen saturation in the older adult population. *Journal of the American Geriatrics Society, 61*(12), 2238–2240.

Stupka, E., & deShazo, R. (2009). Asthma in seniors: Part 1. Evidence for underdiagnosis, undertreatment and increasing morbidity and mortality. *American Journal of Medicine, 122*(1), 6–11.

Thomson, A., & Harris, M. (2011). Community-acquired pneumonia in children: What's new? *Throax, 66*(10), 927–928.

U.S. Food and Drug Administration. (2008). Public health advisory: FDA recommends that over-the-counter (OTC) cough and cold products not be used for infants and children under 2 years of age. Retrieved from http://www.fda.gov/NewsEvents/Newsroom/ PressAnnouncements/2008/ucm051137.htm

Watkins, R. R., & Lemonovich, T. L. (2011). Diagnosis and management of community-acquired pneumonia in adults. *American Family Physician, 83*(11), 1299–1306.

Wunderink, R. G., & Waterer, G. W. (2014). Community-acquired pneumonia. *New England Journal of Medicine, 370*(6), 543–551.

CHAPTER 8

CARDIOVASCULAR DISORDERS

Mary Elizabeth Duffy, DNP, FNP-BC, ACNP-BC, DCC

GENERAL APPROACH

▶ Heart disease and stroke continue to be the leading causes of death in the United States for both men and women.

▶ Systolic blood pressure greater 140 mm Hg is a more important risk factor than elevated diastolic blood pressure in people over 50 years of age.

▶ Primary and secondary prevention strategies are essential to reducing the risk of heart disease and stroke. Identification of high-risk patients through screening is critical to providing preventive education, early treatment, and appropriate referral.

▶ Evidence-based national guidelines such as the "2014 Evidence-Based Guideline for the Management of High Blood Pressure in Adults: Report from the Panel Members Appointed to the Eighth Joint National Committee (JNC 8)" and *2013 ACC/ AHA Guideline on the Treatment of Blood Cholesterol to Reduce Atherosclerotic Cardiovascular Risk in Adults: A Report of the American College of Cardiology/ American Heart Association Task Force on Practice Guidelines*

▶ Patients should be assessed according to risk stratification and treated to obtain optimal control with individualized drug therapy guided by each patient's clinical profile.

▶ Problems related to myocardial infarction are 1 of the 4 leading causes of malpractice lawsuits.

▶ The clinician must assess each patient with chest pain and determine whether the condition is life-threatening or safe to manage on an outpatient basis.

Note: The Test Reference List issued by ANCC for the current exam references the "2014 Evidence-Based Guideline for the Management of High Blood Pressure in Adults: Report from the Panel Members Appointed to the Eighth Joint National Committee (JNC 8)." However, the JNC 8 is not all-inclusive and the author has chosen to reference the JNC 7 for those subjects not covered in the JNC 8 since many practitioners still follow these guidelines.

▶ Nonpharmacologic measures are often effective; educate patients to modify lifestyle risk factors.

▶ Compliance can be a major problem because of health beliefs, cost of medications, side effects, dosing regimens, and difficulty making lifestyle changes; individualize and simplify treatment and continue to re-educate and support.

▶ It is important to maintain knowledge of drugs from each class to reduce the potential for medication errors, interactions, and complications.

▶ Individuals understanding health practices and adhering to therapeutic regimes is critical to reducing health disparities and reducing the risk of heart disease.

▶ Based on survey responses from 2003 to 2012, researchers found that 1 in 3 adults aged 20 years or older has metabolic syndrome. Overall, metabolic syndrome is more common in women than in men and is most common among Hispanic people. Researchers also found that risk of metabolic syndrome increases with age. According to National Health Statistics (2009), only 18% of young adults aged 20–39 years have metabolic syndrome, while 47% of adults over 60 years old are affected by this condition.

▶ The clinician should apply the new American Heart Association/American Stroke Association guidelines on the early management of acute ischemic stroke.

▶ The clinician should consider cardiovascular disease potential in children and apply the 2011 Integrated Guidelines for Cardiovascular Health and Risk Reduction in Children and Adolescents.

RED FLAGS

▶ *Chest pain* should be triaged and evaluated promptly to rule out any life-threatening conditions. An immediate brief history will include the age of patient; past medical history focused on cardiac and pulmonary problems; and onset, location, radiation, quality, intensity, and duration of pain. Determine associated symptoms, relieving and aggravating factors, pattern of pain, risk factors for cardiac disease, and family history of hypertension or cardiac disease. Assess vital signs, lung and heart sounds, obtain 12-lead ECG and pulse oximetry, and integrate assessment findings and risk factors to determine the best management plan. If there are no ECG changes, perform a right-sided 12-lead ECG (and if there is ST depression, leads V1 and V2), obtain a posterior 12-lead ECG, then continue to monitor for 10 minutes. If patient has right-sided ECG changes or known aortic stenosis *do not* give nitroglycerin. Nitroglycerin should not be given to someone who has recently received a phosphodiesterase inhibitor (i.e., sildenafil, vardenafil, or tadalafil)

▶ Myocardial infarction (MI) patients may present with severe ischemic pain lasting more than 20–30 minutes; is not relieved with nitroglycerin; and may be accompanied by nausea, vomiting, anxiety, diaphoresis, pre-syncope, syncope, and dyspnea. (MI patients may also have atypical presentation with pain in the arm, jaw, neck, or back without chest pain. Atypical presentation in women includes fatigue without pain.)

▶ If there is an acute episode of chest pain, administer oxygen and nitroglycerin, call 911, and transport to emergency facility. For nonacute episodes, consult with a physician, refer to a cardiologist, or pursue workup based on history and physical.

▶ Sudden, spontaneous tachycardia of 140–220 beats per minute is known as *paroxysmal atrial tachycardia* (PAT) and may occur in healthy individuals, older adults, those with chronic obstructive pulmonary disease (COPD), and as a sign of digitalis toxicity. Patients may report that it starts and ends abruptly, lasts minutes to several hours, and may be accompanied by anxiety, dizziness, mild chest pain, and shortness of breath. Rhythm is regular and ECG shows P waves characteristically different than before it started. If asymptomatic and nonrecurrent in healthy individuals, it does not need treatment. If of long duration and symptomatic, patient should be referred to the emergency department (ED) for treatment. If recurrent, refer to a cardiologist.

▶ Signs and symptoms associated with pneumothorax or pulmonary emboli include sudden onset of chest pain, hypotension, syncope, dyspnea, tachypnea, and tachycardia. If patient has a risk for thrombophlebitis (recent surgery, immobility, oral contraceptive use) or a recent fracture, consider pulmonary emboli. Some patients with pulmonary emboli may be asymptomatic. Acute presentation requires transfer to an emergency facility.

▶ A hypertensive patient with sudden onset of knife-like or tearing pain in the chest or upper abdomen may have a dissecting aneurysm. Initiate emergency transport system immediately. *Do not* give aspirin if you suspect dissecting aneurysm.

▶ When using statin medications and fibric acids, be alert for signs and symptoms of rhabdomyolysis (muscle pain or weakness) that can lead to renal failure.

▶ Metabolic syndrome, with its constellation of hypertension, diabetes mellitus, hyperlipidemia, and abdominal obesity, is associated with increased risk for heart disease and stroke.

HEART SOUNDS

▶ Evaluation of heart sounds is an important part of the assessment of any patient with a cardiovascular problem.

▶ S_1 = closure of the tricuspid and mitral valves (atrioventricular [AV] valves); heard best at the fifth left interspace medial to the midclavicular line at the left lower sternal border (LLSB)

▶ S_2 = closure of the aortic and pulmonary valves (semilunar valves); best heard at the second left interspace close to the sternal border

  ▷ Normal splitting of S_2 during inspiration is due to greater negative pressure in thoracic cavity = increased systemic venous return = increased blood volume in the right ventricle (RV) = delayed closure of the pulmonary valve

  ▷ Abnormal splitting of S_2 (wide splitting, narrow splitting, or single S_2) is seen in conditions where the RV ejection time is prolonged (atrial septal defect, pulmonary stenosis, right bundle branch block [RBBB]) and the pulmonary valve closes early (pulmonary hypertension), or where only one semilunar valve is present (pulmonary atresia, aortic atresia, truncus arteriosus)

▶ S_3 = low-frequency sound heard early in diastole; related to the rapid filling of the ventricles

  ▷ Heard best at apex or LLSB

  ▷ With tachycardia, forms a "Kentucky" gallop

▷ May be normal in children and during pregnancy, except that a loud S_3 is abnormal (usually audible in conditions with dilated ventricles and decreased compliance)

▶ S_4 = low-frequency sound heard late in diastole

▷ Rare in infants and children

▷ Always pathological; seen in conditions with decreased ventricular compliance

▷ With tachycardia, forms a "Tennessee" gallop

▶ Gallop = rapid triple rhythm

▷ Results from the combination of a loud S_3 (with or without S_4) and tachycardia

COMMON CARDIOVASCULAR DISORDERS

Hypertension

Description

Hypertension (HTN) is defined by the "Seventh Report of the Joint National Committee on Prevention, Detection, Evaluation, and Treatment of High Blood Pressure" (JNC 7) in 2003 as a persistent elevation of blood pressure measured on three separate occasions with a systolic blood pressure (SBP) >140 mm Hg and/or diastolic blood pressure (DBP) >90 (see Table 8–1). It is further classified as either primary (essential, about 95% of cases) or secondary.

The most recent "Report From the Panel Members Appointed to the Eighth Joint National Committee (JNC 8)" in 2014 does not define HTN but recommends blood pressure treatment thresholds, goals, and medical management and lifestyle goals (continued throughout management; see Table 8–2). JNC 8 recommendations are limited to evidence derived from randomized controlled trials (RCTs) alone (systematic reviews or other trials were not reviewed) in an effort to answer the following three questions:

1. In adults with hypertension, does initiating antihypertensive pharmacologic therapy at specific BP thresholds improve health outcomes?

2. In adults with hypertension, does treatment with antihypertensive pharmacologic therapy to a specified BP goal lead to improvements in health outcomes?

3. In adults with hypertension, do various antihypertensive drugs or drug classes differ in comparative benefits and harms on specific health outcomes?

In children, HTN is defined as a systolic or diastolic blood pressure greater than the 95th percentile for gender and age on at least 3 separate occasions (see Figure 8–1).

Etiology

▶ Hypertension is due to an increase in peripheral arterial resistance.

▶ Theories of causation include impaired renin-angiotensin cascade, sympathetic nervous system hyperactivity, defect in natriuresis (sodium excretion), and elevated intracellular calcium (excess arterial constriction).

▶ Essential hypertension is usually idiopathic or may be due to renal retention of salt and water, increased endogenous pressure activity, or both. Essential hypertension accounts for most high blood pressure (HBP).

TABLE 8–1.
JNC 7 CLASSIFICATION OF BLOOD PRESSURE AND RECOMMENDATIONS FOR TREATMENT FOR HYPERTENSION

BP CLASSIFICATION	WITHOUT COMPELLING INDICATION	WITH COMPELLING INDICATION
Prehypertension 130–139/85–89	Lifestyle modification	Drugs for compelling indication
Stage 1 140–159/90–99	Diuretic for most; may consider ACEI, ARB, BB, CCB,* or combination	Drug(s) for the compelling indications; other antihypertensive drugs (diuretics, ACEI, ARB, BB, CCB) as needed
Stage 2 160+/100+	Two-drug combination for most (usually diuretic and ACEI, ARB, BB, or CCB)	Drug(s) for the compelling indications; other antihypertensive drugs (diuretics, ACEI, ARB, BB, CCB) as needed

ACEI = ACE inhibitor, ARB = angiotensin II receptor blockers, BB = beta-blocker, CCB = calcium channel blocker

Adapted from "Seventh Report of the Joint National Committee on Prevention, Detection, Evaluation, and Treatment of High Blood Pressure," by A. V. Chobanian et al. (2003), *Hypertension, 42*(6), pp. 1206–1252.

TABLE 8-2.
JNC 8 SUMMARY OF BP GOAL, TREATMENT GUIDELINES, AND MEDICATION FOR BLOOD PRESSURE FOR ADULTS AGED 18 YEARS AND OLDER

CATEGORY	BLOOD PRESSURE GOAL IN MM HG SYSTOLIC	DIASTOLIC	INITIAL DRUG TREATMENT OPTIONS
Age >60 years	<150	<90	*Non-Black people*: thiazide-type diuretics, ACEI, ARB* or CCB *Black people*: thiazide-type diuretic or CCB
Age <60 years	<140	<90	*Non-Black people*: thiazide-type diuretics, ACEI, ARB* or CCB *Black people*: thiazide-type diuretic or CCB
All Ages +Diabetes Mellitus (DM) Present No Chronic Kidney Disease (CKD)	<140	<90	*Non-Black people*: thiazide-type diuretics, ACEI, ARB* or CCB *Black people*: thiazide-type diuretic or CCB
All Ages CKD present with or without DM	<140	<90	ACEI or ARB*

*Do not use ACE inhibitor in conjunction with ARB in same patient.

If goal BP is not achieved within 1 month of treatment, increase the dose of initial medication or add one form a different drug class. If two drug therapies are unsuccessful in lowering to target BP add a third agent from recommended drug classes. In patients whose goal BP is not reached with 4 agents from different recommended drug classes, use agents from other drug classes and/or refer the patient. Angiotensin converting enzyme inhibitor (ACEI), angiotensin receptor blocker (ARB), calcium channel blocker (CCB)

Adapted from "2014 Evidence Based Guideline for the Management of High Blood Pressure in Adults. Report from the Panel Members Appointed to the Eighth Report of the Joint National Committee (JNC 8)," by P. A. James et al. (2014), *JAMA, 311*(5), pp. 501–520.

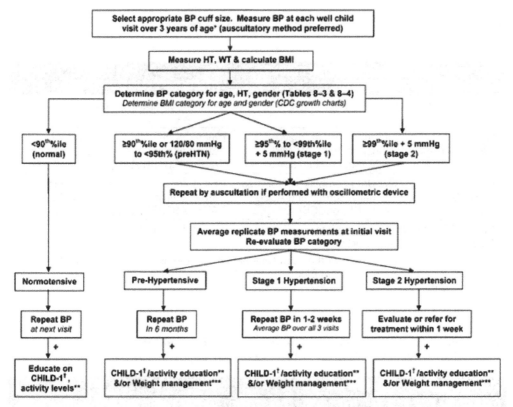

Reprinted from *Expert Panel on Integrated Guidelines for Cardiovascular Health and Risk Reduction in Children and Adolescents: Summary Report,* by the National Heart Lung and Blood Institute, 2012. Retrieved from https://www.nhlbi.nih.gov/files/docs/peds_guidelines_sum.pdf (p. 29)

FIGURE 8–1.
BLOOD PRESSURE EVALUATION FOR CHILDREN 3 TO 18 YEARS OF AGE, MM HG

▶ Secondary hypertension is caused by renovascular disease, vascular problems such as aortic coarctation or renal artery stenosis, endocrine dysfunction such as in Cushing's syndrome and pheochromocytoma, neurologic disorders, and certain medications (oral contraceptives, corticosteroids, sympathomimetics).

Incidence and Demographics (as per National, Heart, Lung, and Blood Institute)

▶ In the U.S. population: approximately 77.9 million (1 out of every 3) adults have high blood pressure:

▷ Non-Hispanic Black people: 42.6% of men and 47% of women

▷ Non-Hispanic White people: 33.4% of men and 30.7% of women

▷ Mexican Americans: 30.1% of men and 28.8 percent of women

▶ In the pediatric population: 1.2%–13%

▶ The younger the child and the higher the blood pressure, the more likely the hypertension is secondary.

▶ Secondary hypertension generally develops before age 35 or after age 55.

▶ More than one third of patients with hypertension remain undiagnosed even though they may have seen a healthcare provider; at least one third of patients who are diagnosed are not treated to goal BP.

▶ Among hypertensive Americans, approximately 82% are aware of their condition and 75% are taking an antihypertensive medication, but only 53% have their blood pressure at target goal.

Risk Factors

▶ *Major*

▷ >45 years of age; men and postmenopausal women or >55 years of age

▷ Family history of cardiovascular disease in women under age 65 or men under age 55

▷ Prehypertension, hyperlipidemia, low HDL cholesterol (<40 mg/dl), hypertriglyceridemia (>200 mg/dl), diabetes mellitus (DM), cigarette smoking

▶ *Other*

▷ Sedentary lifestyle, obesity, metabolic syndrome, stress, excessive intake of sodium, high alcohol intake, pregnancy, renal disease, African American heritage, coronary artery disease, left ventricular hypertrophy, cerebrovascular disease, sleep apnea, some medications (oral contraceptives, corticosteroids, NSAIDs, sympathomimetics)

Prevention and Screening

▶ Patient education for prevention of risk factors (see Box 8–1)

▶ Blood pressure screening (see Table 8–3) and monitoring using proper technique and equipment

Assessment

History

▶ Usually asymptomatic in essential HTN; "silent killer"

▶ Occipital headaches can occur upon awakening with severe HTN, dizziness, rarely epistaxis

▶ Somnolence, confusion, visual disturbances, nausea, vomiting (hypertensive encephalopathy)

▶ Personal history for risk factors; family history for hypertension

▶ Past medical history for comorbid conditions such as gout or sexual dysfunction, or for effects on target organs

Physical Exam

▶ Elevated blood pressure (usually the only sign)

▶ Body mass index (BMI) may be over 30; children may be obese, or thin with failure to thrive

BOX 8–1.

LIFESTYLE MODIFICATIONS FOR PREVENTION AND MANAGEMENT OF HYPERTENSION BASED ON RECOMMENDATIONS OF JNC-8 LIFESTYLE WORK GROUP

- **Stop smoking**.
- Lose weight if overweight, and maintain ideal body weight reduce intake of dietary saturated fat and cholesterol.
- Limit alcohol intake to no more than 1 oz (30 mL) ethanol (e.g., 24 oz [720 mL] beer, 10 oz [300 mL] wine, or 2 oz [60 mL] 100-proof whiskey) per day; 0.5 oz (15 mL) ethanol per day for women and lighter-weight people.
- Moderate to vigorous aerobic activity 40 minutes 3 to 4 times per week. Aerobic physical activity such as brisk walking 30 minutes per day
- Reduce sodium intake to no more than 2,400 mg sodium. If recommended goals for sodium are not attainable, reduce intake by at least 1,000 mg/day, which lowers BP and reduces cardiovascular disease (CVD) by approximately 30%.
- Maintain adequate intake of dietary potassium (approximately 90 mmol or 2 g per day), calcium (approximately 1,000 mg), and 300 mg magnesium daily.

Adapted from "2013 AHA/ACC Guideline on Lifestyle Management to Reduce Cardiovascular Risk: A Report of the American College of Cardiology/American Heart Association Task Force on Practice Guidelines," by RH Eckel, et al. (2014), *J Am Coll Cardiol.*, *63*(25_PA). doi:10.1016/j.jacc.2013.11.003.

TABLE 8–3.
SCREENING TESTS FOR CAUSES OF HYPERTENSION

SUSPECTED HYPERTENSION CAUSE	TEST
Chronic kidney disease	Estimated glomerular filtration rate (GFR)
Coarctation of the aorta	CT angiography
Cushing's syndrome and other glucocorticoid excess states including chronic steroid therapy	History; dexamethasone suppression test
Drug-induced or –related	History, drug screening
Pheochromocytoma	24-hour urinary metanephrine and normetanephrine
Primary aldosteronism and other mineralocorticoid excess states	24-hour urinary aldosterone level or specific measurements of other mineralocorticoids
Renovascular hypertension	Doppler flow study; magnetic resonance angiography
Sleep apnea	Sleep study with O_2 saturation
Thyroid/parathyroid disease	TSH, serum parathyroid hormone (PTH)

Adapted from *Seventh Report of the Joint National Committee on Prevention, Detection, Evaluation, and Treatment of High Blood Pressure* (JNC 7; NIH Publication No. 04-5230), by National Heart, Lung, and Blood Institute. Bethesda, MD: National Institutes of Health, 2004.

▶ Abdominal obesity: waist circumference >40 inches in men and >35 inches in women

▶ S_4 gallop, possible displaced point of maximal intensity (PMI) because of ventricular hypertrophy

▶ Renal artery bruit, carotid bruit, hepatosplenomegaly, edema, decreased peripheral pulses, funduscopic changes (such as AV nicking) with secondary HTN; or target organ damage—angina/MI, transient ischemic attack (TIA), stroke, peripheral arterial disease

Diagnostic Studies

▶ Laboratory tests: urinalysis, urine microalbumin, CBC, blood urea nitrogen (BUN), creatinine, calcium, uric acid, lipid profile, serum electrolytes, glucose

▶ For secondary HTN: chest x-ray; echocardiogram; renal ultrasound; intravenous pyelogram (IVP); 24-hour urine for aldosterone, free cortisol, catecholamines, and creatinine; dexamethasone challenge test; thyroid profile; renal function tests (BUN/CR); screening panels for various endocrine disorders (thyroid-stimulating hormone [TSH]), urine catecholamines, and vanillylmandelic acid)

Differential Diagnosis

Essential vs. secondary causes of hypertension

▶ Pregnancy

▶ Renal artery stenosis

▶ Renal failure

▶ Renal parenchymal disease (polycystic or dysplastic kidneys)

▶ Coarctation of aorta

▶ Patent ductus arteriosus

▶ Aortic insufficiency

▶ Pheochromocytoma

▶ Cushing's disease

▶ Hyperaldosteronism

▶ Hyperthyroidism

▶ Neuroblastoma

▶ Increased intracranial pressure

▶ Hypervolemia

▶ Bronchopulmonary dysplasia

▶ Stevens-Johnson syndrome

Management

Nonpharmacologic Treatment

▶ Lifestyle modification as in Box 8–1; avoidance of oral contraceptives in at-risk individuals

▶ DASH (Dietary Approaches to Stop Hypertension) Diet, decongestants, etc.

▶ Monitor for target organ damage (TOD); target blood pressure according to risk group.

▶ Take part in aerobic activity, such as brisk walking 30 minutes per day or moderate to vigorous activity 3 to 4 days a week averaging 40 minutes each session.

Pharmacologic Treatment

▶ Compelling indications for treating with medications

 ▷ Heart failure (ACEi/ARB, beta blocker [BB], diuretic, spironolction)

 ▷ Post–myocardial infarction (ACEi/ARB and BB)

 ▷ High coronary disease risk (ACEi/ARB, BB)

 ▷ Recurrent stroke prevention (ACEi, diuretic)

 ▷ Diabetes (ACEi/ARB, CCB, diuretic)

 ▷ CKD (ACEi/ARB)

 ▷ Pregnancy (first line is labetolol, then nifedipine, methyldopa)

▶ Children (refer to specialist for treatment)

 ▷ Antihypertensive therapy indicated for HTN treatment in children when the following reasons apply:

   ▶ Family history of early complications of hypertension

   ▶ Presence of coronary artery risk factors

   ▶ Dangerously high blood pressure (>12 mm Hg over the 99th percentile diastolic or >25 mm Hg over 99th percentile systolic) or presence of end-organ damage (ocular, central nervous system [CNS], cardiac, or renal)

 ▷ Medical management begins with a single-drug regimen in combination with nonpharmacologic measures; additional drug therapies are initiated as needed.

 ▷ Diuretics (contraindicated in patients with renal failure)

   ▶ Furosemide (Lasix): 1–8 mg/kg/day divided q 4–12 h

   ▶ Spironolactone (Aldactone): 1–3 mg/kg/day divided q 6–12 h

   ▶ Hydrochlorothiazide (HCTZ): 1–3 mg/kg/day divided q 12 h

 ▷ Vasodilators (use with adrenergic inhibitor to decrease flushing, headache, tachycardia, salt retention)

   ▶ Hydralazine (Apresoline): 0.75–7.5 mg/kg/day divided q 6 h

 ▷ Angiotensin-converting enzyme (ACE) inhibitors (should be used with diuretics to enhance effectiveness; avoid in patients with bilateral renal artery stenosis or transplanted kidney)

   ▶ Captopril (Capoten): 1–3 mg/kg/day divided q 8–24 h

   ▶ Enalapril (Vasotec): 0.1–0.5 mg/kg/day divided q 12–24 h

 ▷ Calcium antagonists of limited use in the pediatric population

   ▶ Nifedipine (Procardia): 0.25–3 mg/kg/day divided q 4–6 h

 ▷ Adrenergic inhibitors (propranolol is contraindicated in patients with asthma)

   ▶ Propranolol (Inderal): 1–8 mg/kg/day divided q 6–12 h

▶ Atenolol (Tenormin): 1–8 mg/kg/day divided q 12–24 h

▶ Adults (see Table 8-4)

▷ Diuretics: first-line therapy; avoid with history of gout, DM, dyslipidemia

▶ Target groups: heart failure (HF), osteoporosis, older patients, African Americans, smokers

▷ Beta-blockers: first-line therapy; avoid with asthma, older White people, conduction disorders, bradycardia

▶ Target groups: young White people, post-MI, angina, migraine, arrhythmias, tremor, hyperthyroid, preoperative; with HF use carvedilol (Coreg); with liver disease use labetalol (Trandate); use with caution in diabetes mellitus, depression

▷ ACE inhibitors (ACEIs)

▶ Target groups: persons with DM, CHF, post-MI; White patients; first-line agent for all adult patients with CKD

▶ Avoid use in Black patients, renal stenosis, elevated creatinine

▷ Angiotensin II receptor blockers (ARBs); avoid in renovascular disease

▶ Target groups: identical to those for ACEIs, with inability to tolerate ACEi because of cough

▷ Calcium channel blockers (CCBs); contraindicated in conduction disorders

▶ Target groups: patients with angina, coronary artery disease (CAD), migraine, arrhythmia (nondihydropyridine CCB); Black people; older persons with isolated systolic HTN

▶ Avoid grapefruit, cimetidine, ranitidine

▶ Avoid beta-blocker and calcium channel blocker combined (nondihydropyridine)

▶ Short-acting nifedipine increases cardiac morbidity

▷ Alpha I adrenergic blockers: second-line therapy

▶ Target groups: benign prostatic hypertrophy, dyslipidemia

▶ First-dose syncope: administer q.h.s.; combination with NSAID may decrease effectiveness

▷ Central alpha 2 agonists; may cause rebound hypertension on withdrawal

▶ Target groups: monotherapy failure

▷ Peripheral alpha 2 agonists; limited use

▷ Renin inhibitors

▶ Direct renin inhibitor. Interferes with conversion of angiotensinogen to angiotensin I. Blocks the renin-angiotensin-aldosterone system

▶ Black box warning in pregnancy—teratogenic

▷ Hyperkalemia, GI disturbance, angioedema

How Long to Treat
▶ Treatment is usually lifelong

TABLE 8–4.
EVIDENCE-BASED DOSING FOR ANTIHYPERTENSIVE MEDICATIONS FOR ADULTS WITH HYPERTENSION BASED ON RANDOMIZED CONTROL TRIALS JNC-8

DRUG	DOSAGES	SIDE EFFECTS
DIURETICS		
Hydrochlorothiazide (HCTZ)	12.5–50 mg	Anorexia, nausea, vomiting, cramping due to potassium and possibly sodium depletion; increased glucose, uric acid levels
Chlorthalidone	12.5–25 mg	
Indapamide (Lozol)	1.25–2.5 mg	
POTASSIUM SPARING DIURETICS		
Spironolactone	25–50 mg	Chlorthalidone and Spironolactone may cause gynecomastia and hyperkalemia. Consider loop diuretic if GFR <40.
Amiloride	5–10 mg	
Triamterene	100 mg	
LOOP DIURETIC		
Furosemide	20–80 mg twice/day	
Torsemide	10–40 mg once or twice daily	
BETA-ADRENERGIC BLOCKERS		
Metoprolol (Lopressor), tartrate or succinate	50–100 mg (1–2x/day)	Not first line agent, target pts with CHF, CAD, post MI. Bradycardia, depression, fatigue, exercise intolerance, asthma
Atenolol (Tenormin)	25–50 mg	
ACE INHIBITORS		
Lisinopril (Prinivil, Zestril)	10 mg	15% have cough, hyperkalemia, ankle swelling, angioedema, leukopenia
Benzepril, fosinopril or quinapril	10 mg	
Captopril (Capoten)	50 mg	
Enalapril (Vasotec)	5 mg	
ANGIOTENSIN RECEPTOR BLOCKERS		
Eprosartan (Teveten)	400 mg	Rare side effects (angioedema, hyperkalemia)
Candesartan (Atacand)	8–32 mg	
Losartan (Cozaar)	50–100 mg	
Valsartan (Diovan)	80–320 mg	
Irbesartan (Avapro)	75 mg	
CALCIUM CHANNEL BLOCKERS		
Dihydropyridines		
Amlodipine (Norvasc)	2.5–10 mg once a day	Peripheral edema, nausea, headache, constipation
Nifedipine	30–90 mg once daily	
Non-dihydropyridines		
Diltiazem (Cardizem)	180–180 mg	Lower HR and proteinuria
Verapamil	80–120 mg 3x/day	
Verapamil ER	ER 240–480 mg once daily	

DRUG	DOSAGES	SIDE EFFECTS
VASODILATORS		
Hydralazine	25–100 mg twice daily	May cause reflex tachycardia and fluid retention
Minoxidil	5–10 mg daily	
ALPHA BLOCKERS		
Terazosin	1–5 mg daily	May cause orthostatic HTN
Doxazosin	1–4 mg once bedtime	
CENTRALLY ACTING AGENTS		
Clonidine	0.1–0.2 mg twice daily	For resistant HTN, clonidine is available in patch form.
Methyldopa	250–500 mg twice daily	

ACEIs = angiotensin converting enzyme inhibitors

Adapted from *2014 evidence-based guideline for the management of high blood pressure in adults*. Report from the panel members appointed to the Eighth Joint National Committee (JNC 8). (2014), Retrieved at https://www.guideline.gov/summaries/summary/48192/2014-evidencebased-guideline-for-the-management-of-high-blood-pressure-in-adults-Report-from-the-panel-members-appointed-to-the-Eighth-Joint-National-Committee-JNC-8.

Special Considerations

▶ Start with low doses for geriatric patients to avoid serious side effects.

▶ Pregnancy: can continue drug(s) used before pregnancy, except ACE inhibitors and ARBs; beta-blockers may cause growth retardation in early pregnancy; if HTN develops during pregnancy, use labetolol, nifedipine, or methyldopa (see Table 8–5).

When to Consult, Refer, Hospitalize

▶ Consult with a physician or specialist when initiating drug treatment for a child with HTN.

▶ Refer as needed for evaluation and treatment of secondary causes of hypertension.

▶ Refer to a specialist (nephrologist, cardiologist, ophthalmologist) for end-organ damage.

▶ Consult physician when no response to first-line therapy, escalating HTN, or HTN emergencies (hypertensive encephalopathy, severe preeclampsia/eclampsia, cerebral hemorrhage, dissecting aortic aneurysm, unstable angina, MI, pulmonary embolism, severe heart failure); hospitalization may be necessary.

Follow-Up

▶ Frequent initial follow-up until normotensive, then routine visits every 3–6 months depending on patient clinical situation; for BP >180 systolic or 110 diastolic, follow-up in 48 to 72 hours

▶ Improve adherence by keeping treatment simple and inexpensive; educate patient and family about hypertension; encourage lifestyle modification along with drug treatment.

Expected Course

▶ Usually requires lifelong treatment; progression depends on ability to control the disease

Complications

▶ Target organ damage includes stroke, coronary heart disease, left ventricular hypertrophy, congestive heart failure, kidney failure, aortic dissection, retinopathy

TABLE 8–5.
TREATMENT OF CHRONIC HYPERTENSION IN PREGNANCY

DRUG	SAFETY INDICATIONS
Labetalol	Preferred to methyldopa owing to reduced side effects
Beta-blockers	Reports of intrauterine growth retardation (atenolol)
	Generally safe
Clonidine	Limited data
Calcium antagonists	Limited data
	No increase in major teratogenicity with exposure
Diuretics	Not first-line agents
	Probably safe
ACEIs, angiotensin II receptor antagonists	Contraindicated
	Reported fetal toxicity and death

ACEIs = angiotensin converting enzyme inhibitors

From "Seventh Report of the Joint National Committee on Prevention, Detection, Evaluation, and Treatment of High Blood Pressure," by A. V. Chobanian et al. (2003), *Hypertension, 42*(6), pp. 1206–1252.

Dyslipidemia

Description

▶ General term used to describe a variety of lipid abnormalities, including low-density lipoproteins (LDL), high-density lipoproteins (HDL), and triglycerides (TGL) that deviate from normal ranges and increase the risk of cardiovascular disease. Elevation in blood lipids is often due to abnormal lipid metabolism (see Tables 8–6 and 8–7).

Etiology

▶ Hyperlipidemias (also called dyslipidemias) are either primary (some genetic forms) or secondary (related to fat, calorie, and alcohol intake; medication use; or caused by metabolic diseases such as hypothyroidism, diabetes mellitus, liver disease, obesity, and nephrosis).

▶ Familial or genetic syndromes include familial hypercholesterolemia, polygenic hypercholesterolemia, familial defective apolipoprotein B-100, familial hypertriglyceridemia, familial combined hyperlipidemia, familial hyperchylomicronemia with marked increase in triglycerides.

▶ Total cholesterol is influenced by 4 major classes of lipoproteins: chylomicrons, very low density lipoproteins (VLDL), LDL, and HDL.

  ▷ HDL carries fat away from blood vessels and prevents or delays atherosclerosis.

  ▷ LDL facilitates forming of cholesterol deposits in the blood vessels.

  ▷ Isolated elevated LDL may be seen in familial hypercholesterolemia.

▶ Other causes include thyroid disease, Cushing's disease, hepatic disease, malignancy, and pancreatitis.

TABLE 8–6.
CLASSIFICATION OF LIPOPROTEINS IN ADULTS

TYPE	LEVEL	STATUS
Low-Density Lipoprotein Cholesterol (mg/dL)	<100	Optimal
	100–129	Near optimal/above optimal
	130–159	Borderline high
	160–189	High
	>190	Very high
Total Cholesterol (mg/dL)	<200	Desirable
	200–239	Borderline high
	>240	High
High-Density Lipoprotein Cholesterol (mg/dL)	<40	Low
	>60	High
Triglycerides (mg/dL)	>150	Increased CHD risk

Adapted from *Third Report of the Expert Panel on Detection, Evaluation, and Treatment of High Blood Cholesterol in Adults* (Adult Treatment Panel III; NIH Pub. No, 01-3670), National Cholesterol Education Program. Bethesda, MD: Author, 2001.

TABLE 8–7.
LDL GOALS AND INITIATION OF TREATMENT

RISK CATEGORY	LDL GOAL	LEVEL TO START TLC**	LEVEL TO CONSIDER DRUG THERAPY
CHD or CHD risk equivalents* (10-year risk† >20%)	<100 mg/dL	>100 mg/dL	>130 mg/dL 100–129: consider initiating therapy, treat other risk factors, or use nicotinic acid or fibrate if high TGL or low HDL
2+ risk factors (10-year risk 10%–20%)	<130 mg/dL	>130 mg/dL	>130 mg/dL
2+ risk factors (10-year risk <10%)	<130 mg/dL	>130 mg/dL	>160 mg/dL
0–1 risk factor (10-year risk assessment not necessary)	<160 mg/dL	>160 mg/dL	>190 mg/dL 160–189 mg/dL: drug therapy optional; consider if single severe risk factor, multiple life-habit or emerging risk factors, or 10-year risk nearly 10%

*CHD risk equivalents: clinical CHD, symptomatic carotid artery disease, peripheral arterial disease, abdominal aortic aneurysm

**TLC: therapeutic lifestyle change

†10-year risk based on clinical conditions such as diabetes, multiple risk factors, age, sex, total cholesterol, HDL, blood pressure and its treatment.

Adapted from *Third Report of the Expert Panel on Detection, Evaluation, and Treatment of High Blood Cholesterol in Adults* (Adult Treatment Panel III; NIH Pub. No, 01-3670), by National Cholesterol Education Program. Bethesda, MD: Author, 2001.

Incidence and Demographics

▶ Some 73.5 million adults (31.7%) in the United States have high low-density lipoprotein (LDL).

▶ Fewer than 1 out of every 3 adults (2.5%) with high LDL cholesterol has the condition under control.

▶ Less than half (48.1%) of adults with high LDL cholesterol are getting treatment to lower their levels.

▶ Some 31 million people in the United States have high total cholesterol (≥240 mg/dL).

▶ Familial combined hyperlipidemia: 1/300 people

▶ Familial hypercholesterolemia: 1/500 people

▶ Between 1999 and 2012, the percentage of American adults with high total cholesterol (TC) decreased from 18.3% to 12.9%.

▶ People with high TC have approximately twice the risk for heart disease as people with ideal levels (CDC, 2015b).

Risk Factors

▶ Obesity, high saturated fat diet, sedentary lifestyle, cigarette smoking, excess alcohol use

▶ More common in males

▶ Elevated plasma fibrinogen, elevated homocysteine

▶ Lipoprotein (a): predictor of premature atherosclerosis

▶ Syndrome X: metabolic syndrome that can involve glucose intolerance, central obesity, hyperlipidemia, and hypertension; people with Syndrome X are at high risk for coronary artery disease

▶ Low HDL is major risk factor for CAD; high HDL (>60) is protective.

Prevention and Screening

▶ Screen for above risk factors.

▶ Encourage interventions for smoking cessation, hypertension, weight management, increasing physical activity, and lipid management.

▶ Treat comorbid conditions.

▶ Measure blood pressure in all adults at least every 2.5 years.

▶ Assess dietary intake with routine evaluations.

▶ Measure lipid profile in adults 20 years of age and older at least every 5 years.

▶ Universal screening for children without risk once at age 9–11 years and again between 17 and 21 years.

▶ Promote the American Heart Association diet for all people.

Assessment

History

▶ Obtain history for other CHD risk factors, family history of hyperlipidemia, dietary and alcohol intake, exercise.

▶ Dyslipidemia rarely produces symptoms unless there are symptoms of related diseases, reactions to medications.

▶ Symptoms predisposing disease: weight gain, cold intolerance, constipation, edema, central obesity, purple striae, fat wasting, hepatomegaly, xanthomas, corneal arcus, earlobe crease, plaques on funduscopic exam, poor wound healing, recurring rashes/pruritus, hypertension

▶ Medications such as thiazide diuretics, treatment for acute pancreatitis, hepatitis, renal disease

Physical Exam

▶ Xanthomas: in familial hypercholesterolemia—papules, plaques, or nodules in the tendons, eyelids, buttocks, knees, and skin folds

▶ Corneal arcus before age 50–60 years, and in young White people

▶ Milky-white serum (hypertriglyceridemia)

▶ Obesity

Diagnostic Studies

▶ Fasting fractionated lipid profile to include total cholesterol, triglycerides, HDL, LDL, VLDL, apolipoprotein

▶ Comprehensive metabolic panel to detect other metabolic abnormalities

▶ Urinalysis to detect kidney disease

▶ Thyroid screening: TSH, FT4

▶ Liver function tests to rule out liver disease and before starting medication

▶ Baseline ECG

Differential Diagnosis

Primary versus secondary causes

▶ Nephrotic syndrome

▶ Chronic renal failure

▶ Diabetes mellitus

▶ Hypothyroidism

▶ Cushing's syndrome

▶ Chronic liver disease

▶ Excessive alcohol intake

▶ Pancreatitis

▶ Obesity

▶ Hyperuricemia

▶ Medications

▶ Pregnancy

Management

Nonpharmacologic Treatment

▶ Lifestyle modifications: smoking cessation, increased physical activity, moderation of alcohol intake, increased use of soy products, diet changes

▶ LDL is primary indicator for treatment.

▶ All patients with hyperlipidemia should be started on the American Heart Association (AHA) Step 2 diet: lean meat, poultry, fish, vegetables, fruits, breads, low-fat dairy products; limit on eggs, fat, sweets, and high-fat desserts for all adults.

  ▷ Step 1 diet reduces serum cholesterol by 3%–14% (maintenance for general public).

  ▷ Step 2 diet confers additional 3%–7% benefit over Step 1 (therapeutic for lipid-lowering).

▶ Guidelines from the National Cholesterol Education Program Adult Treatment Panel (ATP) III: daily intake of less than 7% of calories from saturated fat, less than 35% of calories from total fat provided most from unsaturated fat, less than 200 mg of dietary cholesterol; use of foods rich in soluble fiber; weight control; physical activity that improves HDL

▶ See Table 8–9 for LDL goals and initiation of treatment.

▶ If 3–6 months of diet therapy are not effective in reaching LDL goal, start medications.

  ▷ Saturated fat <10% of total calories

  ▷ Total fat <30% of total calories

  ▷ Dietary cholesterol <300 mg/day

  ▷ Carbohydrates approximately 55% of calories

  ▷ Protein 15%–20% of calories

  ▷ Increase in dietary fiber: oatmeal, oat bran, raw fruits and vegetables

  ▷ Exercise; weight loss in overweight patients

Pharmacologic Treatment (see Table 8–8)

▶ HMG CoA reductase inhibitors (statins)

  ▷ A statin is the drug of choice for all patients with diagnosed CAD.

  ▷ Lowers LDL, increases HDL

  ▷ Evening dosing

  ▷ Atorvastatin (Lipitor), lovastatin (Mevacor), simvastatin (Zocor): metabolized by cytochrome P-450 (CYP)3A4

  ▷ Drug/food interactions: cyclosporine, erythromycin, itraconazole, ketoconazole, fibric acid, diltiazem, verapamil, fluoxetine, nefazodone

  ▷ Contraindicated in liver disease, pregnancy, lactation

  ▷ Rhabdomyolysis may develop if fibrate used in patient with renal dysfunction

  ▷ Monitor liver function tests

TABLE 8–8.
RECOMMENDED DRUG THERAPY FOR HYPERLIPIDEMIA IN ADULTS

DRUG	DAILY DOSAGE RANGE	CLASS
Atorvastatin (Lipitor)	10–80 mg	HMG CoA
Fluvastatin (Lescol)	20–80 mg	HMG CoA
Lovastatin (Mevacor)	20–80 mg	HMG CoA
Pravastatin (Pravachol)	10–40 mg	HMG CoA
Simvastatin (Zocor)	5–80 mg	HMG CoA
Cholestyramine (Questran)	8–24 g	Bile acid sequestrant
Colestipol (Colestid)	5–30 g	Bile acid sequestrant
Gemfibrozil (Lopid)	1,200 mg	Fibrate
Fenofibrate (Tricor)	67–200 mg	Fibrate
Niacin	1.5–3.0 g	Nicotinic acid
Nicotinic Acid (Niaspan)	1–3.0 g	Niacin extended release
Ezetimibe (Zetia)	10 mg daily	Other

▶ Bile acid sequestrants

  ▷ May safely be used in combination with other lipid-lowering medications

  ▷ Used to lower LDL

  ▷ Use with caution if triglycerides >300 (may increase triglycerides 20%–30%)

  ▷ Interference with other drugs (should be taken 1 hour before other medication or 4 hours after) and fat-soluble vitamins

  ▷ Side effects: constipation, flatulence, nausea

  ▷ Cholestyramine (Questran) maintenance dose 2–4 packs a day

  ▷ Colestipol (Colestid) maintenance dose 5 g given q.d. or b.i.d.

▶ Nicotinic acid

  ▷ Lowers total cholesterol and triglycerides, increases HDL

  ▷ Use with caution in DM and gout; monitor liver toxicity.

  ▷ Liver function tests, blood glucose, uric acid before initiation

  ▷ Start with low dose; titrate slowly to avoid flushing; pretreat with aspirin one half hour before dose.

  ▷ Initiate 500 mg q.d., increase by 500 mg q 4 weeks.

  ▷ Side effects: flushing, hypotension, nausea

▶ Fibric acids

  ▷ Lower triglycerides, increase HDL

  ▷ Rhabdomyolysis and renal failure may develop in patients also using statins.

  ▷ Monitor liver function tests.

  ▷ Generally well tolerated

▷ Side effects: dizziness, dyspepsia, diarrhea, blurred vision

▷ Gemfibrozil (Lopid) b.i.d. dosing

▶ Other lipid-lowering drugs—ezetimibe (Zetia)

▷ Decreases cholesterol absorption in the intestine

▷ Lowers LDL

▷ Metabolized in the liver and the small intestine

▷ No dose adjustment needed in patients with renal insufficiency or mild hepatic dysfunction.

▷ Side effects: headache, diarrhea

In 2013 the American College of Cardiology (ACC)/American Heart Association (AHA) developed recommendations on lipid management based on results of RCTs, systemic reviews, and meta-analyses of RCTs; these recommendations are not intended to replace clinical judgment.

Summary of 2013 AHA/ACC Cholesterol Treatment Guidelines

High-dose statin therapy is recommended for the following patients:

1. All patients 21 to 75 years of age with any form of cardiovascular disease (CVD; includes MI, angina, prior arterial revascularization, CVA, TIA, PAD) (Evidence A) or

2. Ages 40–75 with LDL-C ≥190 mg/dL should be treated with high-dose statin (moderate dose if unable to tolerate) i.e.:

   Atorvastatin 40–80 mg or rosuvastatin 20–40 mg

   (Aim to reduce LDL-C by >50% in 4–12 weeks)

Moderate-dose statin therapy is recommended for the following patients:

1. All patients with diabetes (age 40–75 years) with LDL-C 70–189 mg/dl and 10-year CVD risk <7.5% should be treated with moderate-dose statin therapy (Evidence A), i.e.:

   Atorvastatin 10–20mg, or

   Rosuvastatin 5–10 mg, or

   Pravastatin 40–80 mg, or

   Simvastatin 20–40 mg

   (Aim to reduce LDL-C by 30–50%)

2. Consider high-dose statin if such patient's 10-year CVD risk by new risk calculator is >7.5% (many people with diabetes and those with multiple risk factors for CVD may qualify; Evidence E).

3. Use clinical judgment when using high-dose and moderate-dose statins as listed above, a specific target of LDL-C goal (<70 or <100) is *not* recommended.

How Long to Treat

▶ Treatment is usually lifelong.

Special Considerations

▶ In women, using conjugated estrogens reduces LDL approximately 15% and increases HDL approximately 15%; use as adjunct, not as replacement to cholesterol-lowering agents.

▶ Total cholesterol and LDL levels are not measured before 2 years of age; no treatment recommended before that age.

▶ Pregnancy and lactation: levels normally elevated, usually do not test

▶ Older adults: treatment controversial in adults 90 and older, insufficient studies for this age group.

When to Consult, Refer, Hospitalize

▶ Refer all pediatric and adult patients who are not controlled with therapy to a cardiologist and endocrinologist.

▶ Refer if patient is pregnant or has comorbid conditions.

▶ Refer to a dietitian, especially if dietary compliance is poor.

▶ Start immediate treatment for triglycerides >1,000 mg/dL; patient may need to be hospitalized.

Follow-Up

▶ Every 1–2 years with lipid profile for patients not requiring drug therapy

▶ Visits for patients requiring drug therapy should include tolerance of medication (myalgias), diet assessment, compliance with exercise routine, 24-hour recall of diet, and appropriate lab tests.

▶ Inquire about new medications; many medications affect lipid parameters.

▶ For those on drug therapy, monitor lipids and liver function test every 6 weeks until goal is reached.

▶ Visits every 4–8 weeks initially, until lipid control is achieved, then every 6 months; with comorbid conditions, every 3–4 months.

Expected Course

▶ Dependent on etiology, CAD

▶ 1% decrease in cholesterol will decrease risk of CAD by 2%

Complications

▶ CAD progression, stroke

▶ Peripheral vascular disease

▶ Rhabdomyolysis, liver dysfunction secondary to drug treatment

▶ Pancreatitis (with triglycerides higher than 1,000 mg.dL)

Hyperlipidemia Treatment for Children, Adolescents and the Young Adult (see Tables 8-9 through 8-13)

The NHLBI 1992 guidelines for lipid management in children and adolescents focused on identifying children with elevated LDL-C. Since 1992 several critical observational studies demonstrated a correlation between lipoprotein disorders and the onset and severity of atherosclerosis in children, adolescents and young adults. Obesity combined with a moderate to severe elevation in triglycerides (TG), normal to mild elevation in LDL-C, and reduced high-density lipoprotein cholesterol (HDL-C are patterns that have been shown to be associated with the beginning and progression of atherosclerotic plaque in children and adolescents seen on pathology and imaging studies.

TABLE 8-9.
SCREENING FOR HYPERLIPIDEMIA IN CHILDREN AND YOUNG ADULTS

AGE	PROCESS	GRADE
Birth to 12 Months	No screening	Grade C Recommend
2 to 8 Years	No routine lipid screening Measure fasting lipid profile (FLP) × 2*; average results if: • Parent, grandparent, aunt/uncle, or sibling with myocardial infarction (MI), angina, stroke, coronary artery bypass graft (CABG)/stent/angioplasty at <55 years in males, <65 years in females • Parent with TC ≥240 mg/dl or known dyslipidemia • Child has diabetes, HTN, BMI ≥95th percentile, or cigarette smoker • Child has moderate- or high-risk medical condition *Interval between FLP measurements: after 2 weeks but within 3 months.	Grade B Recommend
9 to 11 Years	Universal Screening • Non-FLP: Calculate non-HDL-C: Non-HDL-C = TC − HDL-C* Non-HDL ≥145 mg/dL HDL <40 mg/dL → FLP × 2, lipid algorithms below OR • FLP: LDL-C ≥130 mg/dL, non-HDL-C ≥145 mg/dL HDL-C <40 mg/dL TG ≥100 mg/dL if <10 years, ≥130 mg/dL if ≥10 years → Repeat FLP after 2 weeks but within 3 months → Lipid algorithms below * Disregard TG and LDL-C in nonfasting sample.	Grade B Strongly Recommend
12 to 16 Years	No Routine Screening* Measure FLP × 2,** average results, if new knowledge of: • Parent, grandparent, aunt/uncle or sibling with MI, angina, stroke, CABG/stent/angioplasty, sudden death <55 years old in males, <65 year females • Parent with TC ≥240 mg/dL or known dyslipidemia • Patient has diabetes, HTN, BMI ≥85th percentile, or smokes cigarettes • Patient has moderate- or high-risk medical condition	Grade B Strongly Recommend

*Lipid screening is not recommended for those ages 12–16 years because of significantly decreased sensitivity and specificity for predicting adult LDL-C levels and significantly increased false-negative results in this age group. Selective screening is recommended for those with the clinical indications outlined.

**Interval between FLP measurements: after 2 weeks but within 3 months.

AGE	PROCESS	GRADE
17 to 21 Years	Universal Screening (once during this time)	Grade B Recommend

- Non-FLP:
  Calculate non-HDL-C:
  Non-HDL-C = TC − HDL-C
  17 to 19 years:
  Non-HDL-C ≥145 mg/dL
  HDL-C <40 mg/dL
  →FLP × 2

OR

- FLP:
  LDL-C ≥130 mg/dL
  Non-HDL-C ≥145 mg/dL
  HDL-C <40 mg/dL,
  TG ≥130 mg/dL
  → Repeat FLP after 2 weeks but within 3 months.

- 20 to 21 years:
  Non-HDL-C ≥190 mg/dL
  HDL-C <40 mg/dL*
  → FLP × 2,**, average results
  →*Adult Treatment Panel III (ATP III)* management algorithm

OR

- FLP:
  LDL-C ≥160 mg/dL,
  Non-HDL-C ≥190 mg/dL
  HDL-C <40 mg/dL
  TG ≥150 mg/dL
  → Repeat FLP after 2 weeks but within 3 months, average results
  →*ATP III* management algorithm

*Disregard TG and LDL-C in nonfasting sample.

**Interval between FLP measurements: after 2 weeks but within 3 months.

Grades reflect the findings of the evidence review.

Recommendation levels reflect the consensus opinion of the Expert Panel.

Note: Values given are in mg/dL. To convert to SI units, divide the results for total cholesterol (TC), low-density lipoprotein cholesterol (LDL-C), high-density lipoprotein cholesterol (HDL-C), and non-HDL-C by 38.6; for triglycerides (TG), divide by 88.6.

Retrieved from https://www.nhlbi.nih.gov/files/docs/guidelines/peds_guidelines_full.pdf

TABLE 8–10.
ACCEPTABLE, BORDERLINE HIGH/LOW, AND HIGH/LOW PLASMA LIPID, LIPOPROTEIN, AND APOLIPOPROTEIN CONCENTRATIONS (MG/DL) FOR CHILDREN AND ADOLESCENTS, AND YOUNG ADULTS*

CATEGORY	ACCEPTABLE		BORDERLINE HIGH		HIGH	
Total Cholesterol	<170	(<190)	170–199	(190–224)	≥200	(≥225)
LDL-C	<110	(<120)	110–129)	(120–159)	≥130	(≥160)
Non HDL-C	<120	(<150)	120-144	(150–189)	≥145	(≥190)
Apolipoprotein B (ApoB)	<90		90–109		≥110	
TRIGLYCERIDES						
0–9 years	<75		75–99		≥100	
10–19 years	<90		90–129		≥130	
(Young Adult)		(<115)		(115–149)		(≥150)
CATEGORY	ACCEPTABLE		BORDERLINE LOW		LOW	
HDL-C	>45	(>45)	40–45	(40–45)	<40	(<40)
Apolipoprotein A-1 (ApoA-1)	>120		115–120		<115	

*Young Adults recommendations are in parenthesis.

Adapted from *Expert Panel on Integrated Guidelines for Cardiovascular Health and Risk Reduction in Children and Adolescents Summary Report.* NIH Publication No. 12-7486, October 2012, pp. 38–39. Retrieved from https://www.nhlbi.nih.gov/files/docs/guidelines/peds_guidelines_full.pdf

TABLE 8–11.
AGE AND EVIDENCE-BASED RECOMMENDATIONS FOR PHARMACOLOGIC TREATMENT OF CHILDREN WITH DYSLIPIDEMIA

AGE	RECOMMENDATION	EVIDENCE GRADE
Birth to 10 Years	Medications by lipid specialist only	Grade C Recommend
	Pharmacologic treatment is limited to children with severe primary hyperlipidemia (homozygous familial hypercholesterolemia, primary hypertriglyceridemia with TG ≥500 mg/dL) or a high-risk condition or evident cardiovascular disease	
11 to 21 Years	Detailed family history and risk factor (RF) assessment required before start of drug therapy.* High- to moderate-level RFs and risk conditions (RCs).	Grade C Strongly Recommend
	LDL-C:	
	If average LDL-C ≥250 mg/dL, consult lipid specialist.	Grade B Strongly Recommend
	If average LDL-C ≥130–250 mg/dL, or non-HDL >145 mg/dL:	Grade A Strongly Recommend
	• Refer to dietitian for medical nutrition therapy with Cardiovascular Health Integrated Lifestyle Diet (CHILD 1) CHILD 2-LDL × 6 months, repeat fasting lipid panel (FLP) Repeat FLP:	
	• LDL-C <130 mg/dL, continue CHILD 2- LDL, reevaluate in 12 months	Grade A Strongly Recommend

AGE	RECOMMENDATION	EVIDENCE GRADE
11 to 21 Years (cont'd)	• LDL-C ≥190** mg/dL, consider initiation of statin therapy	Grade A Strongly Recommend
	• LDL-C ≥130–189 mg/dL, (-)FHx, no other RF or RC, continue CHILD 2-LDL, reevaluate q. 6 months	Grade B Recommend
	• LDL-C 160–189 mg/dL with + FHx positive OR at least 1 high-level RF/RC OR at least 2 moderate-level RFs/RCs, consider statin therapy	Grade B Recommend
	• LDL-C ≥130–159 mg/dL + at least 2 high-level RFs/RCs OR 1 high-level + 2 moderate-level RFs/RCs, consider statin therapy	Grade B Recommend
	Children on statin therapy should be counseled and carefully monitored	Grade A Strongly Recommend
	Detailed FH and RF/RC assessment required before initiation of drug therapy***	Grade C Strongly Recommend
	TG:	
	If average TG ≥500 mg/dL, consult lipid specialist	Grade B Recommend
	If average TG ≥100 mg/dL in a child <10 years, or ≥130 mg/dL in a child age 10 to 19 years, or <500 mg/dL:	Grade B Strongly Recommend
	• Refer to dietitian for medical nutrition therapy with CHILD 1 then CHILD 2-TG × 6 months	
	Repeat fasting lipid profile:	
	• TG <100 (130) mg/dL, continue CHILD 2-TG, monitor q. 6 to 12 months	Grade B Strongly Recommend
	• TG >100 (130) mg/dL, reconsult dietitian for intensified CHILD 2 TG diet counseling	Grade C Recommend
	• TG ≥200–499 mg/dL, non-HDL ≥145 mg/dL, consider fish oil ± consult lipid specialist	Grade D Recommend
	NON-HDL-C:	
	Children ≥10 years with non-HDL-C ≥145 mg/dL after LDL-C goal achieved may be considered for additional treatment with statins, fibrates, or niacin in conjunction with a lipid specialist consultation.	Grade D Optional

Grades reflect the findings of the evidence review.

Recommendation levels reflect the consensus opinion of the Expert Panel.

When medication is recommended, this should always be in the context of the complete cardiovascular risk profile of the patient and in consultation with the patient and the family

Table by National Heart, Lung, and Blood Institute. *Integrated Guidelines for Cardiovascular Health and Risk Reduction in Children and Adolescents, The Report of the Expert Panel.* NIH Publication No. 12-7486, p 38-39, October 2012. Retrieved from https://www.nhlbi.nih.gov/files/docs/guidelines/peds_guidelines_full.pdf and http://www.nhlbi.nih.gov/health-pro/guidelines/current/cardiovascular-health-pediatric-guidelines

*Consideration of drug therapy based on the average of ≥2 FLPs, obtained at least 2 weeks but no more than 3 months apart.

**If average LDL-C ≥190 mg/dL after CHILD 2-LDL and child is age 8 to 9 years with + FH OR ≥1 high-level RF/RC *OR* ≥ 2 moderate-level RFs/RCs, statin therapy may be considered.

***Consideration of drug therapy based on the average of 2 fasting lipid profiles obtained at least 2 weeks but no more than 3 months apart.

Note: If child is obese, nutrition therapy should include calorie restriction and increased activity beyond that recommended for all children.

TABLE 8-12.
MEDICATIONS FOR MANAGING HYPERLIPIDEMIA IN CHILDREN AND YOUNG ADULTS

TYPE OF MEDICATION	MECHANISM OF ACTION	MAJOR EFFECTS	EXAMPLES	ADVERSE REACTIONS	FDA APPROVAL IN YOUTHS
HMG CoA reductase inhibitors (statins)	Inhibits cholesterol synthesis in hepatic cells, decreases cholesterol pool, resulting in upregulation of LDL receptors	Mainly lowers LDL-C; some decrease in TG and modest increase in HDL-C	Atorvastatin Fluvastatin Lovastatin Pravastatin Rosuvastatin Simvastatin	Raised hepatic enzymes, raised creatine kinase, myopathy possibly progressing to rhabdomyolysis	All statins listed approved as an adjunct to diet to lower LDL-C in adolescent boys and postmenarchal girls ages 10–18 years (8+ years for pravastatin) with heFH and LDL-C ≥190 mg/dL, or ≥160 mg/dL with FHx of premature CVD and 2+ CVD risk factors in the pediatric patient
Bile acid sequestrants	Binds intestinal bile acids interrupting enterohepatic recirculation, more cholesterol converted into bile acids, decreases hepatic cholesterol pool, upregulates LDL receptors	Lowers LDL-C; small increase in HDL; raises TG	Cholestyramine Colestipol Colesevelam	Limited to gastrointestinal tract: gas, bloating constipation, cramps	No pediatric indication listed for cholestyramine or colestipol; colesevelam indicated as monotherapy or with statin for LDL-C reduction in boys and postmenarchal girls ages 10–17 years with FH after diet trial if LDL-C ≥190 mg/dL or if LDL-C ≥160 mg/dL with FHx premature CVD or 2+ more CVD risk factors in the pediatric patient
Cholesterol absorption inhibitors	Inhibits intestinal absorption of cholesterol and plant sterols, decreases hepatic cholesterol pool, upregulates LDL receptors	Mainly lowers LDL-C; some decrease in TG and small increase in HDL-C	Ezetimibe	Myopathy, gastrointestinal upset, headache	No

	Mechanism	Effect	Agents	Side effects	Comments
Fibric acid derivatives	Agonist for PPAR alpha nuclear receptors that upregulate LPL and downregulate apoC-III, both increasing degradation of VLDL-C and TG. Hepatic synthesis of VLDL-C may also be decreased.	Mainly lowers TG and raises HDL-C, with little effect on LDL-C	Fenofibrate Gemfibrozil	Dyspepsia, constipation, myositis, anemia	No
Nicotinic acid (extended release)	Inhibits release of FFA from adipose tissue; decreases VLDL-C and LDL-C production and HDL-C degradation	Lowers TG and LDL-C and raises HDL-C; can decrease Lp(a)	Niacin, extended release	Flushing, hepatic toxicity, can increase fasting blood glucose, uric acid; hyperacidity	Use not recommended in children age <2 years
Omega-3 fish oil	Decreases hepatic FA and TG synthesis while enhancing FA degradation/oxidation, with subsequent reduced VLDL-C release	Lowers TG, raises HDL-C, increases LDL-C and LDL-C particle size	Omega-3 acid ethyl esters	Occasional gastrointestinal side effects but no adverse effect on glucose levels or muscle or liver enzymes or bleeding	Only one FDA-approved fish oil preparation for adults, but many generic fish oil capsules commercially available

TABLE 8-13.
CLINICAL TRIALS OF LIPID-LOWERING MEDICATION THERAPY IN CHILDREN AND ADOLESCENTS

STUDY	MEDICATION	SUBJECTS/GENDER/ CONDITION	DAILY DOSE	EFFECT ON LIPID PROFILE TC	EFFECT ON LIPID PROFILE LDL-C	EFFECT ON LIPID PROFILE HDL-C	EFFECT ON LIPID PROFILE TG
BILE ACID BINDING RESINS							
Tonstad et al. RCT 1 year	Cholestyramine	72/both/FH (LDL >190 mg/dL without FHx premature CVD or LDL >160 with FHx after 1-year diet; ages 6–11 years)	8 g	–12%	–17%	+8%	NA
McCrindle et al. RCT crossover 2 × 8 weeks	Cholestyramine	40/both/FH (1 parent with FH; LDL-C ≥131 mg/dL; on diet; ages 10–18 years)	8 g	–7 to –11%	–10 to –15%	+2 to +4%	+6 to +9%
Tonstad et al. RCT 8 weeks; open-label 44-52 weeks	Colestipol	66/both/FH (TC ≥239 mg/dL and TG <115 mg/dL; ages 10–16 years)	2–12 g	–17%	–20%	–7%	–13%
McCrindle et al. RCT crossover 2 × 18 weeks	Colestipol	36/both/FH/FCHL (LDL ≥160 mg/dL after 6 months diet counseling; ages 8–18 years)	10 g	–7%	–10%	+2%	+12%
Stein et al.	Colesevelam	191/both/ FH (LDL ≥190mg/dL or LDL ≥ plus 2 additional RFs after 6 months diet counseling; ages 10–17 years.	1.875 g 3.75g	–3% –7%	–6% –13%	+5% +8%	+6% +5%

HMG COA REDUCTASE INHIBITORS (STATINS)

Study	Drug	Sample/Condition	Dose				
McCrindle et al. RCT; open-label 26 weeks	Atorvastatin	187/both/FH/ Severe hyperlipidemia (LDL-C ≥190 mg/dL or ≥160 mg/dL with FHx; and TG <400 mg/dL; ages 10–17 years)	10–20 mg	−30%	−40%	+6%	−13%
Van der Graaf et al. Open-label 2 years	Fluvastatin	85/both/FH (LDL-C ≥190 mg/dL or LDL-C ≥160 mg/dL and 1+ risk factor or LDL receptor mutation; ages 10–16 years)	80 mg	−27%	−34%	+5%	−5%
Lambert et al. RCT 8 weeks	Lovastatin	69/males/FH (LDL-C >95th percentile, FHx atherosclerosis and hyperlipidemia; on diet; mean age 13 years)	10 mg	−17%	−21%	+9%	−18%
			20 mg	−19%	−24%	+2%	+9%
			30 mg	−21%	−27%	+11%	+3%
			40 mg	−29%	−36%	+3%	−9%
Stein et al. RCT 48 weeks	Lovastatin	132/males/FH (LDL 189–503 mg/dL + FHx of high LDL; or 220–503 mg/ dL + FHx CAD death; AHA diet 4+ months; ages 10–17 years)	10 mg	−13%	−17%	+4%	+4%
			20 mg	−19%	−24%	+4%	+8%
			40 mg	−21%	−27%	+5%	+6%
Clauss et al. RCT 24 weeks	Lovastatin	54/females/FH (FHx FH; LDL 160–400 mg/ dL and TG <350 mg/dL; 4-week diet placebo run-in and 20-week tx; ages 10–17 years, postmenarchal)	40 mg	−22%	−27%	+3%	−23%
Knipscheer et al. RCT 12 weeks	Pravastatin	72/ both/FH (FHx hypercholesterol or premature atherosclerosis; LDL >95th percentile; diet × 8 weeks; ages 8–16 years)	5 mg	−18%	−23%	+4%	+2%
			10 mg	−17%	−24%	+6%	+7%
			20 mg	−25%	−33%	+11%	+3%

CONTINUED

STUDY	MEDICATION	SUBJECTS/GENDER/ CONDITION	DAILY DOSE	EFFECT ON LIPID PROFILE TC	EFFECT ON LIPID PROFILE LDL-C	EFFECT ON LIPID PROFILE HDL-C	EFFECT ON LIPID PROFILE TG
Wiegman et al. RCT 2 years	Pravastatin	214/both/FH (LDL-C ≥155 mg/dL and TG ≤350 mg/dL; diet × 3 months; ages 8–18 years)	20–40 mg	–19%	–24%	+6%	–17%
Rodenburg et al. Open-label 2-year RCT; 4.5 year open-label followup	Pravastatin	186/both/FH (LDL-C ≥154 mg/dL and TG <154 mg/dL; 3 months on diet; ages 8–18 years)	20 mg (ages <14 years) or 40 mg (ages >14 years)	–23%	–29%	+3%	–2%
de Jongh et al. RCT 48 weeks	Simvastatin	173/both/FH (LDL-C: 158–397 mg/dL; ages 10–17 years)	10–40 mg	–31%	–41%	+3%	–9%
de Jongh et al. RCT 28 weeks	Simvastatin	50/both/FH (LDL-C >95th percentile, FHx hyperlipidemia, or LDL receptor mutation; ages 9–18 years)	40 mg	–30%	–40%	+5%	–17%
Avis et al. RCT 12 weeks; then, 40 week open label followup	Rosuvastatin	177/both/FH (LDL-C ≥190 mg/dL or LDL-C >160 mg/dL plus (+)FHx of early CVD or ≥2 other RFs for CVD)	5 mg	–30%	–38%	+4%	–13%
			10 mg	–34%	–45%	+10%	–15%
			20 mg	–39%	–50%	+9%	–16%
OTHER AGENTS							
Wheeler et al. RCT 26 weeks	Bezafibrate	14/both/FH (TC >269 mg/dL, nlTG + FHx of FH or premature CAD; ages 4–15 years)	10–20 mg	–22%	NC	+15%	–23%
Colletti et al. Open-label 1–19 months	Niacin	21/both/FH (mean LDL = 243 ± 45 mg/ dL on low-fat diet; mean TG = 87 ± 39 mg/dL; ages 4–14 years)	500–2,200 mg	–13%	–17%	+4%	+13%

Study	Intervention	Criteria	Dose				
McCrindle et al. RCT crossover 2 × 18 weeks	Pravastatin and Colestipol	36/both/FH/FCHL (LDL >160 mg/dL + FHx of FH or premature CAD; TG >177 mg/dL in 10/36; ages 10–18 years)	Pravastatin, 10 mg (with Colestipol, 5g)	−13%	−17%	+4%	+8%
van der Graaf et al. RCT 6 and 27 weeks; open-label to 53 weeks	Simvastatin and Ezetimibe	248/both/FH (LDL >159 mg/dL + genotype-confirmed FH or + parental genotype-confirmed FH or + parental LDL >210 mg/dL or + tendinous xanthomas or LDL >189 mg/dL + FHx of hypercholesterolemia; ages 10–17 years)	Simvastatin 10–40 mg with Ezetimibe 10 mg	−38%	−49%	+7%	−17%
Addendum: Goldberg et al. Omega-3 fatty acid review in adults; no RCTs in children	Omega-3 fish oils** (1 gram/capsule)	—	1–4 g/d	NC	+17% to +31%	+6–17%	−30% to −40%

Table by National Heart, Lung, and Blood Institute. *Integrated Guidelines for Cardiovascular Health and Risk Reduction in Children and Adolescents, The Report of the Expert Panel.* http://www.nhlbi.nih.gov/health-pro/guidelines/current/cardiovascular-health-pediatric-guidelines

ABBREVIATIONS: AHA = American Heart Association; CAD = coronary artery disease; d = day; FHx = family history; g = grams; mg = milligrams; NA = not available; NC = not calculated; TC = total cholesterol; FH = heterozygous familial hypercholesterolemia; FCHL = familial combined hyperlipidemia; RCT = randomized controlled trial; tx = treatment

Definitions of Risk Factors (RFs) for Dyslipidemia Algorithms

▶ (+) Family history: myocardial infarction; angina; coronary artery bypass graft/stent/angioplasty; sudden cardiac death in parent, grandparent, aunt, or uncle; male <55 years old, female <65 years old

▶ High-Level RFs: HTN requiring medication therapy (BP 99th percentile (+5 mmHg)

▷ Current cigarette smoker

▷ BMI 97th percentile

▷ Presence of high-risk conditions

▷ Diabetes mellitus (DM) is also a high-level risk factor and considered a high-risk condition, CVD equivalent by the *Adult Treatment Panel III* recommendations for adults.

▶ Moderate-Level RFs: Hypertension not requiring drug therapy

▷ BMI >95th and <97th percentile

▷ HDL-C <40 mg/dL

▷ Presence of moderate-risk condition

Special Risk Conditions

▶ High Risk: Diabetes mellitus, type 1 and type 2

▷ Chronic kidney disease/end-stage renal disease/post–renal transplant

▷ Postorthotopic heart transplant

▷ Kawasaki disease with current aneurysms

▶ Moderate Risk: Kawasaki disease with regressed coronary aneurysms

▷ Chronic inflammatory disease (systemic lupus erythematosus, juvenile rheumatoid arthritis)

▷ Human immunodeficiency virus infection

▷ Nephrotic syrome

Recommendations for Use of HMG-COA Reductase Inhibitors (Statins) in Children and Adolescents

Patient Selection

1. Use algorithm and risk factor categories to select statin therapy for patients.

2. Include preferences of patient and family in decision making.

3. In general, do not start treatment with statins before age 10 years (patients with high-risk family history, high-risk conditions, or multiple risk factors might be considered for medication initiation at age 10 years or younger.)

4. Precaution/contraindication with potentially interactive medications (cyclosporine, niacin, fibric acid derivatives, erythromycin, azole antifungals, nefazodone, many HIV protease inhibitors).
   Check for potential interaction with all current medications at baseline.

5. Obtain baseline hepatic panel and creatine kinase (CK) before initiating treatment.

Initiation and Titration

1. Choice of particular statin is a matter of preference. Providers are encouraged to develop familiarity and experience with one of the statins, including dosage regimen and potential drug–drug interactions.

2. Start with the lowest dose once daily, usually at bedtime. Atorvastatin and rosuvastatin can be taken in the morning or evening because of their long half-lives.

3. Measure baseline CK, alanine aminotransferase (ALT), and aspartate aminotransferase (AST).

4. Instruct the patient to report all potential adverse effects, especially muscle cramps, weakness, asthenia, and more diffuse symptoms suggestive of myopathy.

5. Advise female patients about concerns with pregnancy and the need for appropriate contraception.

6. Advise about potential future medication interactions, especially cyclosporine, niacin, fibric acid derivatives, erythromycin, azole antifungals, nefazodone, and HIV protease inhibitors. Check for potential interaction whenever any new medication is initiated.

7. Whenever potential myopathy symptoms present, stop medication and assess CK; determine relation to recent physical activity. A CK level that is 10 times above the upper limit of reported normal is cause for concern, considering the impact of physical activity. Monitor the patient for resolution of myopathy symptoms and any associated increase in CK. Consideration can be given to restarting the medication once symptoms and laboratory abnormalities have resolved.

8. After 4 weeks, measure fasting lipid profile (FLP), ALT, and AST

    ▷ The threshold for worrisome levels of ALT or AST is >3 times the upper limit of reported normal.

    ▷ Target levels for LDL-C: Minimal <130 mg/dL; Ideal <110 mg/dL

9. If target LDL-C levels are reached and there are no myopathy symptoms or laboratory abnormalities, continue therapy and recheck FLP, ALT, and AST in 8 weeks and then 3 months.

10. If laboratory abnormalities are seen or symptoms are reported, temporarily withhold the medication and repeat the blood work in 2 weeks. If and when abnormalities resolve, the medication may be restarted with close monitoring.

11. If target LDL-C levels are not achieved, increase the dose by one increment (usually 10 mg) and repeat the blood work in 4 weeks. If target LDL-C levels are still not achieved, dose may be further increased by one increment or another agent (bile acid sequestrant or cholesterol absorption inhibitor) may be added under the direction of a lipid specialist.

Maintenance Monitoring

1. Monitor growth (height, weight, and BMI relative to normal growth charts), sexual maturation, and development.

2. Whenever potential myopathy symptoms present, stop medication and assess CK.

3. Monitor fasting lipoprotein profile, ALT, and AST every 3–4 months in the first year, every 6 months in the second year and beyond, and whenever clinically indicated.

4. Monitor and encourage compliance with lipid-lowering dietary and medication therapy. Serially assess and counsel for other risk factors, such as weight gain, smoking, and inactivity.

5. Counsel adolescent females about statin contraindications in pregnancy and the need for abstinence or use of appropriate contraceptive measures. Use of oral contraceptives is not contraindicated if medically appropriate. Seek referral to an adolescent medicine or gynecologic specialist as appropriate.

CORONARY ARTERY DISEASE (CAD)/ISCHEMIC HEART DISEASE (IHD)
Angina Pectoris
Description

▶ Most common form of heart disease, killing more than 600,000 people each year and costing the United States $108.9 billion each year

▶ High blood pressure, high LDL cholesterol, and smoking are key risk factors for heart disease.

▶ About half of Americans (47%) have at least one of these three risk factors (CDC, 2015a).

▶ Coronary artery disease may develop over years as a result of atherosclerotic lesions that decrease the arterial lumen. Over time, blood flow to the heart may be reduced, producing cardiac ischemic disease.

▶ Angina is a clinical manifestation of ischemic heart disease, occurring when blood flow to an artery is compromised sufficiently to decrease myocardial oxygen and produce subsequent chest discomfort.

   ▷ Classic: substernal pressure or heaviness associated with exertion or anxiety, resolving with rest

   ▷ Women under 50 with angina frequently awaken from sleep with chest pain

   ▷ Types include:

      ▶ Stable: pain duration less than 15 minutes; no change in frequency, severity, or duration of anginal symptoms during the preceding 6 weeks

      ▶ Unstable: recent change in characteristic angina symptoms and may occur at rest

      ▶ Variant (Prinzmetal): transient ST-segment elevation, at rest, with angina symptoms related to coronary spasm usually involving right coronary artery

Etiology

▶ Plaques formed on the intimal lining of artery are composed of lipoproteins, cellular components, and extracellular matrix molecules. Plaque accumulation causes the inner lining of the blood vessels to thicken and blood vessels to lose elasticity.

▶ Atherosclerosis first appears as a fatty streak, which progresses for about 30 years.

▶ Foam cells are macrophages that ingest LDL and the fatty deposits (LDL) cause them to have a foamy appearance, hence the name foam cells. Early in atherosclerosis, foam cells congregate on the fatty lipids on artery walls and plaque begins to form, then develops into a multilayered plaque with a stabilizing fibrous cap.

▶ As early as the fourth decade, the plaque becomes unstable and the foam cells necrose and rupture underneath the fibrous cap.

▶ With progression, the fibrous cap tears and bleeds to produce a thrombus, which occludes the blood vessel either completely or partially and causes decreased blood flow and ischemia or necrosis (myocardial infarction).

▶ The process of atherosclerosis is accelerated by HTN, DM, hyperlipidemia, genetics, coronary artery vasospasm, aortic stenosis, and aortic insufficiency.

Incidence and Demographics

▶ Male prevalence through majority of life span until women reach menopause, when occurrence rises; equal male and female incidence after age 70

▶ Highest incidence in fifth through seventh decade

Risk Factors

▶ Male, HTN, hyperlipidemia, DM, tobacco use, familial history of premature cardiac death (before age 55); menopausal women without estrogen replacement (estrogen treatment for postmenopausal women increases risk of ovarian cancer, however lack of estrogen increases their risk for CAD)

▶ Excessive alcohol consumption

▶ Cocaine

▶ Advancing age

▶ Obesity

▶ Physical inactivity

▶ Poor dietary intake

Prevention and Screening

▶ Modifiable lifestyle changes associated with coronary risk factors

▶ Treatment of comorbid conditions: CAD, HTN, DM, hyperlipidemia

▶ Low-fat and low-sodium diet

▶ Regular aerobic exercise

▶ Avoidance of excessive alcohol intake; smoking cessation

Assessment

History

▶ Classic presentation of substernal pressure or heaviness associated with exertion or anxiety and relieved with rest or nitroglycerin

▶ Arm, back, neck, jaw, or upper stomach pain or discomfort

▶ Each patient has typical pattern: subjective description of tightness, squeezing, burning, pressure, heaviness.

▶ Change in patient's typical pattern indicative of unstable angina

Physical Exam
- ▶ Vital signs: elevation in BP, pulse, and respirations
- ▶ Holosystolic murmur may be present
- ▶ Transient S3 or S4
- ▶ Mitral valve prolapse, intermittent claudication may be present
- ▶ Sparse hair growth on distal extremities with associated peripheral vascular disease

Diagnostic Studies
- ▶ ECG at the time of the pain may show changes; between episodes, ECG may be normal.
- ▶ ECG normal in 25%–50% patients during angina episode; may find evidence of prior MI (Q waves)
- ▶ ECG unreliable in patients with bundle branch block, Wolf-Parkinson-White syndrome
- ▶ Chest X-ray: assess heart size, look for pulmonary edema, pleural effusions, and aortic aneurysm
- ▶ Exercise stress test: S-T segment depression (less accurate in women)
- ▶ Exercise thallium imaging: hypoperfusion found in areas with diminished uptake
- ▶ Used for clarification with ECG abnormalities, often in women and with digoxin and beta-blocker usage
- ▶ CBC, electrolytes, cardiac enzymes, pulse oximetry as indicated
- ▶ Radionuclide ventriculography: left ventricle imaging to differentiate infarction from ischemia
- ▶ Technetium: tagged RBC, highly sensitive for CAD (nonspecific)
- ▶ Coronary angiography: definitive for diagnosis of CAD
- ▶ Rapid sequence MRI: calcified coronary arteries (not sensitive to coronary lesions)
- ▶ CT scan not recommended

Differential Diagnosis

Cardiac
- ▶ Pericarditis
- ▶ Aortic dissection
- ▶ MI
- ▶ CHF

Gastrointestinal
- ▶ Gastroesophageal reflux (GERD)
- ▶ Cholecystitis
- ▶ Esophageal spasm
- ▶ Peptic ulcer

Respiratory
▶ Costochondral pain
▶ Pneumothorax
▶ Pneumonia
▶ Pleurisy
▶ Asthma
▶ Pulmonary emboli

Musculoskeletal
▶ Chest wall syndrome
▶ Shoulder arthropathy

Psychological
▶ Anxiety
▶ Panic disorders
▶ Depression

Management

Nonpharmacologic Treatment
▶ Modification of risk factors: weight, smoking, stress, aerobic activity, diet low in saturated fat and sodium
▶ Cardiac rehabilitation as indicated

Pharmacologic Treatment
▶ Optimal management of comorbid conditions: hyperlipidemia, diabetes, CHF, hypertension, arrhythmias
▶ New guidelines suggest treatment in patients with symptomatic chronic stable angina to prevent MI or death and to reduce symptoms.
  ▷ Aspirin, or clopidogrel when aspirin is absolutely contraindicated
  ▷ Beta-blockers
  ▷ Low-density lipoprotein (LDL) cholesterol-lowering therapy with a statin
  ▷ Angiotensin-converting enzyme (ACE) inhibitor
▶ Agents that should be used in patients with symptomatic chronic stable angina to reduce symptoms only are sublingual nitroglycerin or nitroglycerin spray for immediate relief of angina.
▶ Calcium antagonists (long-acting) or long-acting nitrates when beta-blockers are clearly contraindicated
▶ Calcium antagonists (long-acting) or long-acting nitrates combined with beta-blockers when beta-blockers alone are unsuccessful

Drug-Specific
▶ Nitroglycerin: 0.3 to 0.6 mg sublingual 5 minutes before any activity likely to produce angina

▶ Nitrates (long-acting): used to promote coronary vasodilation

▷ Patient education regarding storage and use of nitroglycerin so it will remain effective; when and how to take it; when to go for medical help

▷ Monitor for hypotension with nitroglycerin use.

▷ Drug tolerance develops rapidly in patients taking nitrogylcerin; patient should have a planned drug-free interval of 10–14 hours on a scheduled basis

▷ Isosorbide dinitrate: 5–40 mg t.i.d.

▷ Isosorbide mononitrate: 10–40 mg p.o. b.i.d. or sustained release 60–120 mg q.d.

▷ Nitro-Dur skin patch 0.2– 0.8 mg/hr, on for 12 hours then off for 12 hours

▶ Aspirin: 81–325 mg q.d.

▶ Hyperlipidemic medication: lower LDL to 100 or lower; see section on hyperlipidemia above

▶ Beta-blockers: decrease heart rate, contractility, and oxygen requirements

▷ Monitor bradycardia, fatigue, depression, CHF, asthma

▷ Metoprolol 25–200 mg b.i.d., atenolol 25–200 mg q.d.

▶ Calcium channel blockers: coronary vasodilation with reduction myocardial oxygen

▷ Best drug for vasospasm

▷ Monitor headache, pedal edema, constipation

▷ Avoid verapamil and diltiazem in patients with arrhythmias

▷ Coronary spasm: nifedipine XL (Procardia) 30–120 mg q.d.; verapamil (Calan) 120–320 mg q.d.; diltiazem (Cardizem) 120–480 mg q.d.

▷ Avoid short-acting calcium channel blockers.

How Long to Treat

▶ Depends on etiology

▶ Often until revascularization

Special Considerations

▶ Women often have atypical symptoms.

▶ Geriatric patients: use low therapeutic doses to avoid side effects, monitor closely.

▶ Pregnancy: exclude other diagnoses, cardiologist to follow-up

When to Consult, Refer, Hospitalize

▶ Consult with a physician on new and uncontrolled cases.

▶ Refer to cardiologist for invasive procedures; coronary revascularization, intolerable symptoms and medication failure; stenosis of left main artery >50% with or without angina; left ventricular dysfunction and 3-vessel damage; unstable angina with ischemia on exercise stress test; or post-infarction continuing angina or ischemia.

▶ Transfer to the nearest ED and hospitalize for acute angina unrelieved with pharmacologic therapy; patient should crush aspirin 325 mg and swallow en route to medical facility.

Follow-Up

▶ Individualized follow-up is dependent on symptoms and condition; minimum every 3 months.

▶ Patient education regarding storage and use of nitroglycerin so it will remain effective, when and how to take it, when to go for medical help

Complications

▶ MI, cardiac arrest, CHF, death

Acute Coronary Syndrome (ACS)

Description

Some 735,000 Americans have heart attacks each year (CDC, 2015a). Myocardial tissue death (necrosis) results from myocardial oxygen demand severely compromised by thrombus formation, leading to subsequent reduction in coronary blood flow with total coronary occlusion (Q-wave transmural infarction or ST elevation myocardial infarction (STEMI) or nonocclusion (non-Q-wave nontransmural infarction or non-ST-elevation myocardial infarction (NSTEMI).

Etiology

▶ CAD: coronary thrombosis secondary to ruptured atherosclerotic plaque

▶ Coronary spasm

Incidence and Demographics

▶ Global incidence with mortality 30%–40%

▶ Male preponderance fourth through sixth decade, equal by age 70

Risk Factors

▶ See CAD risk factors above.

Prevention and Screening

▶ The U.S. Preventive Services Task Force recommends the use of aspirin for men age 45 to 79 years and women 55 to 79 years for the prevention of heart disease. Evaluate the presence and control status of major risk factors for coronary heart disease (CHD) for all patients approximately every 3–5 years.

▶ Calculate 10-year risk (National Cholesterol Education Program global risk) of developing symptomatic CHD for all patients with 2 or more major risk factors to assess the need for primary prevention strategies.

▶ Patients with established CHD should be identified for secondary prevention efforts, and patients with a CHD risk equivalent (e.g., atherosclerosis in other vascular beds, diabetes mellitus, chronic kidney disease, or 10-year risk greater than 20% as calculated by Framingham equations) should receive risk factor intervention equally intensive as for those with clinically apparent CHD.

History

▶ Presentation in older adults is often nonspecific.

▶ Women may have nonstandard presentation; frequently awakened at night with pain.

▶ Elderly patients may have no symptoms—"silent MI."

▶ Shortness of breath, CHF

▶ Pain radiation at rest or minimal activity

▶ Classic: oppressive retrosternal chest pain, not relieved by nitroglycerin; nausea or vomiting; diaphoresis

Physical Exam

▶ High incidence of mortality within first hour following cardiac event

▶ May have obvious pain; usually reduced sensitivity to pain in elders—"silent MI"

▶ Nonspecific presentation, delirium, syncope, weakness

▶ Vital signs: hypotension, tachycardia, dyspnea

▶ General appearance: apprehensive, appears ill, ashen color

▶ Respiratory: shortness of breath, rales

▶ Heart: S3, S4, new mitral regurgitation murmur, arrhythmia

Diagnostic Studies

▶ ECG diagnostic in 85% of cases with ST segment elevation, Q waves, inverted T waves

  ▷ Subendocardial infarction: note ST segment depression (may be the only finding)

▶ Cardiac enzymes (see Table 8–14)

  ▷ Creatine kinase (CK): CK-MB2 to CK-MB2 ratio >1.5, infarction is suggested (more sensitive early marker before elevation of CK-MβB)

  ▷ Troponin T and troponin I (not found in muscle or blood of healthy person) are more specific than CK-MB; become positive 4–12 hours after onset of MI

  ▷ LDH: LDH1 exceeds LDH2 levels in pathology; less specific than cardiac enzymes

  ▷ Troponin T and troponin I offer greater sensitivity

▶ Cardiac catheterization or angiogram to evaluate for coronary artery occlusion or disease

▶ Myocardial perfusion imaging (MPI)

Differential Diagnosis

▶ Unstable angina

▶ Aortic dissection

▶ Pericarditis

▶ Pulmonary embolism

▶ Esophageal spasm

▶ Biliary tract disease

▶ Gastroesophageal reflux disease

▶ Pancreatitis

▶ Chest wall muscle spasm

TABLE 8–14.
CARDIAC ENZYMES IN THE DIAGNOSIS OF MI

LAB	ONSET	COMMENT
CK: MB 1 and 2	3–4 hours	Sensitive, not specific
Troponin I and T	3.5 hours	Highly specific
LDH 1 and 2	24 hours	Sensitive, not specific

Management

Nonpharmacologic Treatment

▶ Acute: immediate emergency room care for evaluation and stabilization

▶ Post-MI:

▷ diet low in saturated fat and sodium; caloric restriction if appropriate

▷ treat underlying risk factors (hypertension, hyperlipidemia)

Pharmacologic Treatment

▶ Acute

▷ Nitroglycerin SL 0.3–0.6 mg every 5 minutes, total 3 doses

▷ Unrelieved chest pain: transport to nearest emergency room or chest pain center with Primary PCI capability. PCI is the recommended triage strategy for patients with STEMI and ischemic symptoms occurring less than 12 hours duration

▷ Aspirin 160–325 mg, preferably chewable

▷ O_2 via nasal cannula at 2 liters, if available

▷ High dose statin (i.e., atorvastatin 80mg po)

▷ Thrombolytic therapy may confer benefit if initiated within 3–12 hours after onset of pain if PCI unavailable

▶ Postinfarction

▷ Treatment of hyperlipidemia, initial high dose statin

▷ Smoking cessation

▷ Antiplatelet agent

▶ Aspirin 81–325 mg q.d. unless contraindicated

▶ Clopidogrel (Plavix) 75 mg p.o. q.d. if unable to tolerate aspirin

▷ Beta-blockers improve survival rates and should be started within first 24 hours.

▶ Except, do not give to patient with marked CHF, cardiogenic shock or bronchospasm

▶ Monitor bradycardia, fatigue, depression

▶ Metoprolol 25–200 mg b.i.d.

▶ Atenolol 25–200 mg q.d.

▷ Calcium channel blockers are not effective and are indicated for secondary prevention.

▷ ACE inhibitors should be considered for all patients.

▶ In patients with left ventricular dysfunction, reduce morbidity

▶ HOPE study showed reduction of mortality in patients without CHF.

▶ Most effective for patients with diabetes, hypertension

▶ Monitor cough and renal function, including hyperkalemia.

▶ Rare: life-threatening angioedema caused by drug

▶ Lisinopril 2.5–10 mg q.d.; start with small dose, titrate up

▶ PEACE study suggests ACE inhibitors do not lower mortality in stable patients with normal heart function.

▷ Glycosides: consider use in CHF

▷ Nitrates

▶ Effective for residual ischemia and coronary atherosclerosis

▶ Monitor hypotension

Special Considerations

▶ None

When to Consult, Refer, Hospitalize

▶ Patients with symptoms of ACS (chest discomfort with or without radiation to the arm[s], back, neck, jaw, or epigastrium; shortness of breath; weakness; diaphoresis; nausea; lightheadedness) should be instructed to call 911 and be transported to the hospital by ambulance rather than by friends or relatives.

▶ Patients with symptoms that may represent acute coronary syndrome (ACS) should not be evaluated solely over the telephone but should be referred to a facility that allows evaluation by a physician and the recording of a 12-lead electrocardiogram (ECG) and biomarker determination (e.g., an emergency department or other acute-care facility).

▶ Initial post-MI care and evaluation by cardiologist

Follow-Up

▶ Long-term management; see at least every 3 months

Expected Course

▶ Two variables dictate course: status of vessel disease and ventricular damage

▷ Main left CAD: 20% mortality in first year; single-vessel damage has 2% mortality; double-vessel damage has 3%–4% mortality; triple-vessel damage has 5–8% mortality

▷ Left ventricular dysfunction: ejection fraction (EF) <40% doubles annual mortality rate

▶ Overall mortality rate 10% in hospital phase, 10% mortality during first year.

▶ 60% of deaths occur in the first hour.

Complications
▶ Death
▶ Chronic heart failure
▶ Ventricular tachycardia or ventricular fibrillation in first 24 hours
▶ Atrial fibrillation (AF) and flutter, bradycardia, heart block
▶ Deep vein thrombosis
▶ Pulmonary embolism
▶ Mitral regurgitation
▶ Cardiogenic shock

Chronic Heart Failure

Description
▶ A clinical syndrome characterized by insufficient cardiac output to meet the metabolic demands of the body, due to decreased contractility (systolic failure) or decreased ventricular filling (diastolic failure). It is classified as left-heart failure (acute) or right-heart failure (chronic) and may present as acute, pure left-sided failure; chronic, pure right-sided failure; or an acute exacerbation of chronic failure.
▶ Formerly called congestive heart failure; nomenclature has switched to chronic heart failure over the last few years.

Etiology
▶ Most common cause in children is congenital heart disease with volume or pressure overload.
▶ Acquired causes are metabolic abnormalities, severe hypoxia, acidosis, viral infection, myocarditis, acute rheumatic carditis, rheumatic valvular heart disease, cardiomyopathy, prolonged supraventricular tachycardia, complete heart block, severe anemia, acute hypertension, and bronchopulmonary dysplasia.
▶ *Left-sided failure:* An acute process causes abrupt decrease in the output of a previously healthy heart. This might include acute MI, acute papillary muscle rupture, acute dysrhythmia, acute valvular regurgitation, or drug toxicity.
▶ *Right-sided failure:* Chronic strain on compensatory mechanisms finally produces a hypertrophied heart that cannot keep up with metabolic demands. Chronic strain may be caused by chronic hypertension; hypertrophic or restrictive cardiomyopathy; chronic, subclinical sympathetic nervous system stimulation; chronic valvular stenosis/regurgitation causing higher pressure; and drug toxicity.

Incidence and Demographics
▶ Occurs in infants through old age
▶ Male preponderance until age 75, then equal occurrence
▶ Most frequent hospital admitting diagnosis

Risk Factors

► Factors precipitating CHF in patients with underlying heart disease include:

▷ Patient noncompliance with medications

▷ Excess salt intake, stress, obesity, pulmonary infection

▷ Uncontrolled hypertension

▷ Dyslipidemia

▷ Inadequate medical therapy for cardiac risk factor (e.g., hypertension, hyperlipidemia, etc.)

▷ Progression or complications of underlying disorder such as arrhythmias and cardiac muscle damage

▷ Increased or decreased volume, anemia, electrolyte imbalance

▷ Chronic or overuse of drugs such as NSAIDs, acetaminophen, beta-blockers, steroids; digitalis toxicity; alcohol

Prevention and Screening

► Control of underlying disorder

► Monitoring for and treatment of risk factors

Assessment

History (see Table 8–15 for CHF Classification)

► Dyspnea on exertion, diminished exercise capacity, weakness

► Nocturia, orthopnea, paroxysmal nocturnal dyspnea, nocturnal cough

► Edema

► Anorexia

► Infants present with poor feeding, poor weight gain, tachypnea that worsens during feeding, cold sweat

► Older children may complain of shortness of breath (especially with activity), puffy eyelids, swollen feet, exercise intolerance

Physical Exam

► Overall appearance, noting whether short of breath on walking or sitting

► Basilar rales, wheezes, S_3 gallop rhythm, displaced point of maximal impulse (PMI)

► Cool extremities, cyanosis, pallor or grayish blue color

► Change in mental status

► Ascites, hepatomegaly

► Hypotension, pulsus alternans, tachycardia, tachypnea

► Frothy pink sputum

► Edema, rapid weight gain

► Jugular venous distention

TABLE 8–15.
NY HEART ASSOCIATION FUNCTIONAL CLASSIFICATION OF HEART FAILURE

CLASS	FUNCTIONAL CAPACITY: HOW A PATIENT WITH CARDIAC DISEASE FEELS DURING PHYSICAL EXERTION
I	Patients with cardiac disease but resulting in no limitation of physical activity. Ordinary physical activity does not cause undue fatigue, palpitation, dyspnea, or anginal pain.
II	Patients with cardiac disease resulting in slight limitation of physical activity. They are comfortable at rest. Ordinary physical activity results in fatigue, palpitation, dyspnea, or anginal pain.
III	Patients with cardiac disease resulting in marked limitation of physical activity. They are comfortable at rest. Less than ordinary activity causes fatigue, palpitation, dyspnea, or anginal pain.
IV	Patients with cardiac disease resulting in inability to carry on any physical activity without discomfort. Symptoms of heart failure or the anginal syndrome may be present even at rest. If any physical activity is undertaken, discomfort increases.

▶ While elements of both left- and right-sided failure often exist in a patient, it is often possible to identify the etiology of the problem by sorting symptoms into these two categories:

  ▷ *Left-sided failure* produces signs and symptoms of acute low cardiac output and high pulmonary pressures: dyspnea at rest, anxiety, chest discomfort/heaviness, pale skin, murmur of mitral regurgitation, S_3 gallop, crackles through most of the lung field bilaterally, frothy cough.

  ▷ *Right-sided failure* produces symptoms of compensated chronic fluid retention/ overload: dyspnea with exertion, easily fatigued, paroxysmal nocturnal dyspnea, orthopnea, anorexia, basilar rales, abdominal fullness, jugular venous distention, lower extremity edema, hepatosplenomegaly, hepatic/splenic hum, pulsatile chest wall heave, displaced point of maximal impulse, single or multiple murmurs of stenosis or regurgitation.

Diagnostic Studies

▶ CHF is a clinical diagnosis and diagnostic tests are used only to assist in identifying the cause and to determine severity and identify complications.

▶ Chest X-ray: for pleural effusions, pulmonary edema, cardiomegaly, and to rule out pneumonia

▶ Electrocardiogram: identify arrhythmias, type of heart disease, and possible left ventricular strain

▶ Echocardiogram: ejection fraction (EF) determines severity; assists in determining the cause of CHF (type of heart defect, enlarged chambers, decreased left ventricular function)

▶ Electrolytes, BUN, creatinine, cardiac enzymes, urinalysis, arterial blood gases, pulse oximetry

▶ Cardiac catheterization: not routine (important for primary etiology)

▶ Endomyocardial biopsy: useful only for myocarditis or infiltrative disease

Differential Diagnosis

▶ Renal disease

▶ Failure to thrive

▶ Chronic obstructive pulmonary disease

▶ Nephrotic syndrome

▶ Cirrhosis

▶ Pulmonary emboli

▶ Acute MI

▶ Pneumonia

▶ Asthma

▶ Bacterial endocarditis

▶ Chronic venous insufficiency

Management

▶ The severity of the CHF dictates the course of medical/surgical management; the goal is to improve quality of life by reducing symptoms.

Nonpharmacologic Treatment

▶ Identify and treat underlying disease and control precipitating factors.

▶ Control leg edema with elastic pressure stockings and elevation of legs.

▶ Sodium and fluid restriction, daily weight assessment

▶ Patient education, cardiac rehabilitation: goal is to balance activity with metabolic restriction

▶ Oxygen

▶ Other options: surgical—valve replacement and cardiac transplant

Pharmacologic Treatment (see Table 8–16)

▶ Pediatric patients requiring medications should be managed by cardiologists.

▶ Patients frequently need a 3–4 drug regimen to control symptoms of cardiac impairment.

▶ Diuretics reduce preload and left ventricular filling.

▶ ACE inhibitors are the cornerstone of therapy; prevent progression of left ventricular dysfunction.

▶ Beta-blockers improve ventricular function and reduce postinfarction mortality.

▶ Glycoside improves contractility in systolic failure.

▶ Vasodilators reduce afterload.

▶ Anticoagulants prevent thrombus formation; generally used when EF <20%.

How Long to Treat

▶ Acute episodes: until resolution and stabilization of symptoms

▶ Chronic condition: indefinitely

TABLE 8–16.
DRUG TREATMENT FOR ADULTS WITH CHRONIC HEART FAILURE

DRUGS	TREATMENT REGIMEN	COMMON SIDE EFFECTS
CARDIAC GLYCOSIDES		
Digoxin (Lanoxin)	Loading dose 1.0 mg p.o. over 24 hours, starting 0.5 mg rather than 0.25 mg q 12 x 2 Maintenance 0.25 mg q.d., or 0.125 mg q.d. if risk of toxicity	GI—anorexia, nausea CNS—apathy, weakness, headache Cardiac—arrhythmia Not indicated for acute MI Monitor toxicity
DIURETICS		
Furosemide (Lasix)	Initial dose 20–80 mg q.d. Dose dependent on acute vs. chronic management	Electrolyte disturbances, orthostatic hypotension, Dizziness, weakness, GI upset Ototoxicity if rapid IV
Hydrochlorothiazide (HCTZ)	Mild symptoms—25–50 mg q.d.	Anorexia, nausea, vomiting, cramping
Metolazone (Zaroxolyn)	2.5–5 mg 1 hour before furosemide Generally, once or twice a week	Marked electrolyte imbalance, CNS effects
Spirolactone (Aldactone)	25–50 mg q.d. or in divided doses	Hyperkalemia
ANGIOTENSIN-CONVERTING ENZYME (ACE) INHIBITORS		
Captopril (Capoten)	6.25–12.25 mg t.i.d.	Angioedema, hypotension Cough—may be significant Hyperkalemia—use with caution in renal impairment
Enalapril (Vasotec)	2.5 mg b.i.d., titrate to 10 mg b.i.d.	Same as above
Lisinopril (Zestril)	20 mg q.d.	Same as above
Quinapril (Accupril)	10 mg q.d.	Same as above
BETA-BLOCKERS		
Carvedilol (Coreg)	3.25 mg p.o. b.i.d., titrate *slowly* to 25 mg b.i.d. or t.i.d.	Bradycardia, depression, fatigue
Metoprolol (Lopressor)	5 mg b.i.d., titrate to 100 mg b.i.d.	Same as above
VASODILATORS		
Hydralazine (Apresoline)	10 mg q.i.d.; target dose 300 mg daily Requires 8–12-hour nitrate-free period before starting	GI side effects, hypotension, headaches, tachycardia
Isosorbide dinitrate (Isordil)	5–10 mg t.i.d.; target dose 160 mg daily	Same as above

Special Considerations

▶ Geriatric patients: special attention to dosage requirements

▶ Lactation: multiple drug regimen is of concern

When to Consult, Refer, Hospitalize

▶ Consult with a physician for initial diagnosis with management plan.

▶ Refer all pediatric patients and pregnant and lactating women with CHF to a cardiologist for treatment.

▶ Refer if complications or exacerbation does not respond to treatment.

Follow-Up

▶ Every 3 months if stable

▶ Patient education about diet, activity, medication, self-monitoring, what symptoms to report

Expected Course

▶ Chronic: poor prognosis if ejection fraction less than 20% or steady decline after diagnosis

▶ Acute: generally responsive to initial treatment

Complications

▶ Electrolyte disturbances, arrhythmias, digitalis toxicity

Syncope

Description

▶ Temporary loss of consciousness, accompanied by fainting; loss of muscle tone; and possibly brief tonic contractions of the face, extremities, and trunk

Etiology

▶ Systemic hypotension leads to brief cerebral ischemia, causing loss of function.

▶ Simple syncope usually is a vasovagal event, triggered by fear, pain, excitement, or extended periods of standing still, especially in warm environments.

▶ Cough syncope is seen predominantly in asthmatic children.

▶ Long QT syndrome is usually characterized by a loss of consciousness during exercise or emotional stress and is accompanied by cardiac rhythm abnormalities.

▶ Vasomotor syncope due to impaired vasoconstriction results in hypotension with decreased cerebral perfusion; includes vasovagal and carotid sinus syncope.

▶ Postural (orthostatic) syncope: dehydration, autonomic insufficiency, medication

▶ Cardiogenic syncope: disturbances of rhythm, conduction, or hemodynamics

▶ Psychiatric disorders: anxiety, depression, conversion disorder

▶ Neurologic disorders (rare): vertebrobasilar TIAs or migraines

▶ Pathophysiology related to reflex-mediated vasomotor instability; decreased cardiac output or blood flow obstruction; metabolic disruptions (hypoglycemia, hypoxia, hyperventilation); neurologic events (seizures, cerebrovascular diseases)

Incidence and Demographics

▶ 30% of adults will experience at least one episode of syncope.

▶ 3% of all ED visits

▶ Vasomotor syncope or "fainting" is common in young women, and associated with stress or pain.

▶ A diagnosis can be made in 45%–50% of cases.

▶ Syncopal events occur in 10%–15% of all adolescents.

▶ Simple syncope is uncommon before age 10–12 and occurs more frequently in girls.

Risk Factors

▶ Cardiac disease, diabetes

▶ Vasodilators, diuretics, adrenergic blocking agents

▶ Age, family history of sudden death

▶ Prolonged QT syndromes

▶ Asthma and cough

Prevention and Screening

▶ Adequate hydration

Assessment

History

▶ Detailed, including symptoms before and after event (position changes, prolonged standing, exposure to warm environment)

▶ Lightheadedness, diaphoresis, nausea, visual changes before event

▶ Length of loss of consciousness, seizure activity, height of fall, any injuries including to tongue

▶ Confusion or drowsiness after event

▶ Associated cardiac or neurological symptoms: chest pain, diaphoresis, palpitations, headache, diplopia, aphasia, unilateral motor weakness, paresthesia

▶ Incontinence of bladder or bowel

▶ Past medical history: cardiac, neurologic; family history of heart disease, seizures

▶ Medications: vasodilators, beta-blockers, diuretics, anticholinergics

▶ Recent drug or medication use

▶ Interview family member or witness

Physical Exam

▶ Vital signs including orthostatic changes

▶ Cardiovascular: arrhythmia, murmurs, displaced PMI (cardiomegaly), bruits, difference in blood pressure between arms including orthostatic pressures

▶ Neurologic exam for focal deficits

Diagnostic Studies

▶ ECG for arrhythmia and other cardiac disease

▶ Chest X-ray (CXR) if associated coughing

▶ CBC and electrolytes to rule out anemia, metabolic abnormalities

▶ Fasting blood glucose, thyroid function tests

▶ Pregnancy testing in women of childbearing age

▶ Echocardiography to rule out valvular disease, particularly if murmur

▶ If exertional syncope, stress testing to rule out ischemia

▶ Holter or event monitoring to rule out arrhythmia

▶ Tilt table to evaluate autonomic dysfunction

▶ Electrophysiologic studies if recurrent event and still no known etiology

▶ Electroencephalography if seizure history or seizures suspected

▶ Brain imaging if focal neurologic signs (CT or MRI)

▶ Carotid or transcranial Doppler studies if bruits or to rule out vertebrobasilar insufficiency

Differential Diagnosis

▶ Vasomotor syncope

▶ Orthostatic hypotension

▶ Acute myocardial infarction

▶ Sick sinus syndrome

▶ Drug reaction

▶ Cough or micturition

▶ Conduction disorders (AV block)

▶ Arrhythmias

▶ Aortic stenosis

▶ Pulmonary stenosis or hypertension

▶ Congenital anomalies with right–left shunting

▶ Seizure

▶ Vertebrobasilar TIA

▶ Psychogenic cause (hyperventilation)

▶ Metabolic abnormality

Management

Nonpharmacologic Treatment

▶ In cases of benign syncope (vasomotor), explain etiology to patient and advise lying down when prodromal symptoms occur.

▶ Simple syncope can be managed by avoiding triggers, pushing fluids, and salt-loading during hot weather.

▶ The patient also can be taught to contract the calf muscles repeatedly while sitting or standing still.

▶ Long QT syndrome can sometimes be managed by the implantation of a cardiac pacemaker.

▶ Occasionally, a left cervicothoracic sympathectomy is necessary.

Pharmacologic Treatment

▶ Medical management depends on etiology.

▶ Use the smallest doses of antihypertensive medications and eliminate any unnecessary drugs.

▶ Use beta-adrenergic blocking agents for recurrent episodes of simple syncope or prolonged QT syndrome.

▶ Improve management of asthma episodes.

Special Considerations

▶ Further evaluation is necessary in the presence of known heart disease, arrhythmias, pathological murmurs, and exertional syncope.

▶ With geriatric patients, increased risk secondary to comorbidities, polypharmacy, autonomic neuropathy, and dehydration due to decreased fluid intake.

▶ Syncope common in third trimester of pregnancy due to aortocaval compression by the enlarged uterus in the supine position; try left-side lying position.

When to Consult, Refer, Hospitalize

▶ Hospitalize for ventricular tachycardia, sustained supraventricular tachycardia, suspected myocardial infarction, medication that can cause malignant arrhythmias (torsades de pointes with quinidine), or any other high risk for cardiac syncope.

▶ Hospitalize for acute focal neurologic signs.

▶ Hospitalize older people who cannot be safely managed in their present living environments.

▶ Refer to cardiology if prolonged QT syndrome is suspected or if simple syncope is hard to control.

▶ Refer to neurology for new-onset seizures.

▶ Refer for mental health evaluation if psychogenic origin is suspected.

Follow-Up

Expected Course

▶ Depends on etiology; patient may outgrow simple syncope by young adulthood.

Complications

▶ Depends on etiology

▶ Increased risk of complications with heart disease, advanced age, and polypharmacy

Murmurs

Description

▶ Sounds created when there is turbulent forward blood flow because of partial obstruction of a stenotic heart valve or turbulent backward flow through an incompetent valve due to faulty valve closure (regurgitation) that produces an abnormal sound distinguishable from other heart sounds

▶ Innocent (functional, physiologic, benign) murmurs: turbulent flow as blood is ejected from a chamber or from increased or vigorous flow across a valve; associated with no structural abnormality

Etiology

▶ Organic: congenital or acquired (atherosclerosis)

▶ Functional: resulting from another medical condition such as anemia, fever, thyrotoxicosis, pregnancy

▶ Innocent murmurs: no evidence of cardiac pathology

▶ Rheumatic fever is a potential contributor to all murmurs.

▶ Infective endocarditis: regurgitation murmurs

▶ Other contributing factors include:

  ▷ Aortic stenosis: congenital and senile calcifications

  ▷ Aortic regurgitation: high blood pressure, aortic dissection, syphilis, collagen vascular disease

  ▷ Mitral regurgitation: ruptured chordae tendineae, CAD, mitral valve prolapse

  ▷ Tricuspid regurgitation: right ventricular failure, right ventricular infarction

Incidence and Demographics

▶ Murmurs are common and can occur in all ages.

▶ Eighty percent of children have innocent murmurs sometime during childhood, usually beginning at age 3.

▶ An innocent murmur is a frequent finding in the third trimester of pregnancy.

▶ Older adults often have a II/VI systolic ejection murmur because of decreased compliance of the heart.

Risk Factors

▶ Age: Children and older adults have the most murmurs.

▶ Physiologic states of increased metabolic demand: fever, anemia, pregnancy, hyperthyroidism

▶ Heart disease

Prevention and Screening

▶ Prevention through treatment of streptococcal pharyngitis to prevent rheumatic fever

▶ Screening through periodic routine examinations

Assessment

History

▶ Symptoms such as shortness of breath, syncope, chest pain, palpitations, and exercise intolerance indicate pathologic murmur.

▶ Family history of heart disease; prenatal and perinatal history

▶ Signs or history of infections and illness

▶ Activity level and endurance; feeding; crying; cyanosis

Physical Exam

▶ Skin color and moisture; nail clubbing

▶ Vital signs; pulses; posture

▶ Neck for distended veins, bruits, and thyromegaly

▶ Lungs for adventitious sounds

▶ Chest for asymmetry, precordial bulge, thrill, heave, and PMI

▶ Abdomen for organomegaly

▶ Extremities for edema

▶ Assessment of murmurs

　▷ Grading of intensity (see Table 8–17)

　▷ Location: area with greatest intensity

　▷ Radiation: heard in direction of blood flow

　▷ Pitch: high, medium, low

　▷ Quality: soft, harsh, rumbling

　▷ Timing: within the cardiac cycle (systolic between S_1/S_2; diastolic between S_2/S_1)

　　▶ Once auscultated, a murmur must be identified as systolic or diastolic.

　　▶ S_1 is mitral and tricuspid valve closure.

　　▶ S_2 is aortic and pulmonic valve closure.

　　▶ The period between S_1 and S_2 is systole.

　　▶ The period between S_2 and S_1 is diastole.

TABLE 8–17.
GRADING OF MURMURS

GRADE	CHARACTERISTICS
I/VI	Very faint, may not be heard in all positions
II/VI	Quiet but heard immediately upon placing the stethoscope on the chest
III/VI	Moderately loud
IV/VI	Loud accompanied by palpable thrill
V/VI	Very loud, heard with a stethoscope partly off the chest; accompanied by palpable thrill
VI/VI	Heard with the stethoscope entirely off the chest and accompanied by palpable thrill

▶ Murmurs that occur after S_1 and before S_2 are systolic.

　▷ Mitral and tricuspid regurgitation (backflow through an incompetent valve)

　▷ Aortic and pulmonic stenosis (turbulent flow through a tight opening)

▶ Murmurs that occur after S_2 and before S_1 are diastolic.

　▷ Aortic and pulmonic regurgitation (backflow through an incompetent valve)

　▷ Mitral and tricuspid stenosis (turbulent flow through a tight opening)

▷ Placement of murmurs

　▶ Once murmurs are identified as systolic or diastolic, the likely valve of origin must be identified by location (see Figure 8–2 and Table 8-18).

　▶ Murmurs loudest at the second intercostal space, right sternal border, are likely aortic.

　▶ Murmurs loudest at the second intercostal space, left sternal border, are likely pulmonic.

　▶ Murmurs loudest at the fourth intercostal space, left sternal border, are likely tricuspid.

　▶ Murmurs loudest at the fifth intercostal space, midclavicular line, are likely mitral.

▷ *Systolic regurgitant murmur:* begins with S_1 and usually lasts throughout systole (pansystolic or holosystolic); caused by blood flow from a chamber that is at a higher pressure throughout systole than the receiving chamber (associated *only* with ventricular septal defect [VSD], mitral and tricuspid regurgitation [MR and TR])

▷ *Diastolic:* early diastolic (caused by the incompetence of the aortic or pulmonary valve); mid-diastolic (caused by turbulence of the tricuspid or mitral valve); or presystolic (caused by flow through the AV valves during ventricular diastole—tricuspid or mitral stenosis [TS or MS])

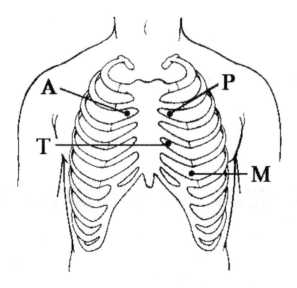

FIGURE 8–2.
STANDARD CHEST AUSCULTATORY POINTS

▷ Continuous murmur: S_1 through S_2; conditions such as patent ductus arteriosus (PDA)

▷ Innocent heart murmurs (functional, physiologic, benign); see Tables 8–19 and 8-20)

▶ Left sternal border (LSB), 2nd through 4th left interspaces and apex

▶ Grade I–II/VI; low pitch; soft, short, nonradiating, midsystolic

▶ Variable loudness; heard best in supine position, diminishes with upright position

▷ Interpretation of murmurs

▶ Once timing and placement are identified, the valvular disorder is evident.

▶ A systolic murmur at the second intercostal space, right sternal border, is an aortic murmur occurring when the aortic valve is open—aortic stenosis.

TABLE 8–18.
HEART SOUNDS AND RELATED HEART VALUES POSITIONS

DIASTOLE	SYSTOLE	DIASTOLE	SYSTOLE
S_2	S_1	S_2	S_1
A/P close	M/T close	A/P close	M/T close
M/T open	A/P close	M/T open	A/P close

TABLE 8–19.
TYPES OF MURMURS

TYPE OF MURMUR	CHARACTERISTICS OF THE MURMUR
Systolic murmur	Occurs between S_1 and S_2
	Systolic ejection murmur: interval between S_1 and onset of murmur (also referred to as crescendo-decrescendo); caused by blood flow through stenotic or deformed semilunar valves or by increased blood flow through normal semilunar valves
	Systolic regurgitant murmur: begins with S_1 and usually lasts throughout systole (pansystolic or holosystolic); caused by blood flow from a chamber at a higher pressure throughout systole than receiving chamber (associated only with VSD, MR, and TR)
Diastolic murmur	Occurs between S_2 and S_1
	Classified as early diastolic and caused by the incompetence of the aortic or pulmonary valve, atrial and pulmonic regurgitation (AR, PR); mid-diastolic, caused by turbulence of the tricuspid or mitral valve; or presystolic, caused by flow through the atrioventricular valves during ventricular diastole (tricuspid or mitral stenosis [TS, MS])
Continuous murmur	Occurs with S_1 and continues through the S_2 into diastole
	Seen with conditions such as patent ductus arteriosus (PDA), pulmonary artery (PA) stenosis, Blalock-Taussig shunt
Innocent heart murmurs (functional murmur) (see also Table 8–20)	Arise from cardiovascular structures in absence of anatomic abnormalities (80% of children have innocent murmurs sometime during childhood, usually beginning at 3 years old); also referred to as functional, benign, or physiological murmurs

TABLE 8–20.
CLASSIFICATION OF INNOCENT MURMURS IN CHILDREN

TYPE OF MURMUR	CHARACTERISTICS OF THE MURMUR
Vibratory murmur (Still's murmur)	Usually detected at 3–6 years of age; uncommon before 2 years of age
	Described as a musical, buzzing, "twanging string," or vibratory sound
	Heard best at middle left sternal border (MLSB) or between left lower sternal border (LLSB) and apex when patient is in supine position; diminishes when patient is upright or does Valsalva maneuver
	Midsystolic and grade II–III/VI in intensity; not accompanied by a thrill
	Intensity may increase with anemia, fever, or exercise; ECG and CXR normal
Pulmonary ejection murmur	Usually detected at 8–14 years of age; heard best at the upper left sternal border (ULSB)
	Early to midsystolic; grade I–III/VI in intensity; not accompanied by a thrill; soft and blowing
	EKG and CXR are normal
Pulmonary flow murmur of the newborn	Blood flow through sharply angulated right and left pulmonary arteries at birth; usually detected in newborns, especially those with low birth weights, and disappears by 3–6 months of age
	Heard best at the ULSB
	Midsystolic and grade I–II/VI in intensity; not accompanied by a thrill
	Transmits well to the right and left chest, back, and both axillae
	Normal EKG and CXR
Venous hum	Originates from turbulence in the jugular venous system
	Usually detected at 3–6 years old
	Heard best at the infraclavicular and supraclavicular areas (disappears when the patient is supine or when the neck veins are gently occluded)
	Continuous humming murmur
	Normal EKG and CXR
Carotid bruit	Originates from turbulence in the carotid arteries; detected at any age
	Systolic ejection murmur; grade II–III/VI in intensity
	Rarely, a thrill is palpable over the carotid artery
	Normal EKG and CXR

▶ A diastolic murmur at the second intercostal space, right sternal border, is an aortic murmur occurring when the aortic valve is closed—aortic regurgitation.

▶ A systolic murmur at the fifth intercostal space, midclavicular line, is a mitral murmur occurring when the mitral valve is closed—mitral regurgitation.

▶ A diastolic murmur occurring at the fifth intercostal space, midclavicular line, is a mitral murmur occurring when the mitral valve is open—mitral stenosis.

Systolic Murmurs

Aortic Stenosis

▶ Second intercostal space (ICS) right of sternum, with patient sitting and leaning forward

▶ Valve is open when stenotic murmur occurs and is caused by forward flow through stenotic valve

▶ Begins after S_1 and is a crescendo-decrescendo or diamond-shaped ejection murmur

▶ Radiation into neck from aortic area

▶ Medium pitch with variable intensity

▶ Harsh, loudest at base; musical at apex

▶ Midsystolic

▶ Systolic thrill may be present

▶ Seen frequently in older adults and associated with a diminished S_2

Tricuspid Regurgitation

▶ Lower LSB

▶ Begins with S_1; high-pitched, smooth, blowing quality

▶ Pansystolic regurgitant murmur, increases in intensity with inspiration

▶ Right ventricular lift

▶ Always associated with pathology, usually diseased right ventricle from rheumatic heart disease

Ventricular Septal Defect

▶ LSB (3rd to 5th ICS)

▶ Radiation wide over precordium but not into axilla

▶ Loud (particularly base), harsh, pansystolic regurgitant murmur with thrill

Hypertrophic Obstructive Cardiomyopathy

▶ LSB

▶ No radiation

▶ Murmur increases with Valsalva maneuver, decreases with patient squatting

▶ Midsystolic

Pulmonic Stenosis

▶ LSB 2nd or 3rd ICS, pulmonary area

▶ Generally no radiation unless loud, then toward left neck

▶ Variable intensity, medium pitch

▶ Midsystolic: begins after S_1 with crescendo-decrescendo contour

▶ Associated with thrill if significant pathology; usually congenital cause

Mitral Regurgitation
- ▶ Location: apex; frequently radiates to wide area of chest and to left axilla
- ▶ Intensity variable, often loud; does not increase with inspiration
- ▶ Pitch is high with blowing quality
- ▶ S_3 usually also heard
- ▶ Pansystolic regurgitant murmur frequently accompanied with thrill
- ▶ Begins with S_1 (which may be decreased)
- ▶ Valve closed when the murmur occurs; noise caused from backflow through incompetent valve
- ▶ Always pathologic

Diastolic Murmurs
- ▶ Always indicative of heart disease
- ▶ Often heard best with the bell of the stethoscope

Mitral Stenosis
- ▶ Listen with patient in left lateral decubitus position; also with exercise.
- ▶ Diastolic rumbling murmur that begins after a short period of silence after S_2
- ▶ Low in pitch, heard best with bell of stethoscope in light skin contact
- ▶ No radiation
- ▶ Loudest at apex; best heard after mild exercise

Aortic Regurgitation
- ▶ Heard at LSB with patient leaning forward and listening with diaphragm of stethoscope pressed firmly on the chest
- ▶ Early diastolic murmur that begins immediately after S_2 and diminishes in intensity
- ▶ Blowing, high-pitched, decrescendo
- ▶ Heard with rheumatic heart disease or syphilis

Pulmonary Valve Insufficiency
- ▶ LSB 2nd ICS
- ▶ Radiates mid-right sternal border
- ▶ High-pitched, loudest base, decrescendo murmur

Continuous Murmurs (Quality Often Varies When Patient Changes Position)
- ▶ Patent ductus arteriosus
- ▶ Coarctation of the aorta
- ▶ Peripheral pulmonary stenosis

Diagnostic Studies
- ▶ ECG to detect underlying heart disease
- ▶ CBC to look for signs of infection, anemia

▶ Chest X-ray to evaluate heart failure, size of heart

▶ Echocardiography for valve pathology and systolic/diastolic function

▶ Angiography for more thorough evaluation

▶ Fluoroscopy to show calcified aortic valve

Differential Diagnosis

▶ See descriptions of systolic and diastolic murmurs above.

Management

Nonpharmacologic Treatment

▶ Patient education on disease entity and lifestyle modifications for underlying disorder

▶ Valvular surgical repair

Pharmacologic Treatment

▶ Stabilize hemodynamic deficiencies.

▶ Antibiotics for endocarditis prophylaxis as indicated

How Long to Treat

▶ Often a chronic condition

Special Considerations

▶ Geriatric patients: aortic stenosis common

▶ Pregnancy: monitor throughout pregnancy with intervention and cardiac consultation for any change in objective findings

When to Consult, Refer, Hospitalize

▶ Consult or refer if symptomatic (signs of heart failure, growth failure, syncope, cyanosis); diastolic murmur; systolic murmur that is loud (grade III/IV or with a thrill), long in duration, and transmits well to other parts of the body; abnormally strong or weak pulses; abnormal cardiac size or silhouette or pulmonary vasculature on CXR.

▶ Refer to pediatric cardiologist for murmur in conjunction with chromosomal abnormalities (especially trisomy 13, trisomy 18, and trisomy 21).

▶ If abnormal ECG and symptomatic, hospitalization may be necessary

Follow-Up

▶ Asymptomatic patients should be assessed at least annually and at every visit.

▶ Innocent murmurs: none necessary

▶ Monitor murmurs associated with pregnancy; if they worsen, refer to cardiology.

Complications

▶ Chronic heart failure

▶ Poor activity tolerance; growth and development problems

▶ Progression of mitral stenosis—potential for thrombus formation and hypoxia

▶ Progression of mitral regurgitation—associated with dyspnea and orthopnea

▶ Atrial fibrillation with mitral stenosis and mitral regurgitation

▶ Stroke or TIA

▶ Bacterial endocarditis

Mitral Valve Prolapse (MVP)

Description

▶ Condition characterized by decreased ventricular load, resulting in prolapse of valve leaflets during systole

▶ Produces a mid-systolic click and late-systolic murmur

Etiology

▶ Strong familial pattern, associated with a connective tissue disorder such as Marfan syndrome and Ehlers-Danlos syndrome (nearly all patients with Marfan syndrome have MVP); systemic lupus erythematosus (SLE)

▶ One-third of patients have congenital heart disease (atrial septum defect, ventricular septum defect, or Ebstein's anomaly).

▶ May be caused by rheumatic endocarditis or ruptured chordae tendineae post-MI

▶ May be idiopathic; 50% of cases are in children

▶ Pathology involves abnormal valvular collagen leading to degeneration. Excessive tissue increases orifice size. Function of the papillary muscle and chordae apparatus is abnormal. MVP is the most common cause of mitral regurgitation.

Incidence and Demographics

▶ Adolescents and young adults; more common in females and thin patients; may be comorbid with minor chest wall deformities

▶ 3% of the general population; 5% of pediatric population; 75% without morbidity/mortality

Risk Factors

▶ Familial history

▶ Connective tissue disorders

▶ Mitral regurgitation

Prevention and Screening

▶ Proper dental care and prophylaxis to prevent endocarditis

▶ Anticoagulation to prevent thrombus/embolus for patients with risk factors

▶ Screening through periodic routine exams

Assessment

History

▶ Frequently asymptomatic

▶ Palpitations, lightheadedness, dyspnea, fatigue, syncope

- ▶ Anxiety, panic attacks
- ▶ Possible chest pain, usually mild

Physical Exam

- ▶ Murmur and clinical findings may vary from visit to visit.
- ▶ Late systolic murmur: begins in mid or late systole and can continue through S_2
- ▶ Mid- and late-systolic clicks may be audible.
- ▶ Positional murmur changes: When standing or with Valsalva, click is closer to the first heart sound (S_1); with squatting, click is farther from first heart sound (S_1).
- ▶ Body build: thin, tall in some cases
- ▶ Autonomic abnormalities: orthostatic hypotension
- ▶ Mitral regurgitation (MR): holosystolic murmur, radiation to axilla, frequent thrill
- ▶ A high incidence of thoracic skeletal anomalies (80%) are seen in association with MVP:
  - ▷ Pectus excavatum (50%)
  - ▷ Straight back (20%)
  - ▷ Scoliosis (10%)

Diagnostic Studies

- ▶ Echocardiogram: diagnostic, should be repeated with significant change in murmur or accompanying clinical findings; will detect and quantify MR
- ▶ ECG: usually normal; possible atrial or ventricular arrhythmias; left atrial/ventricular enlargement
- ▶ CXR: normal
- ▶ Tilt table test to identify autonomic dysfunction
- ▶ Holter monitor to identify arrhythmia

Differential Diagnosis

- ▶ Stenotic mitral or tricuspid valve
- ▶ Pericarditis
- ▶ Tricuspid valve prolapse
- ▶ Papillary muscle dysfunction
- ▶ Hypertrophic cardiomyopathy

Management

Nonpharmacologic Treatment

- ▶ No treatment or activity restrictions in patients with asymptomatic MVP (about 75%)
- ▶ Patients who are symptomatic (palpitations, lightheadedness, syncope) or have arrhythmias should undergo treadmill exercise testing, ambulatory ECG monitoring, or both.
- ▶ Surgery: mitral valve replacement

Pharmacologic Treatment

▶ Prophylactic antibiotics with invasive procedure and dental cleaning if there is MR, to prevent endocarditis

▶ Beta-blockers such as atenolol 25–50 mg if patient has exercise-induced arrhythmias, palpitations, and panic attacks except with asthma

▶ Digoxin with inotropic deficit

▶ Anticoagulation for atrial fibrillation and MR: warfarin (Coumadin) to maintain international normalized ratio (INR) of 2.0–3.0

▶ Sodium chloride tablets for low baseline intravascular volume, abnormal renin-aldosterone response, and abnormal compensatory response

How Long to Treat

▶ Lifelong monitoring and treatment unless patient undergoes surgical valve replacement

Special Considerations

▶ Males over 50 have higher incidence of complications.

▶ Pregnancy may improve symptoms of MVP.

When to Consult, Refer, Hospitalize

▶ Referral to a cardiologist for initial diagnosis, symptomatic patients, arrhythmias, and complications

Follow-Up

▶ Monitor for MR q year with echocardiogram for problems; q 2–3 years for mild/moderate murmur with regurgitation; q 5 years for click only.

Expected Course

▶ 25% function with little problem for several decades; however, with increased decline in valve function, may progress rapidly to more severe symptoms

▶ 75% have stable lifetime function

Complications

▶ Uncommon, usually relate to underlying heart disease

▶ Stroke or TIA from embolus

▶ Progression to or worsening MR

▶ CHF, arrhythmia

▶ Infective endocarditis

▶ Sudden death

Atrial Fibrillation

Description

▶ Common arrhythmia, acute or chronic, characterized by nonsynchronized irregular atrial and ventricular activity

- Untreated rates from atrial 200–600/minute with ventricular rate 80–180/minute
- Difference between apical rate and pulse rate is pulse deficit
- Non–life threatening by itself; however, comes with major risk of embolism

Etiology

- Extra-cardiac causes include pulmonary embolus, surgery, alcohol intoxication and withdrawal, hyperthyroidism
- May be preceded by premature atrial contraction
- May be idiopathic or have a variety of cardiac causes, including rheumatic heart disease, cardiomyopathy, atrial septal defect, mitral valve prolapse, sick sinus syndrome, acute myocardial infarction, heart failure, and pericarditis
- Chaotic electrical activity within the atria; AV node continuously stimulated by atrial impulses, so ventricular rate is irregular and usually rapid
- Ineffective atrial emptying results in hemodynamic instability, poor cardiac output, and stasis of blood

Incidence and Demographics

- According to the Framingham Heart Study (2013), there is a 1 in 4 lifetime risk of developing AF in both men and women 40 years or older.
- Increases with aging
- High recurrence of episodes
- 2%–4% of the adult population

Risk Factors

- Conditions leading to the above etiologies

Prevention and Screening

- Patient should avoid excessive alcohol, caffeine, and nicotine.
- Treat comorbid conditions.
- Assess and aggressively respond to triggers that compromise hemodynamic stability: acute MI, chronic heart failure, or pulmonary embolus.

Assessment

History

- Variable symptoms, from asymptomatic to severe
- Initial presentation may be with paroxysmal rhythm
- Palpitations, angina, fatigue, decline in activity level, marked dyspnea, dizziness, syncope
- Review of systems (ROS) for symptoms of hyperthyroidism, underlying cardiac disease, alcohol use

Physical Exam

- Tachycardia, irregular pulse—marked deficit between apical rate and radial pulse
- Pallor, orthostatic blood pressure changes

▶ Peripheral edema, jugular venous distension

▶ Tachypnea

▶ CNS disturbance: decreased mental acuity

Diagnostic Studies

▶ ECG: confirmatory with absent P waves, irregular ventricular rate, and rhythm 100–160 beats

▶ Cardiac event monitor

▶ Transthoracic or transesophageal echocardiography to assess underlying cardiac dysfunction

▶ Thyroid function tests

▶ Ventilation perfusion scan if pulmonary embolus is suspected (shortness of breath, chest pain)

Differential Diagnosis

▶ Hyperthyroidism

▶ Hypertension

▶ Pulmonary embolus

▶ Atrial flutter

▶ Sinus tachycardia

▶ Alcoholism

Management

Nonpharmacologic Treatment

▶ Treat underlying disorders.

▶ Refer for invasive therapy for refractory cases: cardioversion or radiofrequency catheter ablation of AV node.

▶ Pacemaker implantation

Pharmacologic Treatment

▶ Acute

▷ Hospital setting under care of cardiologist for cardioversion and possible anticoagulation

▷ IV beta-blockers, and calcium channel blockers administered to break arrhythmia (pharmacologic cardioversion), consider digoxin for people who are sedentary

▶ Chronic (rate control)

▷ Digoxin: loading dose 0.25 mg b.i.d. x 2 days or start at maintenance dose; maintenance 0.125–0.25 mg q.d.

▶ Check drug levels 6–8 hours after last dose or before dose.

▶ Monitor toxicity: fatigue, anorexia, weakness, and nausea.

▶ Digoxin ventricular response control is less effective with activity.

▶ Active individual: consider beta-blocker or calcium channel blocker.

▷ Beta-blockers: metoprolol 50–100 mg q.d.; atenolol 25–100 mg q.d. (side effects: bradycardia, fatigue, depression, impotence)

▷ Calcium channel blockers: verapamil 120–480 mg q.d.; diltiazem 90–360 mg q.d. (side effects: constipation, dizziness, headaches)

▷ Use caution with medication; some have a depressing effect on the AV node.

▷ Antithrombotic therapy: warfarin is the drug of choice for chronic atrial fibrillation

  ▸ Aspirin 325 mg q.d. in patients with contraindication to warfarin

  ▸ Arrhythmia > 48 hrs: anticoagulation therapy maintained 3–4 weeks before cardioversion

▷ Profile for those most at risk of stroke secondary to atrial fibrillation includes age over 65 years; previous TIA or stroke; high blood pressure; heart failure; thyrotoxicosis; clinical coronary disease; mitral stenosis; prosthetic heart valve; diabetes

How Long to Treat

▸ Anticoagulation therapy is indefinite unless situations arise that would contraindicate therapy.

▸ The CHA_2DS_2-VASc tool should be used when assessing stroke risk and deciding on the need for oral anticoagulation or antiplatelet therapy or no anticoagulation in the patient with atrial fibrillation (see Table 8-21).

▸ The CHA_2DS_2-VASc score tool should be used when assessing stroke risk and deciding on the need for oral anticoagulation or antiplatelet therapy or no anticoagulation in the patient with atrial fibrillation (from the National Guideline Clearinghouse, 2014).

  CHA_2DS_2-VASc score of 0: No antithrombotic therapy. (Do not offer AC for persons less than 65 with no other risk factor than gender (i.e., woman with score 1—no AC)

  CHA_2DS_2-VASc score of 1: Oral anticoagulation or antiplatelet therapy is recommended but preferably oral anticoagulation.

  CHA_2DS_2-VASc score ≥2: Oral anticoagulation is recommended

▸ See Table 8-21 for assessment of stroke risk using CHA_2DS_2-VASc score and bleeding risk for patients with atrial fibrillation on anticoagulation (AC).

Antiplatelet Agent for Atrial Fibrillation

▸ Aspirin

Anticoagulants for Nonvalvular Atrial Fibrillation

▸ Warfarin—can be used for valvular atrial fibrillation

▸ Dabigatran

▸ Rivaroxaban

▸ Apixaban

▸ When patients are on anticoagulant therapy use the HAS BLED-score to assess their risk for bleeding (see Table 8-22).

TABLE 8-21.
ASSESSMENT OF STROKE RISK USING CHA$_2$DS$_2$-VASC SCORE AND BLEEDING RISK FOR PATIENTS WITH ATRIAL FIBRILLATION ON ANTICOAGULATION (AC)

CHA$_2$DS-VASC	SCORE
Congestive Heart Failure	1
HTN	1
Age >75 years	2
Diabetes Mellitus	1
Stroke/Transient Ischemic Attach (TIA)/Thromboembolic (TE)	2
Vascular disease (prior MI, PAD or aortic plaque	1
Age 65–74 years old	1
Sex, female	1
Maximum Score	**9**

TABLE 8-22
BLED-SCORE TO ASSESS THEIR RISK FOR BLEEDING

HAS-BLED	SCORE
HTN (systolic blood pressure >160 mmHg	1
Abnormal renal and liver function (1 point each)	1 or 2
Stroke	1
Bleeding tendency	1
Labile international normalized ratios (INRs) if on Coumadin (warfarin)	1
Elderly (>65 years old)	1
Drugs or alcohol (1 point each)	1 or 2
Maximum Score	**9**

Special Considerations

▶ Geriatric patients: prevalent problem

▶ Pregnancy (rare): digoxin safe; cardioversion does not affect fetus; anticoagulation may result in spontaneous abortion although heparin does not cross placenta

▷ Recommendations for IV heparin during first trimester, oral warfarin second and third trimester

When to Consult, Refer, Hospitalize

▶ Initially, refer all patients to cardiologist for evaluation and management plan; refer pregnant women for management; and refer patients who are not controlled back to cardiologist for evaluation.

Follow-Up

▶ At least monthly for INR if on warfarin (target 2.5)

Expected Course

▶ Prognosis is dependent on underlying cause.

▶ Exercise and activity levels may be limited because of hemodynamic instability.

Complications

▶ Heart failure

▶ Stroke, peripheral arterial embolism

▶ Bradycardia, torsades de pointes with drug treatment; bleeding with anticoagulants

CONGENITAL HEART DEFECTS

Patent Ductus Arteriosus (PDA)

Description

▶ The ductus arteriosus is a normal fetal structure between the left pulmonary artery and the descending aorta.

▶ Functional closure of the ductus arteriosus usually occurs within 48 hours after birth. Anatomic closure is completed by 2–3 weeks of age.

▶ PDA becomes clinically significant if it persists past the neonatal period; it is unlikely to close spontaneously after that time and may produce signs and symptoms of pulmonary overcirculation.

Etiology

▶ Idiopathic

▶ High altitude

▶ Maternal exposure to rubella during first trimester

▶ Genetic or familial

Incidence and Demographics

▶ Full-term infants: 0.5/1,000 live births; at high altitudes (>4,500 feet), 15/1,000 live births

▶ Premature infants: 8/1,000 live births; prevalence in infants with birth weight <1,750 grams is 45%; <1,200 grams birth weight, 80%

Risk Factors

▶ Genetic predisposition with environmental triggers such as viruses and drugs

▶ Prematurity

Assessment

History

▶ Symptoms dependent on volume of pulmonary blood flow; patients are usually asymptomatic with a small PDA

▶ A moderate to large shunt may cause symptoms of chronic heart failure (tachypnea, sweating, poor feeding/poor weight gain), irritability, and lower respiratory tract infections.

Physical Exam

▶ Classic finding is a "machinery" murmur with continuous systolic and diastolic components, heard best at upper left sternal border (ULSB) and left infraclavicular area; none may be heard with severe left ventricular failure

▶ Patients with small PDAs usually have normal physical growth and normal pulses/pulse pressure.

▶ Tachycardia, tachypnea, crackles in cases of pulmonary overcirculation

▶ Hyperdynamic precordium

Diagnostic Studies

▶ ECG: normal or left ventricular, atrial hypertrophy depending on amount of the shunt

▶ Chest X-ray: normal with a small PDA. Varying degrees of cardiomegaly with enlargement of left atrium, left ventricle, and ascending aorta. Increased pulmonary vascular markings are proportionate to the amount of left-to-right shunting.

▶ Echocardiography: Doppler studies can provide functional information. Dimensions of the left atrium and ventricle can indirectly assess the amount of left-to-right shunting; the greater the dilation of these chambers, the larger the shunt.

▶ Cardiac catheterization: not necessary for diagnostic evaluation

Differential Diagnosis

▶ Arteriovenous malformations (systemic, pulmonary, or coronary)

▶ Venous hum

▶ Ventricular septal defect with aortic regurgitation

▶ Pulmonary atresia

▶ Persistent truncus arteriosus

▶ Aortopulmonary septal defect (AP window)

▶ Peripheral pulmonary stenosis

▶ Total anomalous venous connection

▶ Collaterals in coarctation of the aorta in tetralogy of Fallot/pulmonary atresia

▶ Anomalous origin of the left coronary artery from the pulmonary artery

▶ Ruptured sinus of Valsalva aneurysm

Management

Pharmacologic Treatment

▶ Indomethacin (Indocin; a prostaglandin synthetase inhibitor) during the neonatal period

  ▷ 0.2 mg/kg intravenously every 12 hours for up to 3 doses

  ▷ Contraindications to the use of indomethacin: blood urea nitrogen >25 mg/dL or creatinine >1.8 mg/dL, platelet count <80,000/mm^3, necrotizing enterocolitis, hyperbilirubinemia, and bleeding tendency (including intracranial hemorrhage)

Surgical Treatment

▶ Premature infants

▷ If medical therapy is unsuccessful or indomethacin is contraindicated after 2–3 attempts, surgical repair is indicated.

▷ Percutaneous coil embolization is performed in the cardiac catheterization laboratory. Percutaneous closure is not currently available for very small or preterm infants; new devices under study may make it feasible to close even large PDAs or PDAs in small infants.

▷ Surgical ligation performed by thorascopy with minimal surgical incision is the currently used procedure.

▶ The existence of a PDA, regardless of size, is an indication for surgery.

▶ A PDA ligation is performed between 6 months and 2 years of age; asymptomatic infants may be closed electively at a time chosen by the family and surgeon.

▶ Surgical mortality is less than 1%.

▶ Complications are rare and include injury to the laryngeal nerve (hoarseness), left phrenic nerve (left hemidiaphragm paralysis), or thoracic duct (chylothorax).

Special Considerations

▶ None

When to Consult, Refer, Hospitalize

▶ Refer all patients with PDA-type murmurs to a cardiologist.

Follow-Up

▶ No activity restrictions unless pulmonary hypertension is present

▶ Infective endocarditis prophylaxis for 6 months after surgery/coil embolization

▶ Controversy exists about whether children with silent PDAs, detected by ultrasound but not clinically significant, should be repaired at all

Complications

▶ Complications postsurgery are unusual; may include infective endocarditis, CHF, recurrent pneumonia, pulmonary vascular obstructive disease (PVOD), pulmonary hypertension, and pulmonary or systemic emboli

▶ Rarely, aneurysm of the PDA may occur

Atrial Septal Defect (ASD)

Description

▶ Defect (opening) in the atrial septum

▶ Four types: primum (30%), secundum (50%–70%), sinus venosus (<10%), coronary sinus septal (<10%)

Etiology

▶ No known genetic cause; most are sporadic; primum ASDs associated with trisomy 21

Incidence and Demographics

▶ Isolated cases (those not associated with other cyanotic heart lesions) occur in 0.5–1/1,000 live births (5%–10% of all CHD cases).

▶ ASDs account for <10% of congenital heart disease in infants, but >30% of cases are diagnosed in adults because findings may be subtle and not detected earlier.

Risk Factors

▶ Genetic predisposition with environmental triggers such as viruses and drugs

▶ Prematurity

Assessment

History

▶ Even with moderate to large ASDs, infants and children are usually asymptomatic.

▶ Children with significant defects may be small, but true failure to thrive is rare.

▶ The physiologic impact of the left-to-right shunt increases with age, initially manifests as exercise intolerance, and can lead to overt CHF.

▶ Progressive increase in symptoms in 2nd and 3rd decade of life

Physical Exam

▶ In large defects, height and weight may be slightly below normal.

▶ Heart rate is usually normal; patient may have mild tachycardia; blood pressure is normal.

▶ A prominent precordial bulge or right ventricular heave may be present.

▶ Classic finding is wide, split S_2; may have split S_1 with loud second component.

▶ Grade II–III/VI medium-pitched systolic ejection murmur heard best at ULSB or LMSB secondary to pulmonary valve stenosis

▶ Mid-diastolic rumble at LLSB due to increased flow across the tricuspid valve may be heard with large left-to-right shunts.

Diagnostic Studies

▶ ECG: usually normal sinus rhythm. Right axis deviation and mild right ventricular hypertrophy or right bundle branch block may be seen.

▶ Chest X-ray: may be normal or show cardiomegaly with right atrial enlargement or right ventricular enlargement, prominent main pulmonary artery, increased pulmonary vascular markings. Large pulmonary artery best seen on lateral view.

▶ Echocardiography: transthoracic or transesophageal technique, can identify location of ASD and demonstrate pulmonary venous return

▶ Cardiac catheterization: not necessary for diagnostic evaluation; performed if defect can be closed using an atrial occluder device

Differential Diagnosis

▶ Pulmonary stenosis

▶ Innocent murmur

▶ Physiologic "flow" murmur (e.g., anemia, fever)

▶ Tricuspid stenosis

Management

▶ Patients with isolated defect 3–8 mm in size have a spontaneous closure rate of 80% by 18 months of age.

▶ Patients with an isolated defect <3 mm diagnosed by 3 months of age have a spontaneous closure rate of 100% by 18 months of age.

▶ ASDs >8 mm rarely close spontaneously.

▶ Infective endocarditis does not occur in patients with isolated ASDs.

Nonpharmacologic Treatment

▶ Exercise restriction unnecessary

Pharmacologic Treatment

▶ If signs, symptoms of CHF develop, treatment with digoxin and diuretics indicated

▶ Infective endocarditis prophylaxis unnecessary unless there are associated cardiac lesions

Surgical

▶ High pulmonary vascular resistance (PVR) is contraindication for surgery.

▶ Surgery postponed until 3–4 years of age because of high incidence of spontaneous closure; surgery is performed during infancy, however, if CHF develops and does not respond to medical management

▶ Surgical closure of the ASD

▶ Direct closure of the defect with a patch or stitch closure

▶ Incision made through median sternotomy

▶ Performed under cardiopulmonary bypass through atrial approach

▶ Surgical mortality is less than 1%; mortality rate is higher during infancy and in patients with high PVR.

▶ Complications include postoperative arrhythmias (7%–20%) and cerebrovascular accident.

▶ Placement of atrial occluder ("clamshell" device) to close the ASD (done in the cardiac catheterization laboratory) may be possible for secundum defects.

Special Considerations

▶ None

When to Consult, Refer, Hospitalize

▶ Refer all patients with ASD-type murmurs to a cardiologist.

Follow-Up

▶ Patients without chronic heart failure are managed conservatively; if patient is asymptomatic with small ASD after first year of life, see every 1–2 years to monitor for spontaneous closure of the ASD.

Postoperative Follow-Up

▶ Cardiology visit within one week after discharge and thereafter per cardiologist instructions

▶ No activity restrictions unless complications from surgery have occurred

▶ No infective endocarditis prophylaxis for an isolated ASD

▶ Long-term required for patients with postoperative arrhythmias

Complications

▶ Chronic heart failure and pulmonary hypertension (in third to fourth decade of life)

▶ Atrial arrhythmias (flutter/fibrillation)

▶ Holt-Oram syndrome: tricuspid or mitral insufficiency

▶ Rarely, cerebrovascular accident

Ventricular Septal Defect (VSD)

Description

▶ Defect (opening) in the ventricular septum

▶ VSDs are classified as membranous or muscular, depending on location of defect.

▶ Varied in size, from tiny openings with no hemodynamic compromise to large openings with accompanying pulmonary hypertension and chronic heart failure

Etiology

▶ Unknown

Incidence and Demographics

▶ VSD is the most common form of congenital heart disease (CHD), usually detected by a murmur heard between 2 and 6 weeks.

▶ Isolated cases (those not associated with other cyanotic heart lesions) occur in 1.5–2/1,000 live births (15%–20% of all CHD cases); VSDs are the most common lesion in chromosomal syndromes, although >95% of children with a VSD have normal chromosomes.

▶ 3% of children with a VSD have a parent with a VSD.

▶ 30%–50% of VSDs close in the first 2 years of life.

Risk Factors

▶ Genetic predisposition with environmental triggers such as viruses and drugs

▶ Prematurity

Prevention and Screening

▶ Early referral

Assessment

History

▶ Patients with small VSDs are usually asymptomatic with normal growth and development.

▶ Symptoms vary with the size of the VSD and the degree of left-to-right shunting. Patients with moderate to large shunts show delayed growth and development, increased incidence of respiratory infections, decreased exercise tolerance, and signs and symptoms of chronic heart failure (CHF). CHF usually does not occur until 6–8 weeks of life, after the fall in pulmonary vascular resistance and pulmonary artery pressure.

▶ Infants may have severe dyspnea, feeding difficulties, profuse perspiration, and duskiness with crying or infection.

Physical Exam

Small VSD

▶ Patients are acyanotic and well developed.

▶ Precordial activity is normal; thrill is typically not palpable.

▶ Normal physiologic splitting of S_2

▶ Grade II–VI/VI harsh systolic regurgitant murmur heard best at LLSB

Moderate to Large VSD

▶ Infants may have failure to thrive, show signs of chronic heart failure (usually by 2 months of age).

▶ Hepatomegaly may be present.

▶ Tachycardia

▶ Increased intensity of the precordial impulse

▶ S_2 is narrowly split.

▶ Grade II–VI/VI harsh holosystolic murmur heard best at the LLSB; may obscure 1st and 2nd heart sounds

▶ Apical diastolic rumble

Diagnostic Studies

▶ *ECG*: Normal with small VSD. Left ventricular hypertrophy (LVH) and occasional left atrial enlargement may be seen with moderate VSDs. Combined ventricular hypertrophy with or without left atrial enlargement with large VSDs. Monitor for possible pulmonary hypertension or pulmonic stenosis, which results in right ventricular hypertrophy.

▶ *Chest X-ray*: Normal with small VSD; with moderate to large shunt VSDs, cardiomegaly of varying degrees that involves the LA, LV, and sometimes the RV. Pulmonary vascular markings (PVMs) increased. The degree of cardiomegaly and increased PVMs is directly proportional to the amount of left-to-right shunting.

▶ *Echocardiography:* Two-dimensional echo can determine the anatomical location, size, and number of VSDs. Doppler studies can provide visualization of the shunt and are also used to screen for development of left ventricular outflow tract disease and spontaneous closure

▶ *Cardiac catheterization:* Strongly recommended for critically ill children before surgery. Provides detailed information about the anatomic location of the VSD, quantitative measurements of shunting, and level of pulmonary vascular resistance.

▶ *Selective left ventriculography:* shows "gooseneck" deformity of left ventricular outflow tract

Differential Diagnosis

▶ Tricuspid regurgitation

▶ Mitral regurgitation

▶ Patent ductus arteriosus

▶ Atrial septal defect

▶ Subaortic membrane

Management

▶ Small defects spontaneously close up to 75% of the time; moderate defects close 30%–50%; large defects will decrease in size as the patient grows but have a low spontaneous closure rate. Muscular defects have a higher spontaneous closure rate than membranous defects.

Nonpharmacologic Treatment

▶ Observation only for small to moderate VSDs

▶ Frequent feedings of high-caloric formula, orally or through a nasogastric tube, may help address growth failure in children with moderate to large VSD.

Pharmacologic Treatment

▶ Infective endocarditis prophylaxis, as long as VSD present and until 6 months after surgical correction

▶ If signs and symptoms of CHF develop, treatment includes digoxin and diuretics.

▶ Anemia should be corrected by oral iron therapy.

Surgical Treatment

▶ If growth failure cannot be improved with medical management, the VSD should be closed surgically within the first six months of life. For infants who respond to medical therapy, surgery should be postponed to allow time for spontaneous closure.

▶ Surgical closure of a VSD

▶ Direct closure of the defect with a patch or stitch closure through a median sternotomy

▶ Surgical mortality is 2%–5% after the age of six months; higher in patients less than 2 months of age and those with multiple VSDs or associated defects.

▶ Complications include residual VSD shunt (20% of patients), right bundle branch block (10% of patients), complete heart block (<5% of patients); rarely, cerebrovascular accident.

Special Considerations

▶ None

When to Consult, Refer, Hospitalize

▶ Refer all patients with VSD-type murmurs to a cardiologist.

Follow-Up

▶ Patients without chronic heart failure or pulmonary hypertension are managed con-servatively, with close monitoring of growth. 78%–80% of children with small VSDs will have spontaneous closure during the first 2 years of life.

▶ Patients <6 months with CHF and growth failure should be seen monthly.

Postoperative Follow-Up

▶ Cardiology follow-up as directed by surgery

▶ No activity restrictions unless complications from surgery have occurred

▶ Infective endocarditis prophylaxis may be discontinued 6 months after surgery; how-ever, for residual VSD, continue infective endocarditis prophylaxis indefinitely

▶ Long-term follow-up required for patients who had transient heart block postopera-tively, whether or not a pacemaker was placed

Complications

▶ Subacute bacterial endocarditis

▶ Pulmonary overcirculation/pulmonary hypertension

▶ Left ventricular volume overload

▶ Aortic insufficiency

▶ Eisenmenger syndrome

▶ Acquired left ventricular outflow tract obstruction

▶ Aneurysm of the interventricular septum

▶ Mitral regurgitation leading to valve replacement

▶ Heart block requiring pacemaker placement

Coarctation of the Aorta (COA)

Description

▶ Discrete narrowing of the aorta, just opposite the site of insertion of the ductus arteriosus (juxtaductal position)

▶ Two distinct presentations

▷ Neonatal period: coarctation is usually severe; associated with closing of ductus arteriosus; presents at 4–10 days of life

▷ Infancy, childhood: typically no symptoms; coarctation is less severe; may have good collateral flow to descending aorta

Etiology

▶ Cause unknown

Incidence and Demographics

▶ Occurs in 0.8–1/1,000 live births (8% of all CHD cases)

Risk Factors

▶ Other cardiac defects such as aortic hypoplasia, bicuspid aortic valve (85%), PDA (60%), ventricular septal defect (50%), mitral valve abnormalities, and Shone's syndrome (multiple left-sided obstruction lesions including mitral stenosis, subaortic membrane, valvular aortic stenosis) are often associated with CoA.

▶ Turner syndrome (XO): 30%–35% have CoA

Prevention and Screening

▶ Early referral

Assessment

History

Symptomatic Infants

▶ Poor feeding and weight gain

▶ Dyspnea

▶ Signs of chronic heart failure

▶ Circulatory shock

▶ Normal newborn discharge examination (if PDA did not close and was supplying blood flow to descending aorta)

Asymptomatic Children

▶ Majority of children asymptomatic until late childhood

▶ Occasionally, complaints of pain or weakness in the legs following exercise; headache secondary to hypertension

Physical Exam

Symptomatic Infants

▶ Hallmark is absent or weak femoral pulses

▶ Pale, varying degrees of respiratory distress

▶ Oliguria or anuria

▶ General circulatory shock with severe acidosis

▶ Differential cyanosis (lower part of body appears cyanotic because of right-to-left ductal shunting)

▶ Decreased or absent lower-extremity pulses; qualitative difference between brachial and femoral pulse

▶ Blood pressure discrepancy between the upper and lower extremities (higher in the arms)

▶ Loud single S_2; a gallop usually present

▶ Nonspecific systolic ejection murmur, although 50% of affected infants do not have murmur

Asymptomatic Children

▶ Normal growth and development

▶ Decreased or absent lower-extremity pulses

▶ Hypertension in upper extremities (normally thigh or calf systolic pressure higher than arm)

▶ Systolic thrill may be present in suprasternal notch.

▶ Accentuated A2, normally split S_2

▶ II–IV/VI systolic ejection murmur heard best at the URSB, MLSB, or LLSB that radiates to left interscapular region posteriorly

▶ Ejection click frequently audible

Diagnostic Studies

▶ ECG: Usually normal. RVH or right bundle branch block (RBBB) may be present in infants; LVH can be seen in older children with longstanding CoA.

▶ Chest X-ray: Marked pulmonary edema and cardiomegaly are seen in symptomatic infants. In older children, the heart size is normal or slightly enlarged. A "3 sign" on an overpenetrated CXR (due to a double aortic curve/abnormal contour of the arch) or an E-shaped indentation on a barium-filled esophagus may be seen. Rib notching between the 4th and 8th ribs may be present in older children but is rare before the age of 5 years. Rib notching is erosion of the ribs caused by dilated intercostal collateral vessels.

▶ Echocardiography: Two-dimensional echo and color flow Doppler studies can show the site and extent of coarctation and provide information about left ventricular function and other left-sided lesions.

▶ Cardiac catheterization allows measurement of pressure above and below coarctation.

▶ MRI can be used to further define the location and severity of the CoA and provide data about collateral vessels.

Differential Diagnosis

▶ Aortic stenosis

▶ Pulmonary stenosis

▶ Patent ductus arteriosus

Management

Nonpharmacologic Treatment
Symptomatic Infants

▶ Oxygen

▶ Surgical intervention to follow

Asymptomatic Children

▶ Patients with mild CoA should be followed closely for the development of hypertension or systolic pressure differences between the arms and legs

Pharmacologic Treatment

Symptomatic Infants

▶ Prostaglandin E1 infusion to reopen the ductus arteriosus (0.5 mcg/kg/min)

▶ Correction of acidosis and metabolic disturbances

▶ Inotropic agents (dopamine or dobutamine)

▶ Diuretics

Asymptomatic Children

▶ Patients with mild CoA should be followed closely for the development of hypertension or systolic pressure differences between the arms and legs. Occasionally these children will require chronic antihypertensive therapy, usually with beta-blockers or ACE inhibitors, most commonly if the repair is performed <5 years old.

Surgical Treatment

Symptomatic Infants

▶ Surgery to repair the CoA should be performed urgently on infants with CHF.

▶ Surgical correction of CoA

▶ Surgery is performed without bypass through a left posterolateral thoracotomy.

▶ Types of repair include:

▷ End-to-end anastomosis (area of coarctation resected, distal and proximal aorta anastomosed end-to-end)

▷ Patch aortoplasty (area of coarctation incised, elliptical Dacron patch sutured in place to widen diameter)

▷ Subclavian flap aortoplasty (distal subclavian artery divided, flap of proximal portion of vessel used to expand the coarcted area)

▶ Ductus is always ligated with these surgical techniques.

▶ Surgical mortality is less than 5%.

▶ Complications include residual obstruction or recoarctation (6%–33%) and postoperative renal failure.

▶ Balloon angioplasty may be performed if coarctation recurs.

Asymptomatic Children

▶ Upper-extremity hypertension or a systolic gradient of ≥20 mm Hg between upper and lower extremities is an indication for elective repair of a CoA in children 2–4 years old; mortality less than 1%.

▶ Older children should be operated on as soon as the diagnosis of CoA is made.

▶ Surgical correction of CoA

▶ Surgery performed without bypass through a left posterolateral thoracotomy.

▶ Types of repair are the same as in symptomatic infants.

- ▶ End-to-end is the repair of choice for discrete CoA in older children.

- ▶ Complications include spinal cord paralysis producing paraplegia due to limited collateral circulation during cross-clamping of aorta (0.4%), postoperative rebound hypertension, and post-coarctectomy (reperfusion) syndrome.

- ▶ Balloon angioplasty of native CoA (no history of surgical intervention) is controversial; may be performed if coarctation recurs.

Special Considerations

- ▶ None

When to Consult, Refer, Hospitalize

- ▶ Refer all patients with a CoA-type murmur to a cardiologist.

- ▶ Refer patients with hypertension to a cardiologist if other causes have been ruled out.

Follow-Up

- ▶ Symptomatic infants should be followed every 6–12 months to evaluate for recoarctation.

- ▶ Asymptomatic children can be seen annually to assess for persistent hypertension, recoarctation, subaortic stenosis, and persistent myocardial dysfunction.

- ▶ Require infective endocarditis prophylaxis indefinitely, because of associated bicuspid aortic valve and recoarctation.

CYANOTIC CONGENITAL HEART DEFECTS

Tetralogy of Fallot (TOF)

Description

- ▶ Syndrome of congenital heart defects with 4 components:
    1. Large VSD in the membranous region of the ventricular septum
    2. Pulmonary stenosis
    3. Overriding aorta
    4. Obstructive right ventricular hypertrophy

Etiology

- ▶ Cause unknown

Incidence and Demographics

- ▶ Occurs in 0.2–0.3/1,000 live births (8% of all CHD cases); most common cyanotic CHD beyond 1 week of age

- ▶ Associated defects
    - ▷ Right aortic arch (25%)
    - ▷ Pulmonary atresia (15%)

▷   Abnormal coronary arteries (5%)

▷   Pulmonary branch stenosis

▷   Systemic collateral arteries that feed into the lungs

▷   ASD

▷   Microdeletion of chromosome 22q11 (velocardiofacial syndrome)

Risk Factors

▶   Genetic predisposition with environmental triggers such as viruses and drugs

▶   Prematurity

Assessment

History

▶   Heart murmur audible in the newborn period

▶   Most patients symptomatic with cyanosis present at birth

▶   History of hypoxic spells, especially with crying or exercise

▶   Parents may describe child as squatting while walking.

▶   Patients with acyanotic (pink) TOF asymptomatic

▶   Hypoxic spells ("tet" spells)

▶   Spells usually occur after crying, feeding, or defecation

▶   Spells usually consist of rapid and deep breathing, irritability and prolonged crying, increased cyanosis, and decrease in intensity of murmur.

▶   Severe hypoxic spell may lead to limpness, convulsion, cerebral vascular accident (CVA), or even death

Physical Exam

▶   Varying degrees of cyanosis, with hypercyanosis occurring later in infancy

▶   Growth retardation if cyanosis is severe

▶   Tachypnea

▶   Clubbing may be present if cyanosis has been longstanding (usually >6 months)

▶   Normal S_1 and single S_2 (because aorta is located more anteriorly than normal)

▶   Active precordium, grade III–IV/VI systolic ejection murmur heard best at middle and upper left sternal border (caused by right ventricular outflow tract obstruction); the greater the obstruction, the softer the murmur

▶   Continuous murmur representing PDA shunt may be audible in patients with TOF and pulmonary atresia.

Diagnostic Studies

▶   *ECG:* Normal QRS axis with acyanotic TOF and right axis deviation with cyanotic TOF. Right ventricular hypertrophy (RVH) and right atrial hypertrophy are usually present. Combined ventricular hypertrophy (CVH) may be seen in acyanotic TOF.

▶   *Chest X-ray:* Findings in patients with acyanotic TOF are the same as in those with a small to moderate VSD. With cyanotic TOF, heart size ≤ normal. PVMs are decreased.

Heart may appear "boot-shaped" because of a concave main pulmonary artery with an upturned apex. Right aortic arch (25%) and right atrial enlargement (25%) may be present.

▶ *Echocardiography:* Two-dimensional echo can determine the anatomical location, size, and number of VSDs; assess the anatomy of the right ventricular outflow tract (RVOT), pulmonary valve, and pulmonary arteries; and image the coronary arteries. Doppler studies can visualize the VSD shunt and estimate a pressure gradient across the RVOT obstruction.

▶ *Cardiac catheterization:* Recommended before surgical repair of TOF

Differential Diagnosis

▶ Aortic stenosis

Management

▶ Treatment of cyanotic spells includes knee-chest positioning, oxygen, intravenous fluid bolus, sodium bicarbonate to treat acidosis, morphine sulfate to calm child, vasoconstrictors (epinephrine [Adrenalin] or phenylephrine) to increase systemic vascular resistance, and beta blockers (Inderal) to cause RVOT relaxation.

Pharmacologic Treatment

▶ Treat iron-deficiency anemia, since anemic children are more likely to have a CVA.

▶ Provide infective endocarditis prophylaxis.

Surgical Treatment

▶ Asymptomatic and acyanotic children are repaired at 6–12 months of age.

▶ Asymptomatic and minimally cyanotic children are repaired at 3–24 months of age, depending on the amount of pulmonary artery hypoplasia.

▶ Mildly cyanotic infants who have had a palliative shunt procedure may have a complete repair 1–2 years after the shunt procedure.

▶ Symptomatic infants with a favorable RVOT and pulmonary arteries are repaired at 3–4 months of age.

▶ Surgical repair of TOF

▶ Patch closure of VSD and reconstruction of the RVOT by resection of the infundibular tissue and placement of a transannular patch

▶ Incision is made through a median sternotomy under cardiopulmonary bypass.

▶ Surgical mortality is 2%–5% during the first 2 years of life; higher in patients <3 months of age and >4 years old and those with severe pulmonary hypoplasia, associated defects

▶ Complications include bleeding during the postoperative period, pulmonary valve regurgitation, residual RVOT obstruction, RV dysfunction, residual VSD, right bundle branch block, and, rarely, complete heart block or ventricular arrhythmias.

Special Considerations

▶ None

When to Consult, Refer, Hospitalize

▶ Refer all patients with a TOF-type murmur to a cardiologist

Follow-Up

▶ Symptomatic infants should be seen monthly until surgical repair. Asymptomatic children can be seen every 3–6 months until surgical repair.

Postoperative Follow-Up

▶ Cardiology

▶ Varying levels of activity restrictions

▶ Infective endocarditis prophylaxis indefinitely

▶ Required long term for patients who had sinus node dysfunction, surgical heart block, or ventricular arrhythmias postoperatively, whether or not pacemaker was placed

Complications

▶ Hypoxic spells ("tet" spells)

▶ Right ventricular dysfunction

▶ Ventricular arrhythmias

▶ Rarely, brain abscess and cerebrovascular accident

▶ Infective endocarditis

▶ Polycythemia

PERIPHERAL VASCULAR DISORDERS

Peripheral Arterial Disease

Description

▶ Chronic or acute entity consisting of obstruction or narrowing of the major arteries, commonly affecting the lower extremities and most frequently a result of atherosclerosis

Etiology

▶ Acute thrombus leading to embolus

▶ Chronic atherosclerotic lesions

▶ Inflammatory component in thromboangiitis obliterans (Buerger's disease), giant cell (temporal) arteritis

▶ May also be caused by trauma or entrapment (thoracic, popliteal)

Incidence and Demographics

▶ Older adults

▶ Male preponderance

Risk Factors

- ▶ Age >40 years
- ▶ Tobacco usage
- ▶ Hyperlipidemia, hypertension, atherosclerosis
- ▶ Diabetes mellitus or fasting serum glucose >110 mg/dL
- ▶ Obesity

Prevention and Screening

- ▶ Lifestyle modification
- ▶ Identification and treatment of comorbid conditions

Assessment

History

- ▶ Acute: pain, paresthesia, paralysis, pallor, pulselessness
- ▶ Chronic: lower extremity aching, fatigue occurring with activity and relieved by cessation of activity (intermittent claudication); pain develops at rest as disease progresses
- ▶ Aorta: back or abdominal pain; femoral; hip, buttock, calf pain
- ▶ See Table 8–23 for classification of peripheral vascular disease.

Physical Exam

- ▶ Pale, cool, diminished, or absent pulses in extremity; bruit of femoral artery possible
- ▶ Severity determined by the amount of time required for venous filling and return of color
- ▶ Absent or decreased hair and nail growth of the lower extremities
- ▶ Waxy pallor of affected extremity, or dependent rubor with hyperemia due to compensatory reflex vasodilation of the microvasculature causing bright red distal extremity

Diagnostic Studies

- ▶ Diagnosis is clinical but Doppler ultrasound is used to determine severity.
- ▶ Angiography for acute or surgical candidates

Differential Diagnosis

- ▶ Musculoskeletal strains
- ▶ Osteoarthritis

TABLE 8–23.
FONTAINE CLASSIFICATION OF PERIPHERAL VASCULAR DISEASE

STAGE	CLINICAL FEATURE
1	Silent
2	Intermittent claudication
3	Rest ischemia
4	Ulceration or gangrene

▶ Acute arterial spasm

▶ Deep vein thrombosis (DVT)

▶ Acute embolic conditions

▶ Thromboangiitis obliterans (Buerger's disease)

Management

Nonpharmacologic Treatment

▶ Acute arterial occlusion: Avoid elevating affected extremity; protect extremity and refer for heparin therapy immediately.

▶ Smoking cessation

▶ Control/treat comorbid diseases: hyperlipidemia, diabetes mellitus, hypertension

▶ Initiate prescribed exercise program: preferably walking to point of pain to develop collateral circulation

▶ Educate patient about signs and symptoms that require immediate attention.

▶ Stage 3: diagnostic testing for possible surgery

Pharmacologic Treatment

▶ Acute: heparin IV, possible embolectomy

▶ Chronic: pentoxifylline (Trental) 400 mg t.i.d.; aspirin or cilostazol (Pletal) 100 mg b.i.d. to decrease platelet aggregation

▶ Aspirin 81–324 mg/day for all patients

Special Considerations

▶ Risk of arterial occlusion increases with age

When to Consult, Refer, Hospitalize

▶ Refer to vascular surgeon for new-onset, severe, and stage 3 or greater symptoms; acute arterial occlusion; or arteriosclerosis obliterans (proliferation of the intima leads to occlusion of lumen of the arteries).

Follow-Up

▶ Every 3 months if stable

▶ Patient education about medications, care of feet

Expected Course

▶ Chronic: symptoms differ, with slow progression to rapid deterioration

Complications

▶ Gangrene

▶ Amputation

Superficial and Deep Venous Thrombosis

Description

▶ Deep vein thrombosis (DVT): acute blood clot formation in the deep lower extremity or pelvic veins with ambiguous presenting signs or symptoms

▶ Superficial: acute inflammation and clot formation with associated redness and tenderness along superficial vein

Etiology

▶ Thrombosis consists of red blood cells, platelets, and fibrin attached to part of the inflamed vessel wall.

▶ DVT caused by:

▷ Immobilization secondary to surgery, prolonged bed rest, prolonged travel by plane or car

▷ Venous incompetence, vascular wall injury

▷ Chronic heart failure

▷ Hypercoagulable states: inherited coagulation deficits, malignancy, and estrogen usage

▶ Superficial thrombosis (saphenous vein frequently involved) caused by:

▷ IV therapy, trauma

▷ Bacterial infection

Incidence and Demographics

▶ Common; approximately 1–2 million cases per year

▶ Female preponderance

▶ High incidence with total hip replacement

Risk Factors

▶ DVT

▷ Obesity

▷ Orthopedic surgery, immobility, trauma

▷ Pregnancy, oral contraceptives

▷ Malignancy, coagulation defects

▷ Venous catheters

▷ Rheumatoid disease, lupus

▷ High altitude elevations, polycythemia vera

▶ Superficial

▷ Aseptic procedures

Prevention and Screening

▶ Limit period of immobility

▶ Prophylactic anticoagulation for associated risk factors

▶ Avoidance of estrogen-containing oral contraceptives, or use low dose

▶ Postsurgical mechanical leg compression

Assessment

History

▶ DVT frequently asymptomatic

▶ Possible unilateral leg pain or tenderness of calf, swelling, and discoloration

▶ With superficial thrombosis: acute episode with definite timeframe, local redness, tender cord, swelling, dull pain over inflamed vein, fever

Physical Exam

▶ DVT: reproducible tenderness with calf compression (Homans's sign), leg circumference greater than uninvolved leg because of swelling; cool extremity with weak distal pulses; however, signs often unreliable

▶ Superficial thrombosis: isolated induration, redness, and tenderness along vein, but no significant swelling of the extremity

Diagnostic Studies

▶ Anticoagulation therapy baseline: platelets, PT, PTT, CBC, LFTs, occult blood; monitor platelets daily with heparin treatment

▶ B-mode ultrasound combined with Doppler flow detection: highly sensitive and specific for popliteal and femoral thrombi

▶ Impedance plethysmography: more accurate than duplex ultrasound, which is less precise in the detection of calf vein thrombi

▶ Nuclear scanning: iodine 125–labeled fibrinogen detects active clot formation

▶ Contrast venography: the most sensitive and specific contrast venography; most effective

Differential Diagnosis

▶ Cellulitis

▶ Musculoskeletal strain

▶ Lymphedema

▶ Acute arterial occlusion

▶ Ruptured Baker's cyst

Management

Nonpharmacologic Treatment

▶ DVT

▷ Initially hospitalize with bed rest and leg elevation, anticoagulation

▷ After stabilization, prompt mobilization

- ▷ Intermittent pneumatic compression followed by graded pressure stockings
- ▷ Calf DVT as outpatient
- ► Superficial
  - ▷ Bed rest with leg (or extremity) elevated, local heat
  - ▷ If sepsis, hospitalization often required

Pharmacologic Treatment

- ► Anticoagulation therapy for DVT, as acute treatment and prophylaxis
  - ▷ Heparin: IV 5,000 units titrated to PTT 2–5 seconds above control; subcutaneous 5,000 units 2–3 times day (stops propagation of thrombus; allows fibrinolysis)
    - ► Plethysmogram or ultrasound before discontinuation to ascertain resolution
    - ► Heparin and warfarin concurrent, with heparin starting day 3; heparin discontinued day 5 or 6
    - ► PT therapeutic INR 2.5–3.0 with warfarin therapy
  - ▷ Thrombolytic agents: streptokinase and urokinase; aspirin not beneficial
  - ▷ Filtering devices: umbrella in vena cava traps emboli, useful if anticoagulants are contraindicated
  - ▷ For superficial thrombosis: NSAIDs; appropriate antibiotic if septic

How Long to Treat

- ► Treat single-episode DVT for 3 months; longer if recurrent, associated with pulmonary embolus
- ► Aseptic inflammation of superficial thrombosis subsides in 1–2 weeks

Special Considerations

- ► Geriatric patients: common because of predisposing factors, age-related coagulation deficiencies
- ► Pregnancy: Use heparin—warfarin is a teratogen.
- ► Lactation: unknown if heparin and warfarin are secreted in breast milk
- ► Oncology patients—risk of hemorrhage with heparin

When to Consult, Refer, Hospitalize

- ► Consult with physician for evaluation and management, possible hospitalization.
- ► Refer to vascular specialist for recurrences or complications.

Follow-Up

- ► Monitor oral anticoagulation and for signs of recurrence.
- ► Provide patient education about wearing support hose, warfarin complications, and symptoms of pulmonary embolism (PE).

Expected Course

- ► Prognosis is good once the danger of PE has passed.

Complications
▶ Pulmonary embolism
▶ Chronic venous insufficiency
▶ Septic thrombophlebitis, osteomyelitis with superficial thrombosis

Venous Insufficiency

Description
▶ Chronic condition characterized by noninflammatory incompetence of the venous backflow valves in the veins of the lower extremities. Blood is regurgitated through the valves, resulting in engorgement and secondary edema of the lower leg.

Etiology
▶ Venous valves become incompetent, unable to maintain efficient flow of blood back to heart
▶ May be caused by leg trauma, prior thrombophlebitis, or conditions that cause abnormally high venous pressure

Incidence and Demographics
▶ Female predominance
▶ Onset in late adulthood

Risk Factors
▶ Trauma, obesity, pregnancy, history of thrombophlebitis
▶ Prolonged immobility, particularly standing
▶ Familial tendency, increases with age

Prevention and Screening
▶ Early aggressive treatment of thrombophlebitis
▶ Avoidance of prolonged standing and immobility
▶ Weight loss if appropriate
▶ Avoidance of restrictive lower-extremity garments

Assessment

History
▶ Pain varies from minimal discomfort to marked pain with ulcers.
▶ Lower-extremity edema worsens with prolonged standing.
▶ Mild pruritus of lower extremity, scratching
▶ Recurrent stasis ulcers, weeping, crust formation
▶ Previous history of thrombophlebitis at site
▶ Bilateral aching in the lower extremities—typically worse at night

▶ Bilateral lower-extremity edema with prolonged standing; relieved when legs are elevated

Physical Exam

▶ Hyperpigmentation of distal extremity; appears brown or reddish; brawny, hyperpigmented thick skin

▶ Wet ulceration may be present distally, often over medial aspect of lower leg.

▶ Edema of lower extremity

▶ Varicosities may be present.

▶ Check femoral, popliteal, dorsalis pedis, and posterior tibial pulses.

Diagnostic Studies

▶ Stasis ulcer: culture and sensitivity

▶ Doppler studies: assess vascular status

Differential Diagnosis

▶ Cellulitis

▶ Chronic renal disease

▶ Lymphedema

▶ Acute phlebitis

▶ Fungal infection

▶ Atopic dermatitis

▶ Severe contact dermatitis

▶ Neurodermatitis

Management

Nonpharmacologic Treatment

▶ Elastic stockings before ambulation

▶ Elevation of foot of bed

▶ Avoid prolonged positions or inactivity.

▶ Weight reduction for obese patients

▶ Refer for wound debridement and management.

▶ Treat ulcers with antimicrobial dressing or Unna boot.

Pharmacologic Treatment

▶ Diuretic therapy

▶ Corticosteroid creams such as hydrocortisone cream, triamcinolone 1% for itching

▶ Oral antibiotic for positive wound culture

▶ Broad-spectrum antifungal (clotrimazole)

How Long to Treat
- ▶ Chronic condition
- ▶ Treat exacerbations until resolution

Special Considerations
- ▶ Control edema—venous ulcer will not heal or remain healed with edema.

When to Consult, Refer, Hospitalize
- ▶ Refer to vascular specialist or wound care center for refractory ulcers.

Follow-Up
- ▶ Depends on clinical situation; usually every 3 months if stable
- ▶ Patient education about use of support hose, weight loss, sitting whenever possible

Expected Course
- ▶ Chronic, recurrent with frequent exacerbation if compliance to preventive measures is poor

Complications
- ▶ Bacterial infection
- ▶ Stasis ulcers
- ▶ Thrombus

Varicose Veins
Description
- ▶ Superficial, dilated, tortuous veins arising from incompetent valves and high venous pressure in the lower extremities, usually distant and involving the saphenous vein

Etiology
- ▶ Congenitally incompetent valves
- ▶ Prior thrombophlebitis
- ▶ Pregnancy, obesity, ascites
- ▶ Idiopathic, may have familial tendencies

Incidence and Demographics
- ▶ Female preponderance
- ▶ 20% of adult U.S. population

Risk Factors
- ▶ Prolonged weight bearing, standing
- ▶ Pregnancy, obesity
- ▶ Clothing that causes vasoconstriction of lower extremities

Prevention and Screening
- ▶ Weight control
- ▶ Elevation of lower extremities
- ▶ Elastic support when ambulatory
- ▶ Avoidance of restrictive clothing

Assessment

History
- ▶ Fatigue, aching, heaviness, and cramping, primarily of lower extremities
- ▶ Menses may be a precipitating factor

Physical Exam
- ▶ Dilated and tortuous veins
- ▶ Standing: gravitational advantage to visualize veins
- ▶ Hyperpigmentation of distal leg
- ▶ Veins palpable

Differential Diagnosis
- ▶ Chronic venous insufficiency
- ▶ Peripheral neuropathy
- ▶ Nerve root compression
- ▶ Osteoarthritis—hip
- ▶ Arterial insufficiency
- ▶ Lymphedema
- ▶ Postphlebitic syndrome

Diagnostic Studies
- ▶ Not indicated unless unusual presentation or complications such as DVT

Management

Nonpharmacologic Treatment
- ▶ Elastic compression stockings up to the knee before ambulation
- ▶ Patient should avoid prolonged weight-bearing and standing and not cross legs when sitting.
- ▶ Weight loss; elevation of leg when sitting
- ▶ Avoidance of restrictive garments
- ▶ Low-sodium diet in salt-sensitive persons
- ▶ Sclerotherapy, laser surgery, or ligation and stripping of saphenous vein for severe, refractory cases

Pharmacologic Treatment
▶ Hydrochlorothiazide (HCTZ) 12.5 mg q.d. p.r.n. with fluid retention

How Long to Treat
▶ Chronic problem

Special Considerations
▶ Pregnancy: frequent problem

When to Consult, Refer, Hospitalize
▶ Referral to surgeon if severe and refractory

Follow-Up
▶ If symptomatic

Expected Course
▶ Improvement with surgery
▶ Usually worsens with dependent positions such as standing

Complications
▶ Thrombophlebitis, varicose ulcers
▶ Secondary fungal and bacterial infection
▶ Eczema
▶ Neuritis from scarring secondary to stripping surgery

CASE STUDIES

Case 1

Lori is a 44-year-old White female who presents to the clinic for a well-woman exam. She works as a telephone operator in a busy law firm office. Lori voices no complaints today. Diet recall indicates high-fat meals, including junk foods. She states that she loves cheese.

PMH: Smokes 2 packs per day for 15 years; past medical history significant for hypertension; drinks 3 beers daily

Medications: hydrochlorothiazide 50 mg q.d.
1. What additional history would you ask regarding her cardiovascular status?

Exam: vital signs: BP 128/84; wt: 133 lbs, ht: 64 inches, eyes: yellow-orange raised lesions on eyelids; remainder of exam is unremarkable

2. Would you order any diagnostic test on this patient?
3. If your suspicions are correct, what actions would be required?
4. When Lori returns to the clinic 6 months later with total cholesterol 252, HDL 30, and LDL 170, how will you intervene?
5. What complications can occur with this problem and the treatment regimens?

Case 2

Baby Joe is 1 month old and presents to the clinic because he is not feeding well and his mother states he is losing weight. Baby Joe was delivered vaginally at 36 weeks gestation. His birth weight was 4 lb, 9 oz. The baby is taking 2 oz of formula over a 55-minute period.

Medications: None
1. Are there any other history questions you would like to ask?

Exam: vital signs: temp: 98.0° F/ear, resp: 60, HR: 180, wt: 5 lb, 2 oz. Crying and irritable, sweating; systolic thrill, II/VI continuous murmur at the upper LSB, rate 180; respiratory rate 60 with bilateral crackles; hepatomegaly noted.

2. What are your differential diagnoses?
3. What is your management plan?

Case 3

Mr. Jones is 56 years old and presents to the clinic complaining of decreased appetite, shortness of breath, and swelling in his feet. He is unable to perform normal activities without becoming winded and has a productive cough.

PMH: 6 lb weight gain in the past 7 days. Past medical history significant for hypertension, hyperlipidemia, and MI.

Medications: atorvastatin 20 mg/day, lisinopril 40 mg/day
1.   What additional history would you ask?

Exam: vital signs: BP 90/40; pulse 120; resp 24; skin: cyanotic; CV: S3 gallop, jugular distention; lungs: basilar rales and wheezing; abdomen: hepatomegaly, ascites; extremities: 3+ pedal edema bilaterally

2.   What diagnostic studies would you order?

3.   What is your differential diagnosis?

4.   What is your management plan?

CASE STUDIES DISCUSSION

Case 1

1. What additional history would you ask regarding her cardiovascular status?

    Personal and family history of CHD, DM, hyperlipidemia; any previous lipid evaluation; history of activity/exercise; comprehensive health maintenance history; previous attempt at smoking/alcohol cessation; history of psychosocial stressors; any comorbid disease; abdominal pain; rheumatic disorders; medication history including OTCs, pregnancies

2. Would you order any diagnostic test on this patient?

    Baseline ECG; fasting lipid profile (total cholesterol, triglycerides, HDL, LDL, VLDL, risk ratio); apolipoprotein B; comprehensive metabolic panel, U/A, TSH, free T4; possibly CXR, CBC with differential, CMP

3. If your suspicions are correct, what actions would be required?

    Step 2 diet and exercise program; referral to nutritionist for diet counseling; tobacco and alcohol cessation program; counseling for stress reduction

4. When Lori returns to the clinic 6 months later with total cholesterol 252, HDL 30, and LDL 170, how will you intervene?

    Reinforce Step 2 diet and exercise. Start on a statin such as atorvastatin (Lipitor) 10 mg/day; plan on monitoring hepatic function panel every 4–6 weeks after starting therapy x 3 months and again with any dose

5. What complications can occur with this problem and the treatment regimens?

    Hyperlipidemia: CAD progression, stroke, peripheral vascular disease. Drug treatment: pancreatitis, rhabdomyolysis, hepatic dysfunction

Case 2

1. Are there any other history questions you would like to ask?

    Weight history since birth; prenatal/delivery history; voiding/stooling history in past 24 hours; 24-hour intake history; feeding behavior, sleep pattern

2. What are your differential diagnoses?

    Patent ductus arteriosus, arteriovenous malformations, venous hum, ventricular septal defect with aortic regurgitation, pulmonary atresia, persistent truncus arteriosus, aorto-pulmonary septal defect, peripheral pulmonary stenosis, total anomalous venous connection, tetralogy of Fallot.

3. What is your management plan?

    Refer child to emergency room for admission and evaluation with cardiologist.

Case 3

1. What additional history would you ask?

    Characteristics of cough and sputum; need for additional pillows to sleep—orthopnea; fever; detailed history on comorbid diseases.

2. What diagnostic studies would you order?

    CXR, ECG, echocardiogram, electrolytes, U/A, pulse oximetry, cardiac enzymes, BUN, arterial blood gases.

3. What is your differential diagnosis?

    CHF, renal disease, COPD, nephrotic syndrome, cirrhosis, pulmonary emboli, MI, pneumonia, asthma, chronic venous insufficiency.

4. What is your management plan?

    Give O_2 and consult with physician to plan hospital admission to stabilize; identify and treat underlying disease. At follow-up, educate about sodium and fluid restriction, control leg edema with elastic pressure stockings and elevation of legs, record daily weights; multiple medications needed to treat—diuretics, ACE, beta-blocker, glycoside, vasodilators, and anticoagulants.

REFERENCES

Ahmed, A. (2003). American College of Cardiology/American Heart Association chronic heart failure evaluation and management guidelines: Relevance to the geriatric practice. *Journal of the American Geriatric Society, 51,* 123–126.

ALLHAT Collaborative Research Group. (2002). Major outcomes in high-risk hypertensive patients randomized to angiotensin converting enzyme inhibitor or calcium channel blocker vs. diuretic: The antihypertensive and lipid lowering treatment to prevent heart attack trial. *Journal of the American Medical Association, 288,* 2981–2997.

American Academy of Family Physicians. (2004). Risk classification for stroke, death, and atrial fibrillation. *American Family Physician, 6*(7), 1739–1740.

American Heart Association. (2010). *Classes of heart failure.* Retrieved from http://www.heart.org/HEARTORG/Conditions/HeartFailure/AboutHeartFailure/Classes-of-Heart-Failure_UCM_306328_Article.jsp

American Heart Association. (2008). *Metabolic syndrome.* Retrieved from http://www.american-heart.org/presenter.jhtml?identifier=4756

American Heart Association/American Stroke Association. (2013). Guidelines for the early management of patients with acute ischemic stroke: A guideline for health professionals from the American Heart Association/American Stroke Association. Retrieved at http://stroke.ahajournals.org/content/44/3/870.long

Anderson, J. L., Adams, C. D., Antman, E. M., Bridges, C. R., Califf, R. M., Casey, D. E. Jr., ... Wright, R. S. (2007). ACC/AHA 2007 guidelines for the management of patients with unstable angina/non ST-Elevation myocardial infarction. *Circulation, 116*(7), 148–304.

Boudi, F. B., Ali, Y. S. (2014). *Risk factors for coronary artery disease.* Retrieved from http://emedicine.medscape.com/article/164163-overview

Bret, S., & Lutsep. H. L. (2013). New stroke management guidelines: A quick and easy guide. Retrieved from http://www.medscape.com/viewarticle/779968?src=wnl_edit_specol&uac=105268AK

Centers for Disease Control and Prevention. (2003a). *A public health action plan to prevent heart disease and stroke.* Retrieved from http://www.cdc.gov/dhdsp/library/action_plan/pdfs/action_plan_3of7.pdf

Centers for Disease Control and Prevention. (2003b). State-specific trends in high blood cholesterol awareness among persons screened—United States, 1991–1999. *MMWR: Morbidity and Mortality Weekly Report, 50*(35), 754–758.

Centers for Disease Control and Prevention. (2015a). *Heart disease facts.* Retrieved from http://www.cdc.gov/heartdisease/facts.htm

Centers for Disease Control and Prevention. (2015b). *High cholesterol facts.* Retrieved from http://www.cdc.gov/cholesterol/facts.htm

Chen J. Y., Zhang A. D., Lu H. Y., Guo J., Wang F. F., Li Z. C. (2013). $CHADS_2$ versus CHA_2DS_2-VASc score in assessing the stroke and thromboembolism risk stratification in patients with atrial fibrillation: a systematic review and meta-analysis. *J Geriatr Cardiol,* (10), 258–66.

Chobanian, A. V., Bakris, G. L., Black, H. R., Cushman, W. C., Green, L. A., Izzo, ... Wright, J. T. (2003). Seventh report of the Joint National Committee on Prevention, Detection, Evaluation, and Treatment of High Blood Pressure. *Hypertension, 42*(6), 1206–1252.

Dickerson, L. M., & Gibson, M. V. (2005). Management of hypertension in older persons. *American Family Physician, 17*(3), 469–476.

Ervine, R.B., Division of Health and Nutrition Examination Surveys (2009). National Health and Statistics Reports. Prevalence of Metabolic Syndrome Among Adults 20 years of Age and Over, by Sex, Age, Race and Ethnicity, and Body Mass Index: United States, 2003–2006. Retrieved at http://www.cdc.gov/nchs/data/nhsr/nhsr013.pdf

Expert Panel on Integrated Guidelines for Cardiovascular Health and Risk Reduction in Children and Adolescents (2012). Retrieved at https://www.nhlbi.nih.gov/files/docs/guidelines/peds_guidelines_full.pdf

From the Panel Members Appointed to the Eighth Joint National Committee (JNC 8). (2014). Evidence-based guideline for the management of high blood pressure in adults report. *Journal of the American Medical Association (JAMA), 311*(5), 507–520. Retrieved from http://jama.jamanetwork.com/article.aspx?articleid=1791497

Framingham Heart Study. (2013). *Atrial fibrillation.* Retrieved from http://www.framinghamheart-study.org/risk/atrial.html

Go, A. S., Mozaffarian, D., Roger, V. L., Benjamin, E. J., Berry, J. D., Blaha, M. J., ... Turner, M. B.; American Heart Association Statistics Committee and Stroke Statistics Subcommittee. (2014). Heart disease and stroke statistics—2014 update: a report from the American Heart Association. *Circulation, 129*(3), e28–e292. doi:10.1161/01.cir.0000441139.02102.80.

Jauch E.C., Saver J.L., Adams H.P. Jr., Bruno A., Connors J.J., Demaerschalk B.M., ... Yonas H.; American Heart Association Stroke Council; Council on Cardiovascular Nursing; Council on Peripheral Vascular Disease; Council on Clinical Cardiology. (2013). Guidelines for the early management of patients with acute ischemic stroke: a guideline for healthcare professionals from the American Heart Association/American Stroke Association. *Stroke, 44*(3), 870–947. doi:10.1161/STR.0b013e318284056a. Retrieved from http://www.ncbi.nlm.nih.gov/pubmed/23370205

Massie, B. M., & Amidon, T. A. (2003). Heart. In L. M. Tierney, Jr., S. J. McPhee, & M. A. Papadakis (Eds.), *Current medical diagnosis and treatment* (42nd ed., pp. 312–408). New York: Lange Medical Books/McGraw-Hill.

National Guideline Clearinghouse, National Clinical Guideline Center (2006, revised 2014 Jun). *Atrial fibrillation: The management of atrial fibrillation.* Retrieved from https://www.guideline.gov/summaries/summary/48333

National Guideline Clearinghouse (NGC). *Guideline summary: 2013 ACC/AHA guideline on the treatment of blood cholesterol to reduce atherosclerotic cardiovascular risk in adults: A report of the American College of Cardiology/American Heart Association Task Force on Practice Guidelines.* Available from https://www.guideline.gov/summaries/summary/48337/2013-accaha-guideline-on-the-treatment-of-blood-cholesterol-to-reduce-atherosclerotic-cardiovascular-risk-in-adults-a-report-of-the-american-college-of-cardiologyamerican-heart-association-task-force-on-practice-guidelines

National Heart, Lung, and Blood Institute. (2012). Expert Panel on Integrated Guidelines for Cardiovascular Health and Risk Reduction in Children and Adolescents summary report. Retrieved from https://www.nhlbi.nih.gov/files/docs/peds_guidelines_sum.pdf

National Heart, Lung, and Blood Institute. (2013). *Integrated guidelines for cardiovascular health and risk reduction in children and adolescents—2011.* Retrieved from http://www.nhlbi.nih.gov/health-pro/guidelines/current/cardiovascular-health-pediatric-guidelines

National Heart, Lung, and Blood Institute. (2012). *Fact book, fiscal year 2012. 4. Disease statistics*. Retrieved from http://www.nhlbi.nih.gov/about/documents/factbook/2012

Snow, V., Barry, P., Fihn, S. D., Gibbons, R. J., Owens, D. K., Williams, ... Weiss, K. B.;American College of Physicians; American College of Cardiology Chronic Stable Angina Panel. (2004). Primary care management of chronic stable angina and asymptomatic suspected or known coronary artery disease: A clinical practice guideline from the American College of Physicians. *Annals of Internal Medicine, 141*(7), 562–567.

Snow, V., Barry, P., Fihn, S. D., Gibbons, R. J., Owens, D. K., Williams, S. V., ... Mottur-Pilson, C.; ACP; ACC Chronic Stable Angina Panel. (2004). Evaluation of primary care patients with chronic stable angina: Guidelines from the American College of Physicians. *Annals of Internal Medicine, 141*(1), 57–64.

Solenski, N. J. (2004a). Transient ischemic attacks: Part I. Diagnosis and evaluation. *American Family Physician, 6*(7), 1665–1674. Retrieved from http://www.aafp.org/afp/2004/0401/p1665.html

Solenski, N. J. (2004b). Transient ischemic attacks: Part II. Treatment. *American Family Physician, 6*(7), 1675–1681.

Sontheimer, D. L. (2006). Peripheral vascular disease: Diagnosis and treatment. *American Family Physician, 73*(11), 1971–1976.

Unknown. (1996). Update on the report of 1987 task force on high blood pressure in children and adolescents. *Pediatrics, 79*(1), 1–25.

U.S. Preventive Services Task Force. (2002). Aspirin for the primary prevention of cardiovascular events: Recommendation and rationale. *Annals of Internal Medicine, 136*, 157–160.

Van Vlaanderen, E. (2001). Revised guidelines for acute MI. *Clinical Advisor*, 31–34.

Wing, L. M., Reid, C. M., Ryan, P., Beilin, L. J., Brown, M. A., Jennings, G. L., ... West, M. J. (2003). A comparison of outcomes with angiotensin converting enzyme inhibitors and diuretics for hypertension in the elderly. *New England Journal of Medicine, 348*, 583–592.

Yusuf, S., Sleight, P., Pogue, J., Bosch, J., Davies, R., & Dagenais, G. (2000). Effects on angiotensin converting enzyme inhibitor, ramipril, on cardiovascular events in high risk patients: The Heart Outcomes Prevention Evaluation (HOPE) study investigators. *New England Journal of Medicine, 342*, 145–153.

CHAPTER 9

GASTROINTESTINAL DISORDERS

Kara Ventura, DNP, FNP-BC, CPNP, DCC

GENERAL APPROACH

▶ Older adults are less likely to feel pain with abdominal conditions and do not always present with classic symptoms or lab findings, are more likely to have vague diffuse pain, and tend to have less acute presentation than younger patients.

▶ Iron-deficiency anemia in a male, postmenopausal female, or older adult patient always warrants an upper and lower endoscopy to rule out a gastrointestinal source of bleeding or cancer.

▶ Antidiarrheal medications should never be given to patients under 5 years old or any patient with bloody diarrhea, fever, fecal leukocytes, or abdominal pain because of the possible development of a systemic infection from retained toxins. These patients require prompt evaluation and referral.

▶ Every tender, nonreducible hernia must be referred to a surgeon for prompt evaluation.

▶ Careful history-taking of most GI problems will help to determine the location of the problem.

▶ Always repeat abdominal exam before discharging the patient to validate initial results or detect new findings; document assessment.

▶ Always examine the tender area last to avoid referred pain.

RED FLAGS

▶ A patient who presents with fever, chills, leukocytosis (elevated total white blood count [WBC] with increased neutrophils [polys] and bands on the differential), and rebound tenderness warrants rapid assessment and referral to an acute care facility for a surgical consultation.

▶ Abdominal pain lasting more than 6 hours or pain that wakes the patient up at night requires evaluation and possible referral.

▶ New onset constipation over the age of 50 is also a warning sign.

GASTROINTESTINAL SIGNS AND SYMPTOMS

Dysphagia

Description

▶ Difficulty in swallowing (oropharyngeal dysphagia) and having food pass from the mouth down the esophagus to the stomach (esophageal dysphagia); odynophagia—painful swallowing—is an alarm symptom that requires immediate evaluation to determine cause and treatment.

▶ Patients describe oropharyngeal dysphagia as a feeling of food getting stuck, indicative of upper esophageal or pharyngeal disease; may present as difficulty swallowing solids or liquids, described as trouble initiating a swallow; coughing; choking; nasal regurgitation (oropharyngeal dysplasia); sensation of food "sticking" after it is swallowed (esophageal dysphasia).

▶ May be a structural or neuromuscular problem caused by such conditions as gastroesophageal reflux disease (GERD), esophageal spasm, Barrett's esophagus, benign esophageal or peptic stricture, esophagitis, esophageal rings (also webs and diverticula), carcinoma, goiter, myasthenia gravis, multiple sclerosis, hypothyroidism, Parkinson's disease, achalasia, scleroderma, or polymyositis

▶ May present as chest pain

▶ *Not* attributed to normal aging

▶ Diagnostic workup may include:

▷ CBC and stool for occult blood to evaluate for bleeding (carcinoma)

▷ Liver functions tests to evaluate for metastatic process

▷ BUN, albumin to evaluate nutritional status

▷ Thyroid function tests to rule out hypothyroidism

▷ ECG and cardiac workup if chest pain the presenting symptom

▷ Endoscopy: standard test for diagnosis and management of esophageal diseases because it allows for biopsy and definitive tissue diagnosis

▷ Barium swallow or upper GI series: Often done first to differentiate between mechanical lesions and esophageal motility problems. If a motility problem is suspected, barium swallow should be done first. If a mechanical lesion is suspected, an endoscopy is often done first.

▷ Esophageal pH recording to evaluate for GERD if difficulty establishing diagnosis

▷ Video esophagography—esophageal manometry (not a first-line test)

▷ Outpatient treatment if patient not malnourished and not high risk for aspiration

▶ Treat identifiable condition.

▶ Goal is to treat underlying cause and maintain nutritional status during workup; consider liquid supplementation

▶ Older adults may have poor-fitting dentures that contribute to the problem.

▶ Use thickened liquids for people with dysphagia to prevent aspiration.

▶ Refer any patient with new symptoms and no obvious treatable cause to a gastroenterologist—particularly the older patient, and those with weight loss, bleeding, iron-deficiency anemia, history of chronic GERD, or history of heavy alcohol and tobacco use.

Abnormal Liver Function Tests (LFTs)

Description

▶ Serum liver chemistries are useful in evaluating liver function and include: alanine (ALT) and aspartate (AST) aminotransferase (ALT is highest in liver disease and AST is less-specific; elevated in liver, cardiac, skeletal muscle, kidney, brain, pancreas, or lung disease) evaluate hepatic cellular integrity; bilirubin (direct and indirect), alkaline phosphatase (ALP), and gamma-glutamyl trans peptidase (GGT) assess hepatic excretion; and prothrombin time (PT) and serum albumin evaluate hepatic protein synthesis.

Etiology

▶ Elevated aminotransferases (ALT and AST) may be seen in conditions including biliary obstruction, viral hepatitis, cirrhosis, metastatic liver disease, autoimmune disease, and drug-induced liver injury.

▶ These enzymes are found in multiple tissues and are released into the plasma in response to cellular injury.

▶ ALT is found predominately in the liver, so it is more specific than ALT for evaluating hepatocellular damage.

▶ AST is found in liver, cardiac, skeletal, kidney, and brain tissue; elevated levels alone may indicate tissue damage in any of those organ systems (e.g., myocardial ischemia or musculoskeletal injury).

▶ The highest levels of ALT and AST (usually more than 500 units/liter) occur with severe viral hepatitis, drug-induced liver injury (e.g., acetaminophen, phenytoin, rifampin), or ischemic hepatitis. Moderate elevations (usually less than 300 units/liter) are present in mild to acute viral hepatitis, chronic active hepatitis, cirrhosis, and liver metastases. Mild elevation may be present in biliary obstruction, with higher levels suggesting the development of cholangitis (causing hepatic cell necrosis) with also an elevation in ALP. In alcoholic liver disease, the AST/ALT ratio may be more than 2. A ratio of AST/ALT more than 1 may be seen with fatty liver as seen associated with pregnancy and metabolic syndrome.

▶ An elevated bilirubin (a degradation product of heme) should be fractionated to determine if it is predominantly conjugated (direct, processed by the liver) or unconjugated (indirect, not processed by the liver).

▶ Elevations in direct bilirubin are usually caused by impaired excretion of bilirubin from the liver because of hepatocellular disease, biliary tract obstruction, drugs, or sepsis.

▶ Indirect bilirubin elevation is caused by hemolysis or ineffective erythropoiesis (increased bilirubin production); neonatal jaundice, Gilbert's or Crigler-Najjar syndromes (impaired bilirubin conjugation because of enzyme deficiency); or when hepatic bilirubin uptake is decreased because of drugs, heart failure, or portosystemic shunting.

▶ Alkaline phosphatase is an enzyme found in various tissues, including the liver, bone, intestine, and placenta (more than 80% from liver and bone).

▶ Elevated ALP levels (in the absence of bone disease or pregnancy) usually represent impaired biliary tract function.

▶ Fractionation of an elevated serum ALP can be done to determine the source; however, elevation of other liver function tests is helpful in establishing a hepatic cause.

▶ Mild to moderate increases (usually one to two times normal) occur with hepatocellular disorders such as hepatitis or cirrhosis.

▶ High serum elevations (up to 10 times normal or greater) can occur with extra hepatic biliary tract obstruction (usually a gallstone blocking the common bile duct) or intrahepatic cholestasis (bile retention in the liver) as seen with drug-induced cholestasis and biliary cirrhosis.

▶ The ALP is usually mildly elevated in incomplete biliary tract obstruction and in metastatic and infiltrative liver disease (e.g., leukemia, lymphoma, and sarcoidosis).

▶ An elevated ALP is also present in nonhepatic disorders, with the most common being bone disease (Paget's disease and bone metastases).

▶ Elevated GGT in liver disease is useful in differentiating the origin of an elevated ALP (hepatic vs. bone), as they both tend to increase in similar hepatic diseases.

▶ GGT is also a highly sensitive indicator of acute alcohol ingestion and of other agents that stimulate the hepatic microsomal oxidase system, such as barbiturates and phenytoin.

▶ The GGT enzyme is also present in the pancreas, kidney, heart, and brain, and elevations may occur in disorders involving those organ systems.

▶ A prolonged PT is caused by impaired hepatic synthesis of coagulation factors seen in significant liver disease and/or with vitamin K deficiency that may occur with malnutrition, malabsorption (e.g., cholestasis, steatorrhea, pancreatic insufficiency), and warfarin use. If administration of vitamin K corrects the PT, a deficiency was present.

▶ Decreased serum albumin, the primary protein synthesized by the liver, may be caused by chronic liver disease, or by other nonhepatic factors such as malnutrition, hormonal factors, or excessive protein loss (nephrotic syndrome or protein-losing enteropathy).

Risk Factors

▶ Alcohol

▶ Drugs metabolized by liver

▶ Genetic predisposition

Assessment

History

▶ Many patients are asymptomatic with mild, transient elevations.

▶ Generalized symptoms of fever, anorexia, malaise, weight loss, jaundice, arthralgias, myalgias, rash, and pruritus may be present.

▶ Gastrointestinal symptoms include anorexia, nausea, vomiting, abdominal pain, dark urine, and pale stools.

▶ Additional history is aimed at identifying potential risk factors: history of hepatitis exposure, gallstones, transfusions, previous surgery, medications (including vitamins and herbs, OTCs, acetaminophen), alcohol and drug use, sexual practices, occupational exposure, and travel history.

Physical Exam

▶ Skin exam: jaundice (include sclera), spider angiomas, palmar erythema, gynecomastia, caput medusae (annular purple discoloration around umbilicus or ostomy), and ecchymosis

▶ Abdominal exam: ascites, tenderness (usually right upper quadrant), enlarged gallbladder, hepatomegaly, and splenomegaly; liver may be smaller than normal in advanced liver disease

▶ Extremities: asterixis, temporal and proximal muscle wasting, and peripheral edema

Diagnostic Studies

▶ If the patient is asymptomatic, repeat liver function tests before ordering any other tests. If normal, repeat testing in 3 to 6 months is suggested.

▶ If repeat is abnormal, obtain hepatitis serologies to exclude viral hepatitis A, B, and C (see section on Viral Hepatitis).

▶ If the patient is symptomatic, further tests are guided by history and physical exam (see Table 9–1); consider:

  ▷ Mono spot and CMV IgG, IgM titers

  ▷ Abdominal ultrasound: best screening test to evaluate for gallstones; can also detect biliary tree dilation, biliary obstruction, cholecystitis, fatty liver, and liver parenchymal disease

  ▷ Computed tomography (CT) scan (with IV contrast): best test to evaluate liver parenchymal disease and space-occupying lesions (tumor or abscess); can also assess biliary tree dilation and identify obstructing lesion

  ▷ Magnetic resonance imaging (MRI): similar to CT scan but can better visualize vessels without the use of IV contrast

  ▷ Endoscopic retrograde cholangiopancreatography (ERCP) and percutaneous transhepatic cholangiography (PTC): usually done after screening with ultrasound, CT, or MRI to further assess cause, location, and extent of biliary tree abnormalities

  ▷ Liver biopsy: definitive study to determine the cause and extent of hepatocellular and infiltrative liver disease; biopsy may be guided using ultrasound or CT

TABLE 9-1.
INTERPRETING LIVER FUNCTION TESTS

LIVER FUNCTION TEST	ENZYME FOUND IN	CAUSE OF ELEVATION	CONDITIONS WHERE SEEN	COMMENTS
Bilirubin: direct (conjugated, processed by liver)	Liver, blood, urine	Impaired excretion of bilirubin from the liver	Hepatocellular disease, biliary tract obstruction, drugs, sepsis	
Bilirubin: indirect (unconjugated, not processed by the liver)	Liver, blood, urine	Hepatic bilirubin uptake is decreased	Hemolysis or portosystemic shunting, drugs, heart failure, ineffective erythropoiesis, neonatal jaundice	
Alkaline phosphatase	Bone, liver, intestine, placenta	Impaired biliary tract function (cholestasis) or infiltrative liver disease hepatic excretion	*Mild:* hepatitis, cirrhosis, early cancer	Increases with age, women > men
			High: biliary tract obstruction, cholestasis	Also elevated in bone disease, bony metastasis, and Paget's
GGT	Liver, pancreas, kidney, heart, brain	Hepatic excretion	Sensitive for acute alcohol ingestion, drugs such as barbiturates and phenytoin	Differentiates the origin of an elevated ALP between bone and liver
Transaminases	Many tissues	Acute hepatocellular injury—from necrosis or inflammation	*Mild:* biliary obstruction, mild viral chronic or active and alcoholic hepatitis, cirrhosis, and liver metastases	Do not indicate severity of liver injury; most common cause of elevation is alcoholic hepatitis
ALT	Predominantly liver, more specific test	Celiac disease	*High:* viral hepatitis, drug-induced liver injury	
AST	Liver, cardiac, skeletal, kidney, brain			AST twice as high as ALT typical of alcoholic liver injury
Prothrombin time	Blood	Impaired hepatic synthesis of coagulation factors	Significant liver disease	If vitamin K corrects the PT, a deficiency was present
Albumin	Blood serum	Impaired hepatic protein synthesis, excess protein loss	Chronic liver disease, \	May decrease with age

Management

▶ Aimed at correcting underlying cause

Nonpharmacologic Treatment

▶ Avoid drugs and other agents that are hepatotoxic.

▶ Management will vary depending on etiology.

Special Considerations

▶ Geriatric patients: higher incidence of neoplasm in this age group

▶ Pregnancy: elevated ALP common because present in placental tissue; CT scans contraindicated

When to Consult, Refer, Hospitalize

▶ Consult with or refer to a physician or specialist when significantly abnormal liver function tests persist without an identifiable cause, or for symptomatic patients in need of specialized diagnostic tests and management.

Follow-Up

▶ Recheck studies every 3 to 6 months.

Constipation

Description

▶ A symptom as well as a diagnosis where there is decrease in frequency of stools, excessive difficulty passing stools, leakage from rectum, and straining with defecation

Etiology

▶ Most common cause: functional etiologies—poor dietary intake of fiber and fluids, behavioral habits such as change in environment with travel or schedule, sedentary lifestyle; occurs in children most often when cereal is first introduced to diet, during toilet training, or entry to school

▶ Psychogenic; chronic constipation can begin in first year of life

▶ Congenital disorders

▶ Medications: opiate analgesics, calcium channel blockers, anticholinergics, diuretics, aluminum-based antacids, calcium and iron supplements, NSAIDs, antihistamines, antipsychotics, anti-Parkinson agents, laxative abuse

Prevention and Screening

▶ Exercise; increase daily fiber and fluid intake

▶ If possible, establish time each day to defecate and do not ignore the urge to defecate.

▶ Provide anticipatory guidance regarding toilet training techniques.

Assessment

▶ Rome III criteria must include at least two of the following for 12 weeks in the previous 6 months:

▷ Fewer than three stools per week

▷ Straining at least one-quarter of the time

▷ Hard stools at least one-quarter of the time

▷ Need for manual assist at least one-quarter of the time

▷ Sense of incomplete evacuation at least one-quarter of the time

Physical Exam

▶ Abdominal and gynecological exam for masses, pain

▶ Rectal exam: sphincter tone, fissures, size of rectal vault, rectal prolapse, presence of stool and consistency, masses

▶ Neurologic exam

▶ In frail older adults, evaluate systemic signs of fever, delirium, urinary retention, arrhythmias, tachypnea.

Diagnostic Studies

▶ American Gastroenterological Association guidelines suggest CBC, BS, TSH, calcium, and creatinine routinely

▶ Sigmoid/colonoscopy if red flags are present

▶ Flat plate and upright abdominal films to evaluate for obstruction

▶ Colonoscopy or barium enema if patient anemic to evaluate for colorectal cancer; consider in any adult with new onset over the age of 50

Management

Nonpharmacologic Treatment

▶ Increase fiber in adults: 20–35 g/day.

▶ Increase fiber gradually, over a two-week period.

▶ Increase fluid intake, particularly water, to 1.5–2 liters per day.

Pharmacologic Treatment

▶ First-line:

▷ Hydrophilic colloids or bulk-forming agents: psyllium (Metamucil, Fiberall) 3.4 grams one to three times daily; methylcellulose (Citrucel) 2 grams one to three times daily; polycarbophil (FiberCon) 1 gram one to three times daily; can be used on long-term basis

▷ Surfactants: used to soften stools; docusate sodium (Colace) 50–200 mg daily; used short term up to 2 weeks; may be used longer and do not induce dependency

▷ Osmotic laxatives: used for acute constipation and should not be used long-term; should result in a bowel movement in 0.5 to 3 hours or longer. Miralax (polyethylene glycol) 17 gm daily, is found to be superior to others in category. Lactulose and Sorbitol, 15–60 mL, at bedtime are equally effective but tend to cause flatulence, bloating, and cramping. Magnesium hydroxide suspension (milk of magnesia) 30–60 mL x 1 dose (should not be given to patients with renal insufficiency).

▶ Second-line:

▷ Stimulants: stimulate fluid secretion, colonic contraction; may cause cramping; use infrequently; include Senokot, Ex-Lax, Dulcolax, and Correctol; Peri-Colace acts as lubricant with mineral oil to coat stool

▷ Lubiprostone (Amitiza) 24 mcg b.i.d. is approved for chronic constipation in adults as well as irritable bowel syndrome.

▶ Constipation with fecal impaction

▷ First removal of impaction by use of sodium phosphate enemas; two to three enemas over a 2-day period

▷ Once impaction removed, begin long-term therapy

▶ Mineral oil: adults 60 mL/dose, max two doses/day; children 1 mL/kg/dose b.i.d., max 90 mL /day *or*

▶ Lactulose: adults 15 mL b.i.d.; children 0.5 mL/kg/dose b.i.d.

▶ Treat for 3 to 6 months along with nonpharmacological treatments.

Special Consideration

▶ Evaluate diet, fluid intake, medications, activity in older adults.

When to Consult, Refer, Hospitalize

▶ Refer to a gastroenterologist if patient fails to respond to treatment; stool positive for occult blood, weight loss is present, and over the age of 50 with sudden, unexplained change in bowel pattern.

Expected Course

▶ With treatment, constipation should resolve in several days if there is no significant underlying problem, such as bowel obstruction.

▶ With exercise, a daily bowel regimen and an increase in fiber and fluids, should, for the most part, resolve permanently.

Diarrhea
Definition

▶ Increased frequency, looseness, and volume of stools; may be either acute or chronic condition; infants 6 to 24 months are at highest risk of morbidity and mortality

Etiology

▶ Produced by one or more of the following: abnormal intestinal motility, decreased water absorption, and/or increased fluid secretion.

▶ *Acute:* most commonly caused by infectious agents, viruses, bacterial toxins, or drug (see Table 9–2)

▶ *Chronic:* can be because of many causes but often from hardy agents spread by fecal-oral route

TABLE 9-2.
COMMON CAUSES OF ACUTE DIARRHEA

ORGANISM	TRANSMISSION	INCUBATION	SIGNS AND SYMPTOMS	TYPE OF STOOLS	LAB DATA	SPECIAL NOTATIONS
VIRAL						
Rota and Norwalk (Noro)	Fecal-oral	24–72 hours	Nausea, vomiting, cramps Fever	Watery	No WBCs in stool	Most common causes: Rotavirus in children (6–24 months) More common in winter Norwalk in all others Vomiting most prominent symptom in children Diarrhea most prominent symptom in adults
Bacterial						
Staphylococcus aureus	Food: ham, poultry, creams, mayonnaise	30 minutes– 6 hours	Nausea, vomiting, cramps	Soft, not watery	No WBCs in stool	Onset abrupt, others with symptoms, look for common source
Clostridium perfringens	Food: beef, ham, Mexican cuisine	8–12 hours	Nausea, vomiting, epigastric pain	Watery	No WBCs in stool	Onset not as abrupt as with *S. aureus*
Campylobacter jejuni	Food: chicken Water Fecal material	1–7 days	Nausea, vomiting, abdominal pain, malaise, fever	Watery, gross and occult blood	WBCs in stool Positive culture	Abdominal pain can mimic appendicitis

Salmonella	Food: poultry, red meat, eggs, unpasteurized milk Water Contact with infected pets (turtles, reptiles) Fecal-oral	6–72 hours	Nausea, vomiting, abdominal cramps, fever	Watery, gross and occult blood	WBCs in stool Positive culture	Common in children <5 and adults >70 years
Shigella	Food Water Fecal-oral	1–7 days	Abdominal pain Fever	Watery, occult blood, No gross blood	WBCs in stool Positive culture	Most common in 1- to 4-year-olds, common in childcare centers
Escherichia coli	Food, water contaminated with feces "Traveler's diarrhea"	10 hours–6 days	Abdominal cramps	Watery	Usually no WBCs Positive culture	History of recent travel
Protozoal						
Giardia lamblia, Cryptosporidium	Fecal-oral Water	1–4 weeks	Abdominal pain, flatulence, distention, anorexia	Soft, pale, watery, foul-smelling	Stool positive for ova and parasites	Acute presentation of chronic or recurrent diarrhea

Incidence and Demographics

▶ Common worldwide; 11% of general population

Risk Factors

▶ Institutional settings such as day care, nursing homes, schools

▶ Travel to area with water and soil contamination

▶ Improper cooking and preparation methods, especially items from street vendors where constancy of temperature is issue

▶ Recent antibiotic use

Prevention and Screening

▶ Handwashing, particularly after using bathroom

▶ Avoid water supply while traveling to endemic areas, including water for tooth-brushing, ice cubes

▶ Proper food preparation and cooking of cold salads and meats

▶ Rotavirus vaccine

Assessment

History

▶ Determine whether symptoms were sudden in onset or chronic.

▶ Anorexia, vomiting, malaise, headache, myalgias

▶ Obtain medication history, including any recent courses of antibiotics plus laxative or antacid use.

▶ Inquire about sexual practices and risk of HIV infection.

▶ Obtain description of bowel pattern; contributing factors such as certain foods or stress, family history; and stool characteristics (bloody, watery, with mucous, fatty, foul-smelling).

▶ Weight loss

▶ Travel history: Incubation period is 2 to 4 days for many viruses.

▶ Surgical history; history of exposure to others with similar illness

▶ Symptoms of hyperthyroidism

Physical Exam

▶ Signs of dehydration: tachycardia, confusion, orthostatic hypotension, poor skin turgor, dry mucous membranes, depressed fontanel, eyes sunken, crying without tears, listless, decreased urine output; fever is variable and ranges from afebrile to significant elevations

▶ Abdominal exam may reveal hyperactive bowel sounds and generalized tenderness.

▶ Signs of peritonitis (rebound tenderness) may be seen with severe inflammatory diarrhea.

▶ Particularly in children, look for other possible causes of diarrhea such as otitis media and urinary tract infection (UTI).

▶ Based on presentation, severity, and duration; test if symptoms severe or diarrhea lasts longer than 7 days

▶ Stool cultures, ova and parasites, *Clostridium difficile* toxin, occult blood

▶ CBC to look for anemia, leukocytosis, and eosinophilia (often seen in parasitic infections and inflammatory bowel diseases)

▶ Electrolytes; evaluate for hypokalemia, hyponatremia

▶ BUN and creatinine; elevations may be indicative of dehydration

▶ Blood cultures if systemic infection is suspected—high fever, chills, leukocytosis

▶ In patients with diarrhea lasting more than 3 weeks:

   ▷ Sigmoidoscopy or colonoscopy to diagnose colitis

   ▷ Evaluate for malabsorption: vitamin B_{12}, folate, vitamin D, albumin, cholesterol, iron, iron-binding capacity, prothrombin time, D-xylose absorption test, 24-hour fecal fat collection to diagnose steatorrhea.

Differential Diagnosis

▶ Appendicitis

▶ Volvulus

▶ Cystic fibrosis

▶ Intussusception

▶ Inflammatory bowel syndrome

▶ Inflammatory bowel disease

▶ Irritable bowel syndrome

▶ Meningitis

▶ Pancreatitis

▶ Pneumonia

▶ Lactose intolerance

▶ Colon cancer

▶ Diverticulitis

▶ Pseudomembranous colitis

▶ Fecal impaction

▶ Malabsorption

▶ Cholinergic drugs and magnesium laxative abuse

Management

Nonpharmacologic Treatment

▶ Adequate hydration with fluids containing electrolytes and carbohydrates

▶ In infants without signs of dehydration, continue with formula or breast milk but increase amount; may change to soy-based formula for diarrhea (Isomil/DF, Enfamil, ProSobee, or Lacto free) while ill.

▶ Normal diet when patient able to tolerate; no longer recommending BRAT diet (bananas, rice, applesauce, toast) because not calorie-dense and not enough fat and protein

▶ In children with signs of mild dehydration, give 50 mL/kg of oral replacement therapy (ORT) such as Pedialyte, plus 10 mL/kg for each stool over a 4-hour period; sports drinks may be used in children over 3 years old.

▶ If vomiting present, start with small volumes: 5 mL q. 2 to 3 minutes and increase gradually if vomiting subsides. Also increase ORT by estimated volume loss with emesis.

Pharmacologic Treatment

▶ Antidiarrheal agents: If no contraindications (fever, bloody stools), may consider using:

▷ Loperamide (Imodium): adults: 4 mg initially followed by 2 mg after each loose stool for a maximum of 16 mg in 24 hours; not recommended in children

▷ Bismuth subsalicylate (Pepto-Bismol): adults: two tablets or 30 mL q. 30 to 60 minutes, max eight doses/day; children 6 to 9 years: 10 mL q. 30 to 60 minutes; 9 to 12 years: 15 mL q. 30 to 60 minutes, max eight doses/day

▶ In adults, empirical antibiotic treatment while awaiting stool culture results for patients with moderate to severe fever, bloody stools, tenesmus, or presence of fecal leukocytes

▷ Fluoroquinolones: drugs of choice, as they provide good coverage for most invasive bacterial pathogens

▷ Ciprofloxacin (Cipro) 500 mg b.i.d. *or* levofloxacin (Levaquin) 500 mg daily

▶ Alternative agents

▷ Trimethoprim-sulfamethoxazole 160/800 (Bactrim DS) b.i.d. *or* erythromycin 250–500 mg q.i.d.

▶ If *Giardia* or *C. difficile* is suspected:

▷ Metronidazole (Flagyl) 250 mg t.i.d. for 7 days (avoid alcohol use during and for 48 hours after); for *C. difficile*, 500 mg t.i.d. for 10 to 14 days

▷ Option for *C. difficile*, oral vancomycin

▶ Generally, antibiotics are not used to treat children until the causative organism is known and then only:

▷ *Campylobacter:* erythromycin 20–50 mg/kg/day divided into four doses for 5 to 7 days

▷ *Shigella:* Bactrim 1 mL/kg/day divided into two doses for 5 days

▷ *E. coli:* Bactrim 1 mL/kg/day divided into two doses for 3 days

▷ *Giardia:* furazolidone 6 mg/kg/day divided into four doses for 7 to 10 days (Furox: 1 5 mg/kg/day in four divided doses)

▷ Alinia: new product for *Giardia*; may be given orally; do not use in children younger than 12 months; suspension for ages 1 to 11 yrs; tablets only; tablets only for 12 years and older

▷　Replace lost fluids and electrolytes.

▷　Probiotics in people on antibiotics to prevent diarrhea

How Long to Treat

▶　Depends on underlying cause; for acute diarrhea because of an infection, generally 5 to 7 days

Special Considerations

▶　For chronic diarrhea, treatment may vary according to underlying cause.

▶　Geriatric patients are at greater risk for dehydration and complications.

▶　Neonates are at greater risk for severe infection and should be referred immediately.

▶　Pregnancy and lactation: If antimicrobials are required, check safety profile for use.

▶　Other: Immunocompromised patients are a greater risk for chronic diarrhea from an infectious process such as cryptosporidium (a common, self-limiting infection that people with an intact immune system are able to clear in a few days without treatment).

When to Consult, Refer, Hospitalize

▶　Consult with physician for any child with significant signs and symptoms of dehydration (more than 10% increased pulse rate, poor skin turgor, depressed fontanel, delayed capillary refill, less than 1 mg/kg/hour urine output).

▶　Consult for possible hospitalization for infants under 3 months with bacterial diarrhea.

▶　Any patient with bloody diarrhea, fever, acute abdominal pain, and leukocytosis should be referred and evaluated immediately in an acute-care setting.

▶　Anyone who has not had resolution of diarrhea within 3 weeks needs to be referred to a gastroenterologist for evaluation.

Follow-Up

▶　Depends on cause and severity; none may be necessary if hydration maintained

Expected Course

▶　Acute diarrhea should resolve in 24 to 48 hours.

Acute Abdominal Pain

Definition

▶　Can be caused by obstruction of hollow viscus, altered bowel motility, capsular distention, peritoneal irritation, mucosal ulceration, vascular insufficiency, nerve injury, abdominal wall injury, or pain referred from an extra-abdominal site

Assessment

History

- ▶ Determine the onset, progression, migration, character and intensity, and localization.
  - ▷ Onset: *sudden, rapid,* or *gradual*
    - ▶ Sudden: patient able to relate time of onset to a precise moment
      - ▷ Most often associated with perforation of the gastrointestinal tract that may be caused by a duodenal or gastric ulcer, diverticulum, or foreign body
      - ▷ Other causes: ruptured ectopic pregnancy, ruptured aortic aneurysm, mesenteric infarction, embolism of the abdominal muscle
    - ▶ Rapid: begins within a few seconds and increases in severity in a short period of time
      - ▷ Often associated with intestinal obstruction, ureteral stone, cholecystitis, pancreatitis, diverticulitis, appendicitis, penetrating duodenal or gastric ulcer
    - ▶ Gradual: pain slowly becomes more severe over a course of hours or days
      - ▷ History of onset vague
      - ▷ Often associated with a chronic inflammatory process, neoplasm, or a large bowel obstruction
  - ▷ Progression
    - ▶ Perforated bowel often presents as a sudden onset of pain that dramatically abates if the perforation seals off and there is no further leakage of bowel content or blood into the peritoneum.
    - ▶ A small bowel obstruction may present as intermittent attacks of pain that progress into a steady constant pain suggestive of vascular compromise.
  - ▷ Migration
    - ▶ Pain that changes from the original site of onset to another location
    - ▶ Acute appendicitis may begin as periumbilical or epigastric pain and then localize to the right lower quadrant.
    - ▶ A perforated duodenal ulcer causes pain initially in the epigastrium (because of leakage of gastric contents) and can migrate to the lower quadrants where the gastric material localizes in the abdominal cavity.
    - ▶ Cholecystitis often causes irritation of the phrenic nerve, resulting in diaphragmatic pain that can radiate to the right shoulder, right scapula, or between the shoulder blades (Kehr's sign).
  - ▷ Character and intensity
    - ▶ Cramping, dull, or aching and either constant or intermittent
    - ▶ Cramping (or colicky) abdominal pain increases in intensity in short waves, with intermittent periods of complete absence of pain. Often associated with mechanical small bowel obstruction. Short pain-free intervals may

    indicate a more proximal bowel obstruction; longer pain-free intervals may indicate a more distal obstruction.

▶ Dull or aching abdominal pain that is constant is often caused by distention or edema of the abdominal wall, bowel wall, or inflammation of an abdominal organ (such as the capsule of the liver or spleen).

▷ Localization

▶ Visceral pain due to distension of a hollow viscus is often localized poorly and often perceived in the midline; epigastric, mid-abdominal, or lower abdominal area.

▶ Patients with visceral pain frequently change positions in an attempt to alleviate the pain.

▶ Somatic pain is due to peritoneal inflammation and is usually sharper and more localized to the diseased area.

▶ Patients with peritonitis often lie still on one side with their knees and hips flexed.

▶ Pain from peritonitis is intensified by jarring motions (bumping into the bed).

▶ In children, the closer the pain is to the umbilicus, the less likely it is to be organic.

▶ Additional information:

▷ Have the patient rate pain on a scale of 1 to 10.

▷ Determine if pain interferes with sleep; factors that precipitate or relieve the pain; relationship of pain to meals, specific foods, menstrual cycle, urination, defecation, exertion, and inspiration.

▷ Fever, chills, nausea, vomiting, diarrhea, constipation, or urogenital symptoms may be present.

▷ Blood in the stool, urine, or emesis may be present.

▷ Social history includes alcohol and intravenous drug use.

▷ Gynecological history: Evaluate for possible pregnancy or sexually transmitted disease (STD).

▷ In children, include questions regarding irritability, ability to console, fussiness with feedings, whether infant clenches fists or draws feet up when crying.

Physical Exam

▶ Assess for fever, tachycardia, orthostatic hypotension, pallor, jaundice, perspiration, restlessness, and body positioning.

▶ Abdominal exam: Perform with knees flexed if in severe pain.

▶ Observe for any surgical scars, distention.

▶ Bowel sounds: High-pitched tinkling sounds suggest a dilated bowel with air and fluid under tension. Rushes of high-pitched sounds indicate intestinal obstruction. Absent bowel sounds indicate an ileus or peritonitis.

▶ Inspect and palpate for hernias: abdominal, inguinal, or umbilical.

▶ Palpate for localized tenderness, rigidity, guarding, and rebound tenderness (an indication of peritonitis). Check for CVA tenderness (with pyelonephritis or urolithiasis). Evaluate for hepatosplenomegaly and fluid wave (ascites from liver disease).

▶ Assess for Rovsing's sign, psoas sign, obturator sign (see the Appendicitis section), and Murphy's sign (see the Cholecystitis section).

▶ Rectal exam: Rectal wall pain can be an indication of appendicitis or abscess.

▶ Pelvic exam: for all women with abdominal pain

▶ In children, assess growth parameters.

▶ Other systems for possible origin because of possibility of referred pain, based on history

Diagnostic Studies
▶ CBC with differential; may show leukocytosis or anemia

▶ Serum electrolytes, glucose, BUN, and creatinine

▶ LFTs may be abnormal with liver involvement (AST, ALT, Alk phos, bilirubin, PT, PTT).

▶ Amylase and lipase may be elevated in pancreatic disease.

▶ Beta HCG: Always obtain in women of childbearing age.

▶ STD testing if appropriate

▶ Urinalysis to rule out infection and hematuria (children with appendicitis may have some RBCs and WBCs in urine)

▶ Check stool for blood.

▶ Abdominal ultrasound or transvaginal ultrasound for possible tubo-ovarian pathology

▶ CT scan for possible appendicitis, abscess, diverticular disease, kidney stones, and enlarged pancreas

▶ Consider if diagnosis unclear
  ▷ ECG: Rule out referred pain from cardiac etiology.
  ▷ Chest X-ray to evaluate for heart, lung, and mediastinal disease
  ▷ Flat-plate and upright abdominal film
  ▷ Abdominal MRI
  ▷ Upper and lower GI barium studies
  ▷ Endoscopy, colonoscopy, sigmoidoscopy
  ▷ ERCP
  ▷ Hydroxy-iminodiacetic acid (HIDA) gallbladder scan

Differential Diagnosis

Diffuse Pain
▶ Generalized peritonitis

▶ Metabolic disturbances

▶ Psychogenic illness

▶ AAA

▶ Gastroenteritis

▶ Pancreatitis

Right Upper Quadrant

▶ Cholecystitis

▶ Cholelithiasis

▶ Hepatitis

▶ Hepatic abscess

▶ Right lower lobe pneumonia

▶ Subphrenic abscess

Right Lower Quadrant

▶ Appendicitis

▶ Cecal diverticulitis

▶ Ectopic pregnancy

▶ Ovarian cyst/torsion

▶ Endometriosis

▶ Pelvic inflammatory disease

▶ Ureteral calculi

▶ Mittelschmerz (colicky pain associated with ovulation)

Left Upper Quadrant

▶ Splenic enlargement/hematoma

▶ Left lower lobe pneumonia

▶ Cardiac disease

▶ Pancreatitis

Left Lower Quadrant

▶ Diverticulitis

▶ Ectopic pregnancy

▶ Ovarian cyst/torsion

▶ Endometriosis

▶ Mittelschmerz

▶ Ureteral calculi

▶ Pelvic inflammatory disease

Epigastric or Midline

▶ Gastritis

▶ Cardiac disease

▶ Peptic ulcer disease

▶ Pancreatitis

▶ Abdominal aortic aneurysm

Management

▶ Varies depending on underlying cause of the abdominal pain (see specific gastrointestinal problems discussed in this chapter)

Special Considerations

▶ Geriatric patients: Presentation may be subtle, without classic symptoms.

When to Consult, Refer, Hospitalize

▶ Refer for immediate surgical evaluation in cases of acute abdominal pain associated with high fever with leukocytosis, clinical findings suggestive of peritonitis, or evidence of bleeding.

▶ Consult with a physician or refer to specialist if diagnosis is unclear or patient is unstable.

Follow-Up

▶ Varies by etiology

COMMON GASTROINTESTINAL CONDITIONS

Acute Gastroenteritis (AGE)

Definition

▶ General term used for symptoms of nausea, vomiting, and/or diarrhea caused by inflammation from infection of the stomach and intestinal mucosa. Symptoms may be caused by cholinergic hyperactivity or by the gut as it attempts to rid itself of irritating contents.

Etiology

▶ The visceral afferent nerves of the GI tract and the chemoreceptors are stimulated and send messages to the cerebral cortex that induce vomiting.

▶ Diarrhea is produced from the increased fluid secretion caused by inflammation of the bowel lining, or by damage to bowel mucosa, or abnormal intestinal motility.

▶ Most commonly caused by a viral, bacterial, or protozoal/parasitic infection

▶ Also can occur from an allergic or chemical reaction, from swallowed inorganic materials, or emotional stress

▶ Gastric distress is one of the most common adverse reactions to medication.

Incidence and Demographics

▶ Very common worldwide

Risk Factors

▶ Foreign travel, ingesting contaminated food or water

▶ Exposure to others who have an infectious gastroenteritis

▶ Day care or institutional living

▶ Medication adverse effects

▶ Recent course of antibiotics

▶ Lactose intolerance

Prevention and Screening

▶ Careful food preparation, good handwashing, properly cleaning fresh fruits and vegetables before eating; drinking bottled water and cooked foods when traveling to foreign countries; using bottled water for ice in drinks and tooth-brushing

Assessment

History

▶ Acute onset of nausea, vomiting, and/or diarrhea; usually multiple episodes; symptoms may vary from mild to severe

▶ Fever, abdominal pain, anorexia, malaise, myalgia, and headache may be present.

▶ Characteristics of diarrhea: watery, soft, with mucus or blood

Physical Exam

▶ With severe AGE, may see symptoms of dehydration and electrolyte imbalance including dry, flushed skin; dry mucous membranes; poor skin turgor; decreased urine output; rapid pulse; and orthostatic blood pressure

▶ Bowel sounds may be hyperactive.

▶ There may be diffuse abdominal tenderness and distention or abdominal exam may be unremarkable.

▶ Significant localized rebound tenderness is unusual; if present, especially with a fever and an elevated WBC, suspect other cause, acute surgical abdomen

Diagnostic Studies

▶ Obtain laboratory work if no spontaneous resolution of symptoms within 72 hours; usually not necessary

▶ Stool for culture and ova and parasites to identify a causative organism if present: *Shigella, Salmonella, E. coli*

▶ Stool for *C. difficile*, especially if recent course of antibiotic

▶ Stool for leukocyte and occult blood to rule out bacterial infection

▶ CBC with differential to evaluate for leukocytosis and eosinophilia (increased number of eosinophils commonly seen in parasitic infections)

▶ Electrolytes to evaluate for dehydration and electrolyte abnormalities

Differential Diagnosis

► Acute appendicitis

► Cholecystitis

► Fecal impaction

► Ileus

► Inflammatory bowel disease

► Irritable bowel syndrome

► Bowel obstruction

► Pelvic inflammatory disease

► Diverticulitis

Management

Nonpharmacologic Treatment

► Often initial treatment is supportive: bed rest, fluid replacement, and advancing the diet as tolerated

► Clear liquid diet advance as tolerated using BRATY diet: bananas, rice, applesauce, toast, yogurt

► Children age 5 years to adults: no solid foods; give clear liquids in small amounts (15 mL q 10 min) and gradually increase if no vomiting occurs. If no vomiting for 4 hours and tolerating 8 oz./hour, may begin small amount of regular foods as tolerated. If vomiting reoccurs at any point, let stomach rest (approximately 1 hour), then restart small amounts of clear liquids.

► In younger children aged 1 month to 5 years, give ORT at 50 mL/kg over 4 hours; start with sips and gradually increase; may continue formula or regular diet if able to tolerate it.

Pharmacologic Treatment

► Antidiarrheal agents are controversial in acute gastroenteritis because the causative pathogen needs to be eliminated from the body. In mild to moderate diarrheal illness, antidiarrheal medications can be used with caution (but not if fever and blood in stool).

► If vomiting continues despite slow intake of fluids, consider use of antiemetic.

► Chemoreceptor trigger zone suppressors will suppress vomiting; antihistamines more effective for nausea than for acute vomiting; antimotility agents to suppress diarrhea prolong absorption time of water in the gut but also may cause retention of organism/toxin.

► Antibiotics are used only when an organism is isolated and symptoms are not resolved; when leukocytes or dysentery are present, for treatment of *Shigella*, when there are 8 to 10 stools per day, if patient is immunocompromised. Consider metronidazole (Flagyl), trimethoprim-sulfamethoxazole (Bactrim), fluoroquinolones (Cipro).

Special Considerations

▶ Geriatric and pediatric patients are at higher risk for dehydration

▶ Pregnancy and lactation: If antimicrobials are required, check safety profile before use.

▶ Hospitalization required with severe dehydration, electrolyte imbalance, and/or metabolic acidosis; in older adults or the immunocompromised; for severe abdominal pain, rebound tenderness, or neurological symptoms

Follow-Up

▶ None may be necessary if patient remains hydrated.

Expected Course

▶ Usually self-limiting with vomiting limited to 24 to 48 hours, diarrhea may last 3 to 5 days; inflammation of the bowel due to a drug reaction may last for several weeks

Gastroesophageal Reflux Disease (GERD)

▶ Symptomatic condition characterized by reflux or retrograde passage of low pH gastroduodenal contents into the esophagus, larynx or lungs causing pain, irritability, or vomiting; in children—poor weight gain, respiratory disorders

▶ In infants, regurgitation of some of a feeding; 47% of all infants under 2 months of age display normal physiologic gastroesophageal reflux without associated symptoms at least two times daily and outgrow by 10 months to 1 year

▶ May cause damage to esophageal mucosa with or without failure to thrive, occult blood loss, anemia, and possibly aspiration pneumonia with or without wheezing

Etiology

▶ Inappropriate lower esophageal sphincter (LES) relaxation allows for gastric contents to be refluxed into esophagus. The turgor of the lower esophageal sphincter is influenced by age, intra-abdominal pressure, length of esophagus below diaphragm, hormones, food, and neurologic innervations.

Incidence and Demographics

▶ Affects up to 10% to 20% of the U.S. adult population; 65% of adults have had heartburn, 15% with weekly symptoms

▶ 47% of all infants younger than 2 months display physiologic reflux, outgrown by 18 months in 90% of cases

Risk Factors

▶ Smoking, obesity, alcohol use, caffeine use, position of acid pocket above diaphragm in patients with hiatal hernia

Prevention and Screening

▶ Avoid spicy foods, caffeine, smoking, mints.

Assessment

History

▶ Typical symptoms: heartburn (pyrosis) described as a burning retrosternal discomfort radiating upward toward the neck that occurs 30 to 60 minutes after meals

▶ Symptoms are exacerbated by lying supine or bending over and improve with sitting up or taking antacids.

▶ Excessive salivation, regurgitation, halitosis, sour or bitter taste into the mouth is common.

▶ In children, inquire about type, amount, and frequency of feedings and regurgitation; choking during feedings; any bile or blood in regurgitation; any fevers, diarrhea; upper respiratory infection (URI) symptoms, history of respiratory illnesses, otitis media; and any developmental delays.

▶ Atypical symptoms: dysphagia, odynophagia (painful swallowing), chest pain, hoarseness, cough, sore throat, nausea, and asthma

Physical Exam

▶ Exam often normal; assess hydration status

▶ Adults: weight; children: plot height/weight on growth curve

▶ Respiratory and cardiac exam; abdominal exam to check for tenderness and masses; stool for occult blood

▶ Mental status, irritability, lethargy

▶ Asses developmental milestones in infants; neurologic exam if presents as unexplained vomiting

Diagnostic Studies

▶ Diagnosis can be made without further diagnostic tests in children if typical symptoms of heartburn and regurgitation are present, history and physical exam are normal, and child is developmentally on track and growing appropriately.

▶ Diagnostic studies are recommended when the diagnosis of GERD is uncertain, when symptoms not resolved with 4 weeks of empiric treatment, or if complications are suspected as indicated by atypical symptoms (listed above); symptoms that indicate a more serious etiology such as a cardiac cause for chest pain; evidence of bleeding (guaiac-positive stools or hematemesis); anemia; weight loss; symptoms that persist despite treatment, or daily symptoms.

▶ Barium swallow/upper GI study is usually the first test ordered, but is the least sensitive for diagnosing GERD; its main value is to assess anatomy and rule out malrotation and obstruction. It is useful as a screening test to exclude complications of GERD (mucosal irregularities and ulcer) and evaluate dysphagia (caused by stricture).

▶ Fluoroscopy can demonstrate presence of reflux, as well as rule out other causes of vomiting, such as gastric outlet obstruction.

▶ Esophageal pH monitoring can measure the number of acid reflux events, as well as the duration of each event in a given period of time. A pH probe is indicated to tailor medical management but not necessary in those infants who present with pathologic reflux that has caused a life-threatening event.

▶ Esophagogastroduodenoscopy (EGD) aids in the evaluation of the degree of esophagitis from reflux. Biopsies are obtained to assess mucosal integrity. Evaluation of other disorders such as Crohn's disease, eosinophilic or infectious esophagitis, peptic ulcers, stricture or webs, and bleeding points can also be made.

▶ Stool for occult blood; CBC to rule out anemia

Differential Diagnosis

Infants

▶ Overfeeding

▶ UTI

▶ Pyloric stenosis

▶ Partial upper intestinal obstruction

▶ Otitis media

▶ Pneumonia

Older Ages

▶ Cardiac spasm or MI

▶ Peptic ulcer disease

▶ Esophageal tumor/stricture

▶ Esophagitis, infectious, chemical

▶ Esophageal motility disorders

▶ Esophageal structural disorders

▶ Hiatal hernia

All Ages

▶ Gastroenteritis

▶ Milk/soy intolerance

▶ Celiac disease

▶ Infections

▶ Hepatitis

▶ Drug-induced

Drugs Affecting the Lower Esophageal Sphincter

▶ Nitrates

▶ Nicotine

▶ Narcotics

▶ Theophylline

▶ Anticholinergics

▶ Estrogen

▶ Somatostatin

▶ Prostaglandins

Management

▶ Goals are to relieve symptoms, heal esophagitis, and prevent complications.

Nonpharmacologic Treatment

▶ Lifestyle modification is step 1 therapy and the key component to management.

▶ In adults, elevate head of bed on 6-inch blocks or use wedge under mattress.

▶ Avoid eating 2 to 3 hours before lying down and eat smaller, more frequent meals.

▶ In infants, hold infant upright for 15 to 30 minutes after feeding; prop upright in infant seat/car seat.

▶ In infants, also recommend smaller and more frequent feedings.

▶ Lose weight if overweight; avoid tight-fitting clothing.

▶ Avoid substances that cause symptoms, including foods high in fat, citrus and spicy foods, mint, chocolate, caffeine, and alcohol; patients with GERD and breastfeeding mothers of infants with GERD should stop smoking.

▶ If taking medications that decrease LES tone, seek appropriate alternatives.

Pharmacologic Treatment

▶ Pharmacological treatment in children under the age of 2 years is discouraged.

▶ Acid-neutralizing drugs may be initiated if nonpharmacologic treatment is not effective.

　▷ In mild symptoms, use over-the-counter antacids (also used for breakthrough symptoms of PPIs and H2 antagonists).

　▷ Liquid more effective than tablet form

　▷ Antacids can decrease absorption of other medications (e.g., fluoroquinolones, tetracycline, ferrous sulfate); separate dosing by 2 hours.

　▷ Aluminum or magnesium hydroxide: adults: 10–30 cc p.o. q.i.d.; children: 0.5–2 mL/kg/dose three to six times/day

▶ Step 2 therapy involves adding histamine-2 (H2) receptor antagonists if symptoms not relieved by lifestyle modification or antacids within 2 to 3 weeks.

▶ H2 receptor antagonists suppress gastric acid secretion; symptomatic improvement occurs in approximately 80% within 6 weeks.

　▷ Cimetidine (Tagamet): adults: 400 mg q.i.d., maximum 800 mg b.i.d.; children: 10 mg/kg/dose q.i.d.

　▷ Potential drug interactions with theophylline, warfarin, nifedipine, propranolol, and phenytoin

　▷ Ranitidine (Zantac): 150 mg b.i.d.; famotidine (Pepcid) 20 mg b.i.d.; nizatidine (Axid) 150 mg b.i.d.

▶ Reevaluate 2 weeks after starting therapy with H2 antagonists; if effective, continue for 8 to 12 weeks.

▶ If symptoms do not resolve, go to step 3 therapy: Add a prokinetic agent, use higher-dose H2 antagonist for an additional 8 to 12 weeks, or change from H2 antagonist to a proton pump inhibitor for 4 to 8 weeks.

▶ Prokinetic agents increase LES tone and promote gastric emptying; used for mild-moderate symptoms, typically in combination with H2 receptor antagonists or proton pump inhibitors

  ▷ Metoclopramide (Reglan): adults: 5–10 mg q.i.d.; children: 0.1 mg/kg/dose 20 to 30 min ac and hs

  ▷ Used less frequently because of its potential for dopamine blocking. Side effects such as drowsiness, confusion, depression, and extrapyramidal reactions of dystonia and tardive dyskinesia can occur.

▶ Proton pump inhibitors suppress gastric acid secretion to a greater degree than H2 blockers and are the initial treatment in patients with erosive esophagitis confirmed by endoscopy; take 1 hour before meal—PPIs should ideally be administered 15 to 30 minutes before the first meal of the day.

  ▷ Omeprazole (Prilosec): adults: 20 mg q. a.m.; children: 0.7–3.3 mg/kg/day in one to two doses

  ▷ Lansoprazole (Prevacid): 30 mg q.d.; esomeprazole (Nexium) 40 mg q.d.; or rabeprazole (Aciphex) 20 mg q.d. (1 to 11 yrs., under 30 kg, 15 mg daily; over 30 kg, 30 mg daily)

  ▷ Reports of blood dyscrasias with PPIs and H2 blockers. H2 blockers need to be renally dosed. B_{12} levels should be checked in people on PPIs. B_{12}, iron, and calcium absorption compromised with PPIs.

  ▷ PPIs and H2 antagonists: multiple cytochrome P450 interactions with drugs such as warfarin, phenytoin, and antifungals

How Long to Treat

▶ Reconsider diagnosis if there is no response to proton pump inhibitors after 8 weeks.

▶ Treat erosive esophagitis with proton pump inhibitors for 8 to 12 weeks—more effective than H2 antagonists.

▶ 85% of infants with GERD improve with age as they become more erect and advance to more solid diet.

▶ If patient has a good response to therapy, gradually withdraw medication while continuing lifestyle modifications.

▶ Maintenance therapy with H2 blockers (continue usual treatment dosage) or proton pump inhibitors (omeprazole 20 mg or lansoprazole 30 mg daily) should be considered to prevent relapse that occurs in 80% within 6 months; lifestyle modification should continue throughout treatment and indefinitely to prevent relapse.

Special Considerations

▶ Pregnancy: predisposition due to elevated hormone levels and increased intra-abdominal pressure from pregnant uterus; antacids generally safe

▶ Lactation: antacids generally safe

▶ Consult with, or refer to, a physician or gastroenterologist when the patient does not respond to treatment or has symptoms of dysphagia, evidence of blood loss, iron-deficiency anemia, or significant weight loss, or for pediatric patients with anatomic abnormalities suspected or if there is poor weight gain or developmental delay.

▶ Refer for surgery (gastric fundoplication; step 4 therapy) when all other approaches have failed.

Follow-Up

▶ 2-week intervals until improvement noted, then monthly

Expected Course

▶ In infants, 85% will have resolution when able to sit/stand and have begun on solids

▶ Often a chronic, relapsing condition in adults; however, majority of patients with GERD respond well to medical therapy without developing complications or requiring surgery

▶ Annual endoscopy with biopsy indicated in patients with Barrett's esophagus

Peptic Ulcer Disease (PUD)

Definition

▶ Ulceration in the gastric or duodenal mucosa caused when the normal protective coating of the stomach is penetrated and irritated by acid secretion, causing pain

Etiology

▶ Nonsteroidal anti-inflammatory drugs (NSAIDs)

▶ *H. pylori* infection associated with 95% of duodenal ulcers

▶ Acid hypersecretory states (e.g., Zollinger-Ellison syndrome, caused by a gastrin-secreting tumor)

▶ Ulceration extends through the muscularis mucosa, usually 5 mm or greater in diameter.

Incidence and Demographics

▶ In the United States, approximately 500,000 new cases and 4 million occurrences per year

▶ Duodenal ulcers five times more common than gastric ulcers; more than 95% occur in duodenal bulb or pyloric channel; occur more often between ages of 25 and 64

▶ Benign gastric ulcers commonly occur in antrum on lesser curvature; occur more often between ages of 55 and 70

▶ Geriatric patients: increased mortality with initial attack over 60 years old

Risk Factors

▶ Aging (decrease in gastric mucosal protective mechanisms)

▶ Corticosteroid use, stress; aspirin (ASA) and chronic NSAID use increase risk of gastric ulcers

▶ Smoking, alcohol use do not appear to be causes

Prevention and Screening

▶ Consider using COX2 inhibitor type of NSAIDs (e.g., celecoxib [Celebrex]) to reduce incidence of ulcer, spare gastric mucosal prostaglandin synthesis

▶ Misoprostol (prostaglandin analog) 100–200 mcg t.i.d.–q.i.d., or a proton pump inhibitor b.i.d., given prophylactically in combination with NSAIDs, to prevent NSAID-induced ulcers, for increased risk with age over 70, use of anticoagulants or corticosteroids, and previous history of peptic ulcer and/or complications

▶ Smoking cessation; stress management

▶ NSAIDs with food, only when needed; avoid chronic use

Assessment

History (Diagnosis Often Made by Clinical Presentation)

▶ Classic symptom is epigastric pain (dyspepsia) described as a gnawing or dull ache that fluctuates throughout the day.

▶ With duodenal ulcer, discomfort occurs 1 to 3 hours after meals and may awaken patient at night. Pain is relieved by eating, antacids, or vomiting.

▶ With gastric ulcers, symptoms are more variable; food may increase or decrease symptoms; and anorexia, nausea, vomiting, and weight loss are more common.

▶ Melanotic stools: In older adults and NSAID-induced ulcers, there may be no symptoms until bleeding or perforation occur.

Physical Exam

▶ Abdominal exam may reveal mild, localized epigastric tenderness to deep palpation.

▶ Stool may be positive for occult blood.

Diagnostic Studies

▶ *H. pylori* detection by serum antibodies or endoscopic biopsy (see below) should be evaluated in all patients with diagnosed PUD.

▶ CBC to exclude anemia from GI blood loss and leukocytosis because of ulcer perforation; stool occult blood

▶ Amylase in patients with significant epigastric pain to exclude pancreatic disease

▶ Fasting serum gastrin level to screen for Zollinger-Ellison syndrome; consider in patients with multiple recurrent ulcers, and in those with ulcer and no *H. pylori* or NSAID use (hold H2 receptor antagonists for 24 hours and proton pump inhibitors for 1 week because they may falsely elevate levels.)

▶ Upper endoscopy is best test to diagnose peptic ulcer disease; allows for biopsy to detect malignancy (more than 5% of gastric ulcers are malignant at time of presentation) and *H. pylori* infection (through rapid urease test or histology). Recommended in patients who test positive for *H. pylori* infection (serum antibody) under age 45 and for all patients over age 45.

▶ Barium upper GI series may be used to screen uncomplicated symptoms of dyspepsia; however, cannot distinguish between benign and malignant gastric ulcers

▶ Urea breath test (*H. pylori* generates urease) diagnoses active *H. pylori* infection; useful in evaluating symptomatic patients who have been previously treated for *H.*

pylori (if breath test positive, indicates unsuccessful eradication). The serum *H. pylori* antibody may persist for up to 18 months after treatment, even in those patients who have been successfully treated. Proton pump inhibitors should be held for 7 days before test to avoid a false negative result.

Differential Diagnosis

▶ Gastroesophageal reflux

▶ Cholecystitis

▶ Pancreatitis

▶ Diverticulitis

▶ Biliary tract disease

▶ Gastric carcinoma

▶ Cardiovascular disease

▶ Angina/MI

▶ Gastritis

▶ Functional dyspepsia

Management

Goal: Eradicate bacteria, provide environment for ulcer healing.

Nonpharmacologic Treatment

▶ Stop NSAIDs.

▶ Maintain well-balanced diet.

▶ Smoking should be discouraged as it slows ulcer healing and increases risk for reoccurrence.

▶ Stress management

▶ Surgery for refractory ulcers is rarely performed.

Pharmacologic Treatment (see Table 9–3)

▶ In patients who do not need an endoscopy, have normal CBC, and test negative for *H. pylori:*

  ▷ Proton pump inhibitors (omeprazole and lansoprazole) suppress gastric acid secretion to a greater degree than H2 receptor antagonists. Give 1 hour before meals.

  ▷ H2 receptor antagonists suppress basal and nocturnal gastric acid secretion; less effective inhibition of meal-stimulated acid production

    ▶ Cimetidine (Tagamet), ranitidine (Zantac), famotidine (Pepcid), or nizatidine (Axid)

    ▶ Cimetidine has potential drug interactions with theophylline, warfarin, nifedipine, propranolol, and phenytoin

  ▷ Sucralfate (Carafate) enhances mucosal defenses; efficacy is equal to H2 receptor antagonists in treating duodenal ulcers. Inhibits the absorption of certain medications (i.e., digoxin) and dosing should be separated by 2 hours and taken 1 hour before meals.

TABLE 9–3.
DRUG DOSAGES IN ACTIVE PEPTIC ULCER DISEASE

DRUG	PPIS	H2 BLOCKERS
Omeprazole (Prilosec)	20 mg q.d.	Ranitadine 150 mg b.i.d., 300 mg HS
Lansoprazole (Prevacid)	30 mg q.d.	Nizatidine 150 mg b.i.d., 300 mg HS
Rabezprazole (Aciphex)	20 mg q.d.	Cimetidine 400 mg b.i.d., 800 mg HS
Esomeprazole (Nexium)	40 mg q.d.	Famotidine 20 mg b.i.d., 40 mg HS
Pantoprazole (Protonix)	40 mg q.d.	
All PPIs before breakfast		H2 blockers before meals
Sucralfate (Carafate)	1g q.i.d.	Used as adjunct

NSAID-induced Ulcer Disease

▶ Antibiotic therapy not necessary

▶ Discontinue NSAID if possible.

▶ Substitute COX2 inhibitor when possible.

▶ Once-daily proton pump inhibitor

▶ Prostaglandin analog (misoprostol) used if NSAID continued

▶ Proton pump inhibitor for acute ulcer for 4 to 8 weeks, or indefinitely for prophylaxis

▶ Antacids no longer used as first-line treatment because of newer agents; commonly used to provide symptom relief in addition to other therapies on as-needed basis

H. pylori Ulcer Disease

▶ Triple therapy with 2 antibiotics and a PPI for 14 days is recommended to treat *H. pylori*. Omeprazole 20 mg b.i.d., lansoprazole 30 mg b.i.d., pantoprazole 40 mg b.i.d., rabeprazole 20 mg b.i.d. or esomeprazole 40 mg b.i.d. in combination with clarithromycin 500 mg b.i.d. + amoxicillin 1 GM b.i.d. or metronidazole 500 mg b.i.d. (penicillin-allergic patients) is the currently recommended regimen. Studies have not concluded that quadruple therapy is any more effective than triple therapy and compliance is more difficult.

▶ Either a proton pump inhibitor or a histamine 2 receptor antagonist is required to provide an environment for healing of existing ulcer.

▶ In patients with complicated ulcers (bleeding, nausea, and significant pain), initiate treatment with proton pump inhibitor first to relieve symptoms, followed by treatment regimen for *H. pylori* if test is positive.

How Long to Treat

▶ Active peptic ulcer: Reevaluate in 2 weeks; if symptoms improving, continue treatment.

▶ With proton pump inhibitors, treat uncomplicated duodenal ulcer for 4 weeks, gastric or complicated ulcer for 6 to 8 weeks.

▶ With H2 antagonists, treat uncomplicated duodenal ulcer for 6 weeks, gastric ulcer for 8 to 12 weeks.

▶ With *H. pylori*, give medications for 10 to 14 days minimum; may require retreatment if symptoms recur.

Special Considerations

▶ Pregnancy: Misoprostol may cause uterine contractions, resulting in abortion.

▶ Refer to a gastroenterologist for endoscopic evaluation in patients with symptoms of GI bleeding (iron-deficiency anemia, hematemesis, or melena), persistent vomiting, and weight loss; severe epigastric pain that may suggest ulcer penetration or perforation; patients over the age of 50 with new onset of dyspepsia; persistent symptoms after several weeks of treatment or for recurrent symptoms after finishing treatment; all gastric ulcers.

Follow-Up

▶ Evaluate effectiveness of therapy 2 weeks after initiation and again after completion (4 to 12 weeks).

▶ Using a urea breath test, confirm eradication of *H. pylori* in patients who continue to have symptoms or relapse (may require retreatment with different antibiotic regimen).

▶ Successful *H. pylori* eradication decreases peptic ulcer recurrence to 20% per year.

▶ All gastric ulcers should be reevaluated by endoscopy with cytology after treatment to document resolution and exclude malignancy.

Complications

▶ Hemorrhage, ulcer perforation or penetration, gastric outlet obstruction

Irritable Bowel Syndrome (IBS)

Definition

▶ American Gastroenterological Association: combination of chronic and recurrent GI symptoms not explained by structural or biochemical abnormalities

▶ Rome III criteria for diagnosis: 12 or more weeks in the last 12 months of abdominal pain or discomfort that has 2 of 3 features: relieved by defecation, onset associated in change of frequency of stool, onset associated with change in form of stool

Etiology

▶ Pathophysiology is unknown but may be related to an increase in 5-HT, a neurotransmitter controlling intestinal motility and visceral afferent responses. This increase may be caused by normal or noxious stimuli.

▶ Specific food intolerance (lactose; high fat; citrus or spicy foods; dietetic sweeteners; and gas-producing foods such as beans, cabbage, and raw onions)

▶ Malabsorption of bile acids

▶ Heightened visceral pain perception, especially with stress or around menses

▶ May have history of abuse or depression

Incidence and Demographics

▶ Common, occurs in 15% of the population, but only 15% seek treatment; median age 35; also occurs in children and older adults

Risk Factors

▶ Familial history

▶ Presence of other functional disorders, history of childhood sexual abuse

▶ Emotional and physical stress (e.g., anxiety, excessive worry, major loss, improper diet, overwork, decreased sleep, and poor physical fitness) can exacerbate symptoms.

Prevention and Screening

▶ Stress reduction

▶ Maintain healthy lifestyle by eating a well-balanced, high-fiber, low-fat diet; taking regular exercise; and getting adequate sleep.

▶ Avoid foods or other substances that exacerbate symptoms (see specific foods listed above).

▶ Avoid caffeine, tobacco, and alcohol.

Assessment

History

▶ IBS can present as predominantly constipation, predominantly diarrhea, or mixed.

▷ Constipation is described as small, infrequent, hard stools or straining to defecate.

▷ Diarrhea (usually four to six stools a day) is described as watery, ribbon-like, with clear mucous in the stool.

▶ Blood in stool and waking at night to defecate is more likely inflammatory bowel disease.

▶ Often alternates between both constipation and diarrhea. Increased flatulence and bloating may be present. Symptoms are exacerbated by meals and stress, and are usually relieved by defecation.

▶ History of increased emotional or physical stress, depression, or preoccupation with bowel habits

▶ Weight loss—none with IBS

▶ Diet, eating patterns, medications, treatments tried, family history (colon cancer)

▶ In women, take menstrual history and any association of symptoms with menstruation.

▶ Abdominal pain relieved by defecation; preoccupation with bowel symptoms

Physical Exam

▶ Usually normal; no weight loss

▶ Lower abdominal tenderness or distension may be present but not pronounced; a tender cord may be palpated over the sigmoid colon (left lower quadrant), which indicates the presence of stool; abdominal tympany if air trapping is present; mildly hyperactive bowel sounds may be present.

▶ Digital rectal exam is normal, although may have discomfort on exam

Diagnostic Studies

▶ CBC with differential, erythrocyte sedimentation rate (ESR), and thyroid function tests are normal, tissue transglutaminase; stool test for occult blood negative

▶ In patients with diarrhea, stool studies negative (culture, ova and parasite, and *C. difficile*, WBCs, and fat)

▶ Flexible sigmoidoscopy, colonoscopy, barium enema when symptoms are severe or prolonged, to exclude inflammatory or malignant disease; indicated for patients older than 40

▶ Small bowel series to rule out Crohn's disease when diarrhea predominates

▶ Abdominal plain radiograph during acute episode of abdominal pain to exclude bowel obstruction

Differential Diagnosis

▶ Inflammatory bowel disease

▶ Thyroid disease

▶ Celiac

▶ Diverticulitis

▶ Giardiasis

▶ Celiac disease

▶ Endometriosis

▶ Cystic fibrosis

▶ Lactose intolerance

▶ Colon cancer

▶ Malabsorption

Management

Nonpharmacologic Treatment

▶ Patients should keep a diary in which foods, symptoms, and daily events are recorded to identify possible exacerbating factors.

▶ Dietary changes: Avoid foods and other agents that worsen symptoms.

▶ A lactose-free diet should be tried for 2 weeks in all patients to exclude lactose intolerance.

▶ A high-fiber diet (20–30 g/day) is recommended; may cause bloating and flatulence initially, but usually resolves in few weeks (increase gradually). Add 1 teaspoon bran powder two to three times/day to food or in 8 oz. liquid.

▶ Management of stress through relaxation techniques and behavior modification, emotional support, addressing patient fears

Pharmacologic Treatment

▶ Medications required only in severe cases

▷ Bulk-forming agents may be better tolerated than bran, used in mixed IBS

▶ Psyllium (Metamucil) 1 tablespoon in 8 oz. of fluid up to three times a day

▶ Methylcellulose (Citrucel) 1 tbsp. in 8 oz. of fluid up to three times a day

▷ Anticholinergic agents: relieve spasm and abdominal pain.

▶ Dicyclomine hydrochloride (Bentyl) 10–20 mg q.i.d. p.r.n.

▶ Hyoscyamine sulfate (Levsin) 0.125 mg one to two (tabs or tsp.) q.4.h. orally or sublingually prn

▷ Antidiarrheal agents: used on an as-needed basis

▶ Loperamide hydrochloride (Imodium) 4 mg initially, then 2 mg after each loose stool p.r.n. (max 8 mg/day); diphenoxylate with atropine (Lomotil) one to two tablets q.i.d. p.r.n.

▷ If constipation primary problem, may use lactulose 15–30 mL/dose, max 60 mL/day if increased fiber not effective, or lubiprostone (Amitiza) 8–24 mg b.i.d.

▷ Treatment for flatulence

▶ Simethicone (Phazyme, Gas-X) 125 mg q.i.d. p.r.n. with meals and q.h.s.

▷ Antidepressants are controversial but may be effective for some patients with chronic, unremitting abdominal pain.

▶ Tricyclic: amitriptyline (Elavil) 25–50 mg q.h.s.

▶ Serotonin reuptake inhibitors: citalopram 10–20 mg, initially and increase up to 40 mg daily or fluoxetine (Prozac) 20–40 mg, if depression coexists

How Long to Treat

▶ High-fiber diet and avoidance of exacerbating agents should be continued indefinitely.

▶ Use other agents as needed for symptomatic management.

Special Considerations

▶ Symptoms usually decrease with age.

▶ Pregnancy: Check safety profile of all medications.

▶ Refer to or consult, with a physician or gastroenterologist for severe symptoms; symptoms of nocturnal diarrhea, hematochezia, fever, and weight loss; new onset of symptoms in patients over 40 years old; and patients who have persistent symptoms despite treatment with diet, bulking agents, and antispasmodics.

▶ Refer to a psychologist for counseling and stress management if appropriate.

Follow-Up

▶ Every 2 weeks till symptoms improve, then every month for six months if continued improvement

Expected Course

▶ Most respond well to treatment during the initial 12-month period; however, irritable bowel syndrome is a chronic relapsing condition that may require prolonged therapy.

Ulcerative Colitis

Definition

▶ A chronic, relapsing inflammatory disease of the colon and rectal mucosa

▶ May be limited to the rectum (ulcerative proctitis) or involve the entire colon

▶ Characterized by acute exacerbations and remissions

Etiology

▶ Unknown but possibly autoimmune or genetic predisposition

▶ Inflammatory process causes diffuse friability and erosions that result in bleeding.

▶ Abuse of laxatives can weaken the colon wall.

Incidence and Demographics

▶ Usually manifests between ages of 15 and 35, with second smaller peak in 7th decade of life; can occur as early as 5 years old

▶ In the United States, occurs in 5 to 12 per 100,000; females more common than males

▶ Geriatric patients: increased mortality with initial attack if over 60 years old

Risk Factors

▶ Tenfold increased risk of disease if first-degree relatives affected

▶ Jewish and Middle Eastern descent

Assessment

History

▶ Classic symptom is bloody diarrhea; other symptoms include crampy lower abdominal pain (commonly left lower quadrant, relieved by defecation), fecal urgency, tenesmus, nocturnal diarrhea.

▶ More severe cases have fever, anemia, anorexia, and weight loss and arthralgias.

▶ Extraintestinal manifestations such as oligoarticular arthritis, ankylosing spondylitis, uveitis, oral aphthous ulcers, pyoderma gangrenosum, and erythema nodosum occur in about 25% of cases as in Crohn's disease.

▶ In children, growth retardation, delayed puberty

Physical Exam
- ▶ Orthostatic blood pressure and heart rate measurements are done to determine volume status.
- ▶ Abdominal exam may reveal tenderness or signs of peritonitis; digital rectal exam may reveal red blood and mucous.
- ▶ Signs of extraintestinal manifestations such as arthritis, skin rashes, and eye manifestations

Diagnostic Studies
- ▶ CBC to evaluate anemia from bleeding; may show leukocytosis
- ▶ Erythrocyte sedimentation rate and C-reactive protein are increased in active inflammation.
- ▶ Albumin may be low; electrolytes may be distorted.
- ▶ Stool studies to exclude infection (culture, ova and parasites, *C. difficile* toxin)
- ▶ Sigmoidoscopy is diagnostic; mucosa appears friable and inflamed; purulent exudates and ulcers may also be present; biopsy can differentiate ulcerative colitis from specific types of infectious colitis.
- ▶ Colonoscopy should not be performed in severe active disease because of the risk of perforation; may be performed when symptoms improve on therapy to determine the extent of disease.
- ▶ Plain abdominal radiographs are obtained in severe colitis to exclude toxic megacolon (colon becomes atonic and dilated more than 6 cm and is associated with symptoms of toxicity).
- ▶ Barium enemas are not useful during acute disease and may precipitate toxic megacolon.

Differential Diagnosis
- ▶ Crohn's disease
- ▶ Trauma
- ▶ Enterocolitis
- ▶ Infectious colitis
- ▶ Juvenile polyps
- ▶ IBS
- ▶ Ischemic colitis
- ▶ Neoplasms
- ▶ Diverticulitis
- ▶ Radiation induced proctitis
- ▶ Hemorrhoids

Management

Nonpharmacologic Treatment
▶ Maintain well-balanced, high-fiber diet; avoid caffeine and gas-producing foods.
▶ Surgical intervention: curative with total colectomy; indications include severe colitis that does not respond to steroid treatment, patients with toxic megacolon that fail to improve after 48 to 72 hours (before perforation occurs), and high-grade dysplasia

Pharmacologic Treatment
▶ Fiber supplements or bulk-forming agents if not achieved through diet
  ▷ Bran powder 1 to 2 tbsp. b.i.d., or psyllium (Metamucil) 1 tbsp. in 8 oz. of fluid up to 3 times day, *or*
  ▷ Methylcellulose (Citrucel) 1 tbsp. 8 oz. of fluid up to three times day
▶ Anti-inflammatory agent in mild to moderate disease, effective in inducing remission
  ▷ Sulfasalazine (Azulfidine) and prednisone tablets or liquid for children over 2 years and adults; mesalamine (Rowasa) suppository for rectal involvement, enema for left-sided colitis; hydrocortisone suppository/enema
▶ Antidiarrheal agents should not be used during acute phase as they may precipitate toxic megacolon, but are safe and beneficial in mild chronic symptoms.
  ▷ Loperamide (Imodium) 4 mg initially, then 2 mg after each loose stool prn (max 8 mg/day)
  ▷ Diphenoxylate with atropine (Lomotil) one to two tablets q.i.d. p.r.n.
  ▷ Immunomodulators for more severe disease

How Long to Treat
▶ Treatment is dictated by symptoms; exacerbations treated several weeks to 2 to 3 months
▶ Establish good working relationship with patient and gastroenterologist as you manage the primary care problems of the patient.

Special Considerations

▶ Pregnancy: Acute exacerbations typically occur in the first trimester; advise to postpone becoming pregnant until after one year of remission; continue sulfasalazine with folic acid supplementation during pregnancy to maintain remission. Prednisone is safe in pregnancy; immunosuppressants are unsafe and should be avoided.

When to Consult, Refer, Hospitalize

▶ Refer to a gastroenterologist for initial diagnostic studies and management and when acute exacerbation does not respond to usual therapy.
▶ Refer to a surgeon for surgical intervention when severe disease is unresponsive to treatment.
▶ Hospitalization is indicated for patients who present with fulminant colitis with symptoms of high fever, sepsis, profuse bloody diarrhea, abdominal pain, and severe dehydration.

Follow-Up

▶ Colon cancer screening with colonoscopy and biopsy every 1 to 2 years, beginning 7 to 8 years after disease onset (colon cancer incidence triple in patients with U.C. for over 10 years)

Expected Course

▶ Acute exacerbations are usually well-controlled with medication and patients do not require surgery.

▶ Most never require hospitalization.

▶ Patients who have more severe disease that is resistant to therapy require surgery (up to 20% of patients), which results in complete cure of the disease.

Complications

▶ Toxic megacolon, perforation, strictures, anemia, colorectal cancer

Crohn's Disease (Regional Enteritis)

Definition

▶ A chronic, relapsing disease characterized by patchy inflammation that occurs anywhere in the gastrointestinal tract, but most commonly the terminal ileum and proximal colon

Etiology

▶ Pathogenesis unknown

▶ Often causes ulcerations, strictures, fistulas, and abscesses because inflammatory process involves all layers (transmural) of intestinal wall

▶ One-third of patients have small bowel involvement only, often of terminal ileum (ileitis); one-half of patients have small bowel and colon involvement, commonly terminal ileum and proximal ascending colon (ileocolitis); 20% of patients have only colon involvement.

▶ Possible genetic predisposition

▶ Possible environmental factors, bacteria, viral, dietary

Incidence and Demographics

▶ Onset usually occurs at 15 to 25 years with a second, smaller peak at 55 to 65

▶ More common in women than men

▶ Incidence 20 to 100/100,000 in the United States

▶ 25% present in childhood with an average age of onset 7.5 years

▶ More common in White people and those of Jewish descent

Risk Factors

▶ First-degree relative has disease.

▶ Anxiety may exacerbate symptoms.

Assessment

History

▶ Findings variable; depend on location and extent of disease

▶ Delayed growth and development in children

▶ Common presentation includes nonbloody diarrhea, abdominal pain (often right lower quadrant or periumbilical), nausea, vomiting, weight loss; low-grade fever and malaise may be present.

▶ More serious disease may present with bowel obstruction, fistulas complicated by infection, and perianal disease (anal fissure, perianal abscess or fistula).

▶ Patients may have high fever, dehydration, severe abdominal pain, significant weight loss, malnutrition, and postprandial bloating.

▶ Extraintestinal manifestations occur in 25% and include oligoarticular arthritis, ankylosing spondylitis, uveitis, oral aphthous ulcers, pyoderma gangrenosum, and erythema nodosum.

▶ If disease is confined to colon, may present with rectal bleeding and diarrhea.

Physical Exam

▶ Abdominal exam may reveal a tender mass, which represents thickened or inflamed intestine; commonly found in the right lower quadrant.

▶ Rectal exam to evaluate for perianal disease (fissures, skin tags, fistulas, abscesses, and "blind" sinus tracts)

▶ Exam for extraintestinal findings

Diagnostic Studies

▶ CBC may reflect leukocytosis from inflammation or abscess, iron-deficiency anemia due to mucosal blood loss, megaloblastic anemia from B_{12} deficiency due to terminal ileum disease and malabsorption, or anemia of chronic disease.

▶ Erythrocyte sedimentation rate (ESR) or C-reactive protein elevated during active inflammation

▶ Decreased albumin levels because of malabsorption, intestinal protein loss, or chronic disease

▶ Stool culture, ova and parasites, and *C. difficile* toxin to exclude infectious cause for diarrhea

▶ Upper gastrointestinal series with small bowel follow-through

▶ Colonoscopy is superior to barium enema in evaluating the colon, as it allows for biopsy.

▶ Serologic testing to distinguish between Crohn's disease and ulcerative colitis

▷ Antineutrophil cytoplasmic antibodies (pANCA) only present in 5% to 10% patients with Crohn's disease—much higher in ulcerative colitis

▷ Antibodies to yeast *S. cerevisiae* (ASCA) present in 60% to 70% patients with Crohn's disease (much lower in ulcerative colitis).

▷ The combination of negative pANCA and positive ASCA is 50% sensitive and 97% specific for Crohn's disease.

Differential Diagnosis

- ▶ Ulcerative colitis
- ▶ Gastroenteritis
- ▶ Hemolytic uremic syndrome
- ▶ Acute appendicitis
- ▶ PUD
- ▶ Henoch-Schönlein purpura
- ▶ IBS
- ▶ Constipation
- ▶ Psychosocial problems
- ▶ Lactose intolerance
- ▶ Infectious diarrhea
- ▶ Lymphoma
- ▶ Ischemic colitis
- ▶ Carcinoma

Management

- ▶ Goals are to treat symptoms and control the disease process.

Nonpharmacologic Treatment

- ▶ Maintain a well-balanced diet high in protein and vitamins, particularly B_{12} and iron.
- ▶ Avoid dairy products that contain lactose if they exacerbate symptoms.
- ▶ A low-roughage diet (no raw fruits or vegetables, nuts, seeds, etc.) may be beneficial during acute exacerbations.
- ▶ Stress management; relaxation techniques
- ▶ Psychosocial support is very important in these patients, given the chronicity of this disease.
- ▶ Surgical intervention: not curative; one-half of patients require at least one surgery

Pharmacologic Treatment

- ▶ Parental vitamin B_{12} and medium-chain triglyceride supplementation are given if malabsorption results (common in patients with extensive terminal ileum disease or resection).
- ▶ Iron supplements are needed in patients with chronic blood loss.
- ▶ Drug of choice: 5-ASA and Prednisone for acute exacerbations: 40–60 mg/day for 2 to 3 weeks; taper to 5 mg week to 20 mg/day; taper to 2.5 mg per week to a maintenance dose required for some persons.
- ▶ Azathioprine (Imuran) and 6-MP are used to sustain remission.
- ▶ Anti-TNF are used first-line in rapidly progressive disease.
- ▶ Loperamide (Imodium) as needed

▶ Enteral therapy (tube feedings) or total parental nutrition (TPN) is indicated when patients are unable to tolerate an oral diet for 5 days.

How Long to Treat

▶ Acute exacerbation: Treatment with sulfasalazine (Sulfazine) or mesalamine (Asacol) for 3 weeks usually improves symptoms; however, some may require 2 to 3 months.

▶ Patients who fail to improve after 3 weeks of mesalamine should have systemic corticoids added.

▶ Work closely with the specialist while providing primary care to this patient.

Special Considerations

▶ Pregnancy: Sulfasalazine and steroids are safe in pregnancy.

▶ Refer to gastroenterologist for treatment of diarrhea with bile acid sequestrants, antidiarrheal medications, sulfasalazine, corticosteroids, some antibiotics, and immunomodulators.

▶ Refer to or consult with a gastroenterologist for initial diagnostic studies and management and for acute exacerbations.

▶ Hospitalization is required in acute exacerbations when symptoms persist.

▶ Surgical intervention may be required to remove severely affected bowel or to provide bowel rest.

Follow-Up

▶ Provide patient education about disease process, medication, diet; colonoscopy screening after 10 years of disease because of increased incidence of colon cancer.

▶ Follow-up according to specialist recommendations and for exacerbation of symptoms.

▶ All patients will require emotional support.

Expected Course

▶ Chronic, with acute exacerbations and periods of remission; progression of disease is common, with the average patient having surgery every 7 years.

Complications

▶ Toxic megacolon fistula, abscess, perforation, bowel obstruction, perianal disease, malabsorption, and colon cancer (increased risk, but not as high as with ulcerative colitis)

▶ From chronic steroid use: aseptic necrosis of the hip, cataracts, osteoporosis, diabetes, and hypertension

▶ Depression in 30% to 50% of patients with severe disease

CONDITIONS THAT MAY WARRANT SURGERY

Appendicitis

Definition

▶ Inflammation of the vermiform appendix (small, blind pouch projecting from the cecum), causing obstruction of the lumen of the appendix. Early diagnosis is key to decreasing both morbidity and mortality associated with rupture.

Etiology

▶ Obstruction is the cause in 30% to 40% of cases and is commonly caused by a fecalith (a hard concentration of fecal matter and calcium salts), foreign body, inflammation, or neoplasm.

▶ Other causes include hypertrophy of the lymphoid tissue associated with a viral infection (e.g., measles), trapped barium after an imaging study, foreign body (e.g., seeds), intestinal worms (e.g., pin worms), tumor, or adhesions that cause obstruction.

▶ Obstruction leads to a build-up of mucosal secretions that cause the appendix to become inflamed and may lead to gangrene or perforation.

Incidence and Demographics

▶ Most common in people age 10 to 30 with peak incidence at 15 to 24

▶ In patients older than 50 years and younger than 5 years, classic symptoms are less frequent, although perforation is more common, with a higher mortality and morbidity.

▶ A ruptured appendix occurs in one half of children under 6 years of age with appendicitis.

▶ Most common cause of abdominal pain requiring surgery in childhood and adolescence

Risk Factors

▶ Family history, intra-abdominal tumors, recent gastrointestinal illness—especially viral or worm infestation

Assessment

History

▶ Classic presentation

▷ Pain begins gradually; usually starts as vague, colicky, cramping, and poorly localized to the periumbilical or epigastric area, often associated with the urge to defecate or pass flatus, which helps to reduce the pain. Pain can vary depending on location of appendix. Migration of periumbilical pain to RLQ is one of the most predictive features of appendicitis.

▷ Lasts approximately 4 to 6 hours, followed by increased, steady pain that is more localized, generally to the right lower quadrant (although site can vary because appendix is not always located in RLQ)

▷ Usually aggravated by motion or coughing; pain during car ride is suspicious of rebound tenderness

▷ Anorexia is a frequent cause; nausea and vomiting can also occur.

▷ May have constipation or diarrhea; fever usually low-grade or absent

▶ Atypical presentation in children

▷ Initial symptom is vomiting

▷ May have GI and genitourinary (GU) complaints

▷ URI symptoms, fever over 101° F

▷ Less likely to exhibit abdominal tenderness, rebound tenderness, anorexia, and altered bowel sounds

▶ Atypical presentation in older adults

▷ Mental confusion, no fever, less abdominal tenderness

Physical Exam

▶ Normal or mild elevation in temperature; if febrile, may also have tachycardia

▶ Patient may be lying with knees flexed, guarding abdomen.

▶ Abdominal exam: RLQ tenderness with rebound and guarding usually present at McBurney's point; positive Rovsing's sign (pain referred to the right when direct pressure applied to LLQ), positive psoas sign (pain when raises right leg against resistance), and positive obturator sign (pain when the right hip and knee are flexed and thigh is rotated inward)

▶ In neonates, a palpable abdominal mass and abdominal wall cellulitis may be evident.

▶ In children under 2 years, fever and diffuse abdominal tenderness are the primary presentation.

▶ In children 2 to 12 years, fever and RLQ tenderness are paramount.

▶ Abdominal tenderness may be absent if appendix located in pelvis or behind cecum.

▶ Involuntary guarding and rebound tenderness are indicative of a ruptured appendix.

▶ May present with tender flank, rectum, or pelvis; therefore, a rectal and pelvic exam plus assessing for CVA tenderness are essential.

▶ Mass from abscess may be palpable if perforation occurred several days before exam.

▶ Serial exams are important until diagnosis is made or ruled out.

Diagnostic Studies

▶ CBC frequently shows a moderate leukocytosis with polymorph nuclear predominance of shift to left (more than 90%).

▶ C-reactive protein, nonspecific inflammatory marker, if elevated and combined with leukocytosis, increases likelihood of appendicitis.

▶ Antibiotics and steroids may alter lab results.

▶ Urinalysis to exclude hematuria and infection

▶ Urine beta-HCG (b-HCG) should be performed in post-menarchal women.

▶ Flat-plate and upright abdominal X-ray to exclude intestinal obstruction, bowel perforation, or ureteral calculus; identification of a fecalith

▶ Abdominal CT preferred over X-ray to detect appendiceal inflammation, free fluid, abscess, or other causes of abdominal pain.

Differential Diagnosis

Life-Threatening

▶ Ectopic pregnancy

▶ Intestinal obstruction

▶ Torsion or perforation of viscus

▶ Abdominal aneurysm

▶ Atypical presentation of MI

Other Possible Differential Diagnoses

▶ Acute gastroenteritis

▶ Ruptured ovarian cyst or follicle

▶ Twisted ovarian cyst and endometriosis

▶ Perforated ulcer

▶ Acute diverticulitis

▶ Pelvic inflammatory disease

▶ Acute pancreatitis

▶ Cholecystitis

▶ Ureteral calculus

▶ Pyelonephritis constipation

▶ Hemolytic uremic syndrome

▶ Henoch-Schönlein purpura

▶ Inflammatory bowel disease (IBD)

▶ UTI

▶ Mesenteric adenitis

▶ Meckel's diverticulum

▶ Pneumonia

▶ Sickle cell

▶ Pharmacologic disease

▶ Pelvic inflammatory disease

▶ Intussusception

Management

Nonpharmacologic Treatment

▶ Surgery (appendectomy) required

▶ Avoid use of cathartics or enemas because of risk of perforation.

▶ Push fluids before appendectomy.

▶ Antibiotics should not be given if the diagnosis of appendicitis is in question, because they can mask the presence or development of perforation.

▶ If perforation or abscess does occur, IV antibiotics are given perioperatively.

Special Considerations

▶ Pregnancy: may present with atypical pain due to displacement of the appendix by the uterus

▶ Acute appendicitis may be the first manifestation of Crohn's disease.

When to Consult, Refer, Hospitalize

▶ Immediate referral to a surgeon for appendectomy

Follow-Up

Expected Course

▶ Recovery from an uncomplicated appendectomy is approximately 1 week

Complications

▶ Abscess and/or perforation of the bowel with subsequent peritonitis—either requires drainage and IV antibiotics

Hernias

Description

▶ A defect in the wall of the abdomen and groin that allows intra-abdominal contents to protrude from the normal location

▶ Can develop at sites of previous surgical incisions (incisional hernia)

▶ Clinically, all hernias can be described as reducible (contents can be pushed back into the abdominal cavity), nonreducible (contents cannot be pushed back into the abdominal cavity), incarcerated (a nonreducible hernia in which the flow of intestinal contents is obstructed), or strangulated (an incarcerated hernia in which the blood supply of the hernia contents is compromised).

Etiology

▶ Congenital or acquired defect in the abdominal wall

▶ Situations or conditions that raise intra-abdominal pressure increase occurrence (e.g., Valsalva, ascites, pregnancy).

▶ Incomplete or poor healing of a surgical incision that can predispose to the development of an incisional hernia

Incidence and Demographics

▶ Umbilical: common in infants; more common in Black children, higher incidence in low–birth weight infants. In adults, occur in middle-age multiparous women, patients with ascites, and older adults

▶ Epigastric: common in men 20 to 50 years old

▶ Incisional: common in peritoneal dialysis patients

▶ Inguinal: herniation into the inguinal canal; direct hernias are acquired, indirect are congenital—most common hernia

▶ Femoral: second-most common in both men and women, rare in children; incidence increases with age

Risk Factors

▶ Congenital defect in abdominal wall

▶ Activities and conditions that increase intra-abdominal pressure, such as constipation, straining during micturition, chronic cough, weight-lifting, ascites, pregnancy, obesity

▶ Postoperative wound infection, dehiscence

Prevention and Screening

▶ Avoid excessive straining and lose weight if overweight; good body mechanics

▶ Screen on physical exams

Assessment

History

▶ Umbilical hernia: in infants, asymptomatic; adults may have vague, intermittent pain and tenderness

▶ Epigastric hernias: present with a small painless mass

▶ Incisional or ventral hernia: recent surgery, smoker, post-op wound infection

▶ Peristomal hernia: patients with ostomy

▶ Strangulated hernias present with severe pain, fever, nausea and vomiting, abdominal distension, and constipation.

Physical Exam

▶ Inspection and palpation in both the supine and standing positions, while the patient performs a Valsalva maneuver; abdominal exam to evaluate tenderness, masses, hepatomegaly, and ascites; digital rectal exam to exclude enlarged prostate

▶ Inguinal hernia may be palpable in scrotal sac; inguinal canal can best be palpated with patient standing and exam performed through scrotal sac.

▶ Umbilical or ventral: Palpate the umbilical region in the supine position while the patient raises head and performs a Valsalva maneuver.

▶ Epigastric: usually a small mass located midline between the umbilicus and xiphoid cartilage

▶ Incisional: Presents as a bulge through a surgical incision

Diagnostic Studies
- ▶ Diagnosed by history and physical exam
- ▶ CBC may show leukocytosis if strangulation present
- ▶ Ultrasound may be helpful to diagnose a hernia in patients who report symptoms but have no palpable mass; can differentiate an incarcerated hernia from an enlarged lymph node or other cause.

Differential Diagnosis
- ▶ Muscle strain
- ▶ Arthritis
- ▶ Lipoma
- ▶ Lymphadenopathy
- ▶ Hydrocele, varicocele

Management

Nonpharmacologic Treatment
- ▶ A patient with a symptomatic, reducible inguinal hernia who has relative contrain-dications to surgery may wear a truss (keeps hernia reduced); however, this is not always effective.
- ▶ Elective herniorrhaphy (hernia repair) is indicated for all abdominal hernias before incarceration and strangulation occurs. Patients with evidence indicating a strangu-lated hernia must undergo emergency surgery.
- ▶ Uncomplicated hernia repair is often done under local or spinal anesthesia on an outpatient basis.

Pharmacologic Treatment
- ▶ None indicated
- ▶ Significant pain, if present, is suggestive of a more serious complication such as incarceration or strangulation, and should not be masked by narcotics.

Special Considerations
- ▶ Geriatric patients: inguinal and umbilical more common with increasing age
- ▶ Diastasis recti is a separation of the two rectus abdominis muscles, causing a ridge of abdominal contents to bulge slightly; it has no clinical consequence.
- ▶ Pregnancy: increases risk for developing a hernia because of increased abdominal pressure

When to Consult, Refer, Hospitalize
- ▶ Refer to a surgeon for evaluation.

Follow-Up

Expected Course
- ▶ Risk of reoccurrence after hernia repair: epigastric up to 10%; non-mesh incisional hernias recur 30% to 50%; mesh-repaired hernias recur 20%

Complications

▶ Ischemic bowel with a strangulated hernia; bowel obstruction

Cholecystitis

Description

▶ Acute or chronic inflammation of the gallbladder

Etiology

▶ Over 90% of cases are because of cystic duct obstruction by an impacted stone.

▶ Formation of gallstones is from supersaturation of products in bile exceeding their maximum solubilities.

▶ Gallstones consist predominantly of either cholesterol or calcium.

▶ Other causes include gallbladder stasis that can occur from prolonged acute illness, fasting and hyperalimentation, gallbladder infection; vasculitis; carcinoma of the gallbladder and/or bile ducts; other tumors that compress the gallbladder and/or bile ducts; or infectious agents in clients with AIDS.

▶ Pain arises from the gallbladder contracting against an obstruction.

Incidence and Demographics

▶ Occurs in 16 to 20 million people in the United States, with 1 million new cases each year

▶ Less common in Black people except those who have sickle cell anemia

▶ Geriatric patients — atypical presentation; at higher risk for developing complications, most common indication for abdominal surgery

Risk Factors

▶ Mnemonic: fat, fair, forty, flatulent, female

▶ Increases with age, body habitus, obesity, or rapid weight loss

▶ Childbearing, pregnancy, being female; family, maternal history of gallstones

▶ Drugs: contraceptive hormones, hormone replacement therapy, ceftriaxone

▶ Ethnicity: Pima Indian, Scandinavian

▶ Hyperalimentation; ileal and other metabolic diseases such as diabetes mellitus, Crohn's disease

▶ Rapid weight loss following bariatric surgery

Prevention and Screening

▶ Low-fat, low-carbohydrate, high-fiber diet and physical activity

Assessment

History
- ▶ Acute
  - ▷ Epigastric or right upper quadrant pain, nausea, vomiting, and fever
  - ▷ Pain may radiate to right shoulder, scapula, or between shoulder blades if there is irritation of phrenic nerve (Kehr's sign)
  - ▷ Pain usually precipitated by a large or fatty meal
  - ▷ Past medical history of biliary colic
- ▶ Chronic
  - ▷ Less severe abdominal pain
  - ▷ Episodes shorter in duration (less than 3 hours) and recurrent

Physical Exam
- ▶ Jaundice may be present if there is biliary obstruction (15% of acute cases).
- ▶ Positive Murphy's sign (sudden intake of breath, inspiratory arrest on palpation of the right upper quadrant due to pain)
- ▶ Guarding and rebound tenderness may be present.
- ▶ Geriatric patients: Localized tenderness may be the only presenting symptom, no fever or pain.

Diagnostic Studies
- ▶ Leukocytosis; elevated ALT (over 300 IU/L), AST, GGT; and alkaline phosphatase usually present
- ▶ Elevated bilirubin may be seen with or without obstruction.
- ▶ Serum amylase may also be elevated, especially if a biliary duct obstruction has occurred at or near the pancreatic duct, causing a concomitant pancreatitis.
- ▶ Ultrasound: 95% sensitivity and specificity for diagnosis of gallstones

Differential Diagnosis

- ▶ Pneumonia
- ▶ Thoracic disease
- ▶ Angina
- ▶ Appendicitis
- ▶ Bowel obstruction/IBD
- ▶ Pancreatitis
- ▶ Hepatitis
- ▶ Peptic ulcer disease
- ▶ GERD
- ▶ Cancer of gallbladder or bile ducts
- ▶ Right kidney disease

Management

Nonpharmacologic Treatment
- ▶ For chronic cholecystitis, decrease fat in diet.

Pharmacologic Treatment
- ▶ For chronic cholecystitis, consider using ursodiol (Actigall) 8–10 mg/kg/day divided b.i.d. or t.i.d. (may also be used prophylactically in patients undergoing bariatric surgery).
- ▶ For acute cholecystitis, refer to surgeon.

Special Considerations

- ▶ In obese, diabetic, older adult, or immunosuppressed patient, severe inflammation of the gallbladder with gangrene, necrosis may occur without obvious signs and symptoms.
- ▶ High risk for gallbladder carcinoma: Pima Indian descent, calcified gallbladder, gallbladder polyps more than 10 mm, gallstones more than 2.5 cm, anomalous pancreaticobiliary duct junction
- ▶ Refer all to surgeon for evaluation; those with acute cholecystitis require hospitalization.

Follow-Up

- ▶ Provide patient education about diet, medications

Expected Course
- ▶ Uncomplicated cholecystectomy usually followed by complete resolution of symptoms

Complications
- ▶ Gangrene, necrosis, cholangitis, other complications of surgery
- ▶ Mortality rate markedly increased for older adults who have cholecystectomy for acute cholecystitis

Colorectal Cancer

Definition

- ▶ Malignancy of the large intestine including the rectum

Etiology

- ▶ Most colon cancers are adenocarcinomas that begin as adenomatous polyps (benign epithelial growths).

Incidence and Demographics

- ▶ Third leading cause of death because of malignancy in United States, with 50,000 deaths occurring annually

▶ Increased prevalence in developed countries, urban areas, and advantaged socioeconomic groups

▶ Higher incidence in people of German, Irish, Czechoslovakian, and French descent

Risk Factors

▶ Incidence increases after age 40, with 90% of new cases occurring over age 50.

▶ Previous history or family history of adenomatous polyps

▶ Family history of colorectal cancer, especially in a first-degree relative diagnosed before age 55

▶ Familial polyposis

▶ Inflammatory bowel disease

▶ History of breast or gynecological cancer

▶ Barrett's esophagus

▶ Obesity

▶ Cigarette smoking

Prevention and Screening

▶ Current American Cancer Society screening recommendations include completing one of the following:

▷ Fecal occult blood testing annually

▷ Fecal immunochemical test annually

▷ Stool DNA test, interval not determined

▷ Flexible sigmoidoscopy every 5 years

▷ Double-contrast barium enema every 5 years

▷ Colonoscopy every 10 years

▷ CT colonography every 5 years, colonoscopy completed if positive

▶ Colonoscopy is the recommended screening test for colorectal cancer beginning at age 50.

▶ High-risk patient with first-degree relative with colon cancer should have a colonoscopy, recommended beginning at 40 (or 10 years before cancer diagnosis in relative, whichever is earlier). Patients with negative screening colonoscopies need future screenings every 3 to 5 years.

▶ Direct effect of diet remains unproven; however, a diet high in fiber, fruits, and vegetables and low in red and processed meats shows promise in decreasing colorectal cancer. Calcium supplementation and a daily aspirin have also been shown to be beneficial.

Assessment

History

▶ Often colorectal cancer reaches advanced stages without symptoms.

▶ Symptoms may include rectal bleeding, and altered bowel habits (constipation, occasional diarrhea, pencil-thin stools).

▶ Signs and symptoms of anemia

Physical Exam

▶ A mass may be palpated in the abdomen.

▶ Rectal mass may be palpated on digital exam.

▶ The liver should be evaluated for enlargement suggesting metastatic disease.

▶ Enlarged inguinal lymph nodes

Diagnostic Studies

▶ Stool for occult blood: False positives can be caused by ingestion of red meat, iron, or aspirin, and from upper GI bleeding; false negatives can occur from vitamin C ingestion and intermittent bleeding.

▶ CBC to evaluate for iron-deficiency anemia

▶ Elevated liver function tests raise concern for possible liver metastasis.

▶ Carcinoembryonic antigen (CEA) has not been shown to be efficacious for colorectal cancer screening; however, useful as a marker for treatment response in patients who have been diagnosed with colorectal cancer; if treatment response occurs, the CEA level should decrease.

▶ Colonoscopy with biopsy confirms diagnosis.

▶ Abdominal CT to evaluate for metastatic disease in patients with colorectal cancer

▶ Chest X-ray to look for metastasis to chest

▶ Endoscopic ultrasound to evaluate the extent of rectal cancers

▶ Intraoperative ultrasound may be used to evaluate solid organ (liver) involvement after colorectal tumor is resected

Differential Diagnosis

▶ Rectal polyps

▶ Hemorrhoids

▶ Rectal fissures

▶ Colorectal strictures

▶ Diverticulosis

▶ Colorectal infections

▶ Inflammatory lesions

▶ Other neoplasms

▶ Inflammatory bowel disease

▶ Masses outside bowel wall

Management

▶ Depends on cancer stage (tumor size and extent of bowel wall invasion, lymph node involvement, presence of metastasis) and type of tumor

▶ Surgery is the treatment of choice.

Nonpharmacologic Treatment

▶ Referral to surgeon for surgery and/or radiation.

Pharmacologic Treatment

▶ Chemotherapy

Special Considerations

▶ None

When to Consult, Refer, Hospitalize

▶ If colon cancer is suspected or diagnosed, refer to a surgeon.

▶ Patients with a family history of colon cancer or a history of adenomatous polyps should be followed regularly by a gastroenterologist.

Follow-Up

Expected Course

▶ Depends on stage of the cancer and type of tumor

Complications

▶ Complications associated with chemotherapy, radiation, surgery, and/or metastasis

Acute Pancreatitis

Description

▶ Inflammation of the pancreas causing release of pancreatic enzymes into the surrounding tissue. With acute pancreatitis, there is usually complete restoration of pancreatic function; when recovery is incomplete, the patient develops chronic pancreatitis.

Etiology

▶ Most cases are related to biliary tract disease from a large gallstone causing a blockage of the pancreatic duct or from excessive alcohol consumption.

▶ This causes the release of pancreatic enzymes that cause local and systemic symptoms.

▶ Other causes include hypercalcemia, hyperlipidemia, viral infections (e.g., mumps), renal failure, certain medications, and abdominal trauma.

Incidence and Demographics

▶ Estimated 15 per 100,000

▶ Equal distribution between genders

▶ Acute, no predominant age

▶ Chronic, usually related to alcohol intake, ages 35 to 45

Risk Factors

▶ Alcohol abuse

▶ Gallstones, hyperlipidemia, hyperparathyroidism, hypercalcemia

▶ Abdominal trauma, renal failure, certain viral infections

▶ Certain medications (diuretics, valproic acid, didanosine [ddl], sulfonamides, azathioprine)

▶ Noncompliance with diabetes and hyperlipidemia treatment

Prevention and Screening

▶ Decrease alcohol consumption; a low-fat, low-cholesterol diet

Assessment

History

▶ Abrupt onset of epigastric or left upper quadrant abdominal pain, often radiating to the back, described as steady and severe

▶ Pain worsens with movement or lying supine and improves when sitting or leaning forward.

▶ Nausea and vomiting are generally present.

▶ There may be a history of alcohol intake or a heavy meal before the onset of pain.

Physical Exam

▶ Low-grade fever, epigastric or left upper abdominal tenderness, and distention are usually present.

▶ Occasionally, an upper abdominal mass can be palpated because of pancreatic inflammation or presence of a pseudocyst (a sac of pancreatic enzymes surrounding the pancreas).

▶ Absent bowel sounds may occur if a paralytic ileus is present.

▶ Mild jaundice, tachycardia, hypotension, pallor, and sweating can be seen.

Diagnostic Studies

▶ Serum amylase and lipase will be significantly elevated.

▶ Urinalysis may show proteinuria, increased osmolality, glycosuria, and casts.

▶ CBC may show leukocytosis (10,000–25,000).

▶ Alkaline phosphatase and ALT and ALT may be mildly elevated; elevated bilirubin is more associated with biliary disease.

▶ Serum calcium may be decreased in severe acute disease.

▶ In chronic disease, labs may be normal.

▶ Flat-plate and upright abdominal film rule out perforated ulcer or intestinal obstruction.

▶ Chest X-ray may be needed to rule out chest pathology.

▶ Abdominal CT scan may be used to demonstrate an enlarged pancreas or pseudocyst.

Differential Diagnosis

▶ Acute cholecystitis

▶ Acute intestinal obstruction

▶ Perforated duodenal ulcer

▶ Leaking aortic aneurysm

▶ Renal stone

▶ Acute mesenteric ischemia

▶ Gastroenteritis

Management

Nonpharmacologic Treatment

▶ Referral for hospitalization and treatment of underlying cause, unless mild case and tolerating fluids

Pharmacologic Treatment

▶ Dilaudid is the analgesic of choice in acute pancreatitis. 0.5–1 mg IV every 1 to 2 hours provides adequate pain relief. Morphine causes increased Sphincter of Oddi pressure which can worsen pancreatitis and increase ductal pressure. Demoral causes potential occurrence of toxic metabolites, which can worsen pancreatitis.

▶ Carbapenams are used for prophylaxis in necrotizing pancreatitis if there is more than 30% necrosis on the CT scan. Use of prophylactic antibiotics is still considered controversial.

▶ Zosyn or fluoroquinolones are used if cholangitis is present.

▶ Be vigilant for monilial superinfection with prophylactic antibiotic use.

Special Considerations

▶ Can occur in children secondary to trauma (should increase suspicion of child abuse)

When to Consult, Refer, Hospitalize

▶ Hospitalization required for IV hydration while NPO, pain management, and monitoring response

▶ Surgical consultation is required in all cases of acute pancreatitis with evidence of abscess formation or infected pancreatic tissue.

Follow-Up

▶ For recurrent episodes of pancreatitis

Expected Course

▶ Most uncomplicated cases subside in 3 to 7 days.

Complications
- ▶ Pancreatic pseudocysts, abscesses, necrosis, stricture of the common bile duct, diabetes mellitus, chronic pancreatitis, and occasionally pancreatic cancer

Diverticular Disease

Description
- ▶ Presence of a diverticulum (herniation of mucosa through muscular wall of the colon)
- ▶ Inflammation of a diverticulum, usually caused when undigested food and bacteria remain in the diverticular outpouching and serve as an area where localized abscess and peritonitis begin
    - ▷ Infection can vary from a small abscess to peritonitis.
    - ▷ Size of the inflamed diverticula varies from small to large, and the number can be one to several dozen.
    - ▷ Diverticula are more common in the sigmoid colon (left colon) than in the right colon.

Etiology
- ▶ Diverticula develop from increased intraluminal pressure that results from insufficient intake of fiber.
- ▶ Subsequently, infection and inflammation result from mechanical obstruction from retention of undigested food residues and bacteria in the diverticula.
- ▶ Thought to be a result of poor dietary fiber intake over many years that results in hypertrophy, thickening, and fibrosis of bowel wall from movement of hard stool under increased intraluminal pressures

Incidence and Demographics
- ▶ Common in Western countries; uncommon in developing countries
- ▶ More common in women

Risk Factors
- ▶ Low-fiber diet, increased age, sedentary lifestyle

Prevention and Screening
- ▶ High-fiber diet; avoid foods with small seeds that can become trapped in the diverticula

Assessment
History
- ▶ Complaints vary with severity of the inflammation and infection; diverticulosis is asymptomatic.
- ▶ Crampy left lower or mid-abdominal pain may radiate to the back, or acute pain is localized to the left lower quadrant.
- ▶ Fever, constipation, loose stool, and/or nausea and vomiting may be present.

Physical Exam
- ▶ There may be left lower quadrant tenderness with a palpable mass and hypoactive bowel sounds.
- ▶ Rebound tenderness may also be present and may be suggestive of a perforated diverticulum.
- ▶ Rectal exam may reveal a palpable mass (indicating a pelvic abscess) and heme-positive stool.

Diagnostic Studies
- ▶ CBC shows a mild to moderate leukocytosis; ESR is elevated in diverticulitis; CBC may be normal in diverticulosis; hemoglobin may be low if bleeding is present and causing anemia.
- ▶ Flat-plate and upright abdominal film to look for free air (sign of perforation), ileus, and small or large bowel obstruction
- ▶ Abdominal scan CT with IV and oral contrast to delineate pericolic abscesses
- ▶ Barium enema should not be obtained in the acute phase, because of risk of perforation; perform after patient has responded to medical management to exclude other problems, such as a mass.
- ▶ If a mass or stricture is seen, a colonoscopy should be performed to rule out malignancy after acute episode resolves.

Differential Diagnosis
- ▶ Appendicitis
- ▶ Ruptured ovarian cyst or follicle
- ▶ Twisted ovarian cyst
- ▶ Endometriosis
- ▶ Ruptured ectopic pregnancy
- ▶ Pelvic inflammatory disease
- ▶ Crohn's disease
- ▶ Colon cancer
- ▶ Ischemic bowel
- ▶ Intestinal obstruction

Management

Nonpharmacologic Treatment
- ▶ Outpatient for majority of cases with only mild abdominal tenderness, tolerating fluids, low-grade fever, and leukocytosis less than 12,000; initial liquid diet followed by low-residue diet
- ▶ Gradually increase dietary fiber after acute phase; avoid eating seeds, nuts, and corn.
- ▶ If condition worsens or lacks improvement in 48 to 72 hours, or if peritoneal signs or septicemia, hospitalize.
- ▶ Surgical management is required for signs of abscess or perforation.

Pharmacologic Treatment

▶ Mild symptoms: metronidazole (Flagyl) 250–500 mg p.o. q.8.h. plus either trime-thoprim-sulfamethoxazole 160/180 (Bactrim DS) p.o. q.12.h. or other antibiotic (Cipro, Augmentin) for 7 to 10 days

▶ May treat pain with antispasmodics, opiates (not meperidine—increases intraluminal pressure)

▶ Stool softeners until dietary fiber can be increased

▶ Moderate to severe symptoms require hospitalization, IV antibiotics, and nasogastric intubation

How Long to Treat

▶ Mild symptoms: 14 days

▶ Moderate to severe symptoms: Length of treatment may vary.

Special Considerations

▶ Older adults less likely to have classic symptoms; pursue evaluation despite mild presentation

▶ No alcohol if metronidazole ordered—will provoke severe vomiting

When to Consult, Refer, Hospitalize

▶ Hospitalization with surgical consultation should be obtained in all patients with severe diverticulitis (fever, elevated WBC, rebound tenderness, vomiting, rectal pain) and for those who fail to improve after 48 to 72 hours of medical management.

▶ Hospitalization is often required for older adults with acute diverticulitis and multiple medical problems.

Follow-Up

▶ Within 3 days, sooner if worsens; response to antibiotics should occur in 3 days

Expected Course

▶ Diverticulitis recurs in one-third of patients who receive medical management. Recurrent attacks are an indication for elective surgical resection.

Complications

▶ Perforation, peritonitis, hemorrhage, and bowel obstruction

CONDITIONS OF THE RECTUM AND ANUS

Hemorrhoids

Description

▶ Varicosities of the hemorrhoidal venous plexus that are classified as either internal (above pectinate line) or external (below pectinate line); both may coexist.

▶ Varicosities may be dilated, prolapsed, or thrombosed, often causing painful swelling at the anus.

▶ Forms when vascular anal cushion prolapses through the anal canal and becomes entrapped by the anal sphincter and a hemorrhoid

Incidence and Demographics

▶ Occurs in 50% of adults over age 50

▶ Uncommon under age 25 except in pregnancy

Risk Factors

▶ Constipation, prolonged sitting or standing

▶ Weight-lifting

▶ Pregnancy, obesity

▶ Congestive heart failure, portal hypertension

▶ Rectal surgery, loss of muscle tone

▶ Anal intercourse

▶ Portal hypertension

▶ Pelvic occupying lesions

Prevention and Screening

▶ High-fiber diet

▶ Avoid constipation and straining to defecate.

▶ Proper body mechanics when lifting

▶ Avoid prolonged periods of sitting or standing; change position frequently.

▶ Weight loss if overweight

Assessment

History

▶ Rectal bleeding (usually painless and bright red); rectal discomfort, itching, burning

▶ Inquire about possible risk factors.

▶ Constipation or straining

Physical Exam

▶ External hemorrhoids are a soft and painless mass exterior to the anal verge.

▶ Internal hemorrhoids may be palpated by digital rectal exam or visualized by anoscopy.

▶ If thrombosed, hemorrhoids are bluish in color, firm, and tender to palpation.

Diagnostic Studies

▶ Diagnosed by physical exam; if normal exam but has bleeding, colonoscopy in those over age 40

▶ CBC to rule out anemia

Differential Diagnosis

▶ Anal skin tags

▶ Crohn's disease

▶ Anal fissure

▶ Prolapse of rectal mucosa (common in older adults)

▶ Abscess

▶ Rectal polyps

▶ Rectal or anal carcinoma

▶ Condyloma

Management

Nonpharmacologic Treatment

▶ Eliminate risk factors when possible.

▶ Avoid direct pressure on hemorrhoid while sitting.

▶ Warm sitz baths two to three times daily for 20 minutes, witch-hazel compresses (Tucks) t.i.d.–q.i.d. p.r.n.

▶ High-fiber diet (20–30 g/day) and increased fluid intake (eight 8 oz. glasses/day)

Pharmacologic Treatment

▶ Bulk-forming laxatives to soften stool and prevent constipation

  ▷ Psyllium (Metamucil) 1 tbsp. in 8 oz. of fluid up to three times day

  ▷ Methylcellulose (Citrucel) 1 tbsp. in 8 oz. of fluid up to three times day

▶ Stool softeners to reduce straining during defecation

  ▷ Docusate sodium (Colace) 50–200 mg/day

▶ Topical hydrocortisone preparations to relieve pain, itching, and inflammation; cream, foam, and suppositories are available

  ▷ Anusol-HC, ProctoFoam-HC, Hydrocortisone cream 1% to 2.5% p.r.n.

▶ Local analgesic spray, suppository, or cream provides pain relief

  ▷ Benzocaine (Hurricane), pramoxine (Anusol), or dibucaine (Nupercainal) p.r.n.

How Long to Treat

▶ Use topical hydrocortisone preparations for a maximum of 2 to 3 weeks; stool softeners and bulk-forming laxatives may be used indefinitely to prevent reoccurrence.

Special Considerations

▶ Pregnancy: common, usually resolve spontaneously after delivery

When to Consult, Refer, Hospitalize

▶ Refer to a colorectal surgeon when symptoms do not respond to conservative treatment within 3 to 4 weeks; when patients present with severe pain, thrombosis, strangulation, ulceration, perianal infection, rectal prolapse, or recurrent symptomatic hemorrhoids.

▶ Refer patients over 40 with rectal bleeding, despite hemorrhoids, to a gastroenterologist for sigmoidoscopy and/or colonoscopy to evaluate for other causes of GI bleeding and to exclude cancer.

Complications

▶ Bleeding, thrombosis, strangulation, secondary infection, ulceration, and anemia

Follow-Up

▶ Further evaluation if there is no improvement in symptoms within 2 weeks of initiating treatment, rectal bleeding is excessive or persists, or constipation continues

Anal Fissure

Description

▶ A tear in the lining of the anal canal distal to the dentate line

▶ Most commonly seen in posterior midline (men); anterior midline may occur in women

▶ Once occur, become cyclical in nature

Etiology

▶ Usually associated with the passage of a large, hard stool; can occur with anal stenosis

▶ Trauma to anal wall causing pain and inflammation, but usually no infection due to local defenses

Incidence and Demographics

▶ Incidence unknown, though very common

▶ Typically occur in first 3 to 4 years of life

▶ Can occur in all age groups

Risk Factors

▶ Sexual abuse should be considered in a child with any abnormal findings

▶ Constipation

▶ Trauma

Prevention and Screening

▶ Avoid constipation.

▶ Increase fluids and fiber.

Assessment

History

▶ Passage of a large or hard, dry stool

▶ Crying during defecation, severe pain

▶ Bright-red blood evident on toilet paper

▶ Streaks of blood around stool

Physical Exam

▶ Fissure can often be seen if careful inspection of the anal area is performed.

Diagnostic Studies

▶ Not indicated unless the source of the bleeding cannot be identified; may require anesthesia

Differential Diagnosis

▶ Juvenile polyp

▶ Intussusception

▶ Inflammatory bowel disease

▶ Gastroenteritis

▶ Necrotizing enterocolitis

Management

Nonpharmacologic Treatment

▶ Anal dilatation is necessary if anal stenosis is present, requires referral

▶ High-fiber diet or fiber supplements

▶ Warm sitz baths

Pharmacologic Treatment

▶ Stool softener to facilitate easy passage and prevent stool withholding

▶ Topical antibiotic ointment b.i.d.

▶ Hydrocortisone cream b.i.d. to t.i.d.

▶ Topical anesthetics

▶ Topical nitroglycerin increases local blood flow and reduces pressure in anal sphincter to facilitate healing.

▶ Botulin toxin may be used and has fewer side effects than nitroglycerin therapy.

How Long to Treat

▶ Until soft stool is produced and the fissure is healed

Special Considerations

▶ Suspect sexual abuse when more than one fissure is present or if child

When to Consult, Refer, Hospitalize

▶ Consult or refer to surgeon or colorectal specialist if symptoms persist after 90 days of treatment.

▶ Report to child protective authorities if sexual abuse is suspected.

Follow-Up

▶ 1 to 2 weeks

Expected Course

▶ Uncomplicated; resolves when fissure is healed and constipation resolved

Complications

▶ Recurrence, skin ulceration

▶ Fecal incontinence

CONDITIONS OF THE LIVER

Viral Hepatitis

Description

▶ Inflammation of the liver caused by a viral infection that may be acute (less than 6 months duration) or chronic (over 6 months duration) that produces liver dysfunction with a broad range of severity

▶ Six types of viral hepatitis have been identified: A, B, C, D, E, and G. (Hepatitis A, B, and C are discussed in this chapter.)

▶ Hepatitis B virus (HBV) and hepatitis C virus (HCV) account for 60% to 80% of chronic hepatitis.

Etiology

▶ Hepatitis A virus (HAV): an RNA hepatovirus

▶ Hepatitis B virus (HBV): a DNA hepadnavirus with an inner core protein and outer surface coat component

▶ Hepatitis C virus (HCV): an RNA togavirus

▶ Hepatitis D virus (HDV): a defective RNA virus that only occurs in persons with hepatitis B infection

▶ Hepatitis E virus (HEV): an RNA virus similar to calicivirus

▶ Hepatitis G virus (HGV): a flavivirus

Incidence and Demographics

▶ HAV: 25,000 infections per year since the development of Hep A vaccine; 70% are symptomatic, 33% have serologic evidence for past HAV infection

▶ HBV: 140,000 to 320,000 infections per year, 2 million with chronic infection; more than 500,000 carriers; post-transfusion infection in less than 1%

▶ HCV: 40,000 new infections per year; chronic infection will develop in more than 85% of those infected; approximately 4 million HCV carriers; 10% have no known source of infection

Risk Factors

▶ See Table 9–4.

TABLE 9–4.
COMPARISON OF VIRAL HEPATITIS TRANSMISSION

VIRUS	TRANSMISSION	RISK FACTORS	INCUBATION	CHRONICITY
Hepatitis A	Fecal-oral	Contaminated food and water Common in overcrowded, poor sanitation areas, also close contacts	15–50 days	No
Hepatitis B	Blood Body fluids	Transfusion Needle-sharing Exposure to infected body fluids Sexual activity Perinatal transmission	45–160 days	Yes
Hepatitis C	Blood Body fluids	Transfusion Needle-sharing High-risk sexual behavior Cocaine use Low risk of perinatal transmission	14–180 days	Yes

Prevention and Screening

▶ Healthcare providers need a high index of suspicion.

▶ Universal precautions should be practiced by all healthcare and day care workers when in contact with blood, blood products, or body fluids.

▶ Safe sex practices

▶ Avoid intravenous drug use and sharing of needles.

▶ Screen all blood products for HBV and HCV infection.

▶ Proper hygiene and handwashing by food handlers

▶ Screen all pregnant women for HBV infection.

▶ Vaccinate against hepatitis A and B (see Table 9–5).

▶ Immune globulin to all close personal contacts of those with hepatitis A; traveling to endemic areas; with chronic liver disease or clotting disorders; sewage workers and food handlers, day care workers

Assessment

▶ Symptoms of viral hepatitis are similar, but the severity of symptoms may vary among types, ranging from asymptomatic infection without jaundice to fulminant hepatitis (severe form of acute hepatitis indicated by encephalopathy, hypoglycemia, bleeding, and prolonged prothrombin time).

History

▶ Symptoms vary according to phase of disease:

▷ Pre-icteric: fatigue, malaise, anorexia, nausea, vomiting, headache, aversion to smoking and alcohol

TABLE 9–5.
HEPATITIS VACCINES

VIRUS	VACCINE	TARGET POPULATION	DOSING REGIMEN	DOSE
Hep A	Havrix, Vaqta Twinrix (A and B)	International travelers Children >2 years living in endemic areas Chronic liver disease Men who have sex with men IV drug abusers Occupational risk	*Age 2–18 years:* Havrix, either 2- or 3-dose schedule; Vaqta, 2-dose schedule *Age >18 years:* 2-dose schedule of Havrix; 3–4 dose schedule of Twinrix Second dose given 6–12 months after the first Havrix	*2–18 years:* 0.5 mL *>18 year:* 1 mL IM anterolateral thigh in children, deltoid in adults
Hep B	Recombivax or Engerix-B Pediarix (combination DPT, HepB, and polio) Comvax (combination HIB and HepB)	All infants All children not previously vaccinated Healthcare workers People with high-risk behaviors	3 doses given at 0, 1, and 6 months Many are given in combination with routine pediatric doses in single injection	*0–19 years:* 0.5 mL *>19 years:* 1.0 mL IM in anterolateral thing for children; deltoid for adults
Hep C, D, E, G	None available			

▷ Icteric: weight loss, pruritus, right upper quadrant pain, clay-colored stool; frequently, pronounced jaundice and may appear mildly toxic to acutely ill (see Table 9–6).

Physical Exam

▶ General toxicity varies with disease severity.

▶ Jaundice of the skin, sclera, and mucous membranes

▶ Lymphadenopathy usually present in cervical and epitrochlear areas

▶ Abdominal exam: liver tenderness with hepatomegaly present in more than 50%, splenomegaly present in 15%

▶ Dark urine or clay-colored stools

Diagnostic Studies

▶ ALT and AST may be elevated; levels peak (400 to several thousand U/L) during the icteric phase, then decrease progressively during the convalescent phase.

▶ Serum bilirubin normal to markedly elevated; clinical jaundice evident at levels higher than 2.5.

▶ Alkaline phosphatase may be normal or mildly elevated.

▶ Prothrombin time; if prolonged, may indicate serious disease

▶ CBC may reveal an increased number of atypical-appearing lymphocytes.

TABLE 9–6.
VIRAL HEPATITIS DIAGNOSTIC CRITERIA

VIRUS	SYMPTOMS	CONTAGIOUS INTERVAL	DIAGNOSIS POSITIVE LABS
Hep A	Children either asymptomatic or very mild, nonspecific symptoms Adults usually symptomatic with 1–2 week prodrome of anorexia, nausea, malaise, fever, then jaundice	1–3 weeks before illness lasting through first week of illness	*Acute:* Anti-HAV IgM Anti-HAV IgG develops later in disease and stays for life
Hep B	In young children usually asymptomatic Adult symptoms range from asymptomatic seroconversion to acute illness with anorexia, nausea, malaise, jaundice, arthralgias, arthritis, macular skin rash, to fatal hepatitis	All persons with HbsAG are infectious.	*Acute:* HBsAG HBcAG IgM anti-HBc If HBeAG positive, indication of more serious disease *Recovery:* HBsAG Anti-HBs Anti-HBc *Chronic:* HBsAG Anti-HBc
Hep C	Asymptomatic in children Adults often mild disease, difficult to distinguish from Hep A and Hep B Jaundice in only 25%	All people with HCV antibody or HCV-RNA are considered contagious.	*Acute:* ELISA II RIBA *Chronic:* Serum anti-HCV antibody

▶ Urinalysis may be positive for protein and bilirubin.

▶ Above tests may be normal in patients with chronic hepatitis C.

▶ Serologic tests for viral hepatitis (see Table 9–6)

▶ Liver biopsy if diagnosis is uncertain; gold standard for severity and activity of chronic hepatitis

Differential Diagnosis

▶ Cytomegalovirus (CMV), herpes simplex

▶ Coxsackie virus

▶ Toxoplasmosis

▶ *Candida, Mycobacteria*

▶ *Pneumocystis*

▶ *Leptospira*

▶ Use of hepatotoxic agents

▶ Alcoholic hepatitis

▶ Ischemic hepatitis

▶ Acute cholecystitis

▶ Common bile duct stone

▶ Ascending cholangitis

▶ Cirrhosis

Management

Nonpharmacologic Treatment

▶ Activity as tolerated; high-calorie, small, palatable meals; hydration to 4,000 cc daily

▶ Avoid hepatotoxic agents (i.e., acetaminophen and alcohol)

▶ Colloid baths and lotions to decrease pruritus if present

Pharmacologic Treatment

▶ For acute, uncomplicated hepatitis A and B, no pharmacologic treatment is indicated.

▶ Acute hepatitis C, medications are effective

▶ Antiemetic medications for nausea and vomiting if needed

▶ Use oxazepam if a benzodiazepine is indicated; avoid morphine sulfate.

▶ Both chronic hepatitis B and C are treated with recombinant human interferon Alfa and/or nucleoside analogs (lamivudine and ribavirin) if there is evidence of liver impairment.

▶ Postexposure hepatitis B

▷ Unvaccinated people: immune globulin (HBIG) 0.06 mL/kg IM given as soon as possible (within 7 days of exposure), followed by initiation of HBV vaccination series (above), prevents illness in approximately 75%

▷ Recommended after direct transmucosal or parental exposure with HBsAg-infected blood or body fluids. HBIG (0.5 mL IM) is given to all newborns of HBsAg-positive mothers within 12 hours of birth.

▶ Postexposure hepatitis A

▷ All household and sexual contacts, give 0.02 mL/kg of immune globulin as soon as possible (within 2 weeks) and begin HAV vaccine.

How Long to Treat

▶ In chronic hepatitis B, treatment is continued until loss of HBeAg, loss of HBV-DNA, loss of HBsAg, and normal ALT level achieved.

▶ In chronic hepatitis C, treatment is continued until viral replication is inhibited, normal ALT levels, loss of HCV-RNA, reduction of hepatic inflammation, and improvement in liver histology.

Special Considerations

▶ HBV: transmitted vertically (mother to infant) in less than 10%

▶ HEV: high mortality rate in pregnancy (10% to 20%)

▶ Lactation: HBV transmission uncertain; HCV transmission unlikely

When to Consult, Refer, Hospitalize

▶ Consult with physician or specialist for all cases of hepatitis B, C, or D because of high incidence of chronic hepatitis development.

▶ Refer to a gastroenterologist and/or an infectious disease specialist for uncertain diagnosis, symptoms of fulminant hepatitis, and chronic hepatitis.

Follow-Up

▶ Hepatitis A patients in 2 weeks to reevaluate condition

▶ Hepatitis B,C, D require frequent follow-up during acute stage, then 4 to 8 week intervals if chronic illness develops.

Expected Course

▶ Acute hepatitis usually resolves over 4 to 8 weeks.

Complications

▶ Hepatic necrosis, chronic active or chronic hepatitis, cirrhosis, hepatic failure, hepato-cellular carcinoma (HBV and HCV)

▶ Fatal fulminant hepatitis (HAV)

▶ Chronic hepatitis B and C increase risk for the development of cirrhosis.

GI CONDITIONS FOUND IN INFANTS AND CHILDREN

Physiologic Jaundice in the Healthy Term Newborn

Description

▶ Increased levels of unconjugated serum bilirubin (more than 2.0 mg/dL) that occur 3 to 5 days after birth and cause jaundice

▶ Pathologic jaundice occurs when there is erythrocyte destruction because of ABO or Rh incompatibility, G6PD deficiency, or other pathologic conditions.

▶ Overproduction of bilirubin and delayed conjugation of bilirubin caused by increased rate of hemolysis and inefficient hepatic breakdown of bilirubin

▶ About 60% of infants will have clinical physiologic jaundice with peak bilirubin level 5–6 mg/dL.

▶ Approximately 3% of newborns will have more severe jaundice with serum bilirubin levels in the range of 13–15 mg/dL; 2% of breastfed infants will have a 2 to 8 week course of detectable physiological jaundice with an unconjugated bilirubin level in the range of 10–15 mg/dL.

▶ Parents must be aware that normal physiologic bilirubin levels will not peak until 72 to 96 hours of age for full-term infant.

▶ Teach parents how to assess for the presence of jaundice.

▶ Observe skin color, noting how far down the trunk jaundice has progressed (begins in face and moves downward as bilirubin levels rise).

▶ Blanch the skin to observe jaundice.

▶ Abdominal exam: should have normal liver

Diagnostic Studies

▶ Total bilirubin level, including conjugated, necessary for severe and rapid-onset jaundice

▶ Direct Coombs's test, G6PD enzyme assay done if pathologic jaundice or rapidly advancing physiologic jaundice is suspected

▶ Hematocrit

▶ Blood type, Rh

Differential Diagnosis

▶ Sepsis

▶ Galactosemia

▶ Hemolytic disease

Management

▶ Phototherapy may be necessary: Light enhances bile excretion; home phototherapy can occur in uncomplicated cases.

▶ Guidelines for initiation vary with age of infant, presence of risk factors (i.e., breastfed infants are expected to reach higher levels), hydration status, and gestational age.

▶ Generally, consider in full-term infants with total serum bilirubin levels 12–15 at 24 to 48 hours old, 15–18 at 48 to 72 hours old, or 17–20 over 72 hours old

▶ Breastfeeding can continue and supplementation with water is not necessary, but more frequent feeding should occur.

▶ Monitor total bilirubin levels daily, continue treatment until levels stabilize or begin to fall. When phototherapy is instituted, the infant's eyes must be protected from the light, temperature should be monitored, and extra fluid should be given to replace that lost from evaporation.

▶ Consult with physician or refer to neonatal specialist if pathologic jaundice suspected or feeding difficulty, behavior changes, apnea, fever, or temperature instability.

▶ Suspect pathologic jaundice if t occurs in first 24 hours of life: Total bilirubin rises more than 5 mg/dL per day; total bilirubin exceeds 15 in full-term infants (10 in premature infants); jaundice lasts longer than 10 days in full-term infants (21 days in premature infants); or direct bilirubin exceeds 1.5 mg/dL.

▶ Physiologic jaundice resolves approximately 1 week after birth.

Colic

Description

▶ Excessive crying in an infant who is otherwise well. Crying lasts longer than 3 hours per day, at least 3 days/week, for at least 3 weeks in an infant under 3 months old. Symptoms often peak at 6 weeks.

▶ Exact pathophysiology unknown; historically believed to be problem with interaction between infant and environment, although many researchers question this assumption.

▶ Several possible etiologies: normal variant, maternal/child interaction, family tensions, immaturity of GI tract, stimulus sensitivity, infant temperament, food allergy or intolerance

▶ May be associated with excessive gas, cow's milk, or other food intolerance

▶ Occurs in one-third of all infants

▶ Occurs equally in breastfed and bottle-fed, boys and girls

▶ Discuss crying history, feeding history, elimination patterns, and interventions tried with parents.

▶ Measure growth parameters and developmental milestones.

▶ Careful abdominal examination to assess for masses, tenderness

▶ Observe parent-child interaction.

▶ Diagnostic studies are not necessary if there is adequate weight gain, infant meets developmental milestones, and physical exam is normal.

▶ Reassure parents that no physical problem is present; educate regarding normal infant crying

▶ Soothe infant by providing motion (swing, rocker, car seat), papoose carrier, snug bundling

▶ Ensure adequate burping during feeding.

▶ Encourage and provide support for the mother.

▶ Switching to hypoallergenic formula (casein hydrolysated whey) may be helpful.

▶ Avoiding cow's milk in diet of breastfeeding mothers may also help.

▶ Chamomile tea has been found to decrease the incidence within 7 days.

▶ Colic is a self-limiting condition, which gradually improves.

▶ Virtually gone by the age of 4 months

Pyloric Stenosis

Description

▶ Presents as projectile vomiting in infants between 2 weeks and 5 months of age because of hypertrophy of the pyloric muscle, which causes increasing duodenal obstruction

▷ Infant is hungry, willing to eat after vomiting, but becomes progressively dehydrated.

▷ Fretfulness is common.

▷ There may be visible gastric peristaltic waves from left to right across the abdomen.

> ▷ Palpable pyloric mass, like an olive, best palpable during feeding or immediately after vomiting

> ▷ The infant should be referred to a pediatric surgeon immediately for pyloromyotomy.

▶ Following surgery, nothing by mouth until 12 to 24 hours, then advance to full feeds by 36 to 48 hours

▶ Discharge when tolerating full-strength feeds

▶ Surgery is considered curative.

▶ Gastric spasms cause continued spitting of feeds after surgery. Encourage parents to feed small volumes slowly and frequently reassure the family.

▶ Overfeeding a ravenous baby can lead to regurgitation.

Failure to Thrive (FTT)

Description

▶ General sign characterized by failure of physical growth, malnutrition, and potential retardation of development in children. It is described as a child with any of the following growth abnormalities:

> ▷ Weight for age less than 5th percentile on more than one occasion

> ▷ Weight that drops 2 or more percentile lines on standard growth charts

> ▷ Weight less than 80% ideal body weight based on National Center for Health Statistics growth charts

> ▷ Weight for height less than 10th percentile

> ▷ Height for age less than 10th percentile

▶ Children with various syndromes, premature infants, and intrauterine growth restriction follow different growth patterns.

Risk Factors

▶ Poverty is leading risk factor.

▶ Other risk factors include parents with mental health disorders or cognitive impairment, poor parenting skills, hypervigilant parents, history of physical, emotional, or substance abuse, and social isolation.

Assessment

▶ Labs should be ordered based on history and physical exam findings and age of patient. May include CBC, electrolytes, lead level, LFTs, TSH.

▶ In addition to growth parameters, children should be evaluated for signs of abuse, genetic disorders, hypothyroidism, cystic fibrosis, chronic diarrhea, lactose intolerance, GERD, HIV, and TB.

Management

▶ Treat any underlying conditions that may be identified in the workup.

▶ Parents should be involved in all aspects of the workup and diagnosis, with a focus on building a trusting relationship for future discussions.

▶ More-frequent visits for weight monitoring, weekly until significant weight gain

▶ A multidisciplinary approach to therapy is ideal; parent education and mealtime coaching are paramount.

▶ Provide home resources to evaluate other problems, support and teaching.

▶ High-calorie, high-protein diet calculated to provide 1½–2 times daily caloric needs. Children on this diet should gain significant weight in the first week of therapy.

▶ Vitamin supplementation is warranted.

▶ Close monitoring is warranted for months.

▶ Children who do not respond within 2 to 3 months in the primary care setting should be referred to a pediatric growth specialist or program.

▶ Children who present as severely malnourished, septic, or abused may need to be hospitalized.

▶ Failure to identify at-risk children may result in impaired cognitive and developmental delays, short stature, and chronic medical problems.

Cystic Fibrosis (CF)

Description

▶ Most common lethal genetic disease in the United States

▶ Caused by defect on chromosome 7, autosomal recessive inheritance pattern

▶ Classic diagnostic triad is elevated sweat chloride concentration; production of abnormally tenacious mucus secretion in the gut, pancreas, and hepatobiliary system, resulting in obstruction and chronic pulmonary disease

▶ CF should be considered in any infant with chronic diarrhea and failure to thrive. There is a possible association between GERD and CF. Although CF affects GI system, long-term progressive pulmonary disease leads to mortality.

▶ 1:2,500 White births

▶ Median survival rate is 30 years.

▶ Characterized by poor growth, wheezing, dyspnea and cough, digital clubbing, cyanosis, increased flatulence and foul-smelling, greasy stools, abdominal distention and pain

▶ Diagnosis is made with a positive sweat test: sweat chloride more than 60 mmol/L; may be unreliable in infants under 1 month old therefore confirmation through genetic testing is recommended.

▶ Differential diagnosis includes: failure to thrive, celiac disease, bronchiectasis, reactive airway disease and chronic sinusitis

Management

▶ High-caloric nutritional support, 100–150 Kcal/day

▶ Multidisciplinary team approach

▶ Nighttime nasogastric/gastrostomy/jejunostomy supplementation as necessary

▶ Chest physiotherapy before meals

▶ Pancreatic enzyme supplementation (lipase) 2,500 units/kg/meal or less

▶ Vitamin replacement, particularly A, E, D, K, as these are poorly absorbed secondary to steatorrhea

▶ May need aerosolized bronchodilator therapy

▶ Hospitalization is frequently necessary to treat infection and for pulmonary symptom management.

▶ The average life span is 30 years; with current improved treatment regimens, life expectancy is increasing, challenging adult providers who need to comanage with pediatric consultants.

Intussusception

Description

▶ Telescoping of part of the bowel into another; results in decreased blood flow. Ischemia and infarction of intestine may occur if not treated. Ileocolic intussusception is most common, accounting for 80% of cases.

▶ Idiopathic: most commonly, cause is unknown

▶ Pathologic: lead point found, occurs secondary to an abnormality in the bowel such as Meckel's diverticulum, polyps, intestinal duplication, hematoma, intestinal parasites, or, in older children, a malignancy

▶ Recent history of viral illness postulated to cause an increase in lymph tissue called Peyer's patches, thought to be a lead point for the intussusception

▶ Peak incidence is 3 to 36 months of age; ratio of boys to girls is 2:1

▶ Presents with cramping, intermittent colicky pain

▶ Screaming, pulling legs upward during episode, followed by period of lethargy

▶ Pallor

▶ Bloody stool after the onset of symptoms

▶ "Currant jelly" stool is a late finding.

▶ Sausage-shaped mass may be palpable across the midline.

▶ Bowel sounds may be normal early, hyperactive during painful episodes. Absent bowel sounds are a late finding.

Diagnostic Studies

▶ CBC to rule out infection

▶ Abdominal X-ray reveals staircase pattern due to invagination of intestine.

▶ Ultrasound is diagnostic.

▶ Contrast enema is both diagnostic and therapeutic.

Differential Diagnosis

▶ Gastroenteritis

▶ Tumor

▶ Constipation/impaction

▶ Meckel's diverticulum

▶ Incarcerated inguinal hernia

▶ Malrotation/volvulus

▶ Hirschsprung's disease

Management

▶ Placement of a nasogastric tube and contrast enema reduction done by experienced radiologist is both diagnostic and curative.

▶ Surgery indicated if signs of peritonitis, shock, or incomplete radiologic reduction. Resection of the affected bowel may be indicated.

▶ If reduction complete, restart feedings. Discharge from the hospital takes place after the child has tolerated a full liquid diet.

▶ Radiologic reduction should not be attempted if symptoms present longer than 5 days, in infants under 3 months of age, or in any child with peritonitis or shock, in whom perforation is suspected.

▶ Urgent surgical consultation recommended before radiologic reduction undertaken.

▶ Children are usually discharged from the hospital 24 hours after reduction.

Encopresis

Description

▶ Fecal soiling or staining underwear after 4 years of age because of constipation (retentive) or other factors such as resistance to toilet training or reluctance to leave activities to use toilet

▶ Most common cause is functional etiologies, including poor dietary intake of fiber and fluids, behavioral habits such as change in environment with travel or schedule, sedentary lifestyle. Occurs in children most often when cereal is first introduced to diet, during toilet training, or entry to school.

▶ Psychogenic; chronic constipation can begin in the first year of life

Management

Nonpharmacologic Treatment

▶ Infants under 6 months old

▷ If exclusively on formula or breast milk, continue with same; review formula preparation and fluid intake of breastfeeding mother

▶ Infants 6 to 12 months old

▷ Continue present formula or breastfeeding.

▷ Offer water between feedings.

▷ Add high-fiber food such as prunes, apricots, plums, peas, and beans.

▷ May add apple juice or Karo syrup to diet.

▶ Toddlers and preschoolers

▷ Increase water intake and decrease juice intake.

▷ Offer whole fruits instead of juice.

▷ Increase fiber in diet so child is receiving child's age plus 5 as grams of fiber per day.

▶ All over 5 years of age

▷ Increase fiber; age 3 to 15: age plus 5 equals g of fiber/day; adults: 20–35 g/day

▷ Increase fiber gradually, over a 2-week period.

▷ Increase fluid intake, particularly water; for adults, 1.5–2 liters/day

▷ Physical exercise; bowel training program/behavior modification

▶ Non-retentive encopresis

▷ Increase child's responsibility, provide incentives.

▷ Counsel parents to stop any pressures on child regarding defecation, accidents.

▷ No punishment for defecating in pants

▶ If the nonpharmacological methods are not effective after a month, resort to pharmacologic therapy.

Pharmacologic Treatment

▶ Lactulose, sorbitol, and Miralax are generally well-tolerated in children.

▶ Mineral oil orally 1–3 mL/kg/day (should not be used under a year of age because of risk of aspiration). This has to be disguised to get children to swallow it. Is usually second-line treatment.

▶ Initiation phase: Home colonic clean-out (goal: yellow, liquid stools), often achieved using high doses of Miralax (two to three capfuls for 2 or more days, with dosing more dependent on findings on physical exam than age and weight dosing, or using repeated doses of magnesium citrate [use age-and-weight dosing and repeat b.i.d. to t.i.d. for 2 or more days]). Fleet enemas often needed in this phase. Because this is more invasive and often difficult for parents and child, this decision needs to be made in the context of a physical examination.

▶ Surfactants: used to soften stools; docusate sodium (Colace) for children 3 to 6 years, 20–60 mg/day; 6 to 12 years, 40–150 mg/day; short-term up to 2 weeks; may be used longer and do not induce dependency.

CASE STUDIES

Case 1

A 6-week-old infant presents to the clinic for a well baby exam. The mother tells you the baby is spitting up with every feeding. She has decreased the amount per feeding and increased the frequency, but the child still spits up a large portion of the feeding. He is on Isomil, and Mom is feeding 1–2 oz. every 1 to 2 hours around the clock. There is no weight loss; he has gained 6 oz. since his 2-week visit. Mother denies projectile vomiting.

PMH: He is the product of an uncomplicated pregnancy and term birth. Currently the infant is on no medications.

   1.   What other history would you ask for?

Exam: VS, growth parameters stable. HEENT normal; lungs clear; heart RRR, no murmur; abdomen: normal bowel sounds, soft, no masses, organomegaly.

   2.   What laboratory tests would you order?

   3.   What other studies would you order?

   4.   What is the most probable diagnosis, and what treatment would you provide?

Case 2

An 18-year-old woman presents with abdominal pain. She has had some vague lower abdominal cramping off and on for the last 2 months, but today the pain intensified and she was unable to attend school. She has had episodes of loose stools and that has seemed to ease the pain until today; otherwise, her bowel habits have been normal.

   1.   What other history questions would you ask this patient?

Exam: Alert and oriented woman lying in a fetal position. VSS. Abdomen: increased bowel sounds, softly distended, no masses, organomegaly, diffuse tenderness in R & LLQ, no rebound or guarding. Rectal: no masses or tenderness. Hemoccult: negative. Pelvic: normal.

   2.   What laboratory tests would you order?

   3.   What other studies would you consider?

   4.   What is the likely diagnosis if laboratory tests are normal, and what treatment would you provide?

Case 3

A family of three presents to you complaining of vomiting and diarrhea for 2 days. It started with the 3-year-old son, then the mother, and now the father. They are most concerned about their son because he has not had anything to eat or drink since yesterday and has had a fever of 101°F. He is otherwise healthy and has had no past medical illness other than an occasional cold.

   1.   What other questions would you ask this family?

Exam: 3-year-old Black boy appears lethargic. T101.4°, P120, R22.

HEENT: Normal heart: RRR, no murmur. Lungs: clear.

Abdomen: Increased bowel sounds, soft, no masses or tenderness, organomegaly.

2. What laboratory tests would you order?

3. Are any other diagnostic studies warranted at this time?

4. What is the likely diagnosis, and what treatment would you provide?

CASE STUDIES DISCUSSION

Case 1

1. What other history would you ask for?

    Any choking during feeding (congenital anomalies), any bile or blood in regurgitation (obstruction), fevers, URI symptoms (infection), other illnesses? Are developmental milestones appropriate (smiling, lifting head when prone)? Neurological disorders, stooling pattern, irritability, consolability (intussusception, Hirschsprung's disease), any projectile vomiting (pyloric stenosis), feeding position, and post-feeding position? Family history of food allergies (food intolerances/allergies), sleeping pattern.

2. What laboratory tests would you order?

    CBC, to look for infection, anemia; electrolytes, to evaluate hydration status; U/A, to look for UTI, hydration status

3. What other studies would you order?

    CXR, to look for congenital anomalies, lung status, cardiac enlargement

4. What is the most probable diagnosis, and what treatment would you provide?

    If all studies are normal, would consider change in formula to Nutramigen for possible allergy. Upright with feeding and post-feeding. Review burping techniques and frequency during feedings. Close follow-up and if not resolving referral to pediatric gastroenterologist.

Case 2

1. What other history questions would you ask this patient?

    Stool pattern more than three per day or less than three per week, straining or feeling of incomplete evacuation, mucus in stools, feeling abdominal distention (IBS), any blood in stools, nocturnal diarrhea (UC), fever, anorexia, weight loss (UC), LMP, birth control, history of STIs (PID, ectopic pregnancy), any association with certain foods (lactose intolerance), UTI symptoms, family history of bowel disease, nausea, vomiting, low-fiber diet (diverticulosis)

2. What laboratory tests would you order?

    CBC: infection, anemia, blood loss; ESR: inflammatory process; HCG: pregnancy; stool for WBCs, culture; O&P: infectious etiology; albumin: malabsorption, chronic disease

3. What other studies would you consider?

    Abdominal US: ectopic, ovarian abscess; sigmoidoscopy: UC; colonoscopy: Crohn's disease

4. What is the likely diagnosis if laboratory tests are normal, and what treatment would you provide?

    If all laboratory tests are normal, the most likely diagnosis is IBS. Have patient keep a diary of food intake and symptoms, avoid foods that increase symptoms, trial for 2 weeks on a lactose-free diet, increase fiber. Antidiarrheal or anticholinergic as needed. Close follow-up; if unresponsive refer for further evaluation.

Case 3

1. What other questions would you ask this family?

    ▷ Frequency of vomiting, color of vomitus, waking at night to vomit

    ▷ Frequency of diarrhea, description of stools, blood, mucus

    ▷ Fever, lethargy, urine output, crying with tears

    ▷ Recent travel, camping, day care

    ▷ Any common food source that all members have eaten

2. What laboratory tests would you order?

    ▷ CBC with diff-infection, parasites

    ▷ U/A: hydration status

    ▷ Stool for WBC, culture, O&P

3. Are any other diagnostic studies warranted at this time?

    No

4. What is the likely diagnosis, and what treatment would you provide?

    Acute gastroenteritis

    While awaiting lab results, maintain and improve hydration status. Give oral replacement therapy (ORT) at 50 ml/kg over a 4-hour period, start with sips and gradually increase if no vomiting occurs. If vomiting occurs, either wait an hour and retry or give an antiemetic, then try to rehydrate again with ORT. Once child is rehydrated (crying with tears, alert, good urine output, thirsty), resume regular diet.

REFERENCES

Agency for Healthcare Research & Quality. *Comparing effectiveness of management strategies for gastroesophageal reflux disease: An update of the 2005 report.* Retrieved from http://effectivehealthcare.ahrq.gov

American Cancer Society. *Guidelines for the early detection of cancer.* Retrieved from http://www.cancer.org

American College of Gastroenterology. (2005). Chronic Constipation Task Force: An evidence-based approach to the management of chronic constipation in North America. *American Journal of Gastroenterology, 100*(Suppl. 1), 51–54.

American Gastroenterological Association. (2002). Medical position statement: Irritable bowel syndrome. *Gastroenterology, 123*(6), 2108–2131.

American Gastroenterological Association. (2005). Guidelines: Elevation of liver chemistry tests. *Gastroenterology, 126,* 1364.

Gilbert, D. N., Moellering, R. C., & Eliopoulos, G. M. (2012). *The Sanford guide to antimicrobial therapy 2012.* Hyde Park, VT: Antimicrobial Therapy.

Kornbluth, A., & Sachar, D. B. (2010). Ulcerative colitis practice guidelines in adults (update): American College of Gastroenterology, Practice Partners Committee. *American Journal of Gastroenterology, 105,* 501–523.

Wu, B. U., & Conwell, D. L. (2010a). Acute pancreatitis part I: Approach to early management. *Clinical Gastroenterology and Hepatology, 8*(5), 410–416.

Wu, B. U., & Conwell, D. L. (2010b). Acute pancreatitis part II: Approach to follow-up. *Clinical Gastroenterology and Hepatology, 8*(5), 417–422.